EMERGENCY
FIRST RESPONDER

MAKING THE DIFFERENCE

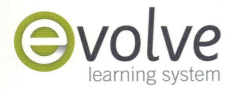

learning system

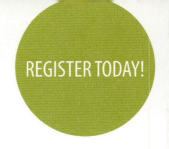

To access your Student Resources, visit:

http://evolve.elsevier.com/Chapleau/EFR/

Register today and gain access to:

- **Anatomy Challenges**
  44 interactive anatomy activities reinforce the anatomy and physiology information provided in the textbook.

- **Body Spectrum Electronic Anatomy Coloring Book**
  80 anatomy illustrations are available to color online or print out for coloring and studying offline. Students can use this interactive format to test their knowledge by completing quizzes after each part is colored.

- **Lecture Notes for PowerPoint Slides**
  Students can view and print these for reference and additional study.

- **Chapter Challenges**
  Multiple-choice questions with immediate remediation and rationale.

- **Weblinks**

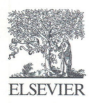

ELSEVIER

EMERGENCY FIRST RESPONDER

MAKING THE DIFFERENCE

SECOND EDITION

WILL CHAPLEAU

Manager
Advanced Trauma Life Support Program
American College of Surgeons

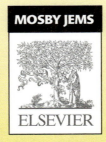

MOSBY JEMS

ELSEVIER

11830 Westline Industrial Drive
St. Louis, Missouri 63146

EMERGENCY FIRST RESPONDER: MAKING THE DIFFERENCE

ISBN-13: 978-0323-05619-9
ISBN-10: 0-323-05619-9

Notice

Emergency medicine is an ever-changing field. As new research and experience broaden our knowledge, changes in practice, treatment and drug therapy may become necessary or appropriate. Readers are advised to check the most current information provided (i) on procedures featured or (ii) by the manufacturer of each product to be administered, to verify the recommended dose or formula, the method and duration of administration, and contraindications. It is the responsibility of the practitioner, relying on their own experience and knowledge of the patient, to make diagnoses, to determine dosages and the best treatment for each individual patient, and to take all appropriate safety precautions. To the fullest extent of the law, neither the Publisher nor the Authors assume any liability for any injury and/or damage to persons or property arising out of or related to any use of the material contained in this book.

Previous edition copyrighted 2004

ISBN-13: 978-0323-05619-9
ISBN: 978-0-323-05619-9

Executive Editor: Linda Honeycutt
Developmental Editor: Kathleen Sartori
Publishing Services Manager: Julie Eddy
Project Manager: Rich Barber
Design Direction: Amy Buxton

Printed in Canada

Last digit is the print number: 9 8 7 6 5 4 3 2 1

Contributors

Diana Cave, RN, MSN, CEN
Emergency Services
Legacy Health System
Portland, Oregon

Ryan S. Stark, Esq.
Associate Attorney
Page, Wolfberg & Wirth, LLC
Mechanicsburg, Pennsylvania

Jamie Temple, BA, NREMT-P, CCP
EMS Coordinator
Eastern Iowa Community College District
Davenport, Iowa

Stephen R. Wirth, JD, BA, MS, EMT-P
Partner, Attorney at Law
Page, Wolfberg & Wirth, LLC
Mechanicsburg, Pennsylvania

Douglas M. Wolfberg, JD
Partner, Attorney at Law
Page, Wolfberg & Wirth, LLC
Mechanicsburg, Pennsylvania

Reviewers

Elizabeth Baggs, BSBM, RN, NREMT-P
Presbyterian Hospital
Albuquerque, New Mexico

Kim Bemenderfer, BS, NREMT-I
North Memorial Medical Center
Rockford Fire Department
Robbinsdale, Minnesota

Joan Curran, CIC
FDNY EMS Academy
Bayside, New York

Steve Dralle, BA, LP, EMSC
Vidacare
San Antonio, Texas

Anne E. Feit, CIC
FDNY EMS Academy
Bayside, New York

Greg Friese, MS, NREMT-P, WEMT
Emergency Preparedness Systems LLC
Plover, Wisconsin

Adam C. Fritsch, NREMT-P, CCEMT-P
City of Delafield Fire Department
Delafield, Wisconsin

Mark Goldstein, RN, MSN, EMT-P I/C
William Beaumont Hospital
Royal Oak, Michigan

Jeff J. Messerole, EMT-P
Clinical Instructor, Spencer Hospital
Spencer, Iowa

Bradford A. Newbury, EMT-P
911 Training Associates
Bridgewater, Massachusetts

Scot Phelps, JD, MPH
Associate Professor of Emergency Management,
School of Health & Human Services
Southern Connecticut State University
New Haven, Connecticut

Jerry Reichel, EMT-P
Emergency Consultants, Inc
Deer Park, Texas

William Edward Rich, AAS, EMT-P, CEM
Centers for Disease Control and Prevention
Atlanta, Georgia

Larry Richmond, AS, NREMT-P, CCEMT-P
Mountain Plains Health Consortium
Fort Meade, South Dakota

Amanda Schmidt, CIC
FDNY EMS Academy
Bayside, New York

John N. Schupra, BS, CCEMTP, EMT-P, EMS I/C
Life EMS Ambulance
Grand Rapids, Michigan

DEDICATION

To Dr. Norman E. McSwain Jr., MD, FACS

I can remember the first time I went to a national conference. It was 1994, and as I was a PHTLS instructor, I attended a PHTLS Division meeting at the annual NAEMT Conference. I had been following Dr. McSwain throughout my career already, as he had written numerous articles and books that were used in my prehospital education. I remember being impressed by how accessible he was and that he truly seemed to feel a part of the prehospital crowd, and treated everyone at the meeting as peers and not subordinates.

Not long after that, I was asked to assist in starting up the PHTLS program in Argentina, and as it turned out, had my first opportunity to work closely with Dr. McSwain for over a week in Buenos Aires. Not only were my initial impressions of him confirmed, but I was consumed by his enthusiasm for prehospital care and the patients who would benefit from their attention. That was the beginning of a professional relationship that has given me many unique opportunities to serve my profession and has certainly influenced my career and the opportunities afforded me.

We have been working together for over two decades now and I am honored to be able to count him as a close friend.

In dedicating this book to him, I am hopefully, in a small way, thanking him for his decades of dedication to care of patients that gives them their best chance of making it safely to the hospital and into the hands of medical professionals that will give them their best outcomes. Dr. McSwain has dedicated his life to trauma patients and has been active in teaching and creating educational material for every level of patient care professionals including prehospital, nursing, and physicians.

I believe that there has been no single person who has had quite the impact on emergency care as he has. Furthermore, in seeking to improve the plight of the injured, he has enhanced my career and countless others by giving them the best tools to do their job and inspiring others to join the fight in getting it right.

About the Author

Will Chapleau has more than 30 years of emergency care experience including 32 years as a paramedic, 20 years as a Trauma Nurse Specialist, and 15 years in the fire service, 6 of those years as chief of the Chicago Heights Fire Department. Currently, he is manager of the Advanced Trauma Life Support Program for the American College of Surgeons.

For more than 25 years, students have had the benefit of Mr. Chapleau's educational expertise in a variety of settings—as an international faculty member for Prehospital Trauma Life Support (PHTLS) since 1984, board member of the National Association of EMS Educators, The National Association of EMTs, and the Society of Trauma Nurses. He also serves on the editorial board for *EMS Magazine*. Mr. Chapleau has contributed to numerous textbooks and journal articles over the course of his career and is well respected by students and peers worldwide.

Will Chapleau has what it takes to bring a project like this together. His experiences lend a perspective and credibility second to none!

How to Use This Textbook

Emergency First Responder: Making the Difference, 2nd edition, focuses on teamwork and the tools you need to be successful in the classroom and in the field:

Lesson Goals are provided at the beginning of every chapter to introduce the chapter's topic, key points, and the learning expectation for the student.

Objectives are listed at the beginning of the chapter. These objectives follow the National Standard Curriculum for the First Responder and the new National Education Standards for the emergency medical responder.

In the Real World case scenarios set the scene for each chapter, giving students a clinical frame of reference. The scenarios are then continued throughout the chapter and resolution is provided at the end.

Caution! boxes featured throughout the text highlight precautions emergency first responders should take when providing care.

Illustrated skill sheets detail easy-to-follow, step-by-step instructions of basic procedures.

Team Work is critical for emergency first responders because working effectively with other emergency personnel is part of the job. This section presents information on how the emergency first responder can assist with more advanced skills, as well as what to expect from interacting with all emergency personnel.

Nuts & Bolts succinctly summarizes the chapter and will help the student review:

Critical Points briefly summarize the take-home message.

Learning Checklists summarize key points in an easy-to-study and review, bulleted format.

Key Terms are highlighted throughout the text and defined at the end of each chapter.

Learning Objectives are presented again for the student to quickly assess his or her retained knowledge from the chapter.

Check Your Understanding is an integrated student workbook that features multiple-choice, matching, labeling, true/false, and fill-in-the-blank questions to test chapter comprehension.

Five Tools for Student Success

Emergency First Responder: Making the Difference, 2nd edition, gives the student three tools to ensure success in the classroom and in the field:

1. Textbook

This textbook is written with a focus on Team Work. Emergency first responders come from all different facets of life, and they must work with many different agencies and individuals to provide excellent patient care.

This textbook is written to follow the current U.S. Department of Transportation National Standard Curriculum for First Responders and the new National Educational Standards for Emergency Medical Responders. However, it goes beyond the curriculum in depth and breadth in areas such as airway management, the human body, and medical emergencies. The unique chapter on Special Populations includes information on such groups as the elderly, patients with disabilities, and those who are critically ill. Two new chapters have been added to this edition. **Communications and Documentation (4)** details how effective communication is absolutely cornerstone to an organized, safe, and successful emergency medical response. **Environmental Emergencies (16)** features descriptions of various environments and the harm they can cause along with the care that can be provided to improve the chances of a positive outcome. It also includes information on allergic reactions and anaphylaxis.

2. Workbook

This revised, integrated workbook makes it easy and inexpensive for students to review material and prepare for tests.

3. RAPID First Responder, 2nd edition

RAPID First Responder, 2nd edition, is included with every textbook. This handy pocket and fluid-resistant pocket guide includes valuable point of care information such as helpful diagnostic tools, assessment sequences, illustrated skills for basic procedures, airway maneuvers, and treatment guidelines. The bulleted format and tabular presentation make for easy access of crucial information.

4. Companion DVD-ROM

This free DVD-ROM features 24 colorful medical animations and skill videos presented in a step-by-step manner. For unmatched visual learning and skills mastery, the Companion DVD complements the text with actual video footage of the procedures explained in the book. You'll see concepts come to life with up-close demonstrations.

5. Evolve Online Resources for Students

Student Resources will include a Spanish/English Glossary, Body Spectrum Coloring Book, PowerPoint Lecture Notes, and Multiple Choice Review questions.

For the Instructor

We include everything instructors may need to teach the emergency first responder. An Instructor's Electronic Resource is available on CD-ROM and on Evolve Online. This resource includes an Instructor's Manual that features Chapter Objectives, Teaching Focus, Instructional Materials, Lesson Checklists, Key Terms, Additional Resources, a Pre-test, Critical-thinking questions, and Classroom Activities. Also on the CD-ROM is a Computerized Test Bank containing approximately 1000 questions in multiple-choice format. Approximately 1000 PowerPoint slides are also available.

The Evolve Course Management System is an interactive learning environment that works in coordination with *Emergency First Responder: Making the Difference, 2nd edition*. It provides Internet-based course content including the Instructor's Manual, Computerized Test Bank, and PowerPoint slides. Learning resources include multiple-choice questions and interactive exercises. Evolve can also be used to publish your class syllabus, outline, and lecture notes; set up "virtual office hours" and email communication; share important dates and information through the online class calendar; and encourage student participation through chat rooms and discussion boards. Contact your Elsevier sales representative for more information about integrating Evolve into your curriculum.

Contents

EMERGENCY FIRST RESPONDER

MAKING THE DIFFERENCE

Chapter 1

Introduction to EMS Systems

LESSON GOAL

This chapter provides a brief introduction to the emergency medical services (EMS) system. You will learn about the administrative elements of EMS and understand that EMS is composed of individuals and institutions that combine various skills and resources to form an effective team with a single purpose—to provide the best medical care for the emergency patient. As an emergency first responder, you have a major role in this system.

OBJECTIVES

1. Define the attributes of emergency medical services (EMS) systems.
2. List the 14 attributes of a functioning EMS system.
3. Differentiate the roles and responsibilities of the emergency first responder from those of other prehospital care providers.
4. Identify how a patient's race, gender, age, and socioeconomic status can affect a First Responder's judgment.
5. Discuss the rationale for maintaining a professional appearance when on duty or when responding to calls.
6. Identify the types of medical oversight and the emergency first responder role in the process.
7. Identify a resource for statutes and regulations pertinent to EMS systems in your state.

In the Real World

While driving down the interstate in your vehicle after work, you notice several motorists pulled over to the side of the road. People are standing on the roadside and pointing to a car resting on its passenger side at the bottom of a small hill. You identify yourself as a member of the local factory's first responder team and ask one of the bystanders what has happened. One young person states that the car had just passed his when the driver apparently lost control of the vehicle and went off the road. You ask if anyone has called for help yet; one person states that he is just now calling 9-1-1. You advise the caller to describe the incident as a single-vehicle crash located just north of mile marker 113 on the interstate.

You return to your car, get your first-aid kit, and head toward the crashed vehicle. As you approach, you notice that the car appears to have left the interstate at a high rate of speed and rolled over once down the embankment.

Few things are more exciting or rewarding than answering a call for help. As an **emergency first responder** in the **emergency medical services (EMS) system,** you will learn skills that will enable you to assist your neighbors, coworkers, friends, and others when they need help the most. By serving your community, you will become a public asset. Strangers will look to you for help in their darkest hours, and years later you may find out how you touched their lives. The lessons you learn while providing prehospital care can benefit you the rest of your life. You will learn to be organized in the face of chaos and to communicate effectively, lead others, and meet challenges. These personal assets are valuable not only at the scene of an emergency but also in most professions and careers. EMS providers occupy a respected and privileged position in our society.

The EMS system comprises a sophisticated team of emergency care providers. An emergency first responder is defined as the first person from that sophisticated team to see a patient with an injury or sudden illness. The EMS system provides a continuation of care from the prehospital into the hospital environment, and each team member has a unique role and contribution. Often, emergency interventions are needed within the first 4 minutes following an emergency. Care given in those first few minutes can be vital to the patient's survival and outcome. The overall goal of this training is to place emergency first responders everywhere in the community to provide this essential emergency care before advanced medical care providers arrive.

Emergencies

When an **emergency** occurs, the first step is for someone to recognize that an emergency has occurred and activate the EMS system. Bystanders at the scene may call 9-1-1, for example, or a family member may call 9-1-1 to seek aid for someone in the home. In many modern EMS systems, the 9-1-1 dispatch personnel are trained to give "prearrival" instructions that will guide bystanders in aiding patients before the arrival of prehospital professionals. As an emergency first responder, you may happen upon the scene first and be the one who calls for additional help, or you may be the first medical responder who is dispatched to a scene.

When you arrive at the scene, you should tell the patient you are a trained EMS provider and ask the patient or bystanders what happened. Unlike other prehospital care providers, emergency first responders face the challenge of providing emergency care without assistance from others who have emergency training. Well-meaning but untrained bystanders may surround you, and sometimes you may need to enlist their help. You should communicate your instructions clearly and then ask the person assisting you to repeat your instructions to make sure he or she understands.

A common role for bystanders is to assist you by calling for additional emergency care personnel if EMS has not yet been contacted when you arrive at the scene. The most important information the emergency operator needs is your location, so ask someone who can give detailed and accurate location information to call. If the scene of the emergency is in a remote or industrial setting or anywhere not easily found from the street, you should ask someone to meet the ambulance at the main road and direct the crew to the scene.

After your arrival, additional emergency first responders may arrive, such as firefighters, law enforcement officers, or an industrial response team. Usually local **emergency medical technicians (EMTs)** arrive next, or

paramedics, whose role is described in greater detail later. They will provide additional emergency medical care at the scene and transport the patient to a receiving facility by ground or air ambulance. The patient will then be transferred to the in-hospital care system *first,* or emergency first responders will assist the transport team and in some cases may accompany the ambulance if their assistance is needed **(Fig. 1-1).**

Emergency Medical Services

As long as 200 years ago, military surgeons were working on care for the injured; their methods would end up setting the pattern for the development of civilian emergency medical services. Battlefield experiences in which soldiers died before getting lifesaving care inspired men like Napoleon's chief surgeon Dominique-Jean Larrey to

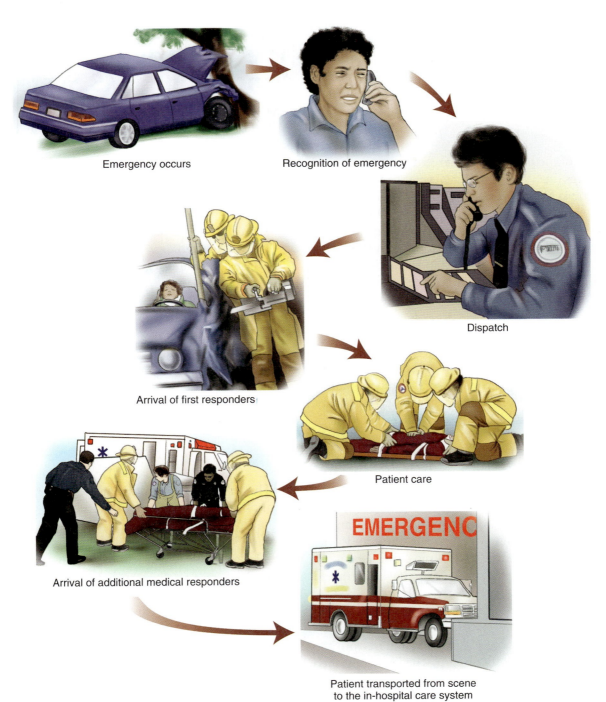

Emergency occurs

Recognition of emergency

Dispatch

Arrival of first responders

Patient care

Arrival of additional medical responders

Patient transported from scene
to the in-hospital care system

Fig. 1-1 Continuation of care in an EMS system.

design ambulances and systems for getting injured soldiers from the front to field hospitals. These early attempts at setting field treatment protocols, providing transport, and designating faculties to receive emergency patients provided a template for the development of EMS systems.

History of EMS in the United States

Ambulances have been in service in the United State since the mid-1800s. Modern EMS can be traced back to the Highway Safety Act of 1966. This act created the National Highway Traffic Safety Administration (NHTSA) within the Department of Transportation (DOT). Also in 1966, the Academy of Sciences National Research Council released the famous white paper, "Accidental; Death and Disability, the Neglected Disease of Modern Society." These events led to the rapid development of today's emergency medical services.

9-1-1

The history of the designated emergency phone number, 9-1-1, begins in 1968 when the American Telephone and Telegraph Company (AT&T) designated 9-1-1 as a national emergency number. Today, nearly all Americans live in areas that have 9-1-1 service to hard lines, cell phones, and Internet-based phones. Modern 9-1-1 dispatch centers include personnel trained to give instructions to bystanders to help them provide some care while waiting for trained prehospital professionals to arrive at the scene.

Standardized Curricula

The NHTSA released the first national standard curriculum for EMS in 1968. The EMT curriculum came first followed by curricula for emergency first responders, EMT-intermediates, and EMT-paramedics. The American College of Orthopedic Surgeons released the first dedicated prehospital textbook in 1969. *Emergency Care and Transportation of the Sick and Injured,* popularly known as the "Orange Book," was written specifically to train EMTs. It was not these events that put prehospital care in public eye, however, but a television program. In 1972, *Emergency* hit the American airways, and long before paramedics were available to most of the country, Americans came to expect a new, higher level of trained prehospital care providers.

Prehospital Legislation

Prehospital care got its biggest federal support with the enactment of the EMSS Act of 1973. The law established EMS regions across the United States and provided funding for planning and implementation. The major components of the EMSS act were as follows:

- To establish a lead agency for EMS in the federal government
- To make grants and contract awards for EMS system development
- To promulgate the Department of Health Education and Welfare EMS system requirements (the original 15 components of a functioning EMS system)
- To provide extensive technical assistance to support EMS system design and development
- To provide leadership to the interagency committee on EMS

The 14 Attributes of a Functioning EMS System

The "EMS Agenda for the Future," published by NHTSA in 1996, revised the original 15 components of an EMS system as published in the 1973 EMSS Act. As a member of the EMS system, you need to understand its fundamental components (Fig. 1-2). The 14 attributes identified by the "EMS Agenda for the Future" are as follows:

- Integration of health services
- EMS research
- Legislation and regulation
- System finance
- Human resources
- Medical direction
- Education systems
- Public education
- Prevention
- Public access
- Communications systems
- Clinical care
- Information systems
- Evaluation

The "EMS Agenda for the Future" made the following recommendations for each of the attributes.

Integration of Health Services

- Incorporate EMS within health care networks' structures to deliver quality care.
- Be cognizant of the special needs of the entire population.
- Incorporate health systems within EMS that dress the special needs of all segments of the population.
- Expand the role of EMS in public health.
- Involve EMS in community health-monitoring activities.

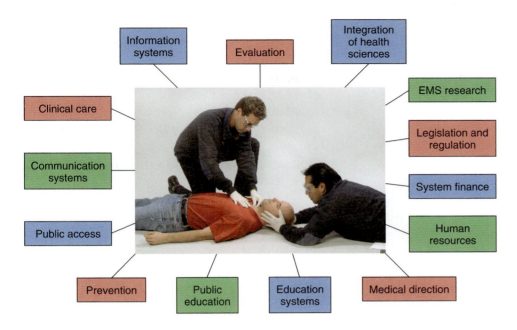

Fig. 1-2 Fourteen attributes of an EMS system. (National Highway Transportation and Safety Administration, EMS agenda for the future, 1996.)

- Integrate EMS with other health care provider networks.

EMS Research

- Allocate federal and state funding for EMS systems research.
- Develop information systems that provide links between various public safety services and other health care providers.
- Develop academic institutional commitments to EMS-related research.
- Develop involvement or support of EMS research by all those responsible for EMS structure, processes, or outcomes.
- Designate EMS as a physician subspecialty and as a subspecialty for other health professions.
- Include research-related objectives in the education processes of EMS providers and managers.
- Enhance the quality of published EMS research.
- Develop collaborative relationships between EMS systems, medical schools, other academic institutions, and private foundations.

Legislation and Regulation

- Authorize and sufficiently fund a lead federal agency.
- Enhance the abilities of state EMS lead agencies to provide technical assistance.
- Pass and periodically review EMS enabling legislation in all states that supports innovation and integration and establishes and sufficiently funds an EMS lead agency.

- Establish and fund the position of EMS medical director in each state.
- Authorize state and local EMS lead agencies to act on the public's behalf in cases of threats to the availability of quality EMS to the entire population.
- Implement laws that provide protection from liability for EMS field and medical direction personnel when dealing with unusual situations.

System Finance

- Collaborate with other health providers and insurers to enhance patient care efficiency.
- Develop proactive financial relationships between EMS, other health care providers, and health care insurers/provider organizations.
- Provide immediate access to EMS for emergency medical conditions.
- Address EMS-relevant issues within governmental health care finance policy.
- Commit local, state, and federal attention and funds to continued EMS infrastructure development.

Human Resources

- Ensure that alterations in expectations of EMS personnel to provided health care services are preceded by adequate preparation.
- Adopt the principles of the National EMS Education and Practice Blueprint.
- Develop a system for reciprocity of EMS provider credentials.

- Develop collaborative relationships between EMS systems and academic institutions.
- Conduct EMS occupational health research.
- Provide a system for critical incident stress management.

Medical Direction

- Formalize relationships between all EMS systems and medical directors.
- Appropriate sufficient resources for EMS medical direction.
- Require appropriate credentials for all those who provide online medical direction.
- Develop EMS as a physician and nurse subspecialty certification.
- Appoint all state EMS medical directors.

Education Systems

- Ensure the adequacy of EMS education programs.
- Update education core content objectives frequently enough so that they reflect patient EMS health care needs.
- Incorporate research, quality improvement, and management learning objectives in higher-level EMS education.
- Seek accreditation for EMS education programs.
- Commission the development of national core content to replace EMS program curricula.
- Conduct EMS education with medical direction.
- Establish innovative and collaborative relationships between EMS education programs and academic institutions.
- Recognize EMS education as an academic achievement.
- Develop bridging and transition programs.
- Include EMS-related objectives in the education of all health professionals.

Public Education

- Acknowledge public education as a critical activity for EMS.
- Collaborate with other community resources and agencies to determine public education needs.
- Engage in continuous public education programs.
- Educate the public as consumers.
- Explore the new techniques and technologies for implementing public education.
- Evaluate public education initiatives.

Prevention

- Collaborate with community agencies and health care providers with expertise and interest in illness and injury prevention.
- Support the safe communities concept.
- Advocate for legislation that potentially prevents injury and illness.
- Develop and maintain a prevention-oriented atmosphere within EMS systems.
- Include the principles of prevention and their role in improving community health as a part of EMS education.
- Improve the ability of EMS to document injury and illness circumstances.

Public Access

- Provide emergency telephone service for those who cannot otherwise afford routine telephone services.
- Ensure that all calls to a public safety answering point (PSAP), regardless of their origins, are automatically accompanied by unique location identifying information.
- Develop uniform 9-1-1 service that reliably reroutes calls to the appropriate PSAP.
- Evaluate and employ technologies that attenuate potential barriers to EMS access.
- Enhance the ability of EMS systems to triage calls, and provide resource allocation that is tailored to patients' needs.
- Implement 9-1-1 nationwide.

Communication Systems

- Assess the effectiveness of various personnel and resource attributes for EMS dispatching.
- Receive all calls for EMS using personnel with the requisite combination of education, experience, and resources to optimally query the caller, make determination of the most appropriate resources to be mobilized, and implement and effective course of action.
- Promulgate and update standards for EMS dispatching.
- Develop cooperative ventures between communications centers and health care providers to integrate communications processes and enable rapid patient-related information exchange.
- Determine the benefits of real-time patient data transfer.
- Appropriate federal, state, and regional funds to further develop and update geographically integrated and functionally based EMS communication networks.
- Collaborate with private interests to effect shared purchasing of communication technology.

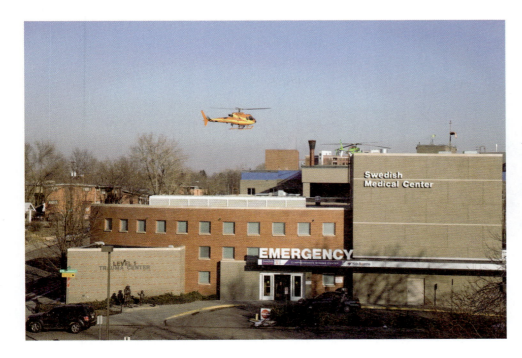

Fig. 1-3 Level 1 trauma center. Trauma centers are specialized hospitals that are ready to care for patients with serious and multiple injuries. (From Henry M, Stapleton E: *EMT prehospital care,* ed 4, St. Louis, 2010, Mosby.)

Clinical Care

- Eliminate patient transport as a criterion for compensating EMS systems.
- Establish proactive relationships between EMS and other health care providers.
- Commit to a common definition of what constitutes baseline community EMS care.
- Subject EMS clinical care to ongoing evaluation to determine its impact on patient outcomes.
- Employ new care techniques and technology only after they have been shown to be effective.
- Conduct task analysis to determine appropriate staff configuration during secondary patient transfers.

Information Systems

- Develop information systems that are able to describe an entire EMS event.
- Adopt uniform data elements and definitions, and incorporate them into information systems.
- Develop mechanisms to generate and transmit data that are valid, reliable, and accurate.
- Develop integrated information systems with other health care providers, public safety agencies, and community resources.
- Provide feedback to those who generate data.

Evaluation

- Develop valid models for EMS evaluations.
- Evaluate EMS effects for multiple medical conditions.
- Determine EMS effects for multiple outcome categories.
- Determine EMS cost-effectiveness.
- Incorporate consumer input into the evaluation process.

Trauma Systems

Another important consideration in EMS systems is participating in a trauma system. Caring for a patient with multiple injuries often requires a variety of health care specialists. Immediate access to surgical care may also be needed. Because few general hospitals can provide these resources, **trauma systems** have been developed. Trauma systems ensure that patients with life-threatening injuries are rapidly transported to the most appropriate hospital or specialized center for life-saving surgical care. Trauma systems will include services ranging from level I trauma centers, where the highest level of care is available, to hospitals that participate in the trauma system by giving immediate care to the trauma patient in preparation for transfer to a higher level of care (Fig. 1-3).

Access to the Emergency Medical System

As an emergency first responder, you may be sent to the scene of an injured or ill patient, or you may be present on the scene and providing patient care before the EMS system is activated. In the latter situation, you or someone else will need to call for additional medical help. The

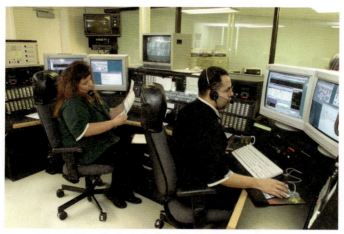

Fig. 1-4 A 9-1-1 dispatch center.

9-1-1 system and the popularity of cell phones have greatly enhanced the ability to call for help. Before the 9-1-1 emergency system was developed, each community had its own separate phone numbers for police, fire, and ambulance services. Currently, many communities have access to either basic or enhanced 9-1-1 systems.

In the basic 9-1-1 system, calls to the emergency number are routed to a central **dispatch center** (Fig. 1-4). The operator must learn the exact location of the emergency from the caller in order to dispatch help. In the enhanced 9-1-1 system, the caller's location is immediately displayed on the dispatcher's computer monitor, so the caller doesn't need to know or provide that information. Modern enhanced 9-1-1 centers can identify the location of the caller's cell phone, which can further assist in getting responders to the scene. Of course, the enhanced system can display only the location of the telephone, not of the emergency. In the opening scenario, for example, if the call were made from a nearby house, the caller would still have to tell the operator the location of the motor vehicle collision in relationship to that house. A caller using a cell phone should also give the dispatcher the details of the emergency location.

In some emergency situations, a patient who calls 9-1-1 might not be able to talk to the dispatcher. The person's injury may affect his or her ability to speak, or the person may feel threatened by a possible attacker present at the scene. In such cases, when the enhanced 9-1-1 system provides the dispatcher with the location, police may be dispatched first to determine the nature of the emergency. The investigating police officer may then request additional medical help.

Not all areas have 9-1-1 dispatch centers, and some may still have different phone numbers for police, fire, and EMS. A nonunified system may cause communication and dispatch delays and ultimately delay patient

care. It is important that you, as an emergency first responder, know and understand the dispatch system used for all of the emergency response agencies in your area.

Levels of Training for Prehospital Care Providers

In the United States, there are four nationally recognized levels of training for prehospital care providers. At each level above the first, additional training is required and the prehospital care provider gains additional skills. In 2005, the National Scope of Practice Document changed the four levels of prehospital care providers to the following:

- Emergency medical responder (formerly first responder)
- Emergency medical technician (EMT) (formerly EMT-basic)
- Advanced emergency medical technician (AEMT) (formerly EMT-intermediate)
- Paramedic (formerly EMT-paramedic)

Emergency Medical Responder

The National Scope of Practice Document recommended changing the title First Responder to emergency medical responder to avoid confusion with the generic first responder term that refers to all responders without regard to training levels. An **emergency medical responder** may be a firefighter, a police officer, a neighbor, a schoolteacher, or an industrial first-aid worker that completes a 40-hour training program. In this text, we will refer to the emergency medical responder as the emergency first responder. The emergency medical responder is the first designated level of professional emergency medical care as outlined by the National EMS Education and Practice Blueprint and the National Scope of Practice. Emergency medical responders are taught the following skills:

- Assessment for life-threatening conditions in both medical and trauma patients
- Provision of initial airway care
- Assistance with breathing
- Provision of cardiopulmonary resuscitation (CPR)
- Control of bleeding
- Stabilization of spinal and extremity injuries

In addition, emergency first responders are taught to use a limited amount of equipment and other skills as determined by local and state regulations. Emergency

In the Real World—continued

About 15 feet from the vehicle you find a young woman on the ground lying on her back. As you approach her you notice that she is not moving, and you see blood coming from a cut on her forehead. As you get closer, you can hear that her breathing is noisy and irregular.

When you finally reach the patient you kneel down and, placing your hands on each side of her head, you hold her head and neck in a stationary position while you open her airway. Once you have the airway open, the patient's breathing improves and becomes less noisy. Just after you open the patient's airway, two law enforcement officers arrive on the scene. One officer positions himself at the roadside and starts to direct traffic. The second officer climbs down the embankment and asks if there is anything she can do to help you. You state that you will stay with this patient but that you need the officer to look for other possible victims.

The officer begins by searching for other victims inside the vehicle but is unable to get a good look inside because the car is still lying on its side and remains unstable. While waiting for the fire and rescue services to arrive, the officer continues to search outside the vehicle for other victims.

first responders are expected to initially control a scene and to activate EMS. Finally, emergency first responders are trained to assist other prehospital care providers.

Emergency Medical Technician (EMT)

The emergency medical technician (EMT) is a progression from skills taught to the emergency first responder with additional skills for managing medical and traumatic emergencies. EMT training programs consist of a minimum of 120 hours of training but may be longer. EMTs learn more advanced airway skills, management of fractures, the administration of some medications, and transport of patients. In most jurisdictions, the EMT is the minimum training level that a person must have to work on an ambulance. EMT skills are the foundation for the more advanced prehospital care levels.

Advanced Emergency Medical Technician (AEMT)

In addition to the skills of an EMT, the AEMT has the skills to establish intravenous (IV) lines and administer IV fluids and certain drugs. AEMTs may also be taught more advanced airway management techniques. Currently, the AEMT level is one of the most variable in EMS. Different jurisdictions have different training and skills expectations.

Paramedic

Paramedics provide the highest level of prehospital care in the United States. Paramedic training programs typically consist of 2,000 hours or more. In addition to having the skills of all other levels, paramedics have training in advanced airway procedures such as endotracheal intubation, medication administration, and management of cardiac emergencies.

Certification or Licensure

Not all states license or certify emergency first responders. In states that do, however, the process is the same as with EMT, AEMT, or paramedic. After completion of a program that uses the education standards and completions of a practical exam that follows the curriculum, the candidate can apply to take the state or national registry exam. Certification or licensure is usually issued for a 2 to 4-year period. For information on licensure or certification in your area, contact your state EMS agency or the National Registry of EMTs at www.nremt.org/about/nremt_news.asp.

Americans with Disabilities Act Compliance

Schools that offer emergency first responder courses will follow the Americans with Disabilities Act and state and local rules, regulations, and policies regarding equal access, harassment, and safe educational environments. Likewise, the National Registry of EMTs makes accommodations for disabled applicants.

Advancement

To advance from emergency first responder to emergency medical technician, the emergency first responder should enroll in a recognized EMT program; candidates who successfully complete the program are allowed to sit for the state or national registry exam.

The Developing Future of EMS

In the United States, federal oversight of EMS is within the NHTSA within the DOT. NHTSA published the "EMS Agenda for the Future" in 1996, which took what earlier national endeavors had done and expanded those methods based on what has been learned in the first 20 years of organized EMS in the United States. These efforts resulted in the "EMS Education Agenda for the Future," which was published in 2000. The National Core Content was published in 2005. This publication listed the skills and knowledge essential to the practice of prehospital care. Also released that same year was "The National Scope of Practice." This document defines the four levels of prehospital care listed earlier in this chapter and the knowledge and skills necessary for each level. The latest release from NHTSA will be the National EMS Standards, which will replace the curricula used in the past. This new approach will delineate standards that academic institutions will use to design individualized curricula to meet those standards.

In-Hospital Care Systems

Most patients who receive EMS care are transported to emergency departments in local community hospitals. Emergency department staff members handle a vast spectrum of emergencies and medical conditions with little or no advance notice. They might go from treating a bleeding nose one minute to managing a major trauma or medical emergency the next (Fig. 1-5).

Because some kinds of emergencies may require more resources than are available in the local emergency department and hospital, specialized emergency centers have been established around the country. A patient might be transported first to the local emergency department, where staff members start treatment and stabilize the patient, and then be transported to a specialized center. In other cases, patients may be directly transported to these specialized centers.

Trauma centers are specialized hospitals committed to maintaining a state of readiness to care for patients with serious multiple injuries (see Fig. 1-3). This type of care is demanding for the hospital staff and requires special resources. Specialized surgeons and nurses must be prepared 24 hours a day to perform complex surgery

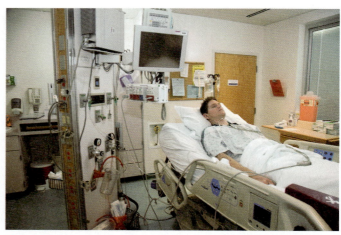

Fig. 1-5 Most patients receiving EMS care are transported to emergency departments in local community hospitals. (From Henry M, Stapleton E: *EMT prehospital care,* ed 4, St. Louis, 2010, Mosby.)

in only a moment's notice. These centers have dedicated intensive care units, computed tomography (CT) scanners, blood banks, specialty physicians, and support staff.

Burn centers provide specialized care for victims of thermal, chemical, electrical, and radiation burns. The staff in these centers also has special expertise for treating smoke inhalation injuries. Because there is only one burn center for every six trauma centers in the United States, a patient might first be transferred to a trauma center and later to a specialized burn center.

Specialty centers cater to specific needs with specialized equipment and trained personnel. We've discussed trauma and burn centers, but some cities may also be served by children's hospitals with specialized facilities and personnel for treating sick and injured children. A poison center is another example of specialty center. Personnel and databases allow these centers to ensure the proper response to patients exposed to poisons. These centers are also accessible via phone or Internet to support poisonings all over the world.

A child with a severe injury or sudden illness also presents unique challenges. It is often said that children are not just small adults, and this is true in important ways. Children's medical emergencies are rarely similar to those seen in adults. Even with the same kind of trauma, the injuries in a child will be different from those in an adult. For the special needs of children, specialized pediatric emergency centers and hospitals have been established.

Complications of childbirth also require specialized care. A woman in preterm labor, for example, may be transported from a community hospital to a center

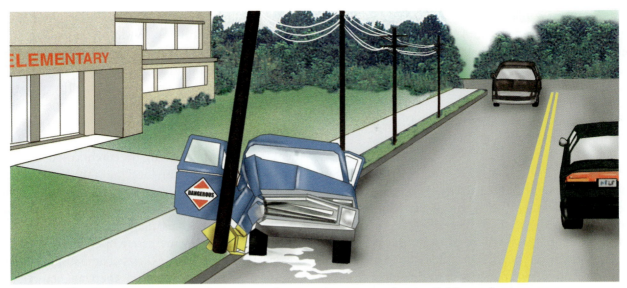

Fig. 1-6 An emergency first responder must be aware of potential hazards at a scene.

specializing in prenatal care (a center that can care for both the mother and the baby).

The **poison control center** for patients who experience a poisoning emergency is another special resource. These centers maintain large databases of information about household and industrial toxins. The people who staff these centers are proficient in toxicology. Poison control centers have a supportive role and can provide information on a particular poisonous substance. There is a nationwide number for poison control (800-222-1212). In addition, each state may have its own poison control center phone number.

Role of the First Responder
Scene Safety

Emergency first responders save lives because, more often than any other emergency care provider, they get to the patient first. A child who chokes on a toy or an elderly man in cardiac arrest has only a few minutes to live unless someone intervenes. A teenager with a head injury after a vehicle collision may experience irreversible brain damage quickly unless someone opens his or her airway. The lifesaving skills that you as an emergency first responder will use with these patients are often simple and do not require specialized equipment. They must, however, be used quickly and effectively.

Emergency first responders programs are therefore designed to teach these skills to people who are most likely to reach the scene before an ambulance arrives, such as police officers, firefighters, teachers, coworkers, factory workers, lifeguards, and other members of the community. When an emergency occurs, the ability to quickly reach the patient's side is vital.

Personal safety, however, must always be a primary responsibility. As an emergency first responder, you should never jeopardize your own security for that of a patient. This principle may at first seem selfish or evenly cowardly. Keep in mind, however, that your objective is to help the patient, and the most immediate threat to the patient is being deprived of your care if you are injured on the scene. If you are injured while rushing to a patient in an unsafe situation, the arriving EMS crew will have two patients and have to divide their efforts and resources between you and the original patient (Fig. 1-6).

In addition to your personal safety, you should also be mindful of bystanders and ensure they are safe. The need to also care for an injured bystander complicates an already difficult task. Bystanders who try to assist you may actually block your access to the patient or they may cause confusion on the scene with emotional outbursts. Relatives are entitled to be anxious and emotional, but when their presence adds chaos or disrupts care, the situation can quickly become ineffective and dangerous. If the presence of family members becomes a problem, you should ask another bystander to help move them out of the immediate area. An emergency first responder should always maintain control of the scene until he or she is relieved by a more advanced health care provider or an incident command officer.

Gaining Access

Sometimes the emergency first responder may have challenges in getting to the patient. Gaining access may be as simple as opening a door or as complex as using special equipment to work in a confined or hazardous space. Emergency first responders should work within the level of their training to ensure that the scene is not made more complex by an injury to an emergency first responder. Many emergency first responders will be trained in extrication or using tools to gain access to an entrapped patient, or they may have technical rescue training for confined spaces and terrain hazards.

Patient Care

In some situations, the patient may not be readily accessible. As a general rule, if the scene is not safe to enter, you must wait for the scene to be made safe. Even if the scene is safe, the patient may need to be moved before patient assessment can begin. Once it is safe to approach the scene, the number of patients should be determined. In multiple patient situations, triage or determining the severity of the patients' injuries ensures that neediest patients are cared for first.

Once at the patient's side, you will perform a systematic evaluation for any life-threatening conditions. Approaching the patient, the emergency first responder should determine the mechanism of injury in injured patients or the chief complaint of ill patients. This will help determine what should be assessed first to determine the presence of any immediate life threats. This is the initial part of patient assessment. In emergency care, patient assessments should always be performed in the same organized manner, as you will learn in the following chapters. No matter how chaotic a situation might become, you can always use the same techniques that you will practice in this course (Fig. 1-7).

The patient is then treated, or managed, based on your assessment findings. Once you have begun treat-

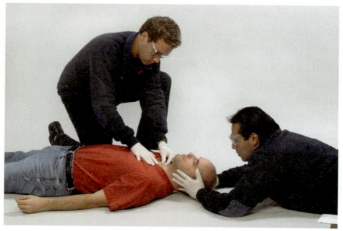

Fig. 1-7 Patient assessment.

ment, you should periodically reevaluate the patient to determine if his or her condition is getting better or worse.

When the ambulance or more advanced medical care arrives on the scene, you should identify yourself as a trained emergency first responder and report the details of the occurrence, your physical assessment, and the treatment you have given. If you are required to document this information in the prehospital care record, you should follow your local or state requirements for documentation. Details about the first few minutes after the occurrence of an emergency can be very important to help physicians diagnose or treat the patient's condition. When emergency personnel with more advanced training arrive, they become responsible for the care of the patient, yet even then an emergency first responder remains a valuable team member and can still render assistance.

In the scenario we have presented in this chapter, the emergency first responder transferred care to the arriving paramedics but remained at the scene and continued to care for the patient by assisting the paramedics as requested.

Personal Traits

As an emergency first responder, your responsibilities involve more than just your actions at the emergency scene.

Personal Health and Well-Being

Emergency care can be physically, emotionally, and psychologically draining. To deal with these stresses, you should strive to maintain your own personal health. Regular exercise will help prevent personal injury and has been shown to be an effective tool for preventing the adverse effects of emotional stress. As a prehospital provider, you can make a positive impact on the lives of people in your community, but only if you stay fit and prevent injury to yourself. Chapter 2 more fully discusses maintaining your own health and well-being.

Personal Behavior

Your personal behavior is also important. Consider for a moment what we do as prehospital providers. People in crisis allow us, strangers, to care for their sick or dying loved ones. Few other individuals in our society share this privilege. You should never betray the public's trust by making rude, crass, or insensitive remarks. You need to remember that what might be a routine situation for you may be frightening and foreign to a patient. Every patient deserves your empathy and compassion; sometimes the most important thing is just to hold the patient's hand and be there to provide emotional support.

It is inappropriate to change your care based on a patient's race, religion, gender, age, or socioeconomic status. All patients have the right to the best care that you can provide.

Self-Composure

Self-composure is essential whenever you are dealing with an emergency. The patient, family members, and bystanders will be focused on you as the emergency first responder and the one in control of the situation. How you react to the emergency will affect how they react. If you panic, bystanders may also panic and the scene may become chaotic. This is a dangerous situation in which either the patient or you may be hurt. It is natural to feel some anxiety when you face a life-threatening situation, but you must contain this anxiety and project calm confidence. One technique you could use to accomplish this is to remember to *stop, think, and act*. Stop for a brief moment to think about what you are doing and what you have been trained to do, and then perform your duties.

Professional Appearance

A professional appearance also contributes to your credibility because people formulate their initial impressions based on your appearance. When you respond to an emergency as part of an EMS agency, you essentially represent that entire service. If your appearance is unprofessional, people may falsely assume that your assessment and care will be below par. Your clothes or uniform should be clean, fit well, and neat. Your shoes should be comfortable yet professional and have good traction for wet surfaces. Remember that you will be kneeling, squatting, and lifting when you wear these clothes, so be sure they are not too tight or constrictive. Health care workers usually refrain from wearing fragrances, which can sometimes aggravate a patient's nausea or allergies. Remember that you are most effective as an emergency first responder when you have total control of the scene. An emergency first responder is a visible individual; you should take advantage of this visibility by making the best possible impression with your behavior and appearance.

Maintain Your Knowledge and Skills

As an EMS professional, you are responsible for the welfare of your patients. The public expects that when they call for help they will receive state-of-the-art emergency care. All prehospital providers therefore have the responsibility to maintain their knowledge and skills by attending continuing education programs and practicing

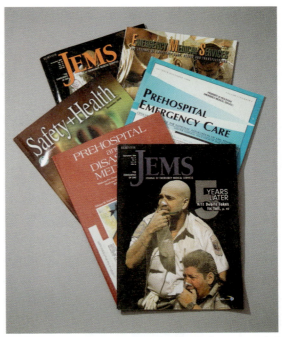

Fig. 1-8 Maintain your knowledge of national issues through subscriptions to EMS magazines.

their skills. Continuing education courses are generally offered at hospitals, fire departments, community colleges, and conferences. Your local EMS system can only be as good as its members, so get involved and take an active role in your continued training. Participation in emergency first responder refresher courses will also help you maintain your skills.

Current Knowledge of Local and National Issues

As an emergency first responder, you should make an effort to stay aware of issues affecting your community. You can maintain your knowledge of national issues through involvement in national or state organizations and subscriptions to EMS magazines (Fig. 1-8). Organizations you can become involved in include the National Association of Emergency Medical Technicians (NAEMT) or your state EMS association.

Medical Oversight

Every EMS system has some form of medical oversight. Usually a physician develops guidelines and protocols for the emergency treatment of patients. This physician is referred to as the **medical director.** The exact responsibilities of medical directors vary in different areas, but the medical director is ultimately responsible for the prehospital medical care delivered by that EMS service. Many

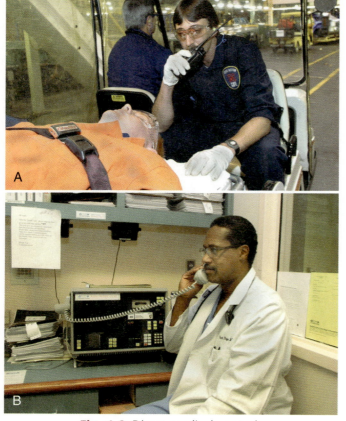

Fig. 1-9 Direct medical control.

states consider that prehospital personnel provide care by acting as an agent for the medical director. Because you as a prehospital provider are a surrogate for the physician, both you and the medical director may be responsible in the event of a problematic outcome.

There are two common types of medical oversight: direct and indirect. **Direct medical control** (also called online, base station, immediate or concurrent control) occurs when the prehospital team communicates with the physician before providing a specific treatment. This communication usually occurs by either radio or telephone (Fig. 1-9).

Indirect medical control (also called offline or prospective control) involves clear protocols, or standing orders, for the treatment of various emergencies. The medical director develops these protocols and ensures that prehospital providers are well trained in them. Prehospital care providers can then provide care in some emergency situations by following these protocols, without first having to communicate directly with the medical director. A continuous quality improvement (CQI) program is needed to evaluate how well the protocols are being carried out. If problems are found, the protocols might need revision or additional training might be required.

Many EMS systems use a combination of these two types of medical control. Written protocols are in place for many emergencies, for example, but the physician's orders might be required to administer a particular medication.

Depending on your state's laws, as an emergency first responder you may be considered an agent of the physician medical director. Frequent and open communication between you and the medical director is in everyone's best interest.

Specific Statutes and Regulations

Every state has its own laws regarding how prehospital care is provided, but the important issues are generally the same. Legal issues affecting EMS include Good Samaritan laws, consent for treatment, and consent for refusal of treatment, abandonment, and confidentiality.

Good Samaritan laws cover the liability of an individual who volunteers assistance in an emergency. These laws protect licensed health care providers who give emergency assistance in good faith as long as they do not commit negligent, willful, or wanton acts of misconduct or omissions, or charge for their services. In general this means that if you volunteer your assistance and act in accordance with your training, you cannot be held liable. If you attempt a technique that you are not trained to perform or intentionally harm a patient, you may be held liable for resulting injuries. Once you start emergency treatment, you are obligated to continue to give care until you have transferred that care to someone of equal or higher training. Failure to continue treatment until you are appropriately relieved is called abandonment.

Before giving treatment, you need consent from the patient. With a minor, consent comes from the child's parent or guardian. Consent need not be written; verbal consent is acceptable. In life-threatening emergencies or situations when the patient is unconscious or otherwise unable to give consent, the consent is said to be implied. Competent patients, however, are allowed to refuse help. If a patient refuses help, you may disagree with that decision but must respect the patient's legal rights. In such a case, you must first ensure that the patient understands the risks of refusing care and explain to the patient what might happen without timely medical attention. You should also inform patients that if they change their minds or their conditions worsen, they should call EMS or go to a local emergency department.

Team Work

As previously discussed in this chapter, emergency first responders perform their work in a variety of settings. You may be on a team at an industrial site or school, or you may be a part of a sophisticated rescue team. Wherever you work, you will be working with police officers, firefighters, rescue teams with specialized training in both medical and nonmedical areas, and others. As an emergency first responder, you will need to familiarize yourself with agencies likely to respond in your service area and have a plan for interaction with them. You will need to work closely with police and fire personnel to ensure the safety of the scene for both you and the patient. Rescue and EMS personnel will depend on you for the initial history of the patient's emergency. It is important to work within the limits of your certification or licensure and to assist other health care providers when called upon. Your patients will certainly benefit from your ability to give an accurate account of their medical histories, the results of your examination, and any treatment you may have provided. Emergency first responders should always remember that they are part of the patient care *team* that *works* toward a positive patient outcome.

In the Real World—Conclusion

Within a few minutes, the fire and rescue services arrive. The rescue service begins the task of stabilizing the vehicle and searching for additional victims. The fire department personnel run a charged line from the pumper to the vehicle for standby in case of fire or the need to isolate and secure gasoline or other hazardous materials.

Soon after the fire and rescue personnel determine that there are no other victims from the crash, the ambulance arrives. Two paramedics ask you for information about the patient, the results of your assessment, and the treatment you have provided. After giving the paramedics a report on the patient, who has remained unconscious, you transfer care of the patient to them. You help the paramedics prepare the patient for transport and load her into the ambulance. The paramedics thank you for your help and head to the trauma center with the patient.

After the ambulance leaves, the law enforcement officers and fire department personnel speak to you about the incident and the patient. After you report to them what you know, they thank you for your help. A wrecker arrives, pulls the vehicle to an upright position, and removes the vehicle as you head back to your own car.

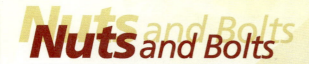

Nuts and Bolts

Critical Points

An emergency first responder should be able to define what an EMS system comprises and what role an emergency first responder plays. An emergency first responder requires adequate training to fulfill his or her role and should know how to interact with other members of the health care team.

Learning Checklist

❑ The steps that occur during an emergency include the initial recognition of the emergency, activation of EMS, arrival of the emergency first responder, patient care, arrival of additional emergency first responders, arrival of EMS, transport of the patient, and the transfer to the in-hospital care system.

❑ As described in "EMS Agenda for the Future," an EMS system has 14 attributes: (1) integration of health services, (2) EMS research, (3) legislation and regulation, (4) system finance, (5) human resources, (6) medical direction, (7) education systems, (8) public education, (9) prevention, and (10) public access, (11) communications systems, (12) clinical care, (13) information systems, and (14) evaluation.

❑ Access to the EMS system is usually achieved through the basic or enhanced 9-1-1 system. In both systems, calls are routed to a central 9-1-1 dispatch center. In the basic system, the caller must identify the location to send help. In the enhanced system, ideally the caller's location is immediately displayed on the dispatcher's computer monitor.

❑ The four levels of training for prehospital care suggested by the 2005 National Scope of Practice are (1) emergency medical responder, (2) emergency medical technician (EMT), (3) advanced emergency medical technician (AEMT), and (4) paramedic.

❑ An emergency first responder is the first to arrive on the scene and provide medical attention to the patient. Skills include immediate assessment and management of life-threatening conditions, control of a scene, activation of EMS, and assistance for other prehospital care providers.

❑ An EMT learns additional airway skills and shock management. The EMT can also administer certain medications and transport patients.

❑ An AEMT has the skills of an EMT and can also establish IV lines and more advanced airways and can administer some medications.

❑ Paramedics are the highest level of prehospital care and are trained, for example, in endotracheal intubation and other advanced airway techniques, and medication administration.

❑ When a patient is transferred to the in-hospital system, he or she may go to a local general hospital or to a specialized center. Specialized centers include trauma centers, burn centers, pediatric emergency centers and hospitals, and perinatal centers.

❑ The responsibilities of an emergency first responder include personal safety, patient care, personal health and well-being, professional and courteous personal behavior, self-composure in an emergency, a professional appearance, current knowledge and practice of skills, and awareness of local and national issues.

❑ The medical director is the physician who maintains medical oversight over an EMS system.

❑ Direct medical control occurs when the prehospital team communicates directly with the physician before giving treatment to a patient. This usually occurs over the radio or the telephone.

❑ Indirect medical control occurs with protocols or standing orders that outline the care to provide a patient in a given situation.

❑ Every state has its own laws regarding prehospital care. It is important for an emergency first responder to find out about and know local laws.

Key Terms

Burn centers Provide specialized care for victims of thermal, chemical, electrical, and radiation burns.

Direct medical control Real-time communication between prehospital care personnel and medical control. This can take place in person, on the phone, or over the radio. Also called online medical control.

Dispatch center A centralized location that obtains information about and assigns resources to an incident.

Emergency An unexpected situation that arises and threatens the life of one or more people.

Emergency first responder One of the four training levels of EMS. The new terminology was created to better describe the position of First Responder as written by the 2005 National Scope of Practice.

Emergency Medical Services (EMS) System The network of services that handles prehospital medical and trauma emergencies. These systems are organized at a local, regional, state, or national level.

Emergency medical technician (EMT) A medical provider who performs prehospital care. Typically refers to the EMT-Basic level but may be used to denote any level of prehospital care. Part of the organized EMS system.

First Responder The initial person at the scene of a medical or trauma emergency trained in medical care. Part of the organized EMS system.

Indirect medical control The use of standing orders or written protocols to provide care. This type of medical control does not involve actual communication with a medical director at the time of the incident. Also called offline medical control.

Medical director A physician who develops guidelines and protocols for the prehospital treatment of patients. The medical director is responsible for the prehospital medical care delivered by the EMS service.

Paramedic The most advanced level of prehospital emergency medical care. Part of the organized EMS system.

Poison control center A service that provides data on all aspects of poisonings, keeps records of poisonings, and refers patients to treatment centers.

Specialty centers Cater to specific needs with specialized equipment and trained personnel.

Trauma center A specialized hospital equipped with personnel and resources to immediately care for a critically injured trauma patient.

Trauma system A system to help identify the appropriate hospital or specialized center for a trauma patient to be transported to.

First Responder NSC Objectives
COGNITIVE OBJECTIVES

- Define the attributes of EMS systems.
- Differentiate the roles and responsibilities of the First Responder from other out-of-hospital care providers.
- Define medical oversight, and discuss the First Responder's role in the process.
- Discuss the types of medical oversight that may affect the medical care that a First Responder provides.
- State the specific statutes and regulations in your state regarding the EMS system.

AFFECTIVE OBJECTIVES

- Accept and uphold the responsibilities of a First Responder in accordance with the standards of an EMS professional.
- Explain the rationale for maintaining a professional appearance when on duty or when responding to calls.
- Describe why it is inappropriate to judge a patient based on a race, gender, age, or socioeconomic model and to vary the standard of care rendered as a result of that judgment.

Check your understanding

Check your understanding

Please refer to p. 439 for the answers to these questions.

1. True or False: All areas of the United States have access to emergency medical care by dialing 9-1-1.

2. True or False: In most cases, an ill or injured person cannot legally refuse the care of an emergency medical responder.

3. The plans, policies, personnel, and resources called upon in a community when there is a medical emergency are part of the _____.

4. The process by which a physician provides guidelines for patient care and reviews the quality of care provided by emergency first responders and other EMS personnel is called _____.

5. The first person with emergency medical training to arrive at the scene of an emergency is a/an _____.

6. A hospital that specializes in maintaining the personnel and resources to care for patients with serious injuries around the clock is a/an _____.

7. A center that maintains a database of information about household and industrial toxins and provides information on toxic substances to medical personnel is a/an _____.

8. The process of finding any immediate life-threatening conditions and evaluating the patient is known as _____.

9. In addition to maintaining medical knowledge and skills and keeping current on local and national issues and trends in EMS, what are four additional responsibilities of an emergency first responder?
   A. _____
   B. _____
   C. _____
   D. _____

10. Leaving a patient after you have started care but before another EMS provider arrives at the patient's side is called _____.

11. State laws designed to protect from liability an individual who volunteers assistance at an emergency are known as _____ laws.

12. Which of the following is among the skills typically taught in an emergency first responder course?
    A. Advanced airway skills
    B. Pneumatic antishock trousers
    C. IVs
    D. Control of bleeding

13. Which of the following is the most highly trained EMT?
    A. Paramedic
    B. EMT-Basic
    C. EMT-Intermediate
    D. Shock-trauma EMT

14. Which of the following is the first, or primary, responsibility of an emergency first responder when responding to an emergency?
    A. Patient care
    B. Assessing the need for additional resources
    C. Personal safety
    D. Determining the number of patients

15. Which of the following individuals may serve as the medical director of an emergency first responder organization?
    A. Physician
    B. Paramedic
    C. EMT at the rank of captain or higher
    D. Emergency department nurse

16. You arrive on the scene where a vehicle has struck a pedestrian. The vehicle is stopped, and the patient is lying in the road about 5 feet from the vehicle. Traffic is stopped. Which of the following should you do first?
A. Check to see if the patient is breathing.
B. Check to see that the vehicle is in *Park*.
C. Ask a bystander to bring blankets to cover the patient.
D. Ask the driver of the vehicle to move the vehicle.

17. You are treating a patient who was involved in an all-terrain vehicle (ATV) collision in a remote area of your region. You are unable to contact the hospital via radio or phone. You are able to perform skills and provide care based on which of the following?
A. Direct medical control
B. Quality assurance
C. Indirect medical control
D. Trauma system

Chapter 2

Well-Being of the Emergency First Responder

LESSON GOAL

Your physical safety and emotional well-being are essential to your effective work as an emergency first responder. This chapter will explore situational risks and challenges and cover methods to maintain your physical and emotional well-being as an emergency first responder.

OBJECTIVES

1. Discuss emotional reactions that may be experienced by emergency first responders, patients, family members, and bystanders when faced with trauma, illness, death, and dying.
2. Discuss the steps in your approach to the family confronted with death and dying.
3. Describe the possible reactions that the family of the emergency first responder may exhibit because of his or her involvement in emergency medical services (EMS).
4. Recognize the signs and symptoms of critical incident stress.
5. State possible steps you may take to help reduce/alleviate stress.
6. Given a scenario, explain how scene safety can be determined.
7. Given a scenario involving the potential for exposure to communicable disease, select the personal protective equipment (PPE) appropriate for body substance isolation.
8. List the PPE necessary for each of the following situations: hazardous materials, rescue operations, violent scenes, crime scenes, electricity, water and ice, and exposure to communicable pathogens.
9. Describe the importance of understanding the response to death and dying and communicating effectively with the patient's family.
10. Demonstrate empathy in all interactions with patients and their family members and friends.
11. Given a scenario, explain the procedures for cleaning, disinfection, or disposal of all items that are potentially contaminated with infectious materials.

In the Real World

You are an emergency first responder on a factory team. You respond to a call and arrive first on the scene. One of the workers on the assembly line has caught his hand on the conveyor belt as it moved by him. You can barely hear him call to you over the noise of the moving line. You survey the scene for safety. You put on safety glasses, gloves, and a hard hat before proceeding. As you approach the victim, you see that he is your sister's husband. He is bleeding heavily from his right arm. You fear that he may lose that arm.

By becoming an emergency first responder you have made a decision to help others even at the potential risk of danger or injury to yourself. This is a commendable decision, but it is also a serious commitment. You must become skilled at coping with the emotional and physical stress of the job. You must also learn to understand and assist others as they endure the stress of an emergency situation. When you arrive at the scene of an emergency, you will assess risks, prepare yourself, and intervene to help victims of injury and illness. You will be able to perform procedures that can save a patient's life. Even in the midst of chaotic situations, you must remember your training. Your first priority must always be to protect your own safety and well-being. You can be the best help to others when you are safe, healthy, and emotionally strong.

The work of an emergency first responder is rewarding but not easy. Sometimes the scene is dangerous and hazards are encountered. You must prepare yourself to minimize the risks. This chapter explores ways to maintain your well-being as an emergency first responder (Box 2-1).

Stressful Situations

Emergency first responders should be prepared to see people at their worst. Sick and injured patients can be stressed and in turn may exhibit irrational behavior. Compassion and professionalism can reassure patients and enable them to manage their stress and assist in their own care.

The horrible things that happen to people can be difficult to witness and live with (Box 2-2). Mass casualty incidents (MCIs), which may involve many people, can be confusing and the cumulative impact of dealing with all of the causalities and pain can be overwhelming. Working with pediatric patients can be particularly difficult because children are expected to be bright and playful, not sick or seriously hurt. Violent situations make little sense, whether the perpetrator is a stranger or a family member. Abuse of children, spouses, or the elderly can evoke your own anger or sadness. Amputations of limbs can be challenging to witness and difficult to explain. The death of a patient can be a jolting experience. When you work hard to keep a patient alive, it may be difficult not to take it as a personal failure if a patient dies. If a coworker or another public safety officer is injured or killed, you may feel the fear or loss more keenly. These are just a few examples of the stressful situations an emergency first responder may face. Everyone has different triggers and thresholds for stress. The trigger that causes you stress may not be the same for someone else.

As an emergency first responder you must be aware of, understand, and plan to manage stress. Stress can come from your patients or from other aspects of your life. The hours and environments of your work can induce stress. You will experience not only your own stress but the stress of patients, families, and bystanders. As an emergency first responder, you must find ways to cope with these stresses or they will have a detrimental effect on your personal and professional life. Recognition of stress and use of coping mechanisms are addressed in greater detail later in this chapter.

Prevention and Promoting Health

As much as this is a stressful business and we need to plan for this stress to stay healthy, overall health and disease prevention will give us our best chances to deal with the physical and mental stresses we can face. Emergency first responders should avoid risks to health such as smoking, being overweight, and using drugs or alcohol inappropriately. Hygiene, healthy diets, and physical exercise have all been shown to contribute to physical and mental health and will enhance our ability to respond to these stresses.

BOX 2-1   Federal Government Begins Mandating High-Visibility Vests for Emergency Responders

On November 24, 2008, a new federal regulation (23 CFR 634) goes into effect mandating that anyone working in the right-of-way of a federal-aid highway must be wearing high-visibility clothing that meets the requirements of ANSI/ISEA 107; 2004 edition class 2 or 3. This requirement will apply to all emergency responders.

The Code of Federal Regulations Title 23 (Highways) Part 634 was originally published in the *Federal Register* Vol 71, No 226, pp 67792-67800. The rule itself (634.3) simply states that:

"All workers within the right-of-way of a Federal-aid highway who are exposed either to traffic (vehicles using the highway for purposes of travel) or to construction equipment within the work area shall wear high-visibility safety apparel."

"High-Visibility Safety Apparel" is defined to mean "personal protective safety clothing that is intended to provide conspicuity during both daytime and nighttime usage, and that meets the Performance Class 2 or 3 requirements of

the ANSI/ISEA 107-2004." ANSI 107 requires that class 2 garments (vests) have at least 775 square inches of high-visibility, fluorescent background material and at least 201 square inches of reflective material.

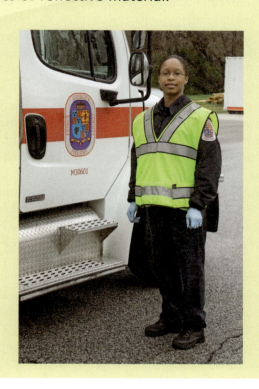

BOX 2-2   Examples of Stressful Situations

- Mass casualty incidents (MCIs)
- Pediatric patients
- Death
- Amputations
- Violence
- Abuse
- Death or injury of a coworker or other public safety worker

Death and Dying

Death affects emergency first responders, other health care team members, family, friends, and bystanders. The way we respond to death is a highly individual matter, shaped by our culture and experience. You may see responses that vary from a family quietly crying, to a room full of inconsolable people wailing and throwing themselves on the floor, to a mob yelling angrily at you. A large part of how we respond to death is learned from our parents and family members or others involved in our upbringing. What you are exposed or not exposed to as you grow up greatly affects your ability or inability to handle the stress of death and dying. Yet no matter what your life experiences may be, as an emergency first responder you must be able to respond professionally and compassionately to dying patients or those affected by death. Some adults may not have experienced the death of someone close to them. Without past experiences from which they have recovered, their sense of loss can be overwhelming. As an emergency first responder, you will probably encounter scenes involving death, treat dying patients, and support the families and friends of those who have died. You must try to understand the concerns of the dying patient, communicate empathetically with family members following the death of a loved one, and manage your own feelings about death and loss.

Signs of Death

Generally, death is defined as the absence of circulatory and respiratory function. Many states have adopted the *brain death* provisions that define death as irreversible cessation of all functions of the brain and brain stem. As an emergency first responder, you may need to determine if a patient is dead or requires emergency medical care. By most current standards, emergency first responders must resuscitate all patients unless they are obviously dead or a do not resuscitate (DNR) order is present. Terminally ill patients may not want to be resuscitated. Chapter 3 discusses your rights and responsibilities related to resuscitation and DNR orders. If a DNR order is unclear or does not seem authentic, or if some other question exists, you should provide emergency medical care in the absence of definitive signs of death until there is clarification or you transfer care to another health care provider.

As a general rule, you should begin emergency medical care if the body is warm and intact. In cases of cold temperature emergencies where the patient may have hypothermia, you should always begin emergency medical care.

Presumptive signs of death are indications of death that, in combination, are accepted by most medical and legal authorities. These presumptive signs have even more weight following severe trauma or the end stages of a long-term illness such as cancer. These signs *are not* considered adequate in cases of extremely cold body temperature (hypothermia), poisonings, or heart attack (cardiac arrest). Box 2-3 includes some of the presumptive signs of death.

The definitive or conclusive signs of death include the following:

- *Clear mortal damage.* This includes such things as the body separated into parts (such as decapitation).
- *Rigor mortis.* Rigor mortis is the stiffening of body muscles caused by chemical changes within muscle tissue. It develops first in the face and jaw and gradually extends downward until the body is in full rigor. The rate of the body's stiffening is affected by the rate at which the body loses heat to the environment. A thin body loses heat faster than one with more body fat. A body on a tile floor loses heat faster than a body wrapped in a blanket in a bed. Rigor mortis can begin 2 to 12 hours after death. At least 2 or more joints should be assessed in order to determine the presence of rigor mortis. The jaw and fingers are usually easily accessible to assess. Postmortem lividity is the term that described the pooling of blood in the lowest parts of the body. This would cause the lower part of the body to appear darker then the higher parts and over more time could have an increasingly mottled or bruised look.
- *Putrefaction.* Putrefaction refers to the decomposition of body tissues. Depending on temperature conditions, this begins 40 to 96 hours after death.

Safety remains a chief determinant as to whether resuscitation should be initiated. If the situation the patient is in is unsafe, the emergency first responder should not attempt resuscitation. Any number of hazards could make it unsafe, such as violent scenes, fire or collapse scenes, or confined spaces.

Emotions of Critically Ill and Injured Patients

Individuals who are dying as a result of trauma, an acute medical emergency, or a terminal disease may experience a wide spectrum of emotions. They may feel threatened, frightened, hopeless, helpless, peaceful, or resigned. Their emotions may also change rapidly. Common emotional states of injured, critically ill, and dying patients include the following:

- Anxiety
- Pain and anger
- Depression
- Dependency
- Guilt
- Behavioral problems

Often these emotions are related to the normal stages of grieving. Your familiarity with these generally recognized stages can help you deal with patients who are

---

BOX 2-3 Presumptive Signs of Death

- Unresponsiveness to painful stimuli
- Absence of breathing
- Absence of a pulse or heartbeat
- Absence of deep tendon or corneal reflexes
- Absence of eye movement
- Lack of blood pressure
- Dependent lividity (blood settling to lowest point of the body, causing discoloration of the skin)
- Profound cyanosis (bluish coloration)
- Lowered body temperature

critically ill or injured. The normal stages of grief are discussed later in this chapter. When patients display emotions related to their critical condition, you should communicate honestly and empathetically as you acknowledge their feelings. Be calm; comfort and reassure the patient while you wait for additional resources to arrive. Your familiarity with common behavioral problems of patients who are critically ill or injured will help you provide effective care.

ANXIETY

Anxiety is a response to the anticipation of danger. These patients are often anxious about what will happen to them—whether they will die or become disabled—and about the care you provide. Patients who are anxious may be as follows:

- Upset
- Sweating and cool (diaphoretic)
- Breathing fast (hyperventilating)
- Tachycardic (have a fast pulse)
- Restless
- Tense
- Fearful
- Shaky (tremulous)

Panic is a severe anxiety reaction that can endanger both patients and emergency first responders. Your calm and confident care can help patients reduce their anxiety and maintain their self-control.

PAIN AND ANGER

Pain often occurs with illness or trauma. Patients may also fear anticipated pain and potential injury. You should encourage patients to express their pains and fears because expression may help them adjust to the pain and accept your emergency medical care.

Patients may also complain, express anger, and be demanding. You should understand that this anger may be a display of their fear or anxiety about emergency medical care. Patients who express anger toward you or other health care providers may express it physically. If a patient or family member gets so emotionally upset that you feel threatened or are physically assaulted, you should remove yourself from the scene and call for law enforcement. Remember, if you cannot make the scene safe, do not enter; if the scene becomes unsafe, leave. Your safety must be your first priority.

DEPRESSION

Most dying patients experience some degree of depression. Some patients have many dissatisfactions and regrets about their lives, whereas others may be concerned about current financial, legal, social, or family problems. You should encourage patients to express their feelings and concerns. Support patients and their families in resolving unsettled matters to help ease their feelings of depression.

DEPENDENCY

When you render emergency medical care to patients, they may develop a sense of dependency on you. As a result, they may become resentful or experience feelings of helplessness, shame, weakness, or inferiority.

GUILT

Many dying patients and their family members feel guilty about what has happened or about what they may or may not have done. Often they cannot explain their feelings. Patients who delayed requesting emergency medical care may also feel guilty.

BEHAVIORAL PROBLEMS

Behavioral problems such as disorientation, confusion, or delusions may develop in a dying patient. The patient may behave in ways that depart from normal patterns of thinking, feeling, or acting. Common characteristics of this behavior include the following:

- Loss of contact with reality
- Distorted perception
- Regressive behavior and attitudes
- Diminished control of basic impulses and desires
- Abnormal mental processes including delusions and hallucinations
- Generalized personality deterioration

Providing Care for Critically Ill and Injured Patients

As an emergency first responder, you should introduce yourself to all patients and let them know your level of training and your motivation—you are there to help. You should let patients know that you are attending to their immediate needs, which are your primary concerns. Also be sure to continually explain what is occurring to decrease patients' confusion, anxiety, and feelings of helplessness. You, other medical providers, and family and friends should not make any grim comments about a patient's condition. Such remarks may depress the patient, reduce hope, and possibly compromise recovery.

Lights, sirens, smells, and unknown personnel can confuse a patient. You should understand this and help the patient stay oriented to the situation. You can give explanations such as "Mr. Smith, you are hurt, the police are here, and I'm now treating your arm. My name is John, and I am an emergency first responder trained in emergency medical care. I'm here to help you and I'll stay with you until the ambulance arrives." You should use your judgment to be honest with patients without unnecessarily shocking or confusing them. If a patient refuses emergency medical care or asks that you leave him or her alone, you should explain the seriousness of the condition and your ability to help. You should not express undue alarm to try to persuade the patient, and you should not say, "Everything will be okay" when it is obvious that it will not. If a patient refuses emergency care, you should document this refusal in your report and, if possible, have the patient sign a refusal of care form (see Chapter 3).

Patients may ask you if they are going to die, and you may feel at a loss for words if you know that the prognosis is poor. You must remember that it is not your responsibility to tell a patient that death is imminent. Instead, you should make honest but helpful statements such as "I don't know if you are going to die, but let's fight this together" or "I'm not going to give up on you, so don't give up on yourself." It is appropriate for an emergency first responder to offer hope and to show conviction about doing everything possible to save a patient's life.

Often patients will ask you to contact a family member or someone else. A patient may or may not be able to assist with phone numbers or other information. In these situations you should assure the patient that you or someone else will attempt to locate the person.

With a critically ill or injured child, you should calm, comfort, and reassure the patient while waiting for additional responders. You can and should enlist the help of a family member, friend, or accompanying adult to relieve a child's anxiety and assist with care as appropriate.

Grieving helps us move through the stages of dealing with death and dying. People progress through these stages to move on with their lives. By becoming familiar with the grieving process, you will be better able to understand and help the people you encounter in each of the phases (Fig. 2-1).

Stages of Grief
DENIAL

The first phase of the grieving process is denial. People try to tell themselves, "This is not happening to me." It is a self-defense mechanism to create a buffer against the shock of death or illness. You may frequently encounter families in the denial stage, and your understanding of this defense mechanism may help you deal with this difficult situation. This stage is often characterized by disbelief at the situation or a "not me" response.

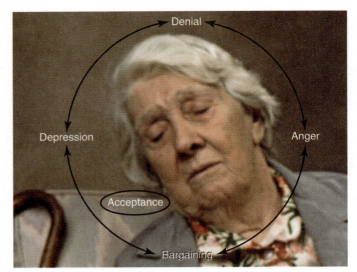

Fig. 2-1 Stages of grief.

ANGER

The next phase of grief is often anger. "Out of all the people in the world, why me?" your patient or their family may ask you. Alternatively, they may make you the target of their disbelief and anger. It is important that you do not take this personally or get defensive. Instead you should try to be tolerant and listen empathetically even if you do not fully understand how the patient feels. People in distress deeply appreciate attentive listening and genuine communication.

BARGAINING

In the next phase of the grieving process, people bargain. For example, a person might think, "Let this person live, and I'll quit smoking," in an attempt to delay death or hold out the chance for a deal to be struck. Again, you can help by listening to the patient and communicating both empathy and clarity. You must be sensitive to the patient and at the same time show strength by conveying the reality of the situation to all involved.

DEPRESSION

In this phase, people may begin to express sadness and despair. Crying followed by silent withdrawal is common. It is difficult to stay involved with desperately sad people, but an emergency first responder must cope with the sorrow and maintain communication with the patient.

ACCEPTANCE

A person may eventually accept his or her approaching death, even while remaining sad or angry. The friends or family will usually require more support during this stage than the patient. Acceptance may or may not be reached during the grieving process. It is important to understand that each of these stages can take time to get through.

Although these have been described as predictable responses to grief, the actual grieving process is highly individualized and may not follow any particular order.

Dealing with the Dying Patient and Family Members

Both the dying patient and the patient's family and friends will go through some or all of the phases of grief. As an emergency first responder, you too may go through a grieving period. It is important to note that different people may be at different stages of their grief. For example, the patient may have had time to accept death but the family may be in denial during your entire experience with them. Another family may have reached acceptance, while the patient struggles with denial. Understanding the process of grief can help you appropriately treat those who deal with death. You will need to express compassion to the patient and family and understanding for their loss.

You must respect a dying patient's emotions. The patient deserves dignity during this ultimate test. You should try to protect the dying patient's privacy and allow him or her any possible control over the care you provide. The patient will want you to listen empathetically and needs you to communicate reassuringly. You should avoid distorting the reality of the situation or making false reassurances. In a gentle tone, you should simply let the patient know that you and others will do everything you can to help. When appropriate, your reassuring touch can be very powerful.

The patient's family and friends may also need to express emotions ranging from rage to despair. In this type of situation, you should also listen empathetically and respond in a gentle tone. You should express your concern for the patient and the family and be honest about the patient's condition. You must be emotionally available to offer comfort to the family.

Stress Management

You may have many sources of stress in your life. Relationships, jobs, and financial situations can all cause stress. Being an emergency first responder will add more stress to your life. The various situations you will be called on to deal with can profoundly affect your life. You must identify the root causes of your stress to effectively manage the resulting feelings, and you should recognize that avoidance of stress is not a solution.

Recognizing Warning Signs

To manage the stress in your professional and personal life, you should be able to detect the warning signs of stress, which include the following:

- Irritability to coworkers, family, and friends
- Inability to concentrate
- Difficulty sleeping and/or nightmares
- Anxiety
- Indecisiveness
- Guilt
- Loss of appetite
- Loss of interest in sexual activities
- Isolation
- Loss of interest in work

The sooner stress and its effects are recognized, the simpler it will be to implement techniques that reduce the impact.

Lifestyle Changes

Once stress is recognized, you can make changes in your lifestyle to help you recover. It is common for emergency first responders to experience "job burnout." If you are unable to find healthy ways of dealing with the natural stress of responding to emergencies, you will likely want to stop experiencing those situations. To help manage stress, you may need to change your diet. Reducing your consumption of caffeine, sugar, and alcohol and balancing your diet will increase your energy level and allow you to think more clearly. Avoiding fatty foods and maintaining adequate protein intake will also increase your stores of energy.

Exercise is also valuable in increasing stamina and energy. You should stay physically active in sports or other recreational pursuits. You can learn and practice relaxation techniques like meditation or visual imagery. These are only a few examples of ways to handle stress; you will need to find ways of distancing yourself from the stress to recharge your emotional batteries.

Balance

The well-being of emergency first responders depends on maintaining a balance of work, family, friends, fitness, and recreation (Fig. 2-2). People who undergo heavy stress often lose the balance important to their physical and emotional well-being. You need to force yourself to make adequate time to balance the elements essential to your well-being. You can, for example, make a schedule and stick to it to ensure time for these activities. After engaging in them, you will be more relaxed and think more clearly.

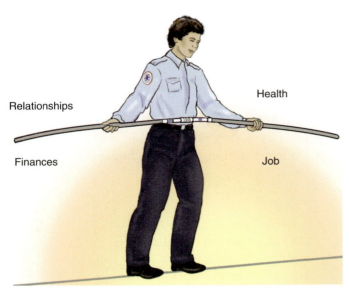

Relationships

Health

Finances

Job

Fig. 2-2 Maintaining balance in your life is an important part of your well-being.

Family and Friends

A common concern of emergency first responders is that friends and families don't understand the nature of being an emergency first responder. Such lack of understanding may cause you to withdraw from your family and friends and delve deeper into work. The need for emergency first responders to be on call can add more stress to family relationships. Coworkers may better understand and share your feelings about the challenging work; your family may feel ignored and fear separation. You may be frustrated by their apparent lack of understanding, whereas they may be discouraged by your distance. You must work to prevent this cycle from starting or getting out of control. You should keep the lines of communication open, share things that are important to you, and take the time to listen to the needs of your family and friends.

Work Environment Changes

Any work environment produces stresses independent of those we expect with EMS work. Your coworkers and supervisors and the way you interact with them can produce work-related stress, which is important to recognize for your well-being. Once identified, improved communication or counseling may help alleviate or otherwise address this type of stress. Shift work is a well-documented cause of stress and can affect your physical health. Changing shifts and working during hours when our bodies are used to sleeping disrupts rest, nutrition, and recreation cycles and can affect our emotional and

physical health. You may need to make compromises to better balance your work and your family. For example, you can request a shift that allows you time to relax with family and friends. If you experience warning signs of excessive stress from your work and your family, you might request a temporary rotation to a less stressful assignment.

Professional Help

You or a coworker at some point may feel unable to juggle the balance and stress of your personal and professional life alone. Mental health professionals, including physicians and social workers, are trained to help you deal with stress and return balance to your life. Clergy may also be helpful. If you had a medical emergency, you would not hesitate to call your EMS system. If you have an emotional problem, call on a mental health professional early to avoid serious disruption to your life. Many employees have access to the confidential services of either an employee assistance program (EAP) or member assistance program (MAP). You should take advantage of the many resources that are out there to help maintain the balance in your life.

Critical Incident Stress Management

An overload of stress can come from a single critical event, an accumulation of incidents, or a mass casualty incident. Whatever the source, it can be overwhelming and damaging to your emotional health. **Critical incident stress** is a normal response to abnormal circumstances. The **Critical incident stress management (CISM)** system is a comprehensive program designed to help people deal with the stress related to work. The system works on the premise that you will stay healthier or recover faster if you can discuss your fears, feelings, and reactions to critical incidents and feel support from coworkers and professionals. Specially trained teams of peer counselors and mental health workers can provide many essential services including the following:

- Preincident stress education
- On-scene peer support
- One-on-one support
- Disaster support services
- Follow-up services
- Family and spouse support
- Community outreach programs
- Wellness programs

Critical incident stress debriefing (CISD) is a function of the CISM system that uses specific techniques to help people express their feelings and recover from a stressful

BOX 2-4   Defusings and Debriefings

Defusings
- Shorter, less formal, and less structured version of CISD
- Used a few hours after the event
- Are 30 to 40 minutes in length
- Allow for initial ventilation
- May eliminate the need for a formal debriefing
- May enhance the formal debriefing

Debriefings
- Held within 24 to 72 hours of the event
- Include open discussion of feelings and fears
- Are not an investigation or interrogation
- Keep all information confidential

incident faster. The CISD team's techniques include **defusings** and **debriefings** (Box 2-4).

CISM leaders and mental health personnel listen to people, evaluate the information, and offer support and suggestions to reduce stress. CISM should be accessed when any of the following occur:

- Line-of-duty death or serious injury
- Multiple casualty incident
- Suicide of a coworker
- Serious injury or death to children
- Events with excessive media interest
- Victims are known to you
- Any event that has unusual impact on personnel
- Any disaster

CISM can provide a team of peers to provide debriefing or defusing sessions according to need.

Debriefings

These are designed to run within 24 to 72 hours of an event and provide an opportunity for open discussion and expression of feelings, fears and reactions. The facilitators will ensure that participants understand that this is not an interrogation or a critique and that all of the exchanges are confidential. Mental health personnel on the team may make suggestions for continued healing after the session ends.

Defusings

These are less formal or structured versions of CISD and are usually held within a few hours of the event. They can eliminate the need for a more formal debriefing or enhance the later debriefing.

As an emergency first responder, you should learn how to access your local critical incident stress response team. For the times when you or a coworker could benefit from their expertise, your team should be within easy reach.

It should be noted that there have been recent challenges in the literature to the effectiveness or even potential harm of these sessions. Proponents of the program still feel strongly about the program's benefits, and in most parts of the United States, EMS systems make CISM available to providers.

Personal Precautions
Risks to First Responders

Some of the most serious hazards you will face as an emergency first responder are invisible. You must be constantly aware of the risks associated with your job, including body substances such as a patient's blood. The **Occupational Health and Safety Administration (OSHA)** has developed guidelines to protect health care workers. The **Centers for Disease Control and Prevention (CDC)** establish protocols for protection against infection from body substances. These guidelines and protocols are referred to as **body substance isolation (BSI)**, standard precautions, or universal precautions. It is necessary to follow the appropriate guidelines for each situation to ensure personal safety.

You can protect yourself from all body substances by using appropriate **personal protection equipment (PPE)**. Whereas gloves and eye protection should always be worn, PPE, depending on the event, may also include a mask and gown (Fig. 2-3) or other specialty equipment. You should always use a pocket-mask with a one-way valve or other barrier device when ventilating or breathing for a patient to prevent your exposure to any diseases the patient may carry. You should always assess the potential risk and be vigilant about taking appropriate precautions. You should know about and use PPE as required by your local system.

You should also review governmental regulations in regard to BSI, including OSHA and state regulations. These regulations should be available through your state EMS office.

In the Real World—continued

As you assess the patient's mental condition, you locate the wound and apply pressure to attempt to slow the bleeding. An EMT arrives on the scene to assist with the care. You relay information and events and step back, ready to assist, as the EMT takes over patient care.

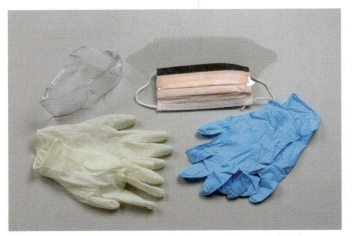

Fig. 2-3 Personal protection equipment (PPE).

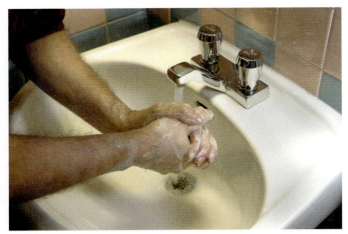

Fig. 2-4 Frequent hand washing is the most important thing you can do to prevent infection.

Infection Control

Many infections and diseases are transmitted by airborne and bloodborne pathogens. Patients may carry minor viruses, such as colds or flu, or dangerous ones such as HIV or hepatitis. These serious viral diseases can result from bloodborne **pathogens**, which are organisms that cause infection. You may also be exposed to bacteria. Tuberculosis (TB) is one example of a disease that is transmitted by airborne bacteria. Another airborne pathogen multiplies on food and, when eaten, causes food poisoning. You can limit your risk of exposure by using PPE and sound infection control practices. Good personal hygiene and frequent hand washing, before and after all patient contact, are simple and effective techniques to prevent disease transmission (Fig. 2-4). *Hand washing is the single most important way of stopping the spread of infection* (Box 2-5). Equipment should always be properly disposed of, cleaned, or disinfected after each use. A common cleaning solution is bleach in water (generally a 1:10 blend of bleach to water) or other commercially prepared solution.

Personal Protection Equipment

Personal protective equipment is used to eliminate any direct contact with patients or their body fluids. Protect-ing ourselves from touching, breathing in, or being splashed by anything coming from the patient is essential to avoid the transmission of disease, which could put us and our families at risk.

Eye Protection

Protective eyewear is used to prevent body substances from reaching the mucous membranes of your eyes. If you wear prescription glasses, goggles may not be required in certain instances if removable side shields are used. However, in situations such as a motor vehicle collision or when there is a high expectation of body fluid exposure (for example, childbirth), goggles are still recommended to be placed over prescription glasses.

Gloves

Before having any physical contact with any sick or injured person, emergency first responders should put on vinyl, plastic, or another type of synthetic gloves. If you are working in an environment where it is likely the gloves may be ripped or punctured, you should wear two layers of gloves or wear them inside work gloves. These

BOX 2-5   Hand Washing

Hand washing should occur in between every patient contact. It is recommended that 10 to 15 seconds of vigorous scrubbing with soap will remove most contaminants. Jewelry should be removed, and you should lather all surfaces of the hands, fingers, and arms. Rinse thoroughly with water and dry off with a disposable towel (if possible). Many medical personnel in the field will use waterless hand cleaners. Water or hand towels for drying are not needed. In fact, in order to get the full sanitizing effect, the waterless hand cleaners should be rubbed in and allowed to air dry.

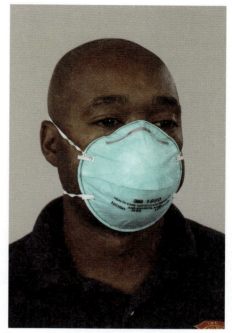

Fig. 2-5 If a patient is suspected of having tuberculosis (TB), a high-efficiency particulate air (HEPA) mask should be worn. (From Chapleau W, Pons P: *Emergency medical technician: making the difference,* St. Louis, 2007, Mosby.)

gloves should be properly disposed of after any use. Wearing gloves does not replace washing your hands. Remember to wash your hands before and after every patient treatment. You should also remember that both patients and health care workers can be allergic to the materials in gloves. Skills 2-1 and 2-2, respectively, illustrate the proper technique to put on gloves and to remove soiled gloves.

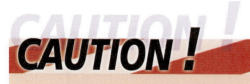

CAUTION!

ALLERGIES

Many of the PPE products we use to protect ourselves are made of latex. A number of health care workers and providers have had serious reactions to latex because of latex allergies. If you have a latex allergy, it is important that you identify latex-containing products that you may be exposed to and replace them with non-latex material.

Gowns

Wearing a gown is recommended if you anticipate the possibility of large splashes of body fluids, such as in childbirth, coughing, spitting, vomiting, or massive bleeding. If a gown is unavailable, you should change your clothes after contact with the patient.

Masks

Several types of masks are available. A surgical type mask will protect your mouth and airway against possible blood splatter. If a patient is suspected of having tuberculosis (TB), a special **high-efficiency particulate air (HEPA) mask** should be worn. HEPA masks are used particularly in enclosed areas (Fig. 2-5). The current standard is the N-95 mask. This standard was revised in response to the anthrax releases that greeted us at the beginning of this new millennium. If you believe a patient has an airborne disease, you can place a paper surgical mask on the patient provided it will not adversely affect the patient's breathing.

MASKS ON PATIENTS

When it can be done without impairing the patient's ability to breathe, patients with known respiratory disease should wear masks to prevent sharing their disease with bystanders or rescuers. Consider their use also in patients with productive coughs when history is not available.

Specialty PPE

There are several types of specialty PPE that are used in situations such as fire, rescue, or violence. Such specialty equipment includes, for example, turnout gear,

Skill 2-1

Putting on Gloves

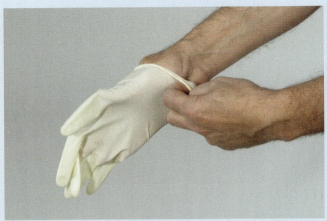

1. Pull glove onto one hand using the fingers of the other hand at the lower cuff area.

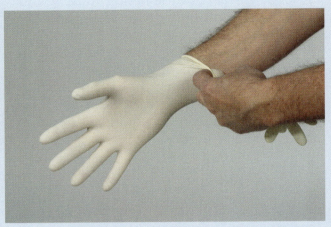

2. Pull glove tight without touching your ungloved hand to the fingers/hand area of the gloved hand.

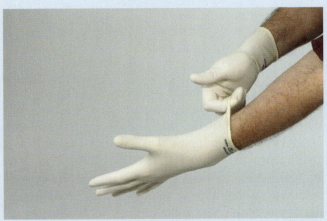

3. Put on other glove using the fingers of the gloved hand.

Skill 2-2

Removal of Soiled Gloves

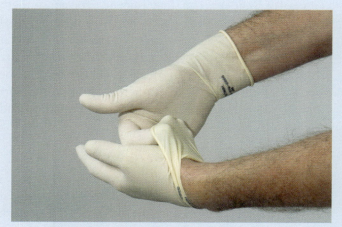

1. Insert a finger from one hand into the glove on the other hand.

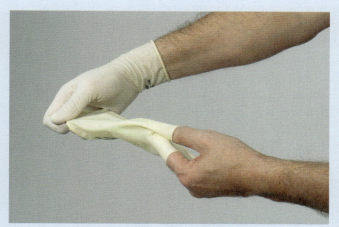

2. Pull the glove off by turning the glove inside out.

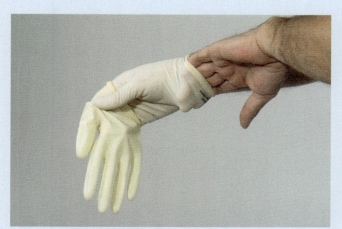

3. Place fingers inside the other glove.

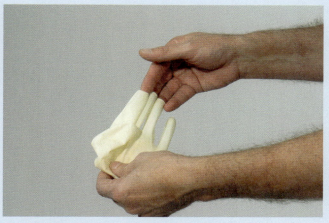

4. Pull the second glove off by turning it inside out.

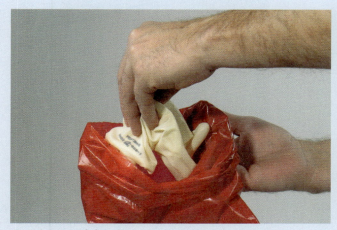

5. Dispose of the gloves in an appropriate container.

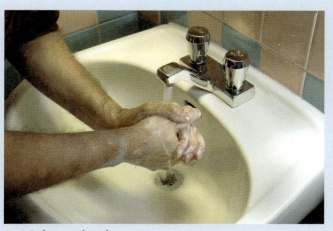

6. Wash your hands.

self-contained breathing apparatus (SCBA), bulletproof vests, and hazardous materials suits.

Contaminated Equipment

Anything used in treating your patient should be considered contaminated. After using equipment, all disposable items should be properly disposed of in the appropriate container. This might include turning any contaminated disposable items to the transport crew or special disposal at your workplace. Your employers or the system you work in should have policies in place that will guide you in the proper procedures for disposing of patient-related disposable equipment.

Cleaning a piece of equipment means washing it with soap and water. **Disinfecting** a piece of equipment refers to cleaning it as well as using something like alcohol or bleach to kill many of the contaminants. **Sterilizing** a piece of equipment involves the use of chemicals and such things as superheated steam to kill *all* contaminants.

Usually your equipment will require only cleaning and disinfecting if it comes into contact with a patient's skin. When cleaning and disinfecting equipment, you should be sure to wear heavy-duty utility gloves. According to the manufacturer's recommendations, some equipment will require sterilization if it comes into contact with a patient's body fluids.

Disposable equipment should be used where possible. After its use, contaminated disposable equipment can be placed in an appropriate plastic bag (usually labeled infectious waste; Fig. 2-6). If your patient is known to have an infectious disease (such as TB, HIV, etc.), disposable items should be double-bagged.

Any equipment, or your vehicle, that does not directly touch a patient should be thoroughly cleaned and disinfected after each patient contact.

Sharps

Needles and contaminated medicine delivery systems are referred to as "sharps" in medicine. Although emergency first responders usually will not have contact with these as a part of their practice, they may be exposed to them in any number of ways. The patient may be using syringes for prescribed or illegal drugs. The emergency first responder may also be working with other health care professionals that use these devices. Sharps need to be disposed of in special (red) puncture-proof containers that when full are taken to special decontamination and disposal facilities.

Specialized Training

Your workplace may have hazards specific to the operations there. It is important to learn all that you can about the materials and activities where you work. If you work in an area that has specific hazards like chemical, electrical, radioactive, biological, poisonous, or explosive materials, special training on additional necessary precautions should be available to you. Take advantage of specialty training to increase your knowledge and decrease your risk. Special PPE may also be required in these situations (Fig. 2-7).

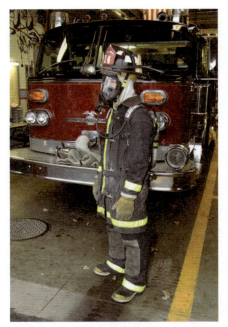

Fig. 2-7 Specialized protective equipment can include turnout gear and a self-contained breathing apparatus (SCBA).

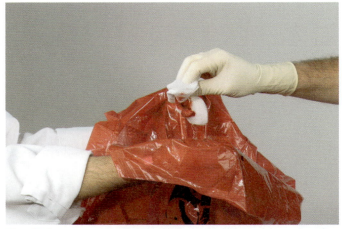

Fig. 2-6 Dispose of contaminated equipment in appropriate places.

Immunizations

Immunizations can protect you from many serious or fatal diseases that your patients may carry. The following immunizations are recommended for all health care providers:

- Tetanus.
- Hepatitis B
- Measles, mumps, and rubella (MMR)
- Chicken pox
- Influenza (flu)
- Others, as currently recommended

Obtain your immunization history and compare it to your department recommendations. Your EMS system can help you access immunizations in your community. In addition, annual TB skin testing is recommended to evaluate for tuberculosis exposure.

Exposure Notification and Testing

In the case of an exposure to body substance, the body areas exposed should be cleaned thoroughly using soap and water. If the eyes are contaminated, they should be flushed continuously for 20 minutes. The agency you are working for should have a policy that includes a plan for responding to exposures that will include access to further evaluation by medical professionals.

You should report any possible exposures to a patient's body fluids to the EMS transport team. They will include the possible exposures in their record and follow up with the EMS system and the patient's hospital. The report should include the date and time you were exposed, the type and amount of body fluid you were exposed to, and the source. You should also know your local and state laws concerning reporting requirements and the transfer of patient information. This information can usually be found through your state EMS office.

Scene Safety

Any time an emergency first responder approaches an emergency, the first priority is to assess the safety of the scene. If the scene is not safe and poses a threat to the responder, the scene should be made safe before the emergency first responder enters. Some of the hazards that might make a scene unsafe include motor vehicle collisions or rescues, hazardous materials, and violence. It is important that emergency first responders recognize the limits of their training and that specialists will need to address hazardous situations before the emergency first responder can assist.

Motor Vehicle Collisions or Rescues

Is there a fire, explosive, or collapse danger at the scene? Is there a hazardous material potential? Motor vehicle collisions present many challenges. The traffic that continues to pass around the collision is a hazard that must be controlled before rescue can be attempted. Safety of the scene first depends on controlling the traffic around the scene. The vehicle itself may also present hazards. Certainly the damaged vehicle with broken glass and jagged metal edges is a hazard to both the patient and the emergency first responder. Emergency first responders on the scene of motor vehicle collisions should wear clothing that protects them from injury caused by these sharp objects. Other professional rescuers with specialized training may need to secure the scene before the emergency first responder can approach the patient. The emergency first responder must understand how to get special rescue teams and equipment to the scene if needed (Fig. 2-8).

Hazardous Materials

Toxic substances or hazardous atmospheres might include dangerous liquids and solids or gaseous chemicals that prevent you from entering the scene. On-site hazardous materials should be identified with placards (Fig. 2-9). These placards identify the type of hazard and will be numbered to guide you to a reference in the *Emergency Response Guidebook,* which is published by the U.S. Department of Transportation (Fig. 2-10). Binoculars may be your most important piece of equipment in identifying hazards because they will allow you to evaluate at a distance the placard or situation before you risk exposing yourself to unseen hazards. Once identified, hazardous materials incidents will be handled by the Office of Hazardous Materials Safety (HAZMAT) teams.

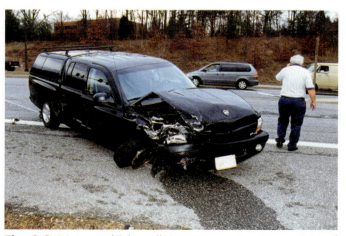

Fig. 2-8 Motor vehicle collisions can present a variety of hazards. Always be sure the scene is safe.

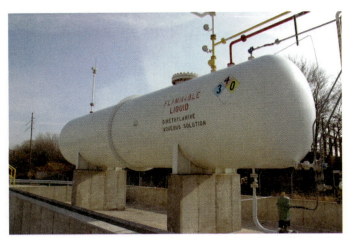

Fig. 2-9 Hazardous materials should be identified with placards.

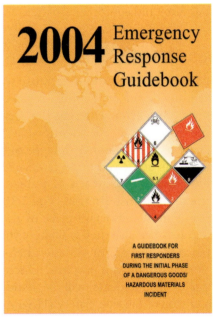

Fig. 2-10 The *Emergency Response Guidebook* is a reference for hazardous materials.

These teams consist of rescuers specially trained in identifying and securing hazardous situations and in decontaminating people exposed to these materials. They may have to decontaminate your patient before they can release him or her to you for treatment. Fire or other hazardous situations may create toxic gasses or insufficient oxygen in the air. This is another situation where rescuers with training specific to these hazards must make the scene safe for the responder to enter. If the scene cannot be made safe, the patient may need to be taken to the emergency first responder by the specially trained

rescuers. It is important that you familiarize yourself with these specialty teams in your area; learn how to contact them and how you might work with them. They probably provide awareness training that will enable you to work with them more closely and prevent you from becoming part of the emergency rather than the rescue.

Violence

Crime scenes or violent scenes present another possible hazardous situation and special concerns that emergency first responders should address. First, the emergency first responder should not enter the scene until the police have secured the scene for safe entry. Second, if a crime has been committed at the scene, the emergency first responder should avoid disturbing possible evidence unnecessarily. Although it is important to preserve the chain of evidence, it is even more important to remember that the patient's needs are the priority after safety of the rescuers. You should never withhold care to preserve evidence. However, you should avoid destroying evidence during the course of care by, for example, cutting around suspected bullet or knife holes in clothing when removing the clothing from a patient.

Physically Unsafe Scenes

The emergency first responder may also be called to assist where the scene is physically unstable. If a patient is found on a slope, or if water or ice presents an unstable surface, the emergency first responder should make sure the scene is stable enough to remove the patient without endangering the rescue team. If this is beyond the emergency first responder's ability, he or she must wait for specially trained rescuers to stabilize the site.

Patient Protection

Patient protection is your priority. You must keep in mind that the environment may pose a threat to your patient. You should shield the patient from extremes of temperature and other environmental factors. You should keep the patient dry and help him or her maintain body heat.

Bystander Protection

Protection of bystanders is also a priority. You should ensure that the cause of your patient's difficulties does not potentially affect others. You should also ensure that your activities in working to help your patient do not harm others who may be crowding around in curiosity or in an attempt to help.

Most important, scene safety must be determined before you enter. If it is unsafe, make it safe. If you cannot make it safe, do not enter.

Team Work

As an emergency first responder, you are an important part of the health care team. As a team member, you must learn to recognize the signs of imbalanced physical and emotional well-being not only in yourself but in your coworkers, family, and friends. A healthy team requires that its members watch out for each other. An emergency first responder who does not understand the importance of being safe, healthy, and emotionally balanced is the weak link in the health care team.

In the Real World—Conclusion

After the patient has been transported, you replay the scene in your mind. You can hear the assembly line, see the blood, and remember the instant you recognized your brother-in-law. You properly dispose of and clean your protective equipment and wash your hands. You are feeling very emotional about it all. Your friend, an EMT on the scene, suggests that you make a call to the CISD team. You know you need a chance to talk about the event.

Nuts and Bolts

Nuts and Bolts

Critical Points

Emergency first responders must understand the probable reactions to death and dying. You should recognize the phases of the grieving process and be able to listen empathetically to and communicate honestly with the patient and his or her friends and family.

As an emergency first responder, you will experience unusual stresses. You need to find healthy ways to manage your stress and balance your personal and professional needs. Use the resources provided by your EMS system and your local mental health professionals. Your emotional well-being is essential to your work and your family.

You must be aware of and protect yourself from the risks associated with emergency medical care. Use the established protocols for protective equipment and practices to reduce your risks. Gloves, mask, gown, and eye protection should be worn to isolate body substances.

The emergency first responder must assess the scene and surroundings of a medical emergency to ensure the safety of all involved. Use your training to protect yourself in scenes involving hazardous materials, motor vehicle collisions, and violence. Remember: if the scene is unsafe, make it safe. Otherwise, do not enter.

Learning Checklist

❑ An emergency first responder will face many stressful situations. These situations may include mass casualty incidents, working with pediatric patients, violent situations, abuse, amputations, death, and injury to or the death of a coworker or close friend or family member.

❑ As an emergency first responder, you will encounter scenes involving death, treat dying patients, and support the families and friends of those who have died. You must try to understand the concerns of the dying patient, communicate empathetically with family members following the death of a loved one, and manage your own feelings about death and loss.

❑ Definitive signs of death include clear mortal damage, rigor mortis, and putrefaction.

❑ Common emotional states of dying, critically ill, and injured patients include anxiety, pain and anger, hostility, depression, and guilt.

❑ To help alleviate anxiety and confusion in patients, you should always introduce yourself to patients, let them know you are there to help them, and continually explain what is happening around them.

❑ You should be honest with patients without unnecessarily shocking or confusing them.

❑ The stages of grief include denial, anger, bargaining, depression, and acceptance.

❑ Different family members, friends, and patients will go through the different stages of grief at different times. As an emergency first responder, you should recognize this fact and the fact that you may also go through periods of grieving.

❑ The warning signs of stress may include irritability, inability to concentrate, difficulty sleeping or nightmares, anxiety, indecisiveness, guilt, loss of appetite, loss of interest in sex, isolation, and loss of interest in work.

❑ To help manage stress, you should reduce consumption of caffeine, sugar, and alcohol and balance your diet. You should avoid fatty foods and maintain an adequate intake of protein.

❑ You should stay physically active in sports or other recreational pursuits to stay healthy and help alleviate stress.

❑ Family members and friends may not understand the nature of an emergency first responder's work. They may feel ignored or fear separation, and you may unwittingly separate yourself from them.

❑ You should recognize the warning signs of stress and make the appropriate changes in your lifestyle or work environment to alleviate it as much as possible. This may include seeking professional help from a mental health worker or a member of the clergy.

❑ Critical incident stress management (CISM) is a comprehensive system designed to help people deal with stress related to work. The services that are offered include preincident stress education, on-scene peer support, one-on-one support, disaster support services, follow-up services, family and spouse support, community outreach programs, and wellness programs.

❑ Critical incident stress debriefing (CISD) is a function of CISM that uses specific techniques to help people express their feelings and recover more quickly from a stressful incident.

❏ CISM should be accessed when any of the following occur: line-of-duty death or serious injury, multiple casualty incident, suicide of a coworker, serious injury or death to children, events with excessive media interest, victims who are known to you, any disaster, or any other event that has an unusual impact on personnel.

❏ Body substance isolation and standard or universal precautions refer to the protocols set by the Centers for Disease Control for protection against infection from body substances.

❏ Good personal hygiene and frequent hand washing before and after all patient contact are simple but effective techniques to prevent disease transmission.

❏ Personal protective equipment includes gloves, eye protection, gowns, masks, or specialty pieces such as turnout gear.

❏ Anything used in treating a patient should be considered contaminated and disposed of or cleaned appropriately.

❏ The following immunizations are recommended for all health care providers: tetanus, hepatitis B, measles, mumps, and flu. Annual skin testing for tuberculosis is also recommended.

❏ You should report any possible exposure to a patient's body fluids to the EMS transport team.

❏ Some of the hazards that an emergency first responder may encounter include motor vehicle collisions or rescues, hazardous materials, violence, and a physically unsafe scene. At any scene your own safety, the safety of your patient, and that the safety of the bystanders are of utmost importance.

Key Terms

Body substance isolation (BSI) An infection control method that is based on the assumption that all body fluids are infectious.

Centers for Disease Control and Prevention (CDC) A federal agency of the U.S. government that provides resources and equipment for the investigation, identification, prevention, and control of infectious disease.

Cleaning Washing something thoroughly with soap and water.

Critical incident stress A stress reaction normally exhibited after experiencing a particularly difficult situation.

Critical incident stress debriefing (CISD) A function of the critical incident stress management system that uses specific techniques such as debriefings to help people express their feelings and recover from a stressful incident faster.

Critical incident stress management (CISM) A comprehensive system devised to help professionals recover from critical incidents.

Debriefing A review of a stressful event to allow discussion between the people involved. Usually held within 24 to 72 hours of the event.

Defusing A shorter and less formal review of stressful events to allow discussion between the people involved. Usually held within a few hours of the event.

Disinfecting In addition to cleaning something, using alcohol or bleach to kill contaminants.

High-efficiency particulate air (HEPA) mask A special mask designed to decrease the spread of infection of airborne diseases such as tuberculosis.

Occupational Health and Safety Administration (OSHA) A federal agency that has developed guidelines to protect health care workers.

Pathogen A microorganism capable of causing disease.

Personal protection equipment (PPE) Equipment used to isolate a health care worker from a patient's body substances. Also refers to specialty equipment that emergency providers use during the course of a rescue or a fire.

Sterilizing The use of chemicals and superheated steam to kill all microorganisms.

First Responder NSC Objectives
COGNITIVE OBJECTIVES

- List possible emotional reactions that the First Responder may experience when faced with trauma, illness, and death and dying.

Nuts and Bolts–continued

- Discuss the possible reactions that a family member may exhibit when confronted with death and dying.
- State the steps in the First Responder's approach to the family confronted with death and dying.
- State the possible reactions that the family of the First Responder may exhibit because of his or her outside involvement in EMS.
- Recognize the signs and symptoms of critical incident stress.
- State possible steps that the First Responder may take to help reduce/alleviate stress.
- Explain the need to determine scene safety.
- Discuss the importance of body substance isolation.
- Describe the steps the First Responder should take for personal protection from airborne and bloodborne pathogens.
- List the personal protection equipment necessary for each of the following situations: hazardous materials, rescue operations, violent scenes, crime scenes, exposure to bloodborne pathogens, and exposure to airborne pathogens.

AFFECTIVE OBJECTIVES

- Explain the rationale for serving as an advocate for the use of appropriate protective equipment.

PSYCHOMOTOR OBJECTIVES

- Given a scenario with potential infectious exposure, the First Responder will use appropriate personal protection equipment. At the completion of the scenario, the First Responder will properly remove and discard the protective garments.
- Given the preceding scenario, the First Responder will complete disinfection/cleaning and all reporting documentation.

Check your understanding
Check your understanding

Please refer to p. 439 for the answers to these questions.

1. List four common emergency situations that are generally stressful for many EMS providers.
   A. _____
   B. _____
   C. _____
   D. _____

2. List five possible emotional reactions experienced by dying patients or their significant others.
   A. _____
   B. _____
   C. _____
   D. _____
   E. _____

3. List two lifestyle changes that can be helpful when coping with stress.
   A. _____
   B. _____

4. Stress that occurs either from a single distressing event, such as the line-of-duty death of a coworker, or an accumulation of incidents is known as _____.

5. Sessions held 24 to 72 hours after an abnormally stressful event in which personnel involved with the event can discuss their feelings confidentially are called _____.

6. The process by which you kill many of the contaminants on surfaces or equipment by using chemicals while cleaning is called _____.

7. The guidelines and protocols for protection against infection that occurs as a result of contact with an infected patient's blood or body fluids are called _____.

8. Gloves, goggles, gowns, and masks are specific examples of _____.

9. List four specific dangers to emergency personnel responding to the scene of a motor vehicle collision.
   A. _____
   B. _____
   C. _____
   D. _____

10. Toxic substances, which may be liquids, powders, solids, or gasses, and require specialized training in identifying and securing, as well as decontaminating people exposed to these substances, are known as _____.

11. In which of the following situations would an emergency first responder most likely be required to begin medical care of a patient who is not breathing and does not have a pulse?
    A. The patient's family shows you a do not resuscitate (DNR) order signed by a physician.
    B. The patient is found outdoors in cold weather.
    C. The patient's blood has settled to the lowest point in the body, causing dependent lividity, or discoloration of the skin.
    D. The patient's muscles are stiff and inflexible.

12. Which of the following is the stage of the grieving process in which the family of a patient who has died refuses to believe that the person is actually dead?
    A. Bargaining
    B. Depression
    C. Anger
    D. Denial

13. Which of the following is NOT a warning sign of stress?
    A. Loss of interest in hobbies or usual activities
    B. Spending more time than usual with friends
    C. Irritability with others
    D. Difficulty sleeping and nightmares

Check your understanding–continued

14. Which of the following is the single most effective way to reduce the spread of infection?
    A. Using eye protection for all patient contact
    B. Frequent hand washing with soap and water
    C. Sterilization of all equipment after each use
    D. Using a high-efficiency particulate air (HEPA) mask for all patient contact

15. For which of the following diseases do health care employers require testing of all patient care personnel on an annual or semiannual basis?
    A. Tetanus
    B. Influenza ("Flu")
    C. Hepatitis B
    D. Tuberculosis (TB)

16. You have responded to the scene of a "sick person" inside a private residence. You find that the patient is a 55-year-old man who has been very ill with cancer. His family states that he just stopped breathing a few minutes ago, but they do not want him to be resuscitated. The family states the patient has a DNR order but that the physician did not give the family a copy of it. Which of the following is the best course of action?
    A. Follow the family's wishes
    B. Call the patient's physician and ask for guidance
    C. Begin your assessment and treatment of the patient while trying to confirm the DNR status
    D. Wait for additional personnel to arrive before making a decision

17. You are on the scene of a serious motor vehicle collision. The driver is a 17-year-old female who is trapped in the vehicle. She appears to be critically injured; she is having great difficulty breathing and appears to have lost a lot of blood. She asks you if you think she is going to die. Which of the following would be the best response?
    A. "I'm going to do everything I can to help you, so hang in there with me."
    B. "You're going to be fine."
    C. "Yes, I think that's a definite possibility from the looks of your injuries."
    D. "I really can't answer that. You'll have to wait until the paramedics get here."

18. You are responding to a report of a "shooting." Upon arrival, your first consideration should be:
    A. Caring for the victim
    B. Ensuring bystander safety
    C. Finding the gun
    D. Personal safety

Chapter 3

Legal and Ethical Issues

LESSON GOALS

As an emergency first responder, you must consider the ethical and legal implications of all your actions while performing emergency first responder duties. Providing medical treatment to patients can only be done within established legal boundaries. Should you stop and treat a motor vehicle collision victim while you are off duty? Should you release patient information to an attorney over the telephone? Can you treat an injured child when the parents are not present? Emergency first responders are faced with these and other issues every day. This chapter highlights the ethical and legal principles you should use to guide your activities as an emergency first responder.

OBJECTIVES

1. Define the emergency first responder standard of care.
2. Discuss the importance of do not resuscitate (DNR) (advance directives) and local or state provisions regarding emergency medical services (EMS) application.
3. Define "consent," and discuss the methods of obtaining consent.
4. Differentiate between expressed and implied consent.
5. Given a scenario involving a minor, discuss how consent would be obtained.
6. Discuss the implications for you of patient refusal of transport.
7. Discuss the issues of abandonment, negligence, and battery and their implications for you.
8. State the conditions necessary for you to have a duty to act.
9. Explain the importance, necessity, and legality of patient confidentiality.
10. List the actions that you should take when providing care at a crime scene.
11. State the conditions that require you to notify local law enforcement officials.
12. Discuss issues concerning the fundamental components of documentation.

In the Real World

Your emergency first responder team is called to the local park where a boy was injured while inline skating. As you approach the patient, you see an approximately 12-year-old male with obvious abrasions to his right shoulder, arm, and both knees. The patient is sitting upright, holding his right arm and crying. After you introduce yourself as an emergency first responder, you ask if you can look at his injuries.

The boy refuses your request and asks that you leave. He goes on to say that he is afraid that his parents will find out that he was at the park while he was supposed to be "grounded." The patient obviously has no life-threatening injuries but has minor injuries that need your attention. You turn to your partner to discuss what you should do now.

Legal and ethical issues have to do with protecting our patients and ourselves from legal complications and protecting the rights of our patients. This chapter will orient you to the legal considerations regarding patients rights, the ethical practice of prehospital medicine, and the laws that determine the manner in which we do our jobs.

Standard of Care

Your primary responsibility as an emergency first responder is to provide for the well-being of your patients. To intervene on their behalf, you must clearly understand what the standard of care is for an emergency first responder in your state. The **standard of care** is what another reasonably prudent emergency first responder with similar training and experience would do in similar circumstances. Although this general definition is clear, the specific actions that make up the standard of care are derived from multiple sources. Individual states regulate who can deliver medical care through statutes and administrative regulations. State laws authorize physicians, nurses, emergency medical technicians (EMTs), and emergency first responders to deliver medical care. Each law defines a scope within which the caregiver must operate. These laws are based on the guidelines developed by the National Highway Traffic Safety Administration of the Department of Transportation (NHTSA/DOT) and by each state's EMS act.

Some states enhance the scope of care through medical oversight. A medical director can relay **protocols, standing orders,** and prescribed actions over a phone or radio to guide the emergency first responder. Other states make your legal right to function contingent upon medical oversight. You may be required to contact your medical director by radio or telephone, or to follow approved

protocols or standing orders for all levels of care. Most states require emergency first responders to be answerable to medical oversight and review through a physician at a local hospital or within the emergency agency. You need to know the state laws that govern the scope of care you give, as well as local protocols and standing orders.

To teach you the emergency first responder standards of care, your instructor may use the following:

- The First Responder National Standard Curriculum
- Materials in emergency first responder training texts and other instructional materials
- Content taught in continuing education curricula
- Local medical protocols and standing orders
- Individual agency requirements

As an emergency first responder, you have a legal duty to act within your state's laws and regulations; to follow local medical control, protocols, and standing orders; and to answer to medical oversight for quality control and training purposes. Failure to do so may mean you are working outside of your scope of practice. You have no legal authority to render medical care outside your scope of practice.

Ethical Responsibilities

The law cannot fully describe the specific responsibilities an emergency first responder has to his or her patients. In addition to legal responsibilities, you have ethical responsibilities as well. The primary ethical responsibility of an emergency first responder is to provide appropriate medical care to a patient for whom the emergency first responder is responsible. This requires timely intervention, in a caring manner, to the level of the emergency first responder's training. This responsibility may be fulfilled while the emergency first responder is on call as a provider or when the emergency first responder acts as a Good Samaritan in an unexpected situation. In other words, you should not only act just because the law requires it—you should act because it is the right thing to do.

The standards are specifically written in formal documents. What you do reflects your personal morality. What would you expect of another emergency first responder if you or your loved one were the victim or patient? The term "standard of care" really implies the prescribed clinical and technical standards you are trained to perform. The standard of "care" defines you as a compassionate human being who has the greater ability to help others.

Ethical decision making can be intimidating and often causes individuals to "shoot from the hip." Although this type of response is common, it can be treacherous. "Because I said so" often does not work. Moreover, legal pronouncements are not always fully understanding of a specific patient's needs. Society expects you to act honorably and morally. Yet where do you really learn right from wrong?

Ethical/Legal Conflicts

Unfortunately, situations in EMS often arise that are not always "black and white" or as well defined as specific laws. Situations may force you to ask yourself how, when, or why to treat a particular patient in a particular way. At times, legal issues will clash with what is best for the patient. What is best for the patient often varies with who is making the decision to treat or not treat: the patient, the patient's family, or you. When faced with an ethical conflict, as the emergency first responder you may be uncertain about what to do or how to act. It is impossible to address every conceivable conflict because no two are exactly alike. However, by adhering to the following basic principles you may, at the very least, gain some guidance in your care:

- Always act in the best interest of the patient.
- Know the laws and protocols in your area as they relate to patient care.
- Respect the patient's autonomy. Patients have rights, and even if those rights conflict with your ideas or opinions, they should be honored within obvious societal norms and constraints.
- Consider the patient's best interest. This may conflict with autonomy, but you should respect the patient's rights.
- "First, do no harm." Don't make the situation worse.

- Practice fairness in your approach to patient care. It is not your place to ration care based on your own social beliefs.
- When in doubt, contact medical control.

If conflict between any of these concepts creates an ethical dilemma, you can approach the situation with understanding and shape a reasonable response. Think of situations you have encountered and what created the ethical dilemma. Now, consider what could have been done to lessen the conflict and help resolve the problem, keeping in mind the rights of the patient and that person's needs. Each time you do this, you will make the next dilemma more understandable and less frustrating for all involved.

Remember, you should never be forced to do something you believe is unethical (political and religious beliefs should be clarified well in advance; patient care is not the arena for debate or action). An example of this situation would be an order from a supervisor not to document a medication error ("no harm, no foul"). A mechanism must be in place for you to report such an occurrence, such as to your EMS coordinator or chief. If this is not possible, your EMS medical director should be available to discuss this situation in a confidential manner.

If you observe an unethical act on the part of a colleague, you have an obligation to report it. Regardless of who the offender is, if you allow this situation to go unnoticed, you are no different from your colleague. Again, the means of reporting this occurrence should be clear and confidential.

Work with your colleagues, administrators, and medical director to encourage an environment of honesty, integrity, and open communication. This is your ethical responsibility, and you and your patients deserve this type of understanding.

Consent

The U.S. Supreme Court has upheld the right of every competent patient to self-determination when it comes to medical care and the application of lifesaving or life-sustaining measures. Put simply, each person has the right to determine whether to accept or reject any type of medical care or treatment (including any form of "laying on of hands" by health care providers) as long as the person is capable of making that decision as a competent adult. Although the fact that a patient can refuse care may be difficult to accept, an emergency first responder can be charged with battery for touching a person without permission or with assault for creating the fear of injury.

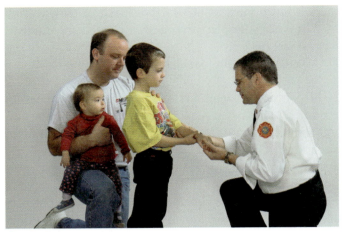

Fig. 3-1 If your patient is a minor, consent must be obtained from a parent or a guardian for medical care.

Individual states have also guaranteed this right through laws and regulations. All health care workers, including emergency first responders, must respect this right. Patients must consent to care before any medical care can be delivered. To give consent, patients must be competent and of legal age (Fig. 3-1). They must understand the type of medical care you are offering and be informed of any significant risks associated with the proposed medical care. You should always know and follow your local protocols.

Expressed Consent

Consent may be expressed or implied. If possible, you should obtain expressed consent from patients. **Expressed consent** means that the patient tells you, the emergency first responder, that he or she consents to medical care. This expressed consent can be written or verbal. Doctors and hospitals usually obtain expressed written consent. A patient must sign consent forms before medical treatment is given. In emergency settings, however, expressed written consent is not always possible.

Emergency first responders usually obtain expressed verbal consent for treatment. To obtain expressed verbal consent, you should first identify yourself and your level of training. You should not mislead the patient about your qualifications or abilities. Most patients are unaware of the various levels of training and the capabilities of EMS personnel. If you arrive in an emergency vehicle or are wearing a uniform, they may assume that you are a paramedic.

You should always explain to the patient what you propose to do and why. Rarely are there significant risks to the medical care you, as an emergency first responder, will give. Nevertheless, if there are risks, you should tell

the patient about them. Expressed verbal consent occurs only when you ask the patient, "May I examine and treat you?" and the patient agrees.

Implied Consent

How is consent obtained with an unconscious or unresponsive patient? Unless such a patient has previously signed a document giving consent to treatment, expressed consent cannot be obtained. Most states allow emergency first responders to give medical care to unconscious or unresponsive patients on the assumption that they would consent to lifesaving medical care. This is termed **implied consent**, based on the patient's condition. Another type of implied consent is consent based on "lack of protest." In this case, a patient who is seriously injured or ill and requires urgent medical care may not be able to directly provide consent. The emergency first responder immediately provides the emergency care if the patient does not protest either verbally or physically. For example, an emergency first responder may apply a pressure dressing on a patient with a significant arm laceration that is bleeding before asking the patient for permission to apply the dressing. If the patient does not protest by pulling his arm away or saying something like, "Leave me alone," the law in many states says that the patient has given consent to the treatment. Further nonlifesaving treatment should be provided only after obtaining expressed consent.

It is important to document the fact that the patient consented to treatment. If you have written consent, that serves as the documentation. If you have obtained expressed verbal consent, you should document the incident in a written statement such as "I explained the benefits and risks of treatment to the patient, and the patient expressed understanding and gave consent." In cases of implied consent, you should carefully document the condition of the patient so it is clear that the care delivered was emergency lifesaving care.

Competence and Capacity

A patient must be legally competent and have the capacity to make an informed decision in order to have the ability to accept or refuse emergency medical care. In other words, even if a patient is legally able to make a decision regarding health care (because he or she is over 18), he or she may still lack decision-making capacity to consent to or refuse medical care.

Competence is a judicial determination, not a medical decision. **Competence** refers to the degree of mental soundness necessary to make decisions about a specific issue or to carry out a specific act. All adults are presumed to be competent unless the law says they are not or a court has made a determination of **incompetence**. Examples of legal disabilities include age (**minors**) and lack of mental capacity (a judge has determined that the patient is incapable of making such decisions). In these cases, even though the patient may understand you and may understand the implications of what you are trying to do, he or she simply cannot legally consent or refuse. Someone else, either a parent or guardian, has the legal authority to consent or refuse for these patients.

Capacity, on the other hand, is a medical determination. It is an individual's ability to make an informed decision (i.e., their decision-making capacity). For example, you arrive on scene to find a highly intoxicated woman who was involved in a motor vehicle collision and she is screaming that she does not need medical treatment. You determine that she is not capable of making this decision because she lacks decision-making capacity. This is a clinical judgment founded on the patient's inability to make a coherent decision. You are making a medical determination that the patient lacks capacity not that the patient is legally incompetent. A patient may lack decision-making capacity and therefore the ability to consent to or refuse care if he or she is (or may be) any of the following:

- Intoxicated
- Under the influence of drugs
- Affected by serious injury
- Someone with a proven medical history of mental incapacity
- Unable to understand your spoken language

Refusal of Care

Competent adult patients have the right to refuse emergency medical care (**refusal**). The same rules that apply to consent also apply to refusals. The law recognizes generally that, subject to certain interests of society, a competent individual has a right to refuse any and all medical care, even if that care would save the person's life. This is embodied in the common law notion of patient self-determination. However, this concept has evolved from a common law notion into a statutory one. More than a decade ago, Congress enacted the Patient Self-Determination Act. Among other things, this law requires most health care facilities in the United States to inform patients upon admission of their right to execute a living will.

The law takes the concept of self-determination by competent patients very seriously. Therefore, a critical element of any refusal situation is an assessment by the EMS providers as to whether their patient is competent. If they determine that the patient is competent, EMS providers should be especially careful to explain fully the specific risks that may result from the patient's refusal

and should make sure the patient is informed of alternatives in the event the person persists in refusing care.

Each person has the right to determine whether to accept or reject any type of medical care or treatment (including any form of "laying on of hands" by health care providers) as long as the person is capable of making that decision as a competent adult. Although the fact that a patient can refuse care may be difficult to accept, an emergency first responder can be charged with battery for touching a person without permission or with assault for creating the fear of a harmful or offensive touching.

This principle of self-determination applies just as clearly in the prehospital environment as it does within the four walls of the hospital. However, in the prehospital setting, the patient is less likely to be competent to make that determination because of a variety of factors, such as shock, alcohol use, and decreased level of consciousness. EMS providers must make sure the patient consents to the assessment and treatment that is to be provided. All competent adults have the right to consent to or refuse care and treatment, even in emergency situations. This includes the right to refuse not just the entire care and treatment package but also portions of it.

Can a patient consent to some treatment and then refuse to consent to certain types of specific treatment? Absolutely. For example, a patient may specifically refuse to consent to the administration of oxygen. What should you do in such cases? First you must make sure the patient understands the importance of the oxygen. A convincing approach usually changes the patient's mind. If not, make sure the patient is competent to make that refusal. All refusals of care must be carefully documented, or you run the risk of a claim of abandonment or negligence. Failure to assess properly the patient's ability to give consent and improper documentation of a refusal of care are crucial areas of liability risk.

A refusal of care can be a complete or a partial refusal. *Complete refusals* are situations in which the patient refuses all aspects of treatment. This is probably the most common type of refusal. A *partial refusal* occurs when the patient agrees to some but not all of the treatment you wish to provide. If a patient refuses a portion of treatment, such as the administration of a specific medication, you can still provide other treatment that the patient agrees to allow. In these situations, you should obtain written documentation of the refusal, even if it is just a partial refusal. Documentation of refusals of care is not limited just to complete refusals.

In all cases, the patient must be informed of and fully understand the risks and consequences of refusing emergency medical care. You should make all reasonable efforts to ensure that any refusal of care is an informed refusal. Informed refusal requires that the patient understand the following:

- What you propose to do and why
- The risks involved
- The alternative treatment possibilities with their potential risks
- The consequences of not being treated and the risks (the worst possible outcomes should be mentioned and documented)

Two additional elements are necessary for informed refusal:

- The patient must comprehend this discussion and demonstrate full understanding.
- The patient's response must be free of coercion.

This process should be well documented and appropriately signed as your local protocol dictates. Of course, you should make all reasonable attempts to convince a patient with decision-making capacity to accept your treatment. The emergency first responder's personal convenience should not be a factor in encouraging a sign-off.

Another consideration is who can sign a refusal of care. A patient with decision-making capacity can; a durable power of attorney for health care can; and a legal guardian can. However, a spouse who is none of these cannot. When the patient lacks decision-making capacity and no legal surrogate exists, you (with the help of medical control if needed) must be an advocate for the patient. A family member should not be permitted to refuse care for a patient.

In reality, a lawsuit is far more likely in cases of improperly obtained refusal than improperly obtained consent. A bad outcome is far more likely with a patient who refuses rather than receives medical care, even if there is some question whether consent was correctly obtained. Therefore, in refusal situations it is even more important to carefully explain the treatment you want to provide and the risks if the patient refuses the treatment. All refusal of care should be thoroughly documented (Fig. 3-2). You should ask a patient who refuses medical care to sign a document outlining the medical care that was offered, the fact that he or she refused medical care,

---

REFUSAL OF TRANSPORT AND TREATMENT
PLEASE READ THIS DOCUMENT

This form has been given to you because you have refused treatment or transportation to the hospital by Emergency Medical Service personnel. Your health and safety are our primary concerns. Even though you have decided not to accept our offer of treatment or transport to the hospital, please remember the following:

1. We recommend that you be evaluated and treated by a physician.

2. Your decision to refuse treatment and transport may result in delay, which may result in worsening of your condition.

3. Medical evaluation or treatment may be obtained by calling your personal physician or by going to any hospital's Emergency Department.

4. You may change your mind abour transport. Please do not hesitate to contact us. We will not hesitate to return to assist you.

5. **Do not wait!** When medical treatment is needed, it is usually better to get it sooner than later.

DIAL 911
IF YOU NEED
EMERGENCY MEDICAL SERVICES

_____   _____
Attending EMS Personnel   Date/Time

_____
Patient Signature

Fig. 3-2 A refusal form. (Courtesy HealthONE EMS, Englewood, CO, in Henry M, Stapleton E: *EMT prehospital care,* ed 4, St. Louis, 2010, Mosby.)

and a description of the risks of refusal you described to the patient. After the patient has signed the document, someone should witness it other than yourself or your partner (if you have one). For example, you could have a police officer who has not been involved in the patient's care witness the form.

You should try to do whatever you can within reason to delay a patient's decision to refuse medical care until additional EMS personnel arrive to help evaluate the patient. In no event should you, as an emergency first responder, decide on your own to accept a refusal to receive medical care. If additional EMS personnel are not present at the scene, local protocols may require radio or telephone contact with a medical supervisor before you have the patient sign a release. While waiting for additional EMS personnel to arrive, you should try to persuade the patient to accept medical care. To determine whether the patient is able to make a rational, informed decision, you should ensure that the patient is not under the influence of alcohol or drugs and does not have an injury or illness that may impair his or her ability to make an informed decision to refuse care.

When it comes to consent issues and refusal of care, a safe philosophy is to err on the side of life. Defending why you cared is always easier than trying to justify why you didn't do something for the patient.

Special Considerations
Children and Incompetent Adults

Obtaining consent or refusal from a minor or an incompetent adult is a more complicated process. A patient is incompetent if he or she has been determined to be incapable of making legal decisions because of a medical or mental condition. As an emergency first responder, you must obtain consent or refusal from the parent or guardian of a minor or from the legal guardian of an incompetent adult. It is important to know your state and local laws because the definition of a minor's age will vary in different jurisdictions. Some states permit emergency care of patients who are minors if a physician determines that delaying care to obtain consent from an absent parent or guardian could harm the patient. In these states, you must contact medical control to obtain a physician's order for treatment. With a minor or an incompetent adult in a life-threatening situation, however, you should provide care based on implied consent.

In some states some minors, called **emancipated minors**, are considered adults in some respects and are legally capable of consenting to or refusing treatment. A minor is emancipated only if a court, after a legal proceeding, makes such a determination. Many emancipated minors carry a copy of the court order declaring them to be emancipated. If you encounter a minor who claims to be emancipated, you should follow your local protocols, which may include contacting law enforcement or medical control.

In some states, minors can consent to or refuse certain types of medical care. For example, in some states minors can refuse or consent to treatment for sexually transmitted diseases, substance abuse, or mental health care. In addition, minors who are parents themselves are allowed to consent to or refuse medical care for their own child, even if they are legally unable to consent to or refuse their own medical care. You must know the laws of your state concerning these issues.

Incompetent adult patients cannot legally consent to or refuse medical care. Consent or refusal must come from the patient's legal guardian. However, if the patient is in a life-threatening situation and you cannot obtain consent, you should treat the patient and seek medical supervision.

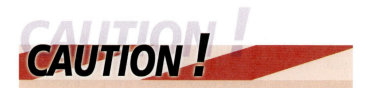

CAUTION !

The golden rule of consent and refusal is: When in doubt, treat the patient.

In the Real World—continued

While discussing the situation with your partner, law enforcement arrives on the scene. You approach the officer and explain the situation. You ask if the officer can place the patient in custody so that you can provide patient care.

The law enforcement officer explains that this is only an option if a patient has broken the law or if the patient's life is in jeopardy.

Advance Directives

An **advance directive** is a document that contains the wishes of the patient and directions to caregivers for the patient's medical care while the patient is alive but incapable of expressing those directions. Advance directives can take various forms such as the living will and the durable power of attorney for health care. All states have living will statutes that allow a person to predesignate the level of medical intervention the person would like to have in the event of a terminal illness. These legal documents provide advance directives, more commonly described as specific orders to the caregiver, as to what level of treatment the patient would like to have in the event of a particular medical situation.

Many advance directives provide limitations on treatment in the event of a cardiac arrest or if the patient lapses into a coma. Typically these directives allow the care provider to treat the patient with palliative or comfort measures and restrict the use of resuscitative measures, such as CPR, endotracheal intubation, or administration of medications.

Most state laws have strict verification requirements to make sure the directive being followed is proper. Some states rely on identification tags that the patient must wear, whereas others require a document signed by the patient's attending physician. Some states require that online medical control be consulted before an advance directive can be recognized. It is important to remember that even if the patient has an advance directive in place, it can be overruled at any time by the patient. A competent patient has the right to void the directive or change his or her mind during the course of treatment.

Living Wills

A **living will** is a legal document that outlines the type of medical care an individual wishes to receive or not receive in certain situations. In most cases a living will does not become effective until the patient has been incapacitated for a defined period of time, sometimes as long as one week. Some states, however, do not permit prehospital care personnel to follow the directions of a living will or the directions of a health care surrogate. You should know your state's laws and regulations regarding use of these directives.

Durable Power of Attorney for Health Care

A **durable power of attorney** for health care is a legal document that gives another individual the right to make health care decisions about another individual. Once the individual has been incapacitated, durable medical power of attorney becomes active. Most states permit emergency first responders and other prehospital personnel to follow the instructions of an agent with a durable power of attorney for health care. The agent speaks for the patient, and in many states this is as powerful and legally binding as the patient's own words. In these states, you are permitted to follow the agent's directions for the patient's health care. What happens if a patient does not have a written advance directive? Most states have a health care surrogate law. This law specifically determines the appropriate person or people empowered to make medical decisions for the patient who lacks that ability. The following is an example of this order of surrogacy:

- Court-appointed guardian
- Spouse
- Adult children (may require majority rule)
- Parent
- Adult siblings
- Adult grandchildren
- Close friend

It is important to remember, however, that if the patient is alert and can competently consent or refuse medical care, you should follow the patient's wishes. An advance directive, living will, or durable medical power of attorney goes into effect only when patients cannot speak for themselves. Emergency first responders should become knowledgeable about the laws of their states as they apply to advance directives.

Do Not Attempt Resuscitation Orders

A **do not attempt resuscitate (DNAR) order** is an order written by a physician, with the consent of the patient and/or family, when death is expected within a relatively short time. The order instructs caregivers not to render medical care to a patient who is clinically dead. In some states, a DNAR order is one of only a few written medical orders prehospital care personnel are allowed to follow outside the orders of their medical control physician.

From an ethical perspective, remember that CPR is presumed for any individual unless specifically declined (DNAR). This means that a DNAR patient, or the person's appropriate surrogate, has thought out the risks versus benefits of resuscitation and has elected, autonomously or by surrogate appointment, not to be resuscitated. This is the patient's right. A patient may still desire aggressive treatment up until the time of cardiopulmonary arrest.

It is important to note that a DNAR order means do not *resuscitate*, it does not mean do not *treat*. DNAR status does not preclude aggressive treatment for other clinical conditions (e.g., infection, transfusion).

Furthermore, an emergency first responder has a responsibility to the patient to make him or her as comfortable as possible within the standard of care when presented with such an order. Both advance directives and the DNAR orders contain a patient's wishes to refuse specified kinds of medical care. However, it can become confusing when encountering advance directives and DNR orders on the scene. As discussed later, whether or not you should follow an advance care directive may depend on your state's laws and regulations. The decision to follow the instructions in a DNAR order depends on whether the patient has a pulse and is breathing. If the patient has a pulse, the DNAR order is not yet in effect, and you should treat the patient.

In some jurisdictions, physicians can write DNAR orders that are almost advance directives. For example, an order can be written requesting that the patient not be ventilated (provided with rescue breathing) even if the patient has a pulse. Such DNAR orders can be confusing and create problems for emergency first responders who do not have the time to calmly contemplate the order as may be possible in a controlled hospital environment. If you encounter such a situation, you should follow established protocols, which usually include contacting medical control for directions. When in doubt, begin resuscitation of the patient.

A patient may be conscious at the time you are presented with a DNAR order. You should then check to be sure that the patient still does not want to be resuscitated. If the patient indicates that he or she wants to be resuscitated, the DNAR order is considered revoked. In this type of situation, you must resuscitate the patient if cardiac arrest occurs.

As an emergency first responder, it is important that you learn the protocols in your jurisdiction for handling DNAR orders and living will procedures. What has been outlined here lays only a basis for the decision-making process. Table 3-1 shows how to respond to advance directives and DNARs.

Medical Examiner Cases

Whether the medical examiner or coroner becomes involved in a patient's death depends on the nature and scene of the death. The medical examiner has a required role in most areas when trauma is a factor, when criminal or suspicious activity is involved, and in unusual situations (e.g., hangings or poisonings). When a medical examiner assumes responsibility for the scene, his or her authority supersedes that of everyone else at the scene, including the family. The following situations are usually medical examiner cases:

- Patient dead on arrival (DOA)
- Death if a patient was not receiving previous medical care
- Physician unable to determine the cause of death
- Suicide
- Violent death
- Known or suspected poisoning
- Death directly or indirectly resulting from unintentional means
- Suspicion of a criminal act

The medical examiner or coroner is usually notified of a death, even in the absence of these criteria, and that person then determines whether an investigation is warranted.

If you have begun emergency medical care, you should keep thorough notes of what you have done or found. Your records may be important in a later investigation. It is important to understand and comply with your local protocols and agreements with law enforcement agencies to record all pertinent information. Typically you would document the following:

- The location of the body
- The body position (e.g., prone, supine, sitting)
- The appearance of the scene, as you may be the only person who can relate these details

TABLE 3-1 Advance Directives and DNAR Orders

PATIENT STATUS	ADVANCE DIRECTIVE	DNAR ORDER
Patient is conscious and can consent or refuse	Obtain consent or refusal directly from patient	Obtain consent or refusal directly from patient
Patient is unconscious or unresponsive and has pulse	Follow advance directive if allowed in your state	Does not apply
Patient has no pulse	Follow advance directive if allowed in your state	Follow DNAR order

Assault and Battery

Touching a person without his or her consent can be considered battery. **Assault** is the threat of touching the person without consent. For example, if someone raises a baseball bat and appears to be ready to strike you, that is an assault. If the person does strike you, he or she has committed **battery**. An emergency first responder who touches a patient without first obtaining the patient's consent could be committing a battery. This is one reason why obtaining proper consent before treatment is so important. You must obtain consent to prevent being accused of assault or battery charges.

Assault and battery are both crimes and civil offenses. Someone who commits an assault or battery may be charged criminally and receive a jail sentence or a fine. They may also be tried in a civil court and sued for damages. Although there is a general application of the terms *assault* and *battery*, each state or jurisdiction has laws that clearly define the local, legal definition.

Negligence

Negligence is the legal claim in this society to seek redress from others who have caused you harm. Ordinary negligence (as basic negligence is called) is defined in most texts as the failure to exercise the degree of care that another reasonable person in a similar position would exercise in the same or a similar situation, resulting in harm to another person. That is the standard to which the average person or professional normally is held to in a negligence lawsuit.

However, most states have laws that protect EMS personnel from liability for ordinary negligence. The Good Samaritan law protects certain care providers if they are delivering care within the scope of their training in good faith. Immunity is an important concept, and you should know your state's laws related to your work. Most states limit immunity to ordinary negligent conduct and do not provide immunity from intentional misconduct or willful and wanton conduct, which some states refer to as gross negligence.

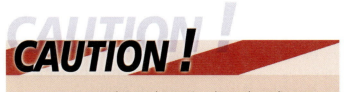

In some areas, the Good Samaritan law only applies to volunteer care providers, whereas other laws protect paid care providers. You must know the local laws that relate to your practice as an emergency first responder.

In any lawsuit for negligence, a patient must prove the following:

- The emergency first responder had a duty to the patient to act.
- The emergency first responder breached his or her duty to the patient.
- The patient was injured.
- The injury to the patient was proximately caused by the emergency first responder's breach of duty.

If the patient successfully proves that the emergency first responder was negligent, damages may be collected from the emergency first responder:

- *Duty to act.* This is generally an easy element for the plaintiff to prove. **Duty to act** is a fairly simple concept: Did you have a duty to provide care to the patient? Because your ambulance service or EMS agency promotes itself to the public as responding to emergency ambulance requests, your agency has a "duty" to respond to the patient and provide the care that a reasonable emergency first responder would be expected to provide. However, the duty to act must be a "legal duty." In other words, you must have a legal obligation to respond and treat and transport the patient before you can breach the duty to act. In most cases, this is a given fact.

  Consider this example. Emergency first responder Waylon Yelp is on his way to start the night shift at ABC Ambulance and Rescue. He hears on his scanner that a serious motor vehicle crash (MVC) has occurred just a few blocks away from his location. Waylon chooses not to respond to that call in his private vehicle. He has no duty to act, because he is not legally obligated to respond. However, if Waylon had been at the station and on duty and had failed to respond, he would have violated the duty to act.

- *Breach of the duty to act.* If you fail in any way to provide the care that your agency requires or local protocols require, you may have breached your duty to act. At this point, the standard of care comes into play. The issue will be this: If you failed to act, was the failure to act inconsistent with local protocol or other direction to provide care? Expert witnesses are used to testify to the standard of care for EMS personnel in the community you serve. The question will be: What would a reasonably prudent emergency first responder do when confronted with the same or a similar situation?

  Consider this example. Waylon is at the end of his shift and is very tired. He is so tired that all he cares about is going home. Right before his shift ends, a call comes in for a possible heart attack. The basic life support (BLS) treatment protocols for the EMT agency require that oxygen be administered in this situation. Waylon simply does not want to turn on the oxygen, because it means he may have to replace the cylinder when the call is over. So he decides not to assist the EMT in administering oxygen, even though it is part of the standard treatment protocol for a heart attack patient. Waylon has breached his duty to act by not administering oxygen in this situation.

- *Causation.* The plaintiff has to prove that your conduct was a substantial factor in bringing about the harm to the patient. This is difficult to prove in most EMS cases, because the wheels of harm to the patient have already been set in motion before EMS is even activated. In other words, you are responding to a patient who has already suffered harm. You are merely trying to intervene to lessen the impact of that harm. The question the jury will have to answer is: Was your conduct the legal cause of the harm to the patient? That is called **proximate cause**. If the harm the patient suffered can be shown to have come from other sources, and not you, this element of proof would not be met.

Consider this example. A patient suffering a heart attack calls 9-1-1. You arrive on scene and decide to wait for the EMT to arrive to begin CPR because you feel as though EMT-Yelp is much more proficient at CPR. EMT-Yelp arrives 4 minutes later and begins CPR on the patient. The patient is unable to be revived and is pronounced upon arrival at the hospital. If it can be shown that the 4-minute delay in delivering administering CPR the patient could have meant the difference between life and death, then proximate causation may be shown.

- *Injury and damages.* A successful lawsuit based on negligence requires that there first must be some harm to the patient. This is usually seen as some sort of physical or emotional injury that has caused some "damage" to the patient. Damage can be shown in the form of the patient's own testimony, the patient's medical records, and the testimony of expert witnesses and other evidence that can show the extent of harm to the patient. The cost of this harm can be translated into medical costs for treatment, recovery, and rehabilitation and for "pain and suffering," as well as other compensatory damages. To prove negligence, the plaintiff typically must show that the harm was the type that could have been caused by the EMS provider.

Consider this example. ABC Ambulance responds to a motor vehicle crash. Upon arrival, EMS personnel find the driver of the vehicle walking around with no apparent injuries. The vehicle suffered minor damage when it struck a parked car. EMT-Waylon approaches the patient, who refuses treatment and says he is fine. Waylon attempts to convince the patient to go to the hospital and explains the risks of refusing treatment and transport. Despite Waylon's efforts, the patient refuses care. Waylon reluctantly asks the patient to sign a refusal of care form, and the patient signs it. The patient goes home and goes to sleep. He sues the ambulance service because he thinks he should have been transported. He alleges that they were negligent because they did not automatically transport him. In this case, it is likely that no harm to the patient has resulted from the acts or omissions of the EMS personnel, as long as the refusal was informed and the EMTs followed proper procedure in obtaining it.

Abandonment

Abandonment is a form of negligence involving willful, wanton conduct. As an emergency first responder, you cannot leave a patient who still needs additional care until someone equally or more highly qualified relieves you. Once you have begun care, you are obligated to continue until another medical professional relieves you. If you do not follow through with your care, you are guilty of abandonment. If you are not aware that the patient needs continued care when he or she does, you are considered negligent. If you know that the patient needs continued care, you must stay with him or her until more help arrives. If you leave, or end required care prematurely, you have committed willful and wanton conduct.

Abandonment can also occur when an emergency first responder leaves a patient who refuses care if he or she has not first obtained a proper refusal. A patient who has a bad outcome from the emergency might later claim he or she was abandoned. Abandonment can also occur in the hospital emergency department if the transporting EMT leaves a patient and that EMT does not first make sure that a nurse or other emergency department staff person has accepted the patient. This is more likely to happen in a busy hospital but can occur in any hospital. If you accompany a patient to the hospital, you should ensure that the patient is accepted and that acceptance of the patient by another health care provider is documented.

Immunity Defense

Many states provide certain "immunities" under the law that makes it more difficult for a plaintiff to prove negligence against an EMS provider. These immunities are based on the age-old Good Samaritan principle. This principle basically is designed to encourage others to assist an ill or injured person to the best of their ability without fear of a lawsuit for mistakes they may make.

Virtually every state has some form of Good Samaritan law. Many of these laws merely protect the bystander or person without medical training from being sued for providing assistance in an emergency. Some of these laws protect physicians and nurses outside their work environment if they provide care at the scene of an emergency. These laws are designed to encourage off-duty health professionals to help out in an emergency without the fear of liability that could cloud their judgment.

Other state laws extend the immunity to EMS personnel and other responders. For example, Pennsylvania's immunity statute for EMS personnel states: "No emergency first responder, emergency medical technician or paramedic, or health professional who in good faith attempts to render or facilitate emergency medical care authorized by this act shall be liable for any civil damages as a result of any acts or omissions, unless guilty of gross or willful negligence."

If these laws apply to you, does it mean you are completely immune from a negligence lawsuit? Not necessarily. The type of immunity that these laws embody is not a full immunity but rather a qualified immunity. The immunity has a restriction: you may not act in a reckless, wanton manner in total disregard of the patient, because acting in this manner would be considered gross negligence. Most immunity statutes provide that you are immune from a negligence lawsuit unless your actions could be shown to constitute gross negligence.

Gross negligence is difficult to prove in many cases. Actions or lack of action must be more than a mere mistake (i.e., more serious than ordinary negligence) to be considered grossly negligent acts. As the Pennsylvania Supreme Court described it, gross negligence is substantially more than "ordinary carelessness, inadvertence, laxity or indifference." It is behavior that is "flagrant, grossly deviating from the ordinary standard of care."

Volunteer EMS personnel often enjoy legal protection for their conduct that may be stronger than the immunity protections for career or paid EMS personnel. The concept is that, if you volunteer to save someone's life or to assist the person in a medical crisis, you should not have to worry about being sued. Otherwise, few "Good Samaritans" would be willing to help in an emergency. In many cases, these state laws require that you at least have some level of training, such as CPR or first aid training, and that you render assistance only within the level of that certification or training.

These immunity protections often apply to all EMS personnel, but some states have limited this protection to volunteer personnel and do not apply it to paid EMS personnel. Why? Because the lawmakers in some states believe that you owe a higher duty to the people you are obligated to serve as part of your profession. This makes some sense, because responding to an emergency is part of your job, and you should be better prepared for these situations than the volunteer Good Samaritan. You should check your state laws carefully to determine whether the immunity statutes apply to paid or career EMS personnel. If the state does not have an immunity statute, the standard for evaluating your conduct likely will be based on ordinary negligence, which is easier to prove than gross negligence.

How do you avoid committing gross negligence? First and foremost, function within your certification level. Don't perform skills that are out of your scope of practice as an emergency first responder, which is the extent to which you can treat the patient as defined in state law. For example, if you are not authorized under state law and by your medical director to administer medications patients, you should administer medication even if it is available to you or is included in your drug box.

Second, always act in good faith. The best way to do this is always to treat patients as if they were your own close relatives. Function in a reasonable and prudent manner with the interest of the patient in your heart and mind. Common sense often helps you in this area. Ask yourself, "Is this the right thing to do in this situation?" If the answer is no, you should reevaluate your plan of action. For example, failure to provide spinal immobilization for an accident victim with neck and back pain clearly is not the right thing to do and is so blatantly wrong that most jurors would find that failure to be outside the bounds of what a reasonable emergency first responder would be expected to do. This failure likely would be seen as an example of not acting in good faith.

Third, don't do things or fail to do things that could be construed as grossly negligent. Function within your scope of practice and do what the public would expect you to do. Don't commit or omit an action that you are under a recognized duty to another to do or not do, knowing or having reason to know that the act or omission could create a substantial risk of harm to the patient. Remember the first rule of medical care: do no harm. If it is likely your actions could harm the patient, you should not initiate them.

Confidentiality

Patient confidentiality in emergency medical services is important; however, it is violated frequently. Virtually everything a patient shares is confidential. However, consider the many ways this information is inadvertently released. An emergency first responder may discuss an EMS run with colleagues. The colleagues can identify the patient from the address of the call. When an emergency first responder arrives at the emergency department with a patient, invariably a nurse or physician asks across the room, "What do you have?" The emergency first responder may then state the chief complaint back to the nurse or physician. Other patients and families often overhear this statement. Do these bystanders need to know that the patient has chest pain or a urethral discharge? What if a bystander knows the patient or the patient's employer? In these examples, medical information has been given away without patient consent.

The legal requirements for maintaining confidentiality are extensive, and an emergency first responder should be familiar with them. Patients trust EMS staff with their innermost feelings and secrets. Beside the legal requirements, you have a solemn ethical obligation to maintain the integrity of your patients' information.

The federal privacy regulations mandated by the Health Insurance Portability and Accountability Act of 1996 (known as HIPAA) went into effect on April 14, 2003. HIPAA is the first comprehensive federal law to protect the privacy of patient information. Its regulations are commonly called the Privacy Rule. These regulations require most health care providers, including ambulance services, to put into place safeguards to protect the use, distribution, and storage of the confidential health information of patients, commonly called protected health information (PHI).

The regulations have some cumbersome aspects. For example, organizations covered by the regulations must appoint a privacy officer, have privacy policies in place, develop a Notice of Privacy Practices to give to patients outlining their rights, obtain acknowledgment that patients received this notice, and train all members of their workforce in the organization's privacy practices. Compliance with HIPAA takes time and effort and requires ongoing work (e.g., training required by the Occupational Safety and Health Administration [OSHA] and fulfillment of other legal requirements).

HIPAA places greater restrictions on the release of health information. PHI is defined as any individually identifiable information about a patient's past, present, or future health care or payment for health care. Under the privacy regulations, EMS personnel are permitted to disclose as much information as necessary and to share that information with other health care providers involved in the patient's care without the patient's specific authorization. Other uses and disclosures of a patient's PHI without an authorization are permitted for billing and for certain quality assurance and health care operations purposes.

State laws also protect the privacy of medical records and in some cases may impose stricter rules than the federal regulations. Patient care reports (PCRs) must be kept strictly confidential. Every ambulance service must protect them to the fullest extent possible. Maintaining patient privacy is an essential legal obligation of an emergency first responder. You should take all reasonable steps to safeguard patient information and to protect it from improper or inadvertent use or disclosure.

Patient Care Report: A Legally Protected Medical Record

The PCR is considered a medical record, and as such the EMS agency that creates it is the owner of the record (Fig. 3-3). As the owner, your service has a duty to safeguard the documents and protect their confidentiality. This means that you may not release the PCR or its contents without the written consent of the patient, a proper subpoena, or a court order. You also should not discuss the contents of the PCR or anything about the patients you treat and transport with individuals outside your organization. Detailed internal discussions about the specific patients you treat should be kept at a professional level, respecting the patient's dignity. Only those with a "need to know" in your organization should be given details about the patient care you provided in a particular case.

The following are the most common examples in which the PCR may be released to others:

- Insurers and third-party payers, for reimbursement purposes, when the patient has given permission to release the information
- Legally authorized research
- Litigation in which the document has been obtained through proper legal process, as during the discovery phase of a lawsuit
- Law enforcement and other investigative agencies pursuant to a subpoena

Whenever your service receives a request for a PCR or any other documents, you should follow these steps:

1. *Verify the request.* Make sure the request is coming from a legitimate source, such as the patient, or from the patient's official representative or attorney with the patient's approval. You should also verify the identity of the person making the request to ensure that this individual is who he says he is. Some private

Patient Case Report

Agency	Unit #	Trip #	Type of incident ☐Medical ☐Trauma ☐No Patient ☐Refusal	# ____ of ____ Patients	Date of service / /

Incident Location	Pt. Destination	Transport By

Attendant	Certification Level	Attendant	Certification Level	Driver	Certification Level

Patient's Age	Sex ☐F ☐M	Chief Complaint	Mechanism of Injury

Narrative

Previous Medical History

Medications

Allergies   Charted By

Patient Vital Signs

Time	Blood Pressure	Pulse Rate	Rhytnm	Respirations Rate Rhythm/Quality	Pupils L R	Movement of Extremities R - arm - L R - leg - L	Glasgow Eyes Verbal Motor	Pulse Oximeter SaO2 O2LPM	Cardiac Rhythm
	/								
	/								
	/								
	/								
	/								

IV Therapy							Medications							
Time	Solution	Site	Size	Rate	Initials	S / U	Medication	Dose	Route	Time	Time	Time	Time	Order From	Response to Treatment
Total Infused		cc	Response											

Times

Tone	Responding	On Scene	ALS On	Departed	Arr Hosp	In Service

Patient Information

Name	DOB / /	S. S #	Telephone

Address	Next of Kin

City, State, Zip	Relationship

Hospital notification	**Assistance**			**Call Outcome**	
Med Channel # _____	Base Physician	☐ Police	☐ Fire	Response Code ☐2 ☐ 3	☐ Transported to Facility
☐ Cellular	☐ Amb Dispatch	☐ Sheriff	☐ Other	Transport Code ☐2 ☐ 3	☐ Care Transferred in Field
☐ Landline	☐ Other	☐ State Patrol	☐ Air Life ☐ Flight for Life	☐ Helicopter transport	☐ Cancelled

White - Agency copy   *Pink - Audit*   *Yellow - Hospital / Medical Records*

Fig. 3-3 A patient care report form. (Courtesy HealthONE EMS, Englewood, CO, in Henry M, Stapleton E: *EMT prehospital care,* ed 4, St. Louis, 2010, Mosby.)

investigators have been known to misrepresent themselves just to get a copy of a PCR.

2. *Consult with counsel.* Before releasing any records, consult with the agency's legal counsel to make sure that proper procedures are in place for the various types of requests for documents.

3. *Get a written release.* Never release a PCR or any other document without a signed authorization from the patient unless it is pursuant to a court order. Also, make sure the individual signs a receipt acknowledging that she received what you provided to her, should there ever be any question as to whether you released the documents in a timely manner. The receipt also documents exactly what you gave the person, because it may appear as evidence at a trial down the road, and remembering exactly what was provided could prove difficult if you are relying simply on memory.

"Superprotection" for Specific Patient Situations

The importance of confidentiality and of protecting the integrity of a medical record, such as a PCR, cannot be overemphasized. Crews must be trained in the importance of not showing or releasing PCRs and other documentation to others. Legal claims for invasion of privacy frequently can arise when a health care organization does not treat medical records and reports with the highest degree of respect. The state and federal governments recently have increased the legal protection and privacy of medical information, and the ambulance industry is not exempt from many of these new requirements.

Some aspects of an individual's medical history have superprotection under the law. For example, a patient infected with the human immunodeficiency virus (HIV) or who has acquired immunodeficiency syndrome (AIDS) is protected from the release of information about the person's medical status in most states. These laws, often referred to as confidentiality of HIV/AIDS information, limit the extent to which health care providers may share information with others about a patient's HIV status. These laws vary from state to state, to an extent. However, most states have adequate safeguards to ensure that ambulance service personnel are adequately informed in case they should come in contact with a patient with HIV or AIDS and exposure to the disease is likely. Beyond that, sharing with others the HIV or AIDS status of a patient you treat or transport generally is improper and may well be illegal.

Does this affect how you document when a person has HIV or AIDS? Absolutely not. The key is to document your observations in an objective way without drawing conclusions. Don't document on the PCR that you *think* the person has AIDS or HIV. However, document it if the patient tells you that he or she has the disease. For example, you can write, "Patient stated, 'I have HIV,' when asked about his past medical history."

As with HIV and AIDS, many states have laws that protect the release of information about an individual's mental health information or past record of drug or alcohol treatment. Many states' laws governing mental health procedures dictate how health care providers may treat this information. In fact, many laws exist to protect individuals from discriminatory treatment based on their particular medical status, such as a history of mental illness or drug or alcohol treatment. In many cases these laws do not specifically include ambulance personnel; however, the general rules of confidentiality should still apply, to minimize your risk of a lawsuit and the inappropriate handling of very sensitive information.

Incident Reporting

Your agency should have a policy on "unusual occurrence reporting." This policy should define what occurrences should be reported and the procedures for reporting them. Once the incident report is completed, it should be submitted to your immediate supervisor. In many cases, it is unwise to attach the incident report to the PCR, because anything attached to that document may become part of the medical record and more easily discovered in litigation. Of course, your PCR should clearly indicate any known errors that occurred in patient care and the steps taken to remedy the errors. However, the details of how the errors occurred are best left for the separate incident report.

Appropriate management personnel and the system medical director should promptly investigate the incident. Depending on the situation, appropriate corrective action should be taken when a medication error has been made. Corrective action may include additional continuing education for the individual, as well as disciplinary action in some cases. Many state EMS laws also require that certain medication errors be reported to the EMS office, and a standard incident report format may be in place.

In many cases of medical errors, problems in the system may have contributed to the occurrence of the error. Every medication error should be reviewed from the quality assurance and risk management perspectives. This helps to ensure that system problems are identified and corrected. Otherwise, the risk of a future error may not be reduced, as another care provider in the system may be just as likely to make the same mistake. System-wide education may be required after the error has been closely reviewed. Obviously medication and other treatment errors are not a good thing to have happen because of the potential for harm to the patient and the risk of a lawsuit. When they do occur, these errors provide an opportunity to review the system critically and to make changes for the betterment of overall prehospital patient care.

Reportable Events

In many states, EMS providers, police officers, and firefighters are mandated reporters of certain crimes that may have been committed against their patients. Mandated reporting requirements typically extend to children, dependent adults, and elderly individuals who have been or may have been neglected or abused. However, in some states the requirements are much broader and include many other crimes. For example, reportable events in some states may include gunshot wounds, stab wounds, and rape or other types of sexual assault. Exposure to a patient's blood or body fluid or certain infectious diseases is also a reportable event. A significant fine or other punishment may be imposed for failure to file a mandated report. As an emergency first responder, you should know what is required of you, both for your protection and that of your patient.

Medical Information Insignia

Medical insignia are commonly present on patients to inform caregivers of preexisting medical conditions such as diabetes, allergies, and epilepsy. You should check for medical insignia devices during your assessment on all patients (Fig. 3-4). Failure to locate a patient's insignia could be considered negligence.

Documentation

The ethical issues involving documentation are rather straightforward:

- Document honestly and in an unbiased manner.
- If you didn't write it, you didn't do it!

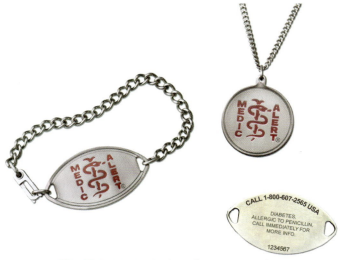

Fig. 3-4 Medical identification jewelry.

The patient care report is the foundation of all that you do in the field. It is the official record of the care you provided. The PCR has significant patient care, billing, and liability ramifications. The basic purpose of the PCR is to provide the reader with a "picture" of the continuum of care provided to the patient, from the arrival of emergency first responders to the transfer of care to hospital staff (see Chapter 4).

In a lawsuit, the PCR becomes your substitute memory, because most liability lawsuits end up in trial years after the harm occurred. Most people have trouble remembering what they did on a particular call a year ago, let alone several years ago. Therefore, you need a complete and "visual" record of what you found and what you did if you expect to come across as a knowledgeable and credible witness before a jury. Sloppy, incomplete, and poorly constructed patient documentation reflects poorly on the individual emergency first responder or paramedic and on the ambulance service itself. Poor documentation may also be used against you in a lawsuit or federal investigation.

Now, more than ever, ambulance services must be vigilant in their documentation efforts. The law of negligence comes into play when a patient sues your service for the care that was provided. The recent focus on the antifraud and abuse laws makes documentation a concern outside of the traditional patient care areas. More than ever, Medicare carriers and the government are closely scrutinizing patient care documentation for false statements, inconsistent information, and other inaccuracies that could lead to a federal false claims act action or other criminal prosecution or civil sanctions.

Clear, accurate documentation is not only required for good patient care, it also is a necessity in this ever-litigious society. Your PCR will be center stage in a malpractice or negligence trial. Therefore, make sure your documentation helps you in your defense rather than hurts you. If you are called to the witness stand, you absolutely will be cross-examined by the plaintiff's counsel about the quality of your documentation. Sloppy, incomplete documentation of the patient care you provide reflects on your credibility as a competent caregiver, even if your documentation has no gross errors.

Bruce, Sones, and Peck pointed out some very important do's and don'ts to consider when documenting patient care.

Do

- Make sure the documentation is an accurate reflection of your prehospital capabilities and your scope of practice.
- Write legibly and in complete sentences, using proper abbreviations so that all personnel can read your report.
- Accurately document the times treatment was provided and give a clear description of that treatment.
- Document any refusal of care by the patient, including instances when a patient refuses only a portion of the treatment you are attempting to provide (e.g., patient refuses oxygen). State why the patient refused the treatment and the steps you took to make this refusal one in which the patient was informed of all the risks of refusing the treatment.
- Document vital signs before and after key treatment and when the patient is moved.
- Document any changes in vital signs, especially if the patient's condition worsens.
- Create a "picture" of the patient's condition so that when others read the PCR, they can actually visualize the patient.

Don't

- Scribble or write illegibly.
- Misspell words or medication names.
- Forget to check the patient's response to any treatments.
- Make up abbreviations or use inappropriate acronyms in your documentation. Use only approved abbreviations.
- Assume that others will take care of your documentation. If you provided the treatment, it is your responsibility to document it.
- Prepare your report late if you can avoid it. Chart any late entries or errors in charting if changes or entries are made after the original report is completed and turned in. And always prepare your documentation as if it will be revealed in a court of law.

Documenting Care Provided to the Patient by Others

A question that often arises is whether an EMT or emergency first responder should document on the BLS patient care report the interventions or assessments performed by the paramedic. This might be an issue in areas where EMS is provided in tiered systems. In other words, it might be an issue in areas where BLS and advanced life support (ALS) are provided by separate organizations. In such systems, BLS providers respond in a transporting ambulance and ALS providers respond in a nontransporting paramedic intercept or "fly car" unit.

In some systems, the practice may be to document that the ALS provider applied a cardiac monitor and to record the electrocardiographic (ECG) rhythm displayed on the monitor. Some emergency first responders also document that the paramedic started an intravenous (IV) line, the number of attempts needed to establish the line, the medications and solutions administered through the IV line, and other such information about the ALS care.

As a general rule, EMS providers should document according to their scope of practice and should not attempt to document skills beyond those for which they are trained and are certified to perform themselves. The risk of inconsistent and inaccurate records is too great when providers document beyond their scope of practice. In addition, such "beyond the scope" documentation may impair the credibility of an EMS provider who ends up on a witness stand defending a lawsuit. For example, emergency first responders who document a particular cardiac rhythm are left wide open to a stinging and damaging cross-examination about their training and qualifications, or lack thereof, to make such determinations and why they would document care beyond their scope of practice. Not being able to answer questions in a deposition or on the witness stand about all the documentation, including the emergency first responder–documented ALS care, could call into question the emergency first responder's quality of BLS treatment by undermining the credibility of the witness.

This is not to suggest that emergency first responders cannot document anything that happens in regard to ALS. The emergency first responder should certainly document the fact that the paramedic provided patient care and should certainly document the emergency first responder's role in the care. For example, if the paramedic intubates the patient and the emergency first responder handles the bag-mask ventilation, the BLS patient care report certainly should reflect that. Other general observations on a BLS patient care report, such as "Paramedic performed a patient assessment," "Paramedic intubated the patient," "Paramedic applied a cardiac monitor," and "IV medications administered by the paramedic," likewise wouldn't create any problems, as long as the emergency first responder refrains from describing details, such as the intubation technique or tube size used, the particular cardiac rhythm displayed on the monitor, or the names and dosages of specific medications administered by ALS providers.

The bottom line is this: In many areas, the provision of emergency medical services is a team effort involving BLS and ALS providers, with each group performing specific responsibilities in patient care. Just as EMS providers must render all patient care within their respective scopes of practice, their documentation shouldn't exceed their scopes of practice.

Changing the Patient Care Report

A common misperception seems to prevail among some EMS professionals—that is, once a PCR is completed, it cannot, under any circumstances, be changed, altered, appended, or amended. As a general rule, this is untrue. Unless your specific state law prohibits it (and we are not aware of any that do), PCRs can be amended to correct erroneous information (e.g., name, address, and insurance information).

You can also add to a PCR after it is completed, using an addendum or second sheet, in the event you later recall important information that was omitted when you completed the initial record. Of course, changing a PCR is improper and illegal if it is done to falsify or misrepresent information for any reason, particularly for billing or reimbursement purposes. Your EMS agency, in conjunction with their legal counsel, should develop a policy regarding the completion and modification of PCRs.

This policy should reaffirm the agency's commitment to honesty, accuracy, and ethics in documentation and should include other specific directions for field personnel. For example, the policy should address issues such as the following: (1) only the original author of the PCR should make modifications; (2) all entries made after the PCR is initially completed should be signed and dated;

and (3) errors on written PCRs should be corrected by striking out the original information, writing the word "error," and entering the correct information. These same principles apply if you complete the PCR electronically (see Fig. 3-3). Most electronic PCR completion software has built-in protections to prevent the original record from being changed without a proper notation. Some programs default to an addendum screen whenever an entry is added after the initial PCR has been completed.

Five Simple Ways to Improve Your Documentation Skills

Good documentation is important to you and your ambulance service for many reasons. Effective documentation can facilitate quality patient care, help protect you from liability, and favorably affect your EMS agency's reimbursement for the services you provide. Here are five quick and easy steps for improving your documentation skills:

1. *Paint a picture.* Think of your documentation as painting a picture of the incident. Instead of using a paintbrush or a camera, you are using words. Set the scene. For instance, at an accident scene, where are the cars? Are there broken glass and tire marks? Is there significant damage to the vehicles and was the passenger compartment compromised? What sights, sounds, and smells are registering on your senses? Documenting these elements can help the reader visualize a patient consistent with the patient about whom you are writing.

2. *Use chronologic narratives.* Avoid the tendency to jump around as things enter your mind. Stay focused; write your narrative so that it flows in chronologic order. Make sure that the steps of your dispatch, assessment, treatment, and transport are documented in a logical fashion. This can be especially problematic when too much time passes between the call and the time the documentation is done. Document when the call is as fresh in your mind as possible.

3. *Stick to the facts.* A well-written PCR is objective rather than subjective. This means that your charts should stick to the facts and should leave out personal interpretations and "spin." For instance, don't simply say that your patient was "intoxicated." Instead, document the facts that led you to that conclusion, such as "Patient's speech was slurred," "Odor of alcohol on patient's breath," "Patient admitted drinking eight beers in the past hour," and other such objective facts.

4. *Do not use "homegrown" abbreviations.* Many EMS providers love to use homegrown abbreviations. Reading their charts is like grading a test—and they're the only ones who have the answer key! Abbreviations are fine, but stick to ones that are common and accepted in the health care professions. Your service can even consider adopting a standard table of abbreviations to be used in your company's PCRs.

5. *Spelling counts.* This can be a tough one. Not everyone has top-notch spelling skills, but proper spelling and good grammar are important. Remember that a jury looks at the PCR you completed, and if it is full of errors, it may lead the jurors to conclude that you are as sloppy at patient care as you are at documentation. That affects your credibility as an EMS professional and could affect the jury's ultimate decision. Nobody's perfect in this department, and medical terms can be especially tricky to spell properly. So, pick up an EMT textbook or get a medical dictionary at the station and commit to learning a new word or two on each shift. This will boost your vocabulary, both in EMS and in life, and also improve your trip sheets.

Crime Scenes

Dispatch should notify the appropriate law enforcement agency when an emergency first responder is sent to a potential crime scene. However, you may unsuspectingly enter a violent crime situation. If violence is occurring or if you recognize a potential crime, law enforcement should be contacted immediately and you should ensure your own safety.

If you are at a crime scene, it is important to focus on your role and provide patient care. The patient's emergency medical care is your primary responsibility. You should assist law enforcement only if this does not compromise patient care. It is important not to disturb any item at the scene unless your emergency care requires you to do so. You should observe and document anything unusual at the scene related to patient care and inform law enforcement officers. If possible, you should avoid cutting through holes in clothing caused by gunshot or stab wounds.

It is important to remember that law enforcement personnel are in charge of the crime scene. You should follow the directions of the police, even if doing so may interfere with patient care. In such a situation, you should tell the law enforcement official how patient care would be compromised and explain the risks. If the official insists, you must follow his or her instructions and return to patient care as soon as you are cleared to do so. The incident should be fully documented.

Organ Donation

An organ donor is any patient who has signed a legal form to donate his or her organs in the event of his or her death. As an emergency first responder, you may find out that a patient is an organ donor through an indication on a driver's license or through family members. It is important to remember that how you treat a patient should be the same whether or not the patient is an organ donor. If you discover that a patient is an organ donor, that information should be included in your report when you turn over patient care.

Team Work

The transfer of care is an important legal and ethical concept. An emergency first responder should understand his or her role as part of the team at an emergency. He or she should render patient care and remain with the patient until someone of equal or higher medical knowledge can assume the care. It is important for transfer of care to occur seamlessly and completely. When giving over care of the patient to another health care provider, such as an EMT, nurse, or physician, you should introduce the patient and report on the patient's medical history, the circumstances of the emergency, your assessment, and any care you have delivered. In addition to giving information to the receiving health care provider, you should also remember to close your relationship with the patient, if appropriate, by taking the time to say goodbye or some other form of "send-off." It may also be appropriate for the transporting EMTs, for example, to follow up with you at a later date and let you know how the patient did during transport. It is important to have circular lines of communication with all health care team members to evaluate the event.

It is also important to realize that you may not always relinquish care to another health care provider. The patient may end up going with law enforcement, or if treatment is refused, back to the care of family or friends. In all cases, you should ensure complete and professional communication. Knowing other agencies and their job roles helps to make a more effective health care team. Other agencies can also be used as a resource for continuing education. There should always be a mutual level of respect for all contributions at the scene of an emergency.

In the Real World—Conclusion

You and your partner decide to explain the situation to the patient. You talk with the patient and explain that he needs some medical attention but you can't help him unless you get approval from one of his parents. After a few minutes of discussion the patient tells you that his name is Peter and that his dad is at work at the local bank. The law enforcement officer takes the information and dispatches another officer to the bank. Within a few minutes, the officer at the bank radios back to his partner at the scene that the father has given permission for treatment. While cleaning the patient's abrasions, the ambulance arrives and you give a detailed report to the EMT. You help prepare the patient for transport to the hospital, where the father will meet the patient.

Reference

Albright v. Abington Memorial Hospital, 696 A. 2d 1159 (Pa), 1997.
   Bruce M, Sones S, Peck P: Medication safety: implications for EMS, *EMS Magazine,* 97-106, 2003.

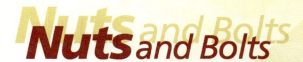

Critical Points

As an emergency first responder, you will deal with legal and ethical issues. You must clearly understand your state and local laws and regulations to make appropriate decisions about patient care. You must understand the scope of care you are legally required to give. You must be able to assess patient competence to give consent or refusal for care. Negligence, advance directives, and DNR orders and documentation are critical issues that affect your job performance and your personal liability.

Learning Checklist

The standard of care is the care that you are expected to give based on your level of training and experience.

- ❑ The standard of care is based on the First Responder National Standard Curriculum, materials in emergency first responder texts and instructional materials, information in continuing education curricula, local medical protocols and standing orders, and individual agency requirement.
- ❑ An emergency first responder has not only a legal obligation to his or her patients but an ethical obligation. You should know your local protocols and laws and always act in the best interest of the patient.
- ❑ Patients must consent to treatment before you provide it. To give consent, patients must be competent and of legal age. They must understand the care you are offering and any consequences if they refuse that care.
- ❑ Expressed consent refers to written or verbal consent to treatment.
- ❑ Implied consent is the assumption that is used to provide lifesaving care to an unconscious patient who is unable to give consent. The consent is implied because you assume that the person would want you to save his or her life. Implied consent can also come from "lack of protest." If you provide a treatment and the patient does not verbally or physically deny that treatment, it is implied that the patient has consented to it.
- ❑ Competence is the patient's ability to make an informed decision about any medical care and any

consequences of the medical care. A patient may be considered incompetent if he or she is (or may be) intoxicated, under the influence of drugs, affected by a serious injury, affected by a legal disability such as age, or has a proven history of mental incapacity.
- ❑ In the case of a patient who does not speak the same language as you, every attempt should be made to find a translator so the patient can make informed decisions.
- ❑ Competent adult patients have the right to refuse medical care. A patient can refuse any or all types of care. If a patient refuses medical care, he or she should sign some type of refusal form that indicates an awareness of the risks of refusing that care. Signing of the refusal form should be witnessed by someone other than yourself.
- ❑ A minor or an incompetent adult cannot legally give consent or refusal for treatment. As an emergency first responder, you must obtain consent from the patient's legal guardian. The age for a minor may vary in different areas so it is important to know your local protocols. With a minor or an incompetent adult in a life-threatening situation, you should provide care based on implied consent.
- ❑ Emancipated minors are considered adults in some respects and can legally consent or refuse medical treatment. A minor is emancipated only if a court, after a legal proceeding, makes that determination.
- ❑ An advance directive is a document that contains the wishes of the patient and directions to caregivers for the patient's medical care while the patient is alive but incapable of expressing those directions.
- ❑ A do not attempt resuscitation (DNAR) order is an order written by a physician with the consent of the patient and/or family when death is expected within a relatively short time. The order is to withhold resuscitative measures if a person has no pulse, for example.
- ❑ Touching a person without his or her consent may be considered battery. Assault is the threat of touching a person without his or her consent.
- ❑ To prove negligence it must be proven that the emergency first responder had a duty to act, the emergency first responder breached his or her duty to the patient, the patient was injured, and the

Nuts and Bolts–continued

injury was proximately caused by the emergency first responder's breach of duty.

❑ As an emergency first responder, you must remain with a patient who still requires medical care until someone at least equally qualified relieves you. If you do not remain with the patient or do not follow through with care, it is called abandonment.

❑ Abandonment can also occur when an emergency first responder leaves a patient who refuses care if the emergency first responder has not first obtained a proper refusal.

❑ Any patient information that you obtain for the purpose of assessment or treatment is considered confidential. This includes any or all information received directly from the patient, through observation and assessment of the patient, or through other health care providers.

❑ Patient information can be released only if the patient has provided written permission for that information to be released or when the information is requested by a subpoena.

❑ Reportable events that require giving information to public health or other officials may include gunshot wounds, stab wounds, sexual assaults, and exposure to a patient's blood, body fluids, or certain infectious diseases.

❑ Part of your assessment should include looking for medical insignia for preexisting medical conditions.

❑ Proper documentation of your involvement in any patient care or emergency situation is important.

❑ If you are rendering patient care at a crime scene, you should focus on patient care and remember that law enforcement personnel are in charge of the scene. If you are requested to stop patient care for some reason, you should explain to law enforcement how or why stopping would be harmful to the patient and allow law enforcement to make an informed decision. If you must stop patient care, you should resume as soon as you have been cleared to do so and you should document the situation.

Key Terms

Abandonment Leaving a patient before another health care provider has assumed responsibility for that patient or before you have delivered the required standard of care.

Advance directive A legal document that contains the wishes of the patient and directions to health care providers for the patient's medical care while the patient is still alive.

Assault The threat of touching someone without his or her consent.

Battery Touching or striking a person without his or her consent.

Capacity A medical determination of a person's ability to make an informed decision.

Competence The ability of a patient to understand your questions and the implications of the decisions he or she might make.

Do not attempt resuscitate (DNAR) order A written order by a physician instructing health care providers not to provide medical care to a patient who is clinically dead.

Durable power of attorney A legal document that designates another individual to make health care decisions for the person who signed the document once that person becomes incapacitated.

Duty to act The legal obligation to provide medical care.

Emancipated minor A minor who has been determined by a court to be legally capable of making adult decisions including consenting to or refusing medical treatment.

Expressed consent Written or verbal consent from a patient that tells you he or she has consented to medical care.

Implied consent A legal definition that assumes a person unable to give expressed consent because of his or her injury would want medical care if he or she could give that consent. Also refers to consent based on "lack of protest" from the patient when medical care is given.

Incompetence The state of a patient who is unable to understand your questions or understand the implications of the decisions he or she may be making.

Living will A written document that describes an individual's wishes for lifesaving measures if certain medical conditions occur.

Medical insignia Any identification device worn by patients to identify certain preexisting medical conditions.

Minor A person not yet of a predefined age to make legal decisions.

Negligence The act of failing to provide the expected standard of care to a patient, which leads to further injury to the patient.

Protocols Written instructions to carry out care for certain medical symptoms or conditions.

Proximate cause A legal term meaning one's actions or inactions were in fact the cause of a patient's injuries.

Refusal Declined medical treatment.

Standard of care The care you are expected to give based on your level of training and experience.

Standing order Patient care instructions, in writing, that authorize specific steps in patient assessment and treatment without contacting medical control.

First Responder NSC Objectives
COGNITIVE OBJECTIVES

- Define the First Responder scope of care.
- Discuss the importance of do not attempt resuscitation (DNAR) (advance directives) and local or state provisions regarding EMS application.

- Define consent and discuss the methods of obtaining consent.
- Differentiate between expressed and implied consent.
- Explain the role of consent of minors in providing care.
- Discuss the implications for the First Responder in patient refusal of transport.
- Discuss the issues of abandonment, negligence, and battery, and their implications to the First Responder.
- State the conditions necessary for the First Responder to have a duty to act.
- Explain the importance, necessity, and legality of patient confidentiality.
- List the actions that a First Responder should take to assist in the preservation of a crime scene.
- State the conditions that require a First Responder to notify local law enforcement officials.
- Discuss issues concerning the fundamental components of documentation.

AFFECTIVE OBJECTIVES

- Explain the rationale for the needs, benefits, and use of advance directives.
- Explain the rationale for the concept of varying degrees of DNAR.

Check your understanding
Check your understanding

Please refer to p. 439 for the answers to these questions.

1. True or False: Whenever there is an ethical duty for the emergency first responder to act, there is also a legal duty to act.

2. According to your training and experience, the level of care expected to be provided to a patient in a given situation is the _____.

3. The range of skills that can be performed by an emergency first responder, which are defined by state laws or rules, are known as the _____.

4. Concerning a patient's ability to consent to medical treatment, his or her ability to understand the questions of the emergency first responder and the consequences of his or her decisions is known as _____.

5. When an emergency first responder treats a patient who is unresponsive, he or she is treating the patient under _____ consent.

6. A document that expresses the wishes of a patient about his or her medical care while he or she is alive is a/an _____.

7. A legal document that gives another person authority to consent to medical care for a patient who is unable to provide consent on his or her own is a/an _____.

8. An emergency first responder provides medical care to a competent adult who is refusing any medical treatment. The emergency first responder may be accused of _____.

9. If an emergency first responder treats a patient in a manner that is not consistent with accepted standards of care and that treatment results in injury to the patient, the emergency first responder may be accused of _____.

10. Written guidelines that outline instructions for caring for patients with certain signs and symptoms are called _____, whereas written authorization to perform certain steps in caring for patients is called _____.

11. Which of the following patients is most likely to be determined competent and able to give legal consent?
    A. Patient in a motor vehicle collision who fails a field sobriety test
    B. Patient who does not know his or her name
    C. Patient is a pregnant 18-year-old patient who is not married
    D. Agitated patient who was hit in the head with a baseball

12. Sharing a patient's information with only those who need to know in order to continue medical treatment of the patient is known as which of the following?
    A. Confidentiality
    B. Privacy
    C. Disclosure
    D. Secrecy

13. You are filling your regular Friday afternoon volunteer shift at your rescue squad. The phone rings and the unfamiliar voice on the other end identifies herself as a paralegal from a large law firm. She states the firm is representing Megan Johnson, a patient you cared for about a month ago. Ms. Johnson is suing the driver of the other vehicle that was involved in the motor vehicle collision in which she was injured. The paralegal states that she needs you to fax a copy of Megan's treatment record to her and that Megan has agreed to this. How should you respond to the request?
    A. Fax the record as requested
    B. Refer the caller to your supervisor
    C. Hang up on the caller
    D. Call Ms. Johnson to get her permission

14. You are caring for a patient with a valid DNAR order who is having severe difficulty breathing and weak pulses. What is your best course of action?
   A. Treat as you would any patient with oxygen and comfort care.
   B. Perform CPR.
   C. Do nothing as there is a valid DNAR.
   D. Wait for ALS personnel to arrive before treating the patient.

15. While you are on scene treating a critically injured patient, an advanced provider tells you to start an IV because he or she needs to do something else. As an emergency first responder, starting the IV would be a violation of:
   A. Scope of practice
   B. Standard of care
   C. Abandonment
   D. Do not attempt resuscitation

Chapter 4

Communications and Documentation

LESSON GOAL

This chapter discusses what effective communication is and how to become a better communicator. We will discuss barriers to effective communication and how to overcome them. We will spend some time identifying the components of today's emergency medical services (EMS) communication systems. We will also discuss the importance of accurate, legible, and organized patient care reporting.

OBJECTIVES

1. Discuss the process of communication and the skills one should use to interact with patients, other agencies, and responders.
2. Describe actions to take to increase the effectiveness of both verbal and nonverbal communications.
3. Discuss various barriers to effective communication and how to overcome those barriers.
4. Describe how to communicate with empathy.
5. Identify a variety of emergency communication equipment, their uses, and their limitations.
6. List the information that is to be included when transferring patient care to another provider.
7. Discuss the uses and critical nature of completing a quality patient care report (PCR).
8. Discuss the absolute need for the confidentiality and privacy of patient health information.
9. List the information required (minimum data set) to be included in each patient care report.

In the Real World

As you grab your coat and stumble out into the night and make your way to the station, something just doesn't seem right. The address that your crew has been paged to just doesn't make sense. You can't stop thinking that those house numbers cannot exist. You arrive at the station and share your concern with your partner, who has the same suspicion. You notify dispatch that you have received the call and are now en route as you pull out of the station and flip the lights. Dispatch then advises that "You are responding to a patient with chest pain."

After a quick check of the map book, you believe you have been given a bad address. You repeat the address back to dispatch, and the dispatcher agrees. You then calmly advise dispatch that that particular street does not have blocks in that number range and ask the dispatcher to check with the caller. Your persistence pays off—the address is corrected and dispatch apologizes. You acknowledge the radio traffic and continue on the call.

Perhaps nothing is more important to the success of an emergency response as clear, concise, and appropriate communication. When you consider all of the communication that must take place to make the proper response happen, you can see how even one single breakdown may have far-reaching effects. If the caller gives the wrong address, the response is delayed. If the dispatcher transposes the numbers incorrectly and gives you 1324 Elm Street instead of 3124 Elm Street, the response is delayed. If the navigator on your crew gives you incorrect directions to the address, the response is delayed. Now that you finally get to your patient, if you are not listening when he or she answers your questions, treatment may be delayed. What if you did not read your patient's nonverbal communication and are now in the middle of a potentially violent situation? This is only a small sampling of how effective communication is absolutely a cornerstone to an organized, safe, and successful emergency response.

Communication

There are many different definitions of the word "**communication.**" Because of the many forms of communication, we will look at it in the following light: *Communication is any act by which one person gives to or receives from another person information about that person's needs, desires, perceptions, knowledge, or affective states. Communication may be intentional or unintentional, may involve conventional or unconventional signals, may take linguistic or nonlinguistic forms, and may occur through spoken or other modes.*[1]

This definition is the foundation of this chapter. Everything you do, say, your tone of voice, your posture, and your general appearance communicates a message to your patient, whether you recognize it or not.

Every communication event starts with a sender, receiver, and a message (Fig. 4-1). As mentioned in the definition, this message may be verbal or nonverbal. As the sender, it is important to put your message into a form the receiver can understand. This process is called **encoding**. We do this each day without even thinking about it. This requires us to have a working knowledge of the receiver and that person's ability to correctly interpret the message. This is the reason we speak differently to small children than we do with adults. We change our voices, make funny faces and noises, and look them right in the eyes, all in an attempt to ensure they get the message. The same message delivered in the same manner to an adult may be cause for concern and may give the impression that you do not respect the other person or their position. We need to be aware that encoding the message properly is paramount to effective communications. Again, take a lesson from the children. A father asks his teenager to clean her room in what he thinks is a clear and easily understood message. Her reply is an appropriate "Yes, sir," but her tone and eye-rolling communicate something else. She got the message, but she sent another with the tone and nonverbals. She encoded her message with a bit of teenage attitude, knowing that her father would understand fully that she was not happy about her task. This show of attitude can be seen as another important component of communication: **feedback**. Feedback lets the sender know the message was received and understood as intended. You know she is not happy about the message but understands just the same. The last example of encoding we will use has to do with crew safety. We have already established that a message must be encoded correctly, but it also must be **decoded**, or understood,

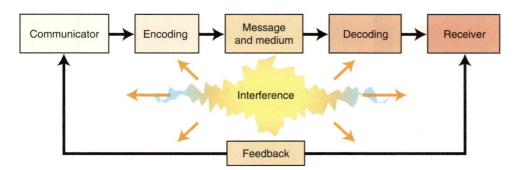

Fig. 4-1 Basic communication model. (From Chapleau W, Pons P: *Emergency medical technician: making the difference,* St. Louis, 2007, Mosby.)

correctly. While on an emergency call, the scene begins to turn violent and unsafe. How do we alert the other crew member of the immediate need to back out of the scene? One technique is to simply call your partner by a different name. This requires the crew to understand what that message means. If the crew has been together for 12 years and are very familiar, the message will be easier to understand and proper action will be taken. If all crew members are new, calling the new guy by the wrong name may truly be a mistake. This lack of experience may be seen as **interference** in the communication process. Interference may be defined as any process that hinders or prevents communication. How is the receiver to decode this message? Hopefully, there has been some preincident communication as to the methods and "buzzwords" that will signal and alert everyone. This preincident briefing would minimize the interference of a new crew.

Importance of Effective Communication
Inter- and Intra-Agency Communication

First, there must be clear communication within each agency. You cannot realistically expect to be able to effectively communicate with other agencies if you cannot communicate within your own. Take the simple example of being asked by a veteran EMS provider for a certain piece of equipment. Before this age of interoperability, you may each have a different name for the same piece of equipment. The focus in today's emergency response environment is on "using plain English" to avoid any confusion. You must take the time to learn these terms, and if you are unsure, by all means, ask someone. You do not want to be the one who did not understand what was meant simply because you did not ask.

Once you can communicate effectively within your organization, you must be able to work with other agencies involved in the response. These agencies each have their own internal language, just as yours does. A good communicator will be able to pick up and correctly translate some of these languages; however, when working with multiple agencies, you can see the benefits of using plain English. Everyone must be reading off of the same

sheet of music, or the result is just noise. You must know which radio system the agency you wish to talk to is using, which channel the agency is on, and even how to get representatives from the agency to your location quickly. These specific issues are addressed at the system or local level. The concept of interoperability is essential in the technologically advancing world of emergency response. Interoperability is a caveat of the National Incident Management System (NIMS). NIMS will be discussed in Chapter 15, Operations.

CAUTION !

"The use of plain language in emergency response is a matter of public safety, especially the safety of emergency first responders and those affected by the incident." . . . "It is critical that all local responders, as well as those coming into the impacted area . . . know and utilize commonly established operational structures, terminology, practice and procedures."

NIMS

Patient Communication

Once you get to the scene of your emergency and gather the necessary resources, it is time to communicate with the patient. As an emergency first responder, you will be present at what may be the worst moments in your patient's life. Your ability to effectively communicate both verbally and nonverbally and to interpret the return messages may have a lasting impact on the patient or the patient's family. There may be situations where you only get one chance to ask a question or listen for the answer before your patient becomes unconscious. We will now look at how to become a more effective communicator, as well as some common barriers you must overcome.

Effective Communication

To improve your ability to better understand the verbal and nonverbal messages you receive, we must approach

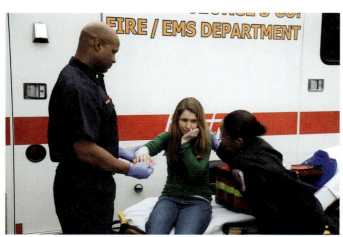

Fig. 4-2 Empathy. (From Henry M, Stapleton E: *EMT pre-hospital care,* ed 4, St. Louis, 2010, Mosby.)

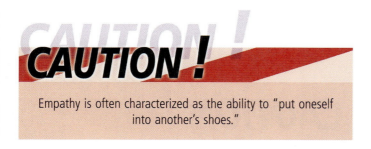

CAUTION !

Empathy is often characterized as the ability to "put oneself into another's shoes."

each patient encounter with **empathy**. Empathy can be considered as one's ability to recognize, perceive, and feel directly the emotion of another (**Fig. 4-2**).

Empathy begins with awareness of another person's feelings. It would be easier to be aware of other people's emotions if they would simply tell us how they felt. But because most people do not, we must resort to asking questions, reading between the lines, guessing, and trying to interpret nonverbal cues.

Once we have figured out how another person feels, we show empathy by acknowledging the emotion with statements such as "I can see you are really uncomfortable about this" or "I can understand why you would be upset."

We can also show empathy through a simple sign of affection such as gesture or a comforting touch, although you must be careful and sensitive to cultural differences in which a touch may be viewed as inappropriate or unacceptable. If you service a culturally diverse population, it would be a good idea to learn about the particular actions that may be interpreted as disrespectful. There are some cultures where touching with the left hand is considered insulting, as the left hand is used for toilet functions. There are also some cultures that make and maintain prolonged eye contact when in conversation. They are showing interest in what you are saying and

judging your trustworthiness. By not returning the same type of eye contact, you are deemed to be untrustworthy. Lastly, you may respond to a situation in which your female patient, by way of cultural heritage, will not allow a male responder to touch her or render care. These are but a few examples, and as populations change and adapt, so will the cultural nuances that we need to keep up with. Though empathy is usually used in reference to sensing someone else's painful feelings, it can also apply to someone's positive feelings of success, pride, or achievement. In this case, a simple "high five" would be an expression of empathy.

Empathy does not involve the statements "I know how you feel" or "I understand." Even though you may have experienced a similar event in your life, it is nearly impossible to fully understand their feelings. By saying, "I understand," you may in fact decrease the level of trust and connection you have worked so hard to forge. A better way to convey your feelings may be "I can imagine that this must be difficult for you." This statement shows genuine concern and honest emotion without running the risk of being perceived as patronizing. Some empathetic statements may include the following:

- "Sounds like you are . . ."
- "I imagine that must be . . ."
- "I can understand that must make you feel . . ."

Sensitivity

As an emergency first responder, you are expected to bring your sensitivity for the human condition to each and every call. A basic guideline for showing sensitivity to someone is to not invalidate him or her. Invalidation is to reject, ignore, mock, tease, judge, or diminish someone's feelings. Try to imagine yourself in the other person's situation. You certainly would not appreciate someone bringing "attitude" or insensitivity to your time of need.

Sensitivity involves being receptive to others' cues, particularly the nonverbal ones such as facial expressions. Sensitivity and empathy are certainly connected at the hip. Remember, you are dealing with people who have varying emotional states, cultural sensitivities, and coping mechanisms. Being sensitive and acting and speaking with empathy gives you the best chance of connecting with your patients and building the bond of trust, which is essential to effective patient care.

Listening

You have no doubt heard the following, probably said by one of your parents: "Are you listening to me?" We know that hearing and listening are different. Hearing is the physical component, which requires an environment conducive to conversation. For example, if your patient is in a loud, thumping nightclub or in a raucous sports arena, hearing is impaired, as is the ability to effectively communicate. The obvious solution is to get the patient into a less distracting environment. Now that you and your patient can hear each other, it is time to begin listening. Listening is the process by which you understand not only what was said but also how it was said and the associated body language. Some of the components of effective listening are as follows:

1. *Use encouraging behaviors.* When speaking, face the other person. By having an open body stance, you are inviting conversation. With your palms open, you are conveying a nonthreatening manner and a sense of honesty, again in an attempt to facilitate open conversation.

2. *Make eye contact.* Looking someone in the eyes tells them you are sincerely interested in what they have to say. Again, pay attention to the nonverbal cues. When we are not interested or feel inconvenienced, we have a tendency to roll our eyes. You patient will pick up this subtle but powerful movement and perceive that you don't really care what he or she has to say. Occasionally nod your head, smile, maybe even raise your eyebrows while listening. You may even interject an encouraging "right," "yeah," or "I see." All of these tell your patient that you are listening and are looking for more information.

3. *Give your full attention.* Emergency situations can be extremely busy with activity, lights, sounds, and other environmental and safety concerns. Let your patient know you are here for him or her and do your best to shut out the scene noise and activity.

4. *Try not to interrupt while the other person is talking.* Your focus is listening to the words and picking up the nonverbal messages, not interjecting your own thoughts. Let your patient express his or her message, then respond.

5. *Summarize.* Sum up what you have heard and seek clarification if required. This helps make sure you understand exactly what your patient was trying to say. Examples of clarifying statements include the following:
   • "Let me see if I've gotten this right . . ."
   • "Tell me more about . . ."
   • "I want to make sure I understand what you've said . . ."

Nonverbal Communication

Whether you realize it or not, your tone of voice and body language can be more important than the actual words spoken. If we don't pay attention to the **nonverbal communication** we see and emit, we are missing a huge portion of the intended message. You must keep in mind that as you are reading the patient's nonverbals, the patient is no doubt reading yours. Let's first examine the nonverbals from the patient's perspective.

How are you dressed? Is your appearance neat and clean? Are you wearing a uniform or other department identifying clothing? Remember, your patients may be complete strangers who willingly and without hesitation allow you into their home or worksite. They have put complete trust in your ability to handle the situation. That bond of trust is the cornerstone of emergency medical care. Understand that your nonverbal communication can help create that trust or lead to the dissolution of that same trust. We have all heard "you cannot judge a book by its cover"; however, we frequently do so. Think about the last time you went out for dinner. If you have two restaurants in mind that serve the same types of food, you will pick the one that seems to be the cleanest, brightest, and may have the better sign or slogan. You have just made a decision about where to eat based on "judging the cover." Remember this analogy when presenting yourself to any patient. Do your best to gain you patient's trust with the first impression.

BODY POSITION

The goal of communication in an emergency response is to create a bond of trust in order to accurately assess and treat you patient. If the patient is sitting in a chair, get down to eye level when speaking with him or her. This shows sincerity and interest. Towering over a patient is intimidating and closes lines of communication. Do your best to foster a sense of equity between yourself and the patient. This will make the patient more comfortable and build the bond of trust. Be aware of personal space. Next time you are at a party or service meeting, take notice of how far people stand from each other while talking. Men usually stand farther apart, whereas women tend to stand closer together. How do you feel when someone "moves into your personal space" or breaches your comfort bubble? We all set up invisible zones of protection around ourselves. The comfortable distance may vary depending on geographical location, cultural differences, and personal experience. Do your best not to burst this safety bubble. The comfortable distance for strangers usually begins at 10 feet. How can you quickly reduce the stranger factor and get right in to the intimate zone for assessment and effective communication? Put the other person at ease with your appearance, tone of voice, body position, and empathetic manner.

In the Real World—continued

Your communication with dispatch has resulted in an address correction and confirmation. As you make your way to the scene, you are running through a mental checklist of possible questions and treatments for a chest pain patient. Upon your arrival at the scene, you survey for hazards and access routes. You notice that the front of the residence sits atop a steep hill with many concrete steps in a state of disrepair. Remembering that safety is your primary concern, you quickly ascend the steps and look at the back side of the house for a better access point. You notice an alley with no steps and no other hazards, and you notify all incoming units to access the residence using the alley behind.

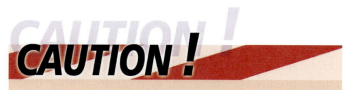

If the patient is threatening violence or the situation is unstable, place yourself in a safe position. This may not be eye level, but be sure you are in a position to quickly take evasive action if necessary.

BOX 4-1 Nonverbal Cues of Aggressive Behavior

- Finger-pointing
- Glaring
- Invasion of personal/intimate space (4 inches and closer)
- Arms crossed
- Widening of stance
- Hands on hips
- Clenched fists
- Increase in volume of voice

Take an open stance, with your palms open. This posture is considered inviting and submissive and tells your patient that you are here to help, not for confrontation. Standing with your arms crossed or hands on your hips sends the message that you really don't care what the patient has to say or about the emergency. Keep in mind, the crisis the patient is experiencing is real to that person. Do your best not to minimize or poke fun at the situation by what you say or your nonverbals (Box 4-1).

Initial Patient Contact

Now that we have discussed the components of effective communication, it is time to put them into practice and look at the actual patient/provider interaction.

As you approach, be aware of the surroundings by scanning for potential hazards or danger and a route of egress. Greet your patient and introduce yourself. Ask the patient's name and then address him or her using the last name and appropriate title, such as "Mrs. Jones" or "Mr. Smith." This shows respect for them as people. If they want to be called by their first name or a nickname, they will tell you. Take into consideration generational and cultural differences when addressing your patients. It may not be necessary to address a small child as "Mr. Nelson." The rule of thumb is never call someone older than you by their first name, at least until given permission. The next step is to ask, "How may I help you today?" or "What can I do for you today?" Notice, this was not "What is your problem?" Again, you are being respectful and honest right away. Stand with your palms open, and get down to eye level. Make and maintain eye contact for comfortable periods of time. Use encouraging statements and begin to ask questions. There are two types of questions at your disposal, open-ended and closed-ended questions.

Closed-Ended Questions

Closed-ended questions are those that require a simple yes or no answer. There are some patients and situations where these are your best option. Be sure to give ample time for an answer. To expand this type of questioning, ask a question and give them answer choices, such as "Is the pain squeezing, sharp, or burning?" This forces the patient to pick one of your answers. This type of question is extremely helpful to the patient who just cannot describe his or her symptoms. The patient may need a little assistance from you in the form of a closed-ended question.

Open-Ended Questions

Open-ended questions are those that cannot be answered with a simple yes or no. These questions allow the patient to describe his or her symptoms and situation in their own words. In keeping with the closed-ended question asked previously, here we would ask the patient, "Describe the pain you are having." Open-ended questions also give you the best opportunity to watch body language and facial expressions and listen to the tone and inflection of voice while the patient is answering. You can learn about the patient's distress level by reading the nonverbal cues. This type of questioning is the preferred method, but it cannot be used in every situation. Take the patient who is having extreme difficulty breathing. Do you want him expending energy and breath giving you his entire story, or can you get your information by asking yes or no questions? You can be sure this patient would prefer to nod or shake his head instead of using precious breath.

Barriers to Effective Communication

Few things can be more frustrating than trying to send or receive a message and not being able to get it right. You know what you want to say, but the other party is not getting the message. We will look at some common barriers to effective communication and suggest some techniques to overcome them.

Language Barriers

When your patient speaks a different language than you do, communication is made significantly more difficult. How will you obtain a patient history or even a chief complaint? If you don't have a field impression, how can you correctly treat the patient? A trained medical interpreter may offer some assistance, but you don't find those folks in the ditch at 4 AM. You can, however, once you know that a language barrier exists, tell dispatch to have an interpreter meet you at the hospital. There are some commercially available cards or pocket references that have some common questions printed in a few different languages, which both parties can use in a point-to-the-question-and-point-to-the-answer format. Another suggestion to overcome a language barrier is to learn a foreign language. If you work among a large population of persons who speak a specific language, it makes sense to learn to communicate with them in their language. Your organization can make pocket cards with familiar phrases or important questions for use in the field. Think of the bond of trust formed if you speak to patients in their own language! Remember, they will be as nervous about the situation as you are. They have a message to send, and they think you will never understand them.

Visual Impairment

When speaking with a visually impaired patient, first understand that just because they are visually impaired does not mean they are necessarily hearing impaired.

Speak in a calm and reassuring voice, and don't be afraid to put your hand on the person's shoulder or if the person seeks your hand with his or her own. The connection contained in the touch may be immeasurable. As with any patient with a disability or impairment, do not patronize these patients. They are very aware of this process and will shut you out if they feel you are not sincere. Again, the light touch lets them know you are still there. Take extra care to tell them everything that is happening and is going to happen. As a rule of safety, do not touch or distract a service dog without asking the owner.

Hearing Impairment

There are many different levels of hearing impairment, ranging from mild, moderate, severe, and profound affecting one or both ears. Regardless of the degree or cause of the impairment, you may need to adapt your communication techniques to get the job done. The most common adaptation is to automatically raise your voice when speaking. Unless the patient specifically tells you to do so, speak normally. These patients may ask you to speak into one ear versus the other or to get their hearing aid so they can put it in. They may ask you to speak slowly and close to them so they cam read your lips. If they are having trouble understanding, find a different way of asking the same question. Don't simply repeat the same words over and over, as this leads to frustration for both parties. Do not assume that a hearing-impaired person is also mentally impaired. Once you fall into this trap, all of the time spent gaining trust is lost, and your job just became more difficult.

Sign Language

If you know how to use sign language, you have a definite advantage in communicating with some hearing-impaired patients. However, not all hearing-impaired folks use or know sign language. If you have some sign skills, by all means use them. If the patient does use sign language, you have immediately gained ground in forming the bond of trust. If you do not know sign language, other methods are available. You may try using gestures. Keep in mind that hearing-impaired people are much more experienced communicating with you than you are with them. They may be able interpret your attempt at a gesture correctly.

Writing

Left with few options, you may need to resort to writing your questions and having the patient write responses. This method is accurate and actually may remove some of the awkwardness of the situation. Don't be shy in resorting to this method. Be sure to write legibly, and allow time for responses.

Lip Reading

Often thought of as the most common and effective way to communicate with the hearing-impaired, lip reading is effective approximately 33% of the time and takes practice to become proficient. If there is no other mode of communication, face the patient on the same level, stop chewing gum, and keep your hands away from your face. Do not shout or overenunciate your words, just speak in a calm tone and at a normal rate.

Barriers Specific to Emergency Response

Any emergency scene is brimming with distractions; from semis and cars speeding by you as you work in the median on the interstate to the sometimes overwhelming smells coming from someone's residence. Noise, weather, traffic, unbelievable stories, profound sadness, and people-watching are just a few of the common barriers to effective EMS communication. Maybe you have been called to an area of poor radio reception. Will your cellular phone work? Are your batteries fully charged? Are you on the correct frequency or radio system? We rely so much on technology for emergency communications that any glitch in that technology may render the communication system momentarily useless. Each organization should have a contingency plan or backup plan for communication breakdowns. Other responders can hinder effective communication. Not everyone understands that radio traffic should be short and sweet. You need to transmit your message concisely and then wait for a response. Do not monopolize the radio! If there are issues that require more time to explain, specific channels may be set aside expressly for that prolonged communication. Don't take up time on the common channel for routine communication. If a large or critical event is happening with a lot of radio communications, you might want to hold your routine traffic communications until the priority traffic is finished (Box 4-2).

Emergency Communications

Think about what happens to your body physiologically when you are on an emergency call. Your heart rate increases, as does your blood pressure and respiratory rate. Suffice it to say your adrenaline is flowing and things are happening faster than usual. Think of it this way: After running the 100-yard dash, how easy is it to speak clearly and slowly? It may take a concerted effort on your part to communicate effectively in an emergent situation. We will now examine who we need to communicate with and how to get the results you want.

Communication between emergency vehicles is obviously necessary, but it maybe not always so simple. On the way to an emergency call, sirens and horns are blaring, crew members are trying to talk over the noise, and now you need to hear that dispatch has changed the address or indicated an unsafe scene. You can see the importance of having good listening skills. It would also be beneficial to you and your crew if you had a good handle on local ten-codes. This way, you can be listening for key words or codes that should prompt you to take notice and alert other incoming units of the changing address or safety concern. Ten-codes are like abbreviations: useful, but not universal. Be sure you are well versed in your local system's use of ten-codes. As always, be sure to use terminology that all parties will easily understand. Avoid agency-specific terms when dealing with a multiagency response.

When communicating with other health care providers, whether they are other emergency first responders, emergency medical technicians (EMTs), paramedics, nurses, or physicians, treat them with respect. Speak to them in language that they can understand. That is your responsibility, to encode the message properly. This communication may be done via radio, cell phone, or face to face. Be clear, accurate, and to the point when providing this information.

Emergency First Responder Patient Hand-off Report

After gathering patient information and then assessing and treating the patient, it is time to transfer care to a transporting agency. The thing to keep in mind here is that the transporting agency may not have the opportunity to view the same scene as you did. Representatives from this agency may benefit to see how much blood was on the floor or the crash dynamics. It is your responsibility to make sure they understand exactly what happened and what has been done. As mentioned earlier, you have the best vantage point and need to be the eyes and ears of the patient care team. Some agencies have formal written documentation that is handed to the transporting agency. Others have a template for verbal hand-off information (see Patient Assessment, Chapter 8). Whichever method your system employs, the information contained within should include the items listed in Box 4-3. *The minimum patient data set works well for a quick reference for a verbal hand-off report.*

BOX 4-2 Radio Procedures

When you need to speak on the radio, remember that interference is inherent on each emergency response. Therefore, speak clearly and slowly, in a calm manner. Remember not to use slang, jargon, profanity, or to state opinion. The following guidelines will help you communicate effectively when using the radio:

- Make sure the radio is on and volume is appropriate. Also, be sure that the channel is clear. Many agencies will be communicating; don't become interference for someone else.
- If using a mobile radio, be sure your portable radio is turned down to avoid annoying microphone feedback. Everyone will appreciate your effort in reducing the "squeal."
- Press the microphone or "PTT" button and wait for 1 to 2 seconds before speaking. This will help ensure that your entire message is transmitted. It takes a little time for the channel to open up and become ready for use.
- Speak in a normal voice and tone, with the microphone 2 to 3 inches from your mouth. With the microphone too close, your transmission may be garbled and hard to understand, whereas if you are too far away from the microphone, the transmission may be hard to hear.
- Most systems prefer to identify who you are calling first, then tell them who is

calling. For the sake of our example, you are responding in Medic 4. The communication would sound something like this: "Dispatch from Medic 4." "Go ahead Medic 4, this is dispatch." Wait until the party you are calling acknowledges you and requests you to proceed.
- Be careful not to "walk all over" someone else who is transmitting. This is why you make sure the channel is clear before attempting your transmission.
- Know your local ten-codes and nomenclature. When all else fails, you may resort to plain English or clear text.
- As mentioned previously, keep your transmissions clear, concise, and brief. You must also be certain that the receiver understood your intended message. If you are unsure, you must seek clarification. Was the address on Shaker or Schafer Court? Both can sound the same on the radio. If you need the information repeated, the sender will do so. Think about what you want to say *before* you key the microphone. Don't think out loud with the mic keyed.
- Watch out for the dreaded "open mic" situation. This happens when a microphone gets keyed accidentally without anyone realizing the channel is transmitting. Private conversations are now broadcast over the radio, leading to a number of potentially embarrassing or even litigious situations.

BOX 4-3 Initial Patient Data

- Current patient condition
- Patient's age and gender
- Chief complaint
- Brief, pertinent history of what happened, how you found the patient
- Major past illnesses
- Current vital signs
- Pertinent findings of the physical exam
- Emergency medical care given and the response to that care

In the Real World—continued

You have made contact with your patient, a 53-year-old hearing-impaired man experiencing chest pain. From his medicines, you suspect a cardiac history. You can tell he is having a difficult time understanding and answering your questions. To more effectively communicate with him, you resort to a pencil and paper and writing questions and answers. You complete the history and gather other important information. You suggest that he post, in an accessible place, such as on the front of the refrigerator, a precompleted information template. After your assessment is complete, you have called for ALS transport because of the patient's cardiac history and complaint of chest pain that is similar to the pain when he had his myocardial infarction. After oxygen has been applied and the patient made comfortable, you consider how you are going to get the patient from his upstairs bedroom down to the waiting ambulance. After a brief discussion, you call and have someone bring in the stair-chair and a few more responders to assist with the carry down the stairs. The ALS transporting service arrives, and the patient is placed on the cot and prepared for transport. Your hand-off report brings no questions from the paramedic, and the patient is transported.

Communication Systems

For all of your communication efforts to be effectively transmitted and received, you need to have a functional communication system or network. You can be the best communicator in the world, but if you don't have the radios and other hardware to make transmission possible, it is to no avail. Here we will discuss some common components of modern EMS communication systems.

Federal Communications Commission (FCC)

This governmental body is responsible for regulating all radio communications in the United States. If you want to use the airwaves to transmit information, the **FCC** must grant you a license to do so. With your license comes your assigned frequency or frequencies. These frequencies must be used for the purpose for which the license was obtained. The FCC is also responsible to monitor the content of what is transmitted. If the content is considered inappropriate or against FCC regulations, the FCC can and will levy fines.

Base Stations

A **base station** is a powerful radio (transmits at a higher wattage output) located at a fixed location such as fire departments, ambulance services, dispatch centers, or hospitals. There are a couple of types of base stations, yet each relies on strategically placed large antennae for increased transmission.

Mobile Radios

Mobile radios are those that are mounted inside emergency response vehicles such as ambulances, fire trucks, and police cruisers. These radios operate with lower power than the base station, an area capable of transmitting about 10 to 15 miles. In today's world, the need for increased range from mobile radios has led many agencies to install **repeaters**. A repeater simply takes a weaker signal broadcast on one frequency and rebroadcasts that signal with the power of the repeater on a different frequency, greatly increasing the ability to communicate over a larger geographic area (**Fig. 4-3**).

Portable Radios

These are usually referred to as "handheld radios." As you would expect, the power output of these **portable radios** is less in comparison to a mobile or base radio. Again, with a repeater system, the range may be enhanced for better communication especially in rural areas (**Fig. 4-4**).

Cellular Phones

A large percentage of the population has access to a cellular phone. Although it is a more secure way of communicating, remember it still transmits over the airwaves and can therefore be monitored. Treat the cell phone conversations with the same care as any other radio transmission. Also, be careful when speaking on the cell phone; don't speak so loudly that you could be overheard by anyone that is not part of the conversation.

Privacy

Don't think just because you transmitted over a wireless radio network that your communications are private. Individuals with the appropriate equipment can find your transmitting frequency and listen to every word you say. With that in mind, here are some things to avoid putting over the air:

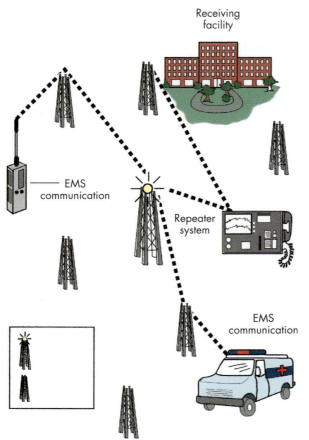

Fig. 4-3 Repeater systems allow EMS systems to overcome poor output capabilities of portable radios. (From Shade B, et al: *Mosby's EMT-intermediate textbook for the 1999 National Standard Curriculum*, ed 3, St. Louis, 2007, Mosby.)

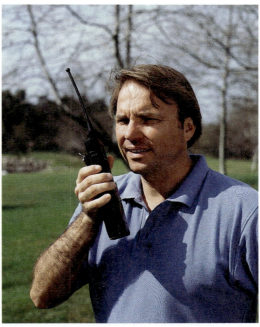

Fig. 4-4 Clear and concise message given over the radio to allow for communication and patient care. (From Shade B, et al: *Mosby's EMT-intermediate textbook for the 1999 National Standard Curriculum*, ed 3, St. Louis, 2007, Mosby.)

1. Do not broadcast patient's names or other identifying information; remember the Health Information Portability and Accountability Act (HIPAA) discussion.
2. Avoid profanity, as it is unprofessional and may bring a hefty fine from the FCC.
3. Avoid graphic descriptions.
4. Keep personal opinions to yourself.

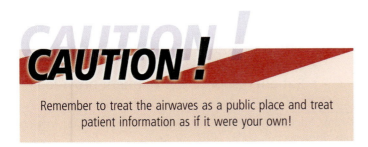

Remember to treat the airwaves as a public place and treat patient information as if it were your own!

Tips for Difficult Communications

- *Be honest.* Nothing destroys trust quicker than a lie.
- *If you don't know the answer, don't make it up.* Tell the other person you don't know, and if you do find the answer, provide it to the person.
- *Speak clearly and slowly.* Make sure the message is completely understood.
- *Watch your body language.* It should match your empathetic speech.
- *Check your own emotions and gather yourself before speaking.* Do your best to put forth an image of confidence. It will help everybody.
- *If you have to deliver bad news or ask private or difficult questions, find the appropriate setting.* This would usually be a quiet, one-on-one environment.

Tips for Pediatric Communications

- *Get down to the child's level.* Do not tower over children. This intimidates them and shuts them down.
- *Do your best to keep a parent, guardian, relative, or friend with the child.* This increases the comfort factor and decreased your degree of difficulty. Separation anxiety is definitely not your friend.

- *If you need to ask private questions, dealing with things like abuse, drugs, or pregnancy, please be discreet.* You may have to do this in a private setting, away from parental influence.
- *Try to keep somewhat up to date on pop culture and what kids are into.* If you can find a common interest such as a game, music, or TV show, trust occurs much more quickly.
- *Remember, a crying child is telling you he has an open airway, he is breathing, and has a pulse.* In our world, a crying child is a good thing, all things considered.

Documentation

It is difficult to overemphasize the absolute importance of complete and accurate documentation. After every emergency response, there must be a written record of what occurred. This documentation serves a number of purposes, none more important than to protect you and your organization during any legal action associated with an emergency response. Here are some of the other functions of documentation:

1. An accurate patient care report (PCR) detailing what was done, when it was done, and who did it is a required part of each emergency response. This report should be completed as soon as possible after the response. As time passes from response to written report, we forget details, and the chance of omitting important information increases greatly. Remember, physicians, lawyers, quality control, and any other number of professional persons may read this patient report. Therefore, pay close attention to aspects like spelling and legibility. In a court of law, a poorly written, poorly spelled, illegible, and incomplete patient care report all may give the impression that you did not deliver care in accordance with the standard of care. You certainly may have given entirely appropriate patient care; however, your poor documentation may lead others to believe otherwise.

2. An accurate and complete report also documents the continuity of patient care. As an emergency first responder, you may be handing your patients off to a transporting service, be it ground or air. It is crucial to ensuring the seamless transfer of care to other patient care providers. You would not want to leave out important information about what you have done for the patient before transferring care. This documentation again protects you and your organization. When you transfer care to a transporting agency, be sure to document who took over your patient and the condition of the patient.

3. Documentation also serves numerous administrative functions. Organizations have quality improvement and quality assurance programs, which rely on the written report for things like statistical reporting, protocol compliance, identifying trends, and proposing solutions. The way to accurately gather this information is a through examination of patient care reports and the minimum data set.

Minimum Data Set

In every patient care report, there are certain required pieces of information. These data are collected from patient information (Box 4-4) and administrative information (Box 4-5). Knowing the importance of such data should ensure the accurate completion of both the patient and administrative data.

Now that we have discussed the importance of accurate documentation, we will look at how to construct the patient care report. There are many different templates or styles to assist in the report-writing process (Box 4-6). You will need to check with your local agencies and quality departments to determine which style is appro-

---

BOX 4-4   Minimum Data Set: Patient Information

- Age and gender
- Chief complaint
- Mechanism of injury or nature of illness
- Level of consciousness (AVPU [alert, verbal, painful, unresponsive], Glasgow Coma Scale)
- Pertinent medical history
- Signs and symptoms
- Vital signs
- Blood pressure (in patients over 3 years of age)
- Pulse
- Respirations
- Skin perfusion
- Treatment provided
- Patient response to treatment provided

(From Chapleau W, Pons P: *Emergency medical technician: making the difference,* St. Louis, 2007, Mosby.)

BOX 4-5 Minimum Data Set: Administrative Information

- Date of call
- Times
- Time dispatched
- Time responded
- Time arrived at the scene
- Time departed from the scene
- Time arrived at destination (health care facility)
- Location of call

- Call type
- Medical or trauma
- Emergent or nonemergent to and from the scene
- Use of lights and sirens
- Care information
- Names of personnel responding
- License or certification number

(From Chapleau W, Pons P: *Emergency medical technician: making the difference,* St. Louis, 2007, Mosby.)

BOX 4-6 Patient Care Report Templates

SOAP Method

S—Subjective. Information that was relayed to you by the patient, bystanders, other EMS providers (chief complaint, history, medications, allergies, etc.).

O—Objective. Information you have gathered through the patient exam, including scene observations.

A—Assessment. Your field impression (this component is sometimes omitted, leaving you with the SOP method).

P—Plan. Your treatment provided in chronological order.

SOP Chart Example

S (Subjective)

Responded to a 53 y/o male with a chief complaint of chest pain. Pt relays his pain began 60 minutes ago while he was mowing the lawn. Pt rates the pain a "6" out of "10," non-radiating and squeezing in nature. Pt does not complain of any difficulty breathing. Pt does have a history of previous cardiac problems, including a bypass 5 months ago. Pt relays that this episode is similar to the last episode, which required bypass surgery. Pt has not taken any nitro since pain began.

History: Bypass, hypertension

Medications: Nitro, metoprolol, cardizem

Allergies: Sulfa

O (Objective)

Pt found CAO × 3 sitting on the couch; physical exam

ABC: Intact × 3 without compromise

SKIN: Pink, warm, dry

HEENT: PERL 3 × 3, no JVD, no 6 of respiratory distress

CHEST: Clear × 4, symmetrical expansion

ABD: Soft, nontender

EXTR: GROM × 4, no deficits, all pulses present

P (Treatment PLAN)

Primary exam

HPI

Oxygen applied via nasal cannula, 4 lpm with a slight decrease in chest pain severity

Vital signs: BP 116/70; pulse 74 strong/regular; respirations 18, nonlabored

Secondary exam

Report given to transport Paramedic J Smith, pt's condition improved, chest pain now "4" out of "10," and he states that he feels much better.

Narrative Method

This style simply tells the story from start to finish, again in chronological order. This chart basically is in paragraph form and reads like a story.

BOX 4-6 Patient Care Report Templates—cont'd

CHART Method

C—Chief complaint. What the patient tells you.

H—History. History of the present illness, and prior events, and current medications.

A—Assessment. Results of the initial and focused exam.

R—Rx (treatment). Any treatment provided at the scene, including and interventions performed before your arrival. Also includes the patient response to the interventions.

T—Transport. Who was the patient transferred to and in what condition.

BOX 4-7 Elements of a PCR

1. *Times.* Accurate reporting of times such as call time, arrival at scene time, patient care times and transfer of care time are just a few examples.

2. *Scene observations.* As a group, emergency first responders often have the best vantage point of anyone involved in patient care. The patient care team members rely on the prehospital observations. Law enforcement also relies on the visual and auditory information that can be gleaned early on in the response. Take special notice of things like where crash victims are positioned, conditions of the environment (house, vehicle, etc.), and what someone may have said. This information may prove critical in the outcome of your patient.

3. *All treatments performed must be documented.* Remember to report not only what was done, but who did it, what time it was done, and the outcome. Was your oxygen therapy effective? This is a necessary component of a properly written patient chart.

priate. Regardless of the style, there are certain elements that must be included in each report (Box 4-7).

In each EMS system, there are certain types of responses or injuries that must be reported to the proper agencies. These may include gunshot wounds, stabbings, abuse of a dependent adult or child, and certain communicable diseases. These are not the only situations requiring special reporting, but they are the most common. Know the guidelines that govern your particular system and what events you are compelled to report.

Confidentiality and Privacy

Any information contained in the PCR is considered protected. This means that the information cannot be shared or released except to those persons directly involved in the patient's medical care. All of the demographic information, such as address, birthday, and social security number, must remain confidential. The Health Information Portability and Accountability Act (or HIPAA) makes provisions for severe financial penalties for both individuals and organizations for anyone found to violate patient confidentiality. The HIPAA applies to the entire medical profession, from pharmacies to physicians' offices, hospitals, and EMS. It is therefore in your best interest to become familiar with how the HIPAA applies to you and your organization and follow the guidelines established.

Just as the written PCR is protected, it is improper to talk about the incident outside of your crew. Be careful as to where you are when talk of the last call comes up. If you are in a public place and someone familiar with your patient overhears your conversation, you could be charged with a HIPAA violation. If you think of this protected information as your own, you should have no trouble maintaining confidentiality.

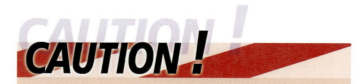

Don't leave protected information out in the open (such as on the table at the station) or take it home with you. Protect it as if it were your own.

Tips for Better Documentation

Every emergency response is an opportunity for learning. That also holds true for every patient care report. The following are just some helpful tips to assist you in writing a quality patient chart:

1. As mentioned, take the time to write the report immediately after the response is finished. The chances of forgetting something important decrease when you complete the report directly.
2. Find a style or template that works for you and stick with it. If all of your charts look and feel the same, you decrease the likelihood of leaving out something important. By knowing how your chart will look and sound, it forces you to seek out the information you will need to complete the chart; that same information is also important to treating your patient correctly.
3. Be careful not to use slang or jargon in your report. Again, remember who may be reading the chart and for what purpose. Call equipment and procedures by their proper names, not the nicknames or "street" names. Remember, local systems may have different terminology. Only state facts, not opinions. If you need to document exactly what the patient said, use quotation marks, but be accurate in your quote. Stay away from judgmental statements, such as "The patient was absolutely hammered." You have no way of factually knowing that was the case. Just report that the patient had the odor consistent with the consumption of alcoholic beverages noted on his breath, and document any strange or erratic behavior.
4. Make sure you are using approved abbreviations. It is acceptable to abbreviate some words, as long as the abbreviation is listed and approved within your system. Some abbreviations may mean two things to different people from different systems. Remember the interoperability concept we spoke of earlier in this chapter.
5. If you are using a computer-based charting program, use the "spell-check" feature. If you are using paper and pen, consult a medical dictionary for any spelling questions. Either way, the effort will be minimal and the reward is great. The more professional the report looks and reads, the more professional the caregiver appears.
6. If your patient care report ends up going to court, this process may take months or even years. Be sure to write your chart well enough that you can easily recall the incident just by reading through it. As time passes, details fade. Document all important details at the time of the incident in order to make your life easier down the road.
7. The catch phrase used in health care documentation is "If you didn't write it down, it didn't happen." This should always be in the back of your mind when completing a patient care report.

Summary

EMS is about relationships. We have only a few short, sometimes intense minutes to connect with our patients. By being an empathetic listener and gaining the patient's trust, those minutes will be much more productive. As noted, there are many barriers to effective communication. Some of those barriers we cannot control, such as the hearing or vision impaired or language. Dealing with or adjusting our own outlooks may be necessary to allow the lines of communication to open and stay open.

As an emergency first responder, each response will require effective communication and quality documentation. To gather the necessary information to correctly assess and treat your patient, you must apply the techniques of effective communication. Interestingly enough, it is that same information that will be used to complete an accurate patient care report. The information gathered may need to be shared with other responders, law enforcement, hospital staff, and a host of other potential players. It is your mission to put the information into understandable and usable terms, taking into consideration the different interpretative modes of each organization. Regardless of the circumstances, you as the emergency first responder must make absolutely sure the intended message gets to the intended receiver, is interpreted correctly, and has the intended result. This holds true for verbal and written (patient care reports) communication. Building proficient communication skills is just as important as any other skill discussed in this book. Remember, you will communicate on every call of your career. Take the time to become an effective communicator.

In the Real World—Conclusion

You put your equipment away and begin to drive back to the station. You notify dispatch that you are finished with this call and available for the next one. Upon arrival back at the station, your partner restocks the truck, and you complete the patient care report (PCR). Your crew has a discussion about how the call went and makes suggestions on how to avoid address confusion in the future. You then deposit the PCR in the appropriate location, remembering the gravity of any HIPAA violations.

Team Work

As an emergency first responder, it makes sense to say you will often be the first and sometimes the only one on an emergency scene. You need to take this perspective seriously and understand that what you see, hear, and do will be the basis for your patient's care. Think for a minute of all of the people who will provide medical care for your patient. They may include emergency field providers, nurses, emergency department physicians, and a multitude of other medical professionals. If you are able to communicate your findings both verbally, such as transferring patient care to a transporting agency, and through the written word as in the patient care report, the patient stands to benefit. Remember, you will work with many different agencies with diverse personnel. Take the time to develop relationships within your system and increase the number of effective tools in your communication toolbox.

TEAMWORK SCENARIO

You are the first unit to arrive on the scene of a multiple vehicle collision. While your partner performs initial triage of the victims, you are surveying the scene to identify what additional resources you will need. Within your jurisdiction, who can help you provide emergency care and transportation for the victims in the most expeditious manner? A response like this runs more smoothly if there has been some preplanning between service providers to do such things as identify resources and special training, as well as create agreements and relationships that will benefit the public. Which departments carry the equipment needed for extrication? You determine you need two ALS ambulances, a helicopter for transport of the most critical patient, numerous law enforcement units for traffic control, and the local utility company to take care of the downed power pole. As you can see, just for this single incident, numerous agencies must have the ability to not only communicate with each other but work quickly and safely toward a positive outcome for the victims of the collision. You identify the needs, contact the appropriate agencies, and have a safe, effective response with all victims receiving swift and appropriate care.

Reference

1. National Joint Committee for the Communication Needs of Persons with Severe Disabilities, 1992, p. 2.

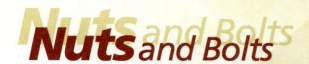
Nuts and Bolts

Critical Points

Your ability to communicate effectively is as important as any other skill your will learn in your EMS career. It becomes extremely difficult to provide quality patient care if you cannot gather the information that is essential for correct decision making. How will you know what treatment to perform if you do not understand the chief complaint or medical history? As we discussed, you will need to communicate with many different agencies in many different situations, all with varying levels of stress and excitement. Therefore, you will need to understand the common barriers to communication and, more important, how to overcome them. Do everything within your ability to allow the bond of trust to be formed in that first 3 minutes of patient contact. You should learn how to communicate with the varying populations you serve. Know how to quickly communicate with the vision impaired, the hearing impaired, children, and those with language barriers. Take time to understand your local communication system. How unfortunate it would be to have a crucial piece of information and not be able to communicate it because you cannot work the radio. Bear in mind that the safety of your crew and proper transport and treatment of the patient may depend on your ability to gather and distribute information quickly and concisely. Each response in your career will require verbal, nonverbal, and written communication. Be sure to document important findings both with your patient and the scene. Your documentation is a legal document that will serve as your event record. Write each report as if it were your sole source of response information.

Learning Checklist

❑ Communication is fundamental to emergency response. Knowing how communication works will help you understand how to become a more effective communicator. You must understand encoding and decoding, as well as feedback and interference.

❑ Always speak and act with empathy. Be aware of your patient's feelings, but do not validate or patronize them. Use statements such as "I imagine that must be . . ." or "I can see that you are really upset." Remember, it is nearly impossible to completely understand their feelings, so don't say that you do.

❑ When having a conversation, work at becoming a better listener. Make and keep eye contact, open your hands, face the other person, and invite the exchange of information. Try to minimize interruptions and use clarifying statements to be sure you understand the information you were given.

❑ Always be aware of your nonverbal communication. Your appearance, body position, tone, and facial expressions can destroy the bond of trust you have worked so hard to create.

❑ You will encounter patients who may become aggressive. Look for nonverbal clues of impending aggression such as finger pointing, counting on fingers, a widened stance, and an invasion of your personal space. There are more, but this short list may just keep you upright!

❑ Upon patient contact, scan the scene for hazards an egress routes. Introduce yourself and address them as Mr. or Mrs. Don't assume familiarity, as it may be perceived as a sign of disrespect.

❑ Use open-ended questions whenever possible. These allow for the most detailed and complete answers. Some patients may require the use of closed-ended questions: questions with "yes" and "no" answers. Be careful not to put words into another person's mouth. You may need to give your patient a few options to pick from based on the information you need to know.

❑ When dealing with a patient who speaks a different language than you do or who is visually or hearing impaired, you can prepare for some of these situations by knowing your population and learning a different language. Take a deep breath and solve the problem. This may require drawing, pointing to a card or picture, or the use of a translator. Make no mistake, you must find a useful medium of communication with all patients, no matter what barriers are placed in your way.

❑ Emergency communication systems range from the very simple to the very complex. It is your responsibility to understand how your particular system functions. Whether you are using the base station, mobile radio, portable radio, fax machine,

Nuts and Bolts–continued

GPS unit or cell phone, each have their own usage procedures and limitations. You never know which component you will use on the next response. As always, professional and appropriate use of the communication system is expected. In the United States, the Federal Communications Commission (FCC) is responsible for regulating radio transmissions.

❑ Respect and maintain the privacy of your patients at all times. Do not put names or other identifying information out over the radio waves.

❑ Emergency first responders must be able to give accurate verbal reports to incoming responders as to the scene dangers, positioning concerns, resource needs, and patient conditions. Each service has the preferred format or method for these reports. Become familiar with procedures and proficient with the delivery of this information.

❑ Each emergency response will involve a number of communication steps with a number of entities. You will have to talk with dispatch and let them know of your receipt of the call, your arrival time, your resource needs, and your route of travel if necessary, just to name a few. You will also have to contact medical control and give patient condition reports. Each agency has their own terminology, so become familiar with the expectations.

❑ Every patient contact will require completion of the patient care report, or PCR. This documentation is absolutely essential to the health care system. You are responsible to document what you saw, heard, and found, as well as any other information that may be pertinent. This is a legal document, so take your time and write a quality, correctly spelled and legible patient care report (PCR). This is your best protection in a legal action, but it could also discredit you if you wrote a poor, incomplete, or illegible report.

❑ HIPAA regulations require you to maintain strict confidentiality in regard to any identifying patient information. Violation of the HIPAA standards may result in legal action against you and your service as well as severe financial penalties. Treat patient information as if it were your own.

Key Terms

Base station A radio located at a fixed location, such as a hospital, dispatch center, or emergency services station. This is usually the most powerful radio within the EMS communication system.

Closed-ended questions Questions that can be answered with a yes or no answer. In other words, these are questions that require specific responses using the answer choices you provide.

Communication Any act by which one person gives to or receives from another person information about that person's needs, desires, perceptions, knowledge, or affective states. Communication may be intentional or unintentional, may involve conventional or unconventional signals, may take linguistic or nonlinguistic forms, and may occur through spoken or other modes.

Decoding The process by which the intended receiver interprets the meaning of a message sent by another.

Empathy One's ability to recognize, perceive, and feel directly the emotion of another.

Encoding The process by which the sender of a message places the message into a format that the receiver can understand.

Federal Communications Commission (FCC) An agency of the federal government that is responsible for governing all radio transmissions in the United States.

Feedback The component of communication that indicates whether the message received was actually the message that was intended.

Interference Any disruption or distraction in the communication process.

Mobile radio A radio that is mounted in a vehicle.

Nonverbal communication A component of communication in which messages are relayed through movements, posture, gestures, and the eyes.

Open-end questions Questions that cannot be answered with yes or no answers. These questions allow patients to put their situations in their own words and provide the most information. These questions also allow an opportunity to identify nonverbal communication clues.

Patient care report (PCR) The standard form used to document patient care in emergency medical systems.

Portable radio A radio that an emergency first responder can carry wherever he or she goes. Although very convenient and necessary, these radios have a limited transmission distance.

First Responder NSC Objectives
COGNITIVE OBJECTIVES

- Discuss the process of communication and the skills one should use to interact with patients, other agencies, and responders.
- Describe actions to take to increase the effectiveness of both verbal and nonverbal communications.
- Discuss various barriers to effective communication and how to overcome those barriers.
- Describe how to communicate with empathy.
- Identify a variety of emergency communication equipment, their uses, and their limitations.

- List the information that is to be included when transferring patient care to another provider.
- Discuss the uses and critical nature of completing a quality patient care report (PCR).
- Discuss the absolute need for confidentiality and privacy of patient health information.
- List the information required (minimum data set) to be included in each patient care report.

AFFECTIVE OBJECTIVES

- Demonstrate a caring attitude toward any patient with illness or injury who requests emergency medical services.
- Show compassion when caring for the physical and mental needs of patients.
- Communicate with empathy to patients being cared for, as well as the patient's family members and friends.

Check your understanding

Check your understanding

Please refer to p. 439 for the answers to these questions.

1. You are standing in a group of fellow emergency first responders while attending training, when your service is toned out for an emergency response. Which of the following allows only your agency to be toned out?
   A. Repeater
   B. Encoding
   C. 10 codes
   D. Base Station

2. The process by which the sender knows their message was heard and understood is called
   _____.

3. List three things you can do to reduce the amount of interference on an emergency response.
   _____
   _____
   _____

4. Give three examples of empathetic statements.
   _____
   _____
   _____

5. Loud noises, inclement weather, and poor radio procedures are just a few common forms of _____ that can hinder or prevent effective communications.

6. List four of the nonverbal clues that your patient may become physically aggressive.
   _____
   _____
   _____
   _____

7. Which of the following nonverbal clues will assist you in building the patient's trust?
   A. Towering over a seated patient
   B. Not looking at them when you are speaking to them
   C. Getting on their level, palms open
   D. Addressing them as "dude" or "sweetie"

8. Your patient is having significant difficulty breathing, and traditional questioning is not working. What type of questions should be used in this situation?
   A. Open-ended questions
   B. Closed-ended questions
   C. Investigative questions
   D. Narrative questions

9. List three things that should be included in the patient hand-off report.
   _____
   _____
   _____

10. You are attempting to communicate with a hearing-impaired patient. Which of the following techniques may prove helpful?
    A. Speaking loudly
    B. Writing responses/questions
    C. Attempting sign language without proficiency
    D. Repeating the same words over and over

11. Telling your neighbor about the call you went on last night, while using the patient's name and other identifying information, would be a violation of which law?
    A. COBRA
    B. Standard of Care
    C. HIPAA
    D. Scope of Practice

12. Characteristics of good, sound EMS documentation include which of the following?
    A. Use of jargon or slang
    B. Opinions
    C. Spelling errors
    D. Objective observations

13. Why it is important to use plain English when working at a multi-agency response?
    _____
    _____

14. During the last 3 weeks, someone has been using your department's radio frequency for casual conversation, even uttering some profanities. Which organization is responsible for "cleaning up" the frequency?
A. DOT
B. FCC
C. OSHA
D. Homeland Security

15. While on scene at a multiple casualty incident (MCI), you need to notify all responding resources with important scene safety information. You are out of your vehicle surveying the scene, which is in an extremely rural location. Which type of radio should you use to reach the most responders?
A. Portable radio
B. Mobile radio
C. Base station
D. FM Radio

Chapter 5

The Human Body

LESSON GOAL

You must be familiar with the anatomy and physiology of the human body to provide accurate assessment and treatment of your patients. This chapter provides essential information and terminology for the anatomy and physiology of the human body. You will rely on this foundation as you build patient care skills throughout your career as an emergency first responder.

OBJECTIVES

1. Describe the anatomy and function of the respiratory system.
2. Describe the anatomy and function of the circulatory system.
3. Describe the anatomy and function of the musculoskeletal system.
4. Describe the components and function of the nervous system.
5. Given a body in a normal anatomical position, use directional terms to identify how body parts are related to one another.
6. Relate a given surface landmark with the appropriate underlying anatomy.
7. Identify the significance of injury to the respiratory system, circulatory system, nervous system, musculoskeletal system, integumentary system, gastrointestinal/genitourinary system, reproductive system, endocrine system, and the lymphatic system.

In the Real World

Your engine company is called to a motor vehicle collision. When you arrive, you assess the scene and make the following observations: You see a single car crashed into a tree and there is steam, but no fire, coming from under the hood. There is extensive frontal damage to the car. The steering wheel is bent under and the lower dash is damaged. You see an unrestrained teenager in the driver's seat. He is complaining of extreme pain in his left thigh and a "stomachache." He is alert and oriented. You put on gloves and goggles and prepare to begin your assessment.

Understanding the basics of anatomy and physiology and being familiar with medical terminology will help you identify life-threatening problems and communicate with other health care professionals. **Anatomy** refers to the structure of the body, while **physiology** refers to the function of the body. The use of a common medical language is essential to describe a patient's condition so that all members of the health care team can understand the location and extent of a patient's injuries. Knowledge of the human body is the cornerstone of the many skills needed to become an excellent emergency first responder.

Body Directional Terms

Medical professionals refer to the body in a **normal anatomical position.** In this position the human body is standing upright, facing you, with arms at the side and palms of the hands turned forward. An imaginary vertical line drawn down the middle of the body is called the **midline.** All references to *right* and *left* refer to the *patient's* right or left. All the following directional terms are based on the normal anatomical position (Fig. 5-1).

Anterior is toward the front of the body, and **posterior** is toward the back of the body. For example, during cardiopulmonary resuscitation (CPR), you perform compressions on the breastbone, located in the anterior chest. With each press downward the heart is squeezed against the backbone, which is in the posterior chest. When the body is in the normal anatomical position, you see the anterior (front) side.

Lateral is away from the midline and **medial** is toward the midline. If you assess a football player who complains of pain on the outside of his or her knee, you report this as pain to the "lateral knee." If your patient has a cut on the inside of his or her knee, you report the injury as a laceration to the "medial knee."

Superior is toward the head, or top, and **inferior** is toward the feet, or below. For example, the nose is superior to the mouth and the chin is inferior to the mouth.

To describe injuries to the extremities, the term **proximal** is used to indicate toward the trunk of the body and the term **distal** is used to indicate away from the trunk. For example, the elbow is at the distal end of the upper arm while the shoulder is at the proximal end of the upper arm. As a First Responder you should always try to use directional terms to explain your assessment. For example, if you are assessing a child who fell from a swing, you may describe an injury such as a deformity to the distal left forearm. This description is an accurate assessment and helps other health care providers prepare to receive the patient and select the appropriate equipment for treatment. As an emergency first responder, however, you may not be dealing with emergencies on a regular basis and get regular practice with medical and directional terms. If you are unsure which term should be used, it is better to use terms such as back or front, for example, to avoid confusion and inaccuracies. Table 5-1 is an overview of directional terms.

Along with the use of specific terms to describe or refer to locations on the human body, medically trained persons speak a language that may seem foreign to most non–medically trained individuals. Understanding this language and proper use of medical terminology will be helpful when providing or receiving patient reports. Most medical terms used to describe components of the body can be understood by breaking the word into the prefix and/or suffix. By combining the prefix *cardio-*(pertaining to the heart) with the suffix *-vascular* (referring to blood vessels) the medical term *cardiovascular* is formed. Cardiovascular system is a medical term used to describe the main organs and structures that support the pumping of

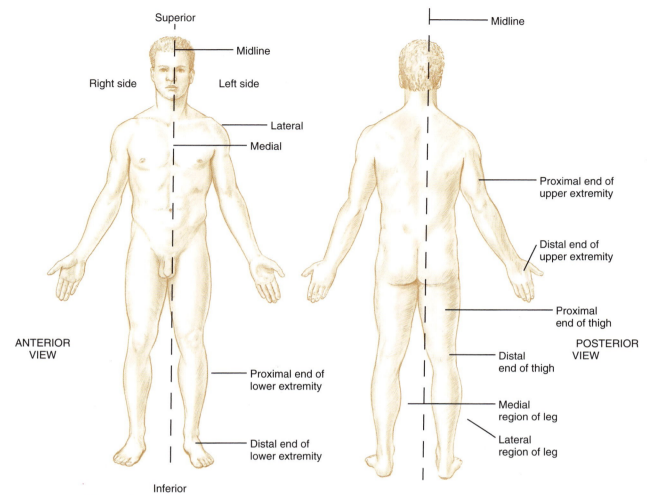

Fig. 5-1 Normal anatomical position. (From Henry M, Stapleton E: *EMT prehospital care,* ed 4, St. Louis, 2010, Mosby.)

TABLE 5-1 Directional Terms

DIRECTIONAL TERM	DEFINITION	EXAMPLE OF USAGE
Left	To the left of the body (the patient's body)	The stomach is to the left of the liver.
Right	To the right of the body (the patient's body)	The right kidney is damaged.
Lateral	Away from the midline of the body	The ears are lateral to the nose.
Medial	Toward the midline of the body	The nose is medial to the ears.
Anterior	Toward the front of the body	The sternum is on the anterior portion of the chest.
Posterior	Toward the back of the body	The spine is located on the posterior portion of the trunk.
Superior	Toward the head or top of the body	The nose is superior to the mouth.
Inferior	Toward the feet or bottom of the body	The chin is inferior to the mouth.
Proximal	Toward the trunk of the body	The shoulder is at the proximal end of the upper arm.
Distal	Away from the trunk of the body	The elbow is at the distal end of the upper arm.

blood through the body. Some additional prefixes that may be helpful to the emergency first responder include the following:

- Arterio-   relating to arteries
- Hemo-   relating to blood
- Hyper-   excessive or above the normal
- Hypo-   beneath something, a deficiency, below the normal
- Naso-   relating to the nose
- Neuro-   relating to the nervous system
- Oro-   relating to the mouth
- Therm-   denoting heat
- Vaso-   relating to a blood vessel

Regions of the Body

The body is also described in terms of body regions. These regions include the head, neck, trunk, and the upper and lower extremities (Fig. 5-2). The head consists of the cranium, which houses the brain, and the face. The head is supported by the neck. Below the neck is the trunk

(also called the torso), which has three parts: (1) the **thorax** (or chest), which contains the heart, the lungs, and the great vessels—which originate from the heart; (2) the **abdomen;** and (3) the **pelvis.** The thorax is divided from the abdomen by a large muscle called the diaphragm. The diaphragm assists in the breathing process and is part of the respiratory system.

The extremities are attached to the trunk. The upper extremity begins at the shoulder and includes the arm, elbow, forearm, wrist, and hand. The hip, thigh, knee, leg, ankle, and foot make up the lower extremity.

This knowledge of basic anatomical terms, body directions, and body areas is the starting point for understanding how the body works. Normal body functions provide a reference point for patient evaluation. For instance, once you know how to locate the radial pulse in the wrist, you can count the heart rate in beats per minute. By monitoring changes in the pulse quality and rate, you can determine if the body is functioning normally. This information is critical to the health care team. Your understanding of the basic anatomy and physiology of the major body systems, covered in the following sections, will help you provide a detailed assessment to other health care providers.

Abdominal Quadrants

The abdomen is further divided into four equal "quadrants" (Fig. 5-3). An imaginary horizontal line is drawn across the abdomen through the umbilicus ("belly-

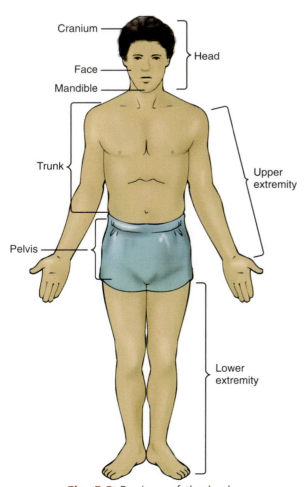

Fig. 5-2 Regions of the body.

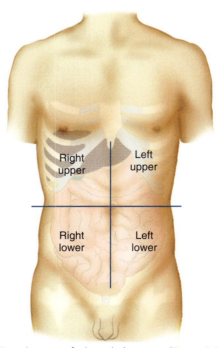

Fig. 5-3 Quadrants of the abdomen. (From McSwain N, Paturas J: *The basic EMT: comprehensive prehospital patient care,* 2003 ed, St Louis, 2003, Mosby.)

button"). Another imaginary line is drawn vertically through the umbilicus to divide the abdomen into four equal parts. The following terms describe these regions: left upper quadrant (LUQ), right upper quadrant (RUQ), left lower quadrant (LLQ), and right lower quadrant (RLQ). As an emergency first responder, you should also have a basic knowledge of organ location within the abdominal quadrants (Fig. 5-4). The RUQ holds the gallbladder and the liver. The LUQ contains the stomach and the spleen. The appendix is within the RLQ. The small and large intestine wind through all four of the quadrants. Pelvic organs such as the bladder and female reproductive organs are also found within the lower quadrants. The kidneys are located behind the abdominal cavity in an area referred to as the retroperitoneal space and just to the side of the spinal column. One kidney is found in the RUQ and the second kidney in the LUQ. Observed trauma to these different areas should alert you to possible underlying injuries. It is also important to note that when injured, these organs can bleed profusely into the abdominal cavity.

Body Systems

It is important to know that the body is divided into separate yet interrelated systems. The body systems include the respiratory, circulatory, nervous, musculoskeletal, integumentary, gastrointestinal, urinary, reproductive, endocrine, and lymphatic systems.

The Respiratory System

Our body tissues require a constant supply of oxygen to produce energy and operate efficiently. Every function of the body, from muscle contraction to food digestion, requires oxygen. During this process of metabolism (producing energy) body tissues give off waste products that need to be released. The respiratory system both delivers oxygen to the blood and removes some waste products, primarily carbon dioxide. A functional respiratory system is essential to survive. Irreversible damage to the brain and other organs can occur as early as 4 minutes without an adequate supply of oxygen. Other body functions may deteriorate if carbon dioxide levels rise above normal. It

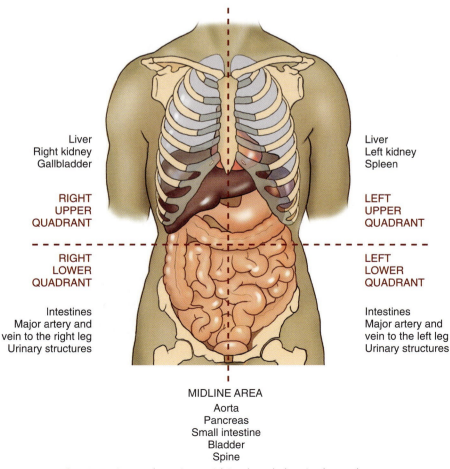

Fig. 5-4 Organ location within the abdominal quadrants.

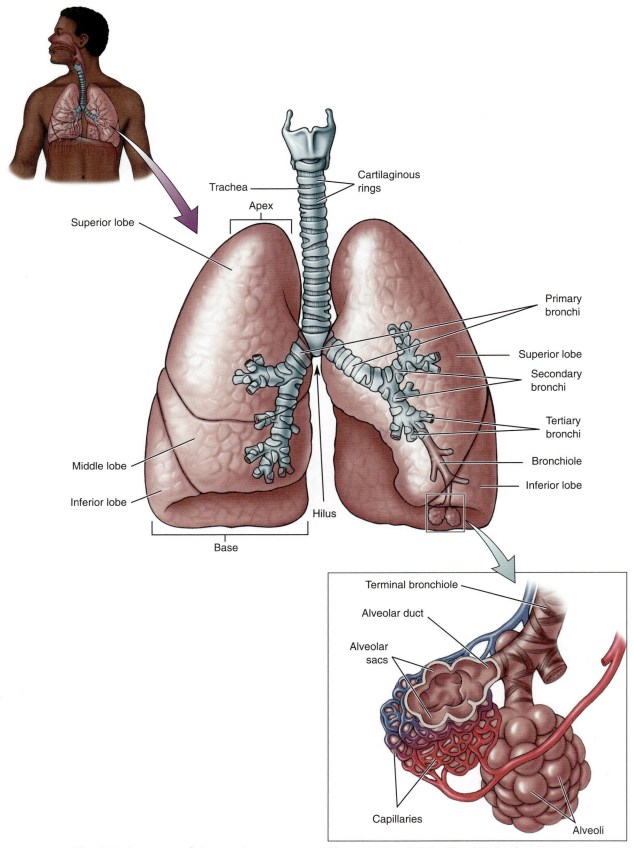

Fig. 5-5 Anatomy of the respiratory system. (From Herlihy B, Maebius N: *The human body in health and illness,* ed 3, St. Louis, 2007, Saunders.)

In the Real World—continued

You assess the patient; he has a deformity to his left thigh and the bone is visible. His right upper quadrant is bruised and tender to your touch, and also feels rigid. You realize his liver and/or gallbladder could be injured. Your partner takes vital signs and finds that the radial pulse is 100, res-pirations are 24 and shallow, and blood pressure (BP) is 104/84. The patient becomes unresponsive. The closest hospital is 10 minutes away, and the trauma center is a 20-minute transport. You check his airway and try to control the bleeding from his thigh.

is for these reasons that emergency care starts with the assessment and management of the respiratory system. Assessment and management of airway and breathing are discussed further in Chapter 7. To provide the best care to your patients, it is important that you, as an emergency first responder, know how the respiratory system works.

All the structures involved in delivery of oxygen to the blood are components of the respiratory system (Fig. 5-5). Room air, which contains approximately 21% oxygen, enters the airway through the mouth and nose. Air entering the mouth passes through the oropharynx. Air that enters through the nose passes through the cavity above the roof of the mouth called the nasopharynx. The oropharynx and nasopharynx cavities are sometimes referred to together as the pharynx. The epiglottis is located in the posterior pharynx. This leaf-shaped flap keeps food and liquid from entering the lungs during swallowing. When the epiglottis opens, air enters the trachea (windpipe), which contains the larynx (voice box). You speak by passing air over the vocal cords in your voice box. Below the larynx, the trachea divides into two bronchi in the lungs. Each bronchus continues to divide into smaller and smaller branches. The air reaches the bronchioles, which finally connect to the alveoli (air sacs). Each alveolus is covered in a net of small blood vessels called pulmonary capillaries. When air enters the alveoli, molecules of oxygen freely cross through a thin membrane into the blood. Carbon dioxide moves from the blood back into the alveoli, to be exhaled from the respiratory system via the lungs.

The mechanical process of moving air in and out of the airways is called **ventilation.** Ventilation is accomplished through the movement of a dome-shaped muscle, the **diaphragm,** and other muscles in the chest wall. As the diaphragm muscle contracts, it moves downward, expanding the lung and causing air to enter the lung (inspiration). The chest muscles assist by contracting to expand the thorax. When the diaphragm relaxes, the lung decreases in size and the air is pushed out (expiration).

The Circulatory System

The circulatory system consists of a pump (the heart), blood, and blood vessels. The heart pushes blood through the blood vessels, resulting in blood flowing to every region of the body. In essence, the circulatory system is a transportation pipeline.

Heart

The heart can be described as two independent pumps, a low-pressure pump and a high-pressure pump, that work together to pump blood through the circulatory system (Fig. 5-6). The right side of the heart, which is the low-pressure pump, receives blood from the vena cava that is low in oxygen levels but high in waste material. The right atrium pumps this waste-laden blood to the lungs, where carbon dioxide waste is removed and oxygen is added through gas exchange as previously described. Because the right side of the heart only has to pump blood to the lungs, the muscle mass on the right side of the heart is smaller in comparison to the muscle mass on the left side of the heart. The oxygen-rich blood from the lungs is now pumped into the left side of the heart. The left side of the heart, which is the high-pressure pump, pumps this oxygen-rich blood out through the aorta to begin its cycle through the body again. The muscles on the left side of the heart are greater in mass than the muscle mass on the right side of the heart because the left side of the heart must pump the blood against great resistance and further distance.

The heart muscle itself consists of four individual chambers (Fig. 5-7), two upper atrium chambers and two lower ventricle chambers. Two valves located between the upper and lower chambers of the heart allow blood to flow only in a one-way direction. Blood that is low in oxygen is pumped from the inferior vena cava and superior vena cava into the right atrium. Blood from the right atrium is now pumped through a one-way valve into the right ventricle. Blood from the right ventricle is pumped out of the heart, through the pulmonary arteries, into the lungs for gas exchange. Blood high in oxygen from the

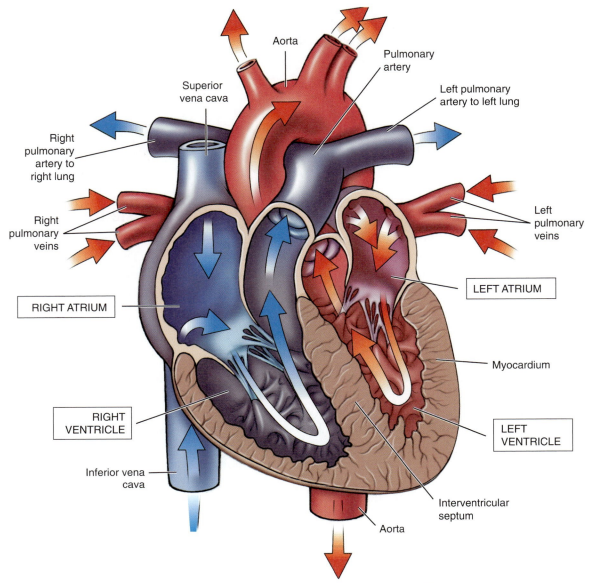

Aorta

Pulmonary artery

Superior vena cava

Left pulmonary artery to left lung

Right pulmonary artery to right lung

Right pulmonary veins

Left pulmonary veins

RIGHT ATRIUM

LEFT ATRIUM

Myocardium

RIGHT VENTRICLE

LEFT VENTRICLE

Inferior vena cava

Interventricular septum

Aorta

Fig. 5-6 Anatomy of the heart. (From Herlihy B, Maebius N: *The human body in health and illness,* ed 3, St. Louis, 2007, Saunders.)

lungs is pumped through the pulmonary veins, into the left atrium of the heart. Blood from the left atrium is pumped through a one-way valve into the left ventricle. Blood from the left ventricle is now pumped from the heart, through the aorta, to the body.

Each time the left ventricle of the heart contracts, it sends a pulse wave of blood into the arteries. The pulse is a reflection of the patient's heart rate. You can palpate (feel) these pulse waves wherever an artery passes near the skin's surface and over a bone. You will often assess a patient's pulse over the carotid, femoral, radial, and brachial arteries.

Blood Vessels

Blood carries oxygen and other nutrients, such as glucose, to the cells and carries carbon dioxide and other wastes away from the cells. Blood is pumped through a closed system of a highly organized network of blood vessels (Fig. 5-8). These blood vessels include arteries, arterioles, capillaries, venules, and veins.

Blood leaves the left side of the heart and enters a system of large-sized vessels called **arteries,** which carry oxygenated blood away from the heart. The aorta leaves the left ventricle of the heart, extending upward, and then arches downward toward the chest and abdomen. Several

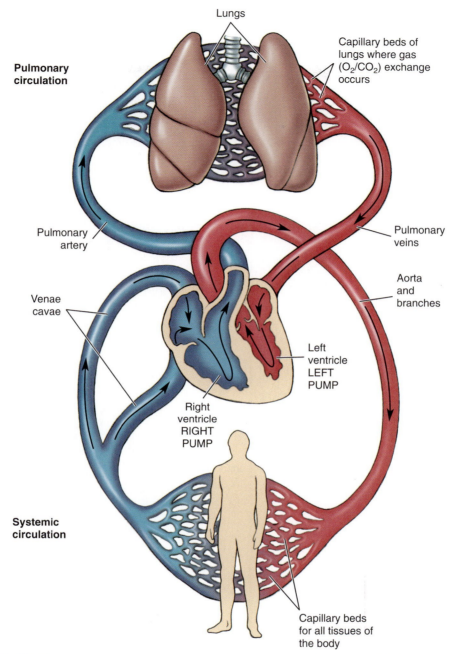

Fig. 5-7 The heart can be described as two independent pumps. (From Herlihy B, Maebius N: *The human body in health and illness,* ed 3, St. Louis, 2007, Saunders.)

major arteries branch from the aorta to supply blood to the heart muscle (coronary arteries), the head (carotid arteries), the upper extremities, and the internal organs. The pulse of the carotid arteries is felt in the neck to the left and the right of the larynx. This pulse is usually stronger than in other arteries because it is close to the heart.

Major arteries to the upper extremities also branch off the aorta to the brachial artery down each arm. Because it is difficult to find the carotid artery in an infant, the brachial artery is felt on the inside of the arm at the elbow to determine if an infant's pulse is present. The brachial artery divides into two smaller arteries that deliver blood

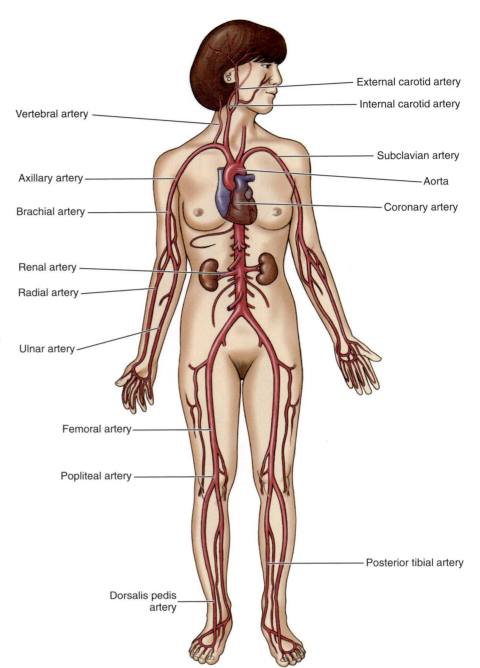

External carotid artery

Internal carotid artery

Vertebral artery

Subclavian artery

Axillary artery

Aorta

Brachial artery

Coronary artery

Renal artery

Radial artery

Ulnar artery

Fig. 5-8 Major arteries of the body. (From Herlihy B, Maebius N: *The human body in health and illness,* ed 3, St. Louis, 2007, Saunders.)

Femoral artery

Popliteal artery

Posterior tibial artery

Dorsalis pedis artery

to the forearm and hand. You frequently palpate the radial artery to count the pulse rate in conscious adult patients. It is located on the lateral (thumb) side of the wrist.

The aorta continues downward through the chest and into the lower abdomen. There it splits into two large arteries that pass through the pelvis to the lower extremities. Each femoral artery is the major artery for the thigh. The femoral artery can be palpated in the groin area near the crease between the abdomen and thigh. The femoral

artery then continues to the smaller arteries of the leg and foot.

As blood continues through the arterial system, the vessels become smaller and are called arterioles. The arterioles connect to tiny capillaries, found in all tissues of the body. Capillaries supply the cells of the body with oxygen and nourishment. The capillaries also carry away carbon dioxide and other waste products from the cells of the body.

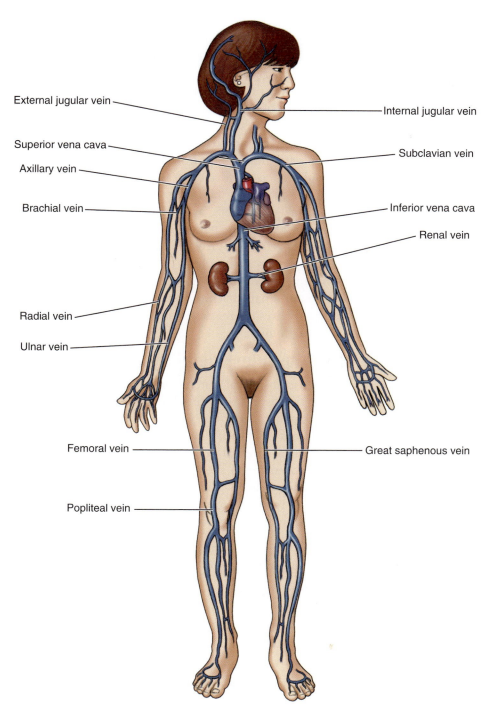

External jugular vein

Internal jugular vein

Superior vena cava

Subclavian vein

Axillary vein

Brachial vein

Inferior vena cava

Renal vein

Radial vein

Ulnar vein

Femoral vein

Great saphenous vein

Popliteal vein

Fig. 5-9 Major veins of the body. (From Herlihy B, Maebius N: *The human body in health and illness,* ed 3, St. Louis, 2007, Saunders.)

As blood leaves tissue capillaries, it enters small vessels called venules. These venules empty into **veins,** which carry blood toward the heart. These small vessels join others to form larger veins as they carry away blood with waste. The largest vein in the body, the vena cava, empties directly into the right side of the heart (Fig. 5-9).

The Nervous System

The nervous system controls the voluntary and involuntary activities of the body. It also provides for higher mental functions such as thought, emotion, and memory. The two main components of the nervous system are the central nervous system (CNS) and the peripheral nervous system (PNS) (Fig. 5-10).

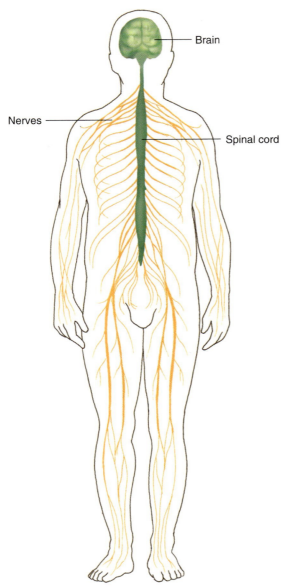

Brain

Nerves

Spinal cord

Fig. 5-10 The nervous system. (From McSwain N, Paturas J: *The basic EMT: comprehensive prehospital patient care,* 2003 ed 2, St Louis, 2003, Mosby.)

is like a high-speed information highway that carries messages between the brain and the rest of the body. Proper functioning of the CNS is vital for the well-being and survival of the whole body.

The PNS is the system of nerves that carry messages between the body and the CNS. Two types of nerves make up the PNS: motor nerves, which carry information from the brain to the muscles of the body, and sensory nerves, which carry information from the body to the brain. For example, when you decide to take a patient's pulse, your brain (CNS) sends a "take the radial pulse" message down your spinal cord (CNS) and motor nerves (PNS) to your fingers to feel for the patient's pulse. The sensory nerves in your fingers (PNS) feel the patient's pulse waves. Your sensory nerves then collect the information about the pulse and deliver that information to your spinal cord (CNS) and finally back to your brain (CNS). Your brain (CNS) receives the message and calculates the number of beats per minute.

The Musculoskeletal System

The musculoskeletal system consists of the bones, joints, connective tissues, and muscles. All of these components work together to give the body form and allow it to move. The bones of the skeletal system provide shape and protect vital internal organs. The muscular system provides movement to the skeletal system and is a part of every body system. The musculoskeletal system is also used as a reference tool to describe other body systems and anatomical parts. For example, the radial artery and radial nerve lie next to the radius bone in the forearm.

The Skeletal System

The skeletal system can be divided into two main sections, the axial skeleton and the appendicular skeleton. The axial skeletal section is the central portion of the skeletal system and consists of the skull, spinal column, and thorax. The appendicular skeleton section "hangs" from the central (axial) skeletal section and consists of the upper extremities, pelvis, and lower extremities (Fig. 5-11). The skull is divided into two parts, the cranium and the face (Fig. 5-12). The cranium houses and protects the brain. The face contains several bones, including the mandible (jawbone). The mandible is an important landmark for learning how to properly open a patient's airway, as you will learn in Chapter 7. Connected to the skull and extending down the length of the back is the spinal column. The spinal column is a collection of 33 individual bones called vertebrae, which are stacked on top of each other (Fig. 5-13). The slightly S-shaped spinal column holds the body upright and

The CNS consists of the brain and spinal cord. The brain is referred to as the control center of the body because it controls everything from muscle movements to emotional response. The brain is thinking and problem-solving as you study this chapter, and it also controls your finger muscles to turn the pages as you read. It controls basic life functions such as breathing and maintaining body temperature.

The spinal cord extends downward from the brain through the center of the spinal column. The spinal cord

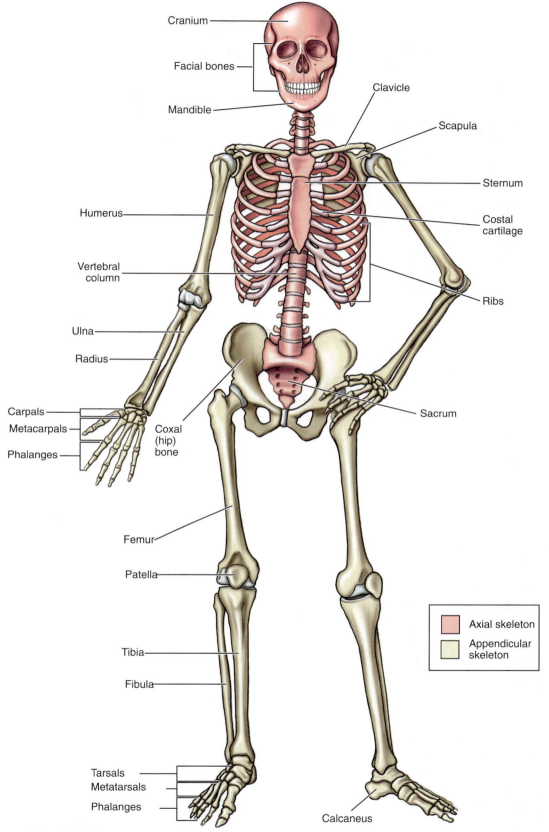

Fig. 5-11 The skeletal system. (From Herlihy B, Maebius N: *The human body in health and illness,* ed 3, St. Louis, 2007, Saunders.)

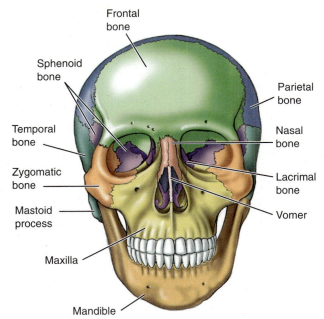

Fig. 5-12 The skull. (From Herlihy B, Maebius N: *The human body in health and illness,* ed 3, St. Louis, 2007, Saunders.)

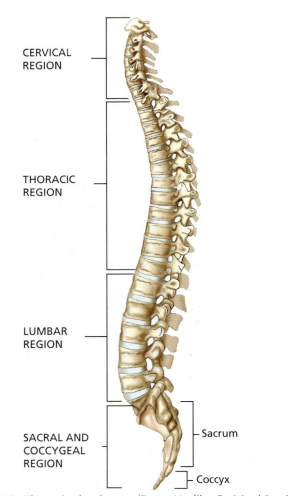

Fig. 5-13 The spinal column. (From Herlihy B, Maebius N: *The human body in health and illness,* ed 3, St. Louis, 2007, Saunders.)

allows for bending and twisting. The spinal column surrounds and therefore protects the spinal cord.

The thorax is composed of 12 pairs of ribs (**Fig. 5-14**). The ribs are connected to the spinal column in the back and some are connected to the sternum (breastbone) in the front. The **xiphoid process** is the lower portion of the sternum. The xiphoid process is an important landmark to know when delivering chest compressions during CPR, as you will learn in Chapter 9. The clavicle (collarbone) connects the upper sternum to the scapula (shoulder blade), located in the posterior chest. The clavicle and scapula form the shoulder joint.

The upper extremity contains the humerus, which connects to the shoulder joint at its proximal end (**Fig. 5-15**). The distal end of the humerus meets the radius and ulna at the elbow. The radius is located on the lateral side of the forearm and the ulna is on the medial side. The wrist is composed of many small bones called carpals. The carpals join with the bones of the hand, the metacarpals, to allow movement. The many small bones of the fingers are called phalanges.

The pelvis is composed of two large bones attached to the lower portion of the spinal column. The pelvis is a large, bony ring and forms a cradle in the lower abdomen (**Fig. 5-16**). It is important to note that this cradle can collect a large amount of blood from internal bleeding.

The lower extremities connect to the pelvis where the head of the femur joins to create the hip joint (**Fig. 5-17**). The femur is the longest single bone in the body. At the distal end of the femur lies the knee joint. The patella (kneecap) covers the anterior knee and helps to protect the joint. Distal to the knee are two bones that compose the leg. The larger tibia, or shin bone, is located in the anterior portion of the leg. The smaller fibula lies posterior and lateral to the tibia. The distal ends of these two bones are connected to the foot at the ankle joint. Bones of the ankle are called tarsals. A similar name, metatarsals, is given to the bones of the foot. Toes are formed by multiple smaller bones called phalanges.

The bones of the human skeleton are held together by connective tissues called ligaments. Where two bones come together a joint is formed, which allows for movement. Fibrous tissue called cartilage lines the surface of joints, allowing smooth movement and providing cushioning between the two bones.

The Muscular System

The human skeleton is much like a locomotive engine sitting at the train station. All the structures and joints are in place to allow movement, but it cannot move unless force is applied. The muscular system provides the force needed to get the work done. It also helps to give

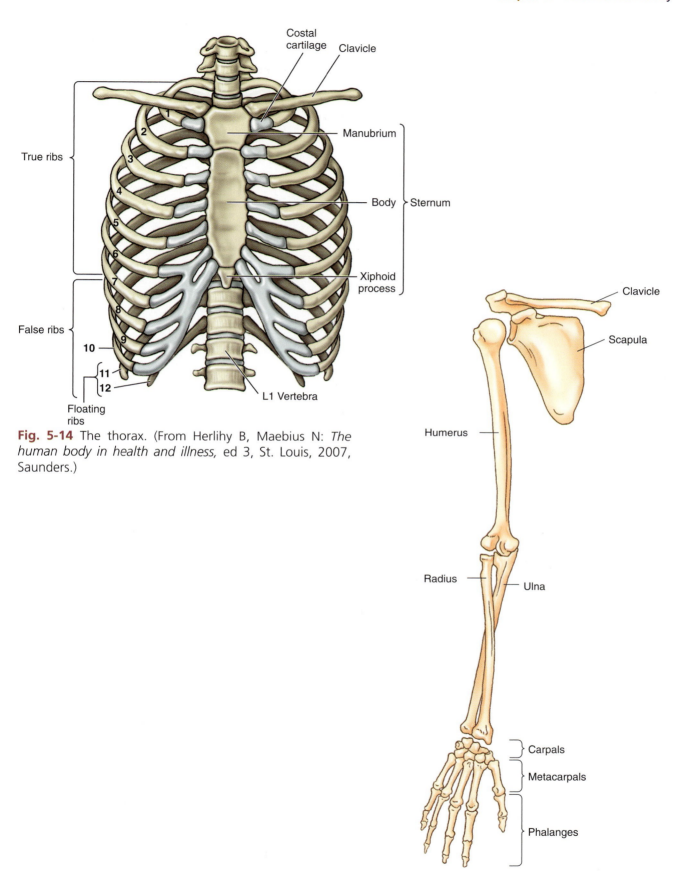

Fig. 5-14 The thorax. (From Herlihy B, Maebius N: *The human body in health and illness,* ed 3, St. Louis, 2007, Saunders.)

Fig. 5-15 Upper extremity. (From McSwain N, Paturas J: *The basic EMT: comprehensive prehospital patient care,* ed 2, St Louis, 2003, Mosby.)

Pelvis

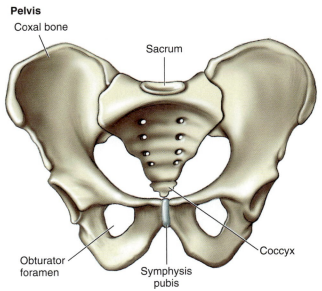

Coxal bone
Sacrum
Obturator foramen
Symphysis pubis
Coccyx

Fig. 5-16 The pelvis. (From Herlihy B, Maebius N: *The human body in health and illness,* ed 3, St. Louis, 2007, Saunders.)

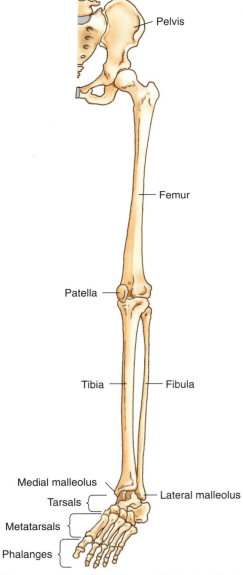

Pelvis
Femur
Patella
Tibia
Fibula
Medial malleolus
Lateral malleolus
Tarsals
Metatarsals
Phalanges

Fig. 5-17 Lower extremity. (From McSwain N, Paturas J: *The basic EMT: comprehensive prehospital patient care,* ed 2, St Louis, 2003, Mosby.)

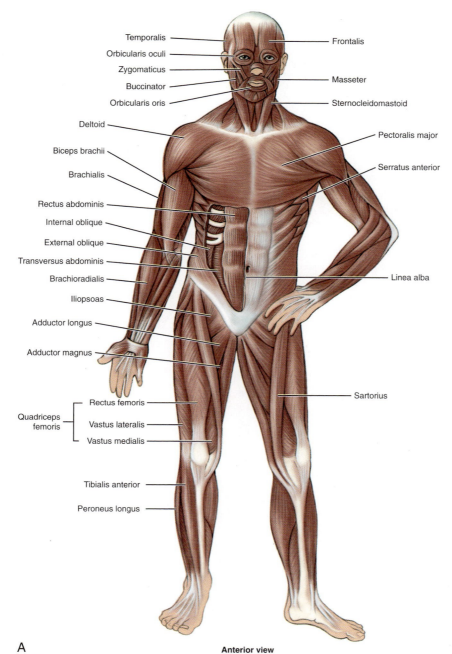

Temporalis
Orbicularis oculi
Zygomaticus
Buccinator
Orbicularis oris
Deltoid
Biceps brachii
Brachialis
Rectus abdominis
Internal oblique
External oblique
Transversus abdominis
Brachioradialis
Iliopsoas
Adductor longus
Adductor magnus
Rectus femoris
Quadriceps femoris
Vastus lateralis
Vastus medialis
Tibialis anterior
Peroneus longus

Frontalis
Masseter
Sternocleidomastoid
Pectoralis major
Serratus anterior
Linea alba
Sartorius

A

Anterior view

Fig. 5-18 The muscular system. (From Herlihy B, Maebius N: *The human body in health and illness,* ed 3, St. Louis, 2007, Saunders.)

the body shape and protect internal organs **(Fig. 5-18)**. The muscular system involves three different types of muscles, as follows:

1. *Voluntary.* Voluntary muscles (also called skeletal muscles) are attached to bones by tendons. Skeletal muscle contraction creates movement. For example, you are using such muscles in your hand, through the voluntary control of your brain, as you take notes in your emergency first responder class.

2. *Involuntary.* Involuntary muscles (also called smooth muscles) are found in the walls of tubular structures such as blood vessels, small airways of the lungs called bronchioles, the gastrointestinal tract, and the urinary system. As the name suggests, these muscles work involuntarily. While you read this page, your stomach and intestines are moving to digest your last meal, and your blood vessels are expanding and contracting to the size needed to keep blood flowing to all body tissues.

B

Posterior view
Fig. 5-18, cont'd

3. *Cardiac.* Cardiac muscle is found only in the heart. It works constantly and automatically and requires a continual supply of oxygen-rich blood as fuel. Cardiac muscle can survive only a very short interruption of blood flow. If cardiac muscle goes too long without oxygen, the muscle will die (infarct).

The Integumentary System

The integumentary system (the skin) protects the body from the environment and harmful substances, helps regulate body temperature, and provides sensory input to the brain. The skin also keeps the body from becoming dehydrated. The body is approximately 60% water and must maintain a specific balance of solutions to support normal body functions. The skin also provides a barrier against the elements, bacteria, and other sources of infection.

The skin plays a major role in regulation of body temperature. It helps rid the body of excess heat and retains heat as needed. When a patient has a severe burn on a large surface area of skin, the damaged skin can no longer retain body heat and the patient's body temperature drops.

Sensory nerves that gather information about temperature, touch, pressure, and pain are located in the skin. These nerves constantly relay information to the brain via the spinal cord.

The skin is divided into three layers (Fig. 5-19). The outermost layer is the epidermis. Cells that give the skin its color are located here. The epidermis is closely adhered to the second layer of the skin, the dermis. These layers are so thin and held so close together that they appear as one. The dermis contains blood vessels, hair follicles, sweat glands, oil glands, and nerves. Below the dermis lies the subcutaneous layer. This is a layer of fatty tissue that

holds water and nutrients and provides insulation and cushioning to the body. The thickness of this tissue varies from body part to body part and from person to person.

The Gastrointestinal and Urinary Systems

The gastrointestinal and urinary systems are responsible for processing food and eliminating waste from the body. The digestive tract begins in the mouth and continues through the esophagus to the stomach and into the small and large intestines. As food moves through the digestive tract, mechanical and chemical processes occur to absorb nutrients and water. The leftover waste is eliminated as fecal material (Fig. 5-20). Blood carrying nutrients and water from the digestive tract also filters through the liver and kidneys, where the nutrients and water are absorbed and any extra water or any waste is eliminated as urine (Fig. 5-21).

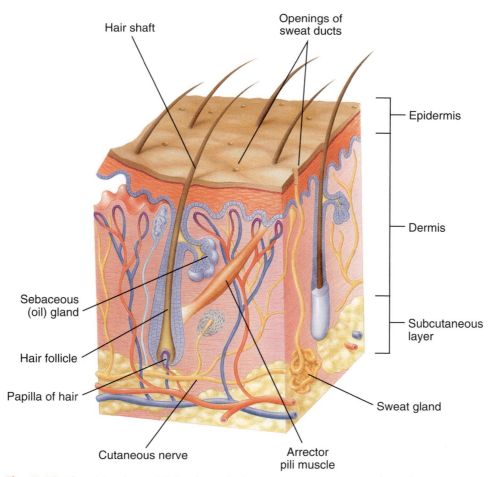

Fig. 5-19 The skin. (From Thibodeau G, Patton K: *Anatomy & physiology,* ed 6, St Louis, 2007, Mosby.)

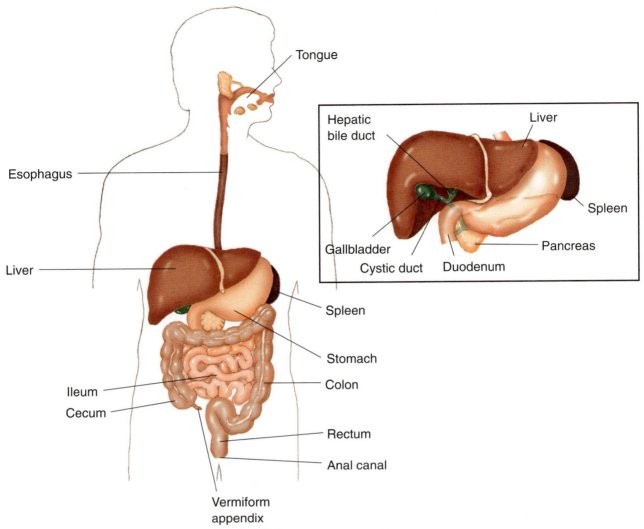

Fig. 5-20 The gastrointestinal system.

The Reproductive System

The reproductive system is the system of structures and hormones required for reproduction **(Fig. 5-22).** This system is closely associated with the urinary system, and together they are sometimes referred to as the genitourinary system. The reproductive system consists of the ducts, glands, and penis in males and the ovaries, fallopian tubes, uterus, and vagina in females. The male testes produce semen, which combines with an egg released from the female ovaries to create a fetus.

The Endocrine System

The endocrine system is composed of glands that produce chemicals known as hormones. Endocrine glands include the pituitary, thyroid, parathyroid, and adrenal glands, and the ovaries, testes, and pancreas **(Fig. 5-23).** Hor-

mones give us strength, endurance, and the ability to move fuel into cells to create energy and to participate in reproduction. The hormone insulin is produced in the pancreas and helps to regulate the amount of sugar (glucose) in the body.

The Lymphatic System

The lymphatic system provides links between the digestive and circulatory systems by transporting vitamins and nutrients from the digestive tract into the blood. It also works as a bridge from tissues to the circulatory system by removing fluid and waste from tissues and transporting them into the circulatory system. Fluid and waste can then be transported to the liver and kidneys to be filtered out and eliminated. The lymphatic system also participates in the immune response by transporting special substances to attack foreign bodies and fight infection.

A

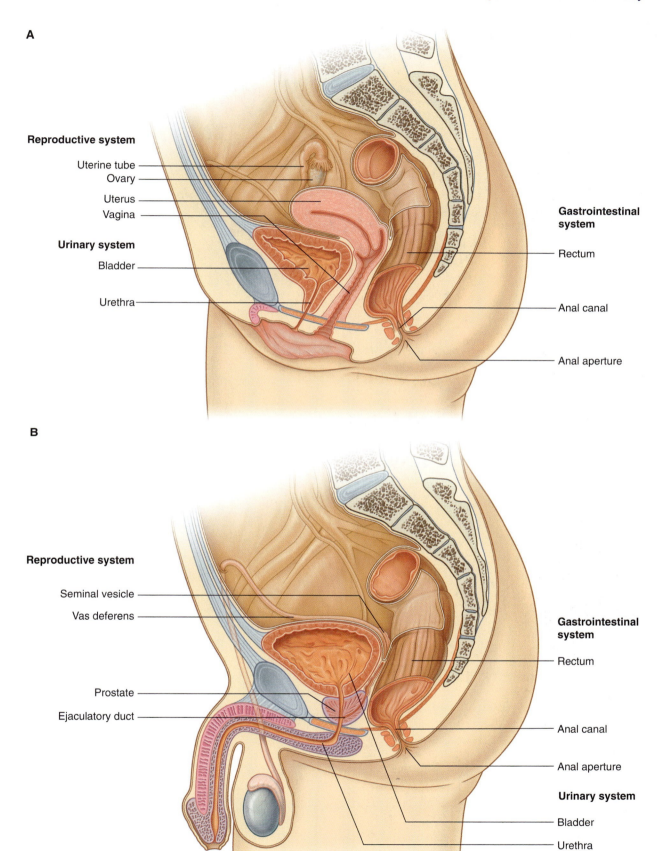

Reproductive system

Uterine tube

Ovary

Uterus

Vagina

Urinary system

Bladder

Urethra

Gastrointestinal system

Rectum

Anal canal

Anal aperture

B

Reproductive system

Seminal vesicle

Vas deferens

Prostate

Ejaculatory duct

Gastrointestinal system

Rectum

Anal canal

Anal aperture

Urinary system

Bladder

Urethra

Fig. 5-21 The reproductive, gastrointestinal, and urinary systems. **A,** In women. **B,** In men. (From Drake R et al: *Gray's anatomy for students,* London, 2005, Churchill Livingstone.)

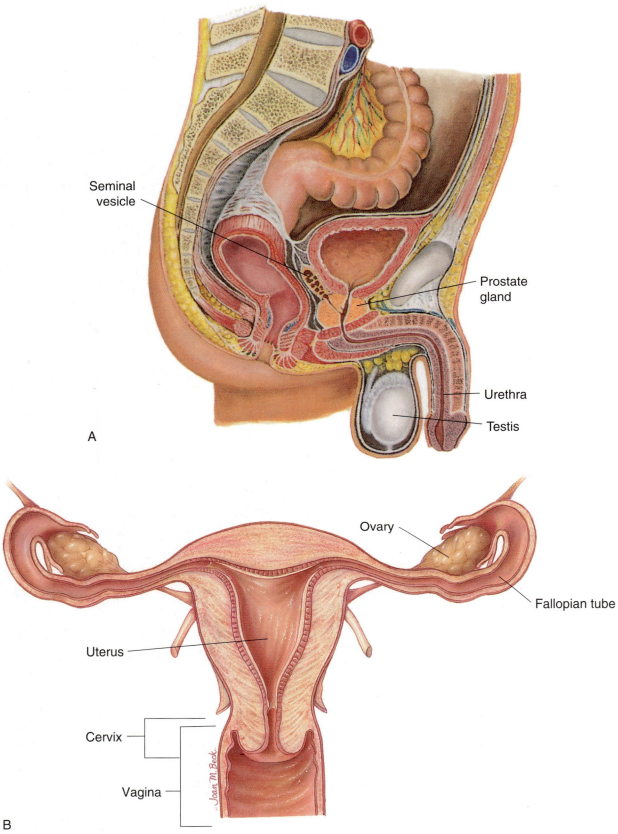

Seminal
vesicle

Prostate
gland

Urethra

Testis

A

Ovary

Fallopian tube

Uterus

Cervix

Vagina

B

Fig. 5-22 The reproductive systems. **A,** In men. **B,** In women. (McSwain N, Paturas J: *The basic EMT: comprehensive prehospital patient care,* ed 2, St Louis, 2003, Mosby.)

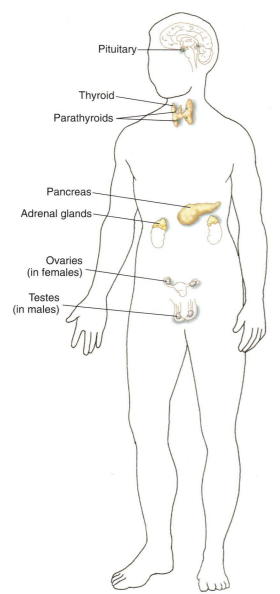

Pituitary
Thyroid
Parathyroids
Pancreas
Adrenal glands
Ovaries
(in females)
Testes
(in males)

Fig. 5-23 The endocrine system. (From McSwain N, Paturas J: *The basic EMT: comprehensive prehospital patient care*, ed 2, St Louis, 2003, Mosby.)

Team Work

As an emergency first responder, it is important that you know and understand the different body systems and how they relate to one another. Understanding, for example, that the circulatory system transports the oxygen received from the respiratory system to critical organs such as the brain will help you do a thorough assessment of a patient and give the appropriate treatment. An accurate assessment and early life-saving care are of utmost importance to the outcome of the patient and the care that the rest of the health care team will provide.

As part of the health care team, it is also important to know how to describe the location of injuries and to identify potential internal injuries from external forces. Correct use of directional terms and surface landmarks is an important tool to communicate your assessment and management to other team members and to document the event. Speaking a common medical language makes assessment and management more efficient.

Your description of the injuries may also help guide the dispatch of appropriate help or the transport decision of the transporting crew. For example, knowing that a burn can take away the protective mechanisms of the skin and lead to many complications can help you to communicate the severity of the burn injury. Your description may enter into the decision to transport the patient to a burn center.

There are certain situations, such as triage during a multicasualty incident, where you may be expected to relate injury to different body systems to a patient's priority for treatment. The rest of the team at the incident will rely on your knowledge of body systems to ensure that the appropriate patients are treated first.

In the Real World—Conclusion

Your knowledge of anatomy leads you to suspect life-threatening abdominal bleeding in this patient that may require early surgical intervention. You and your partner immobilize the patient and provide him with high-concentration oxygen. When the ambulance arrives, you provide a clear and thorough report of your assessment and management of the patient. The EMT radios this information to the trauma center.

Later in your shift you call the trauma nurse to follow up on your patient's condition. The nurse tells you that soon after arrival, the patient's blood pressure dropped. Doctors immediately took him to the operating room to remove his ruptured spleen and repair his fractured femur. They expect him to recover fully.

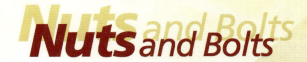

Nuts and Bolts

Critical Points

Knowledge of anatomy and physiology is a solid foundation for learning patient care skills. To communicate with other health care professionals, it is essential to learn a common language. To identify a patient's needs, you must know how major body systems function and work together. As an emergency first responder, it is important to be able to recognize the structure and function of the respiratory, circulatory, nervous, and musculoskeletal systems and to understand the workings of other body systems.

Learning Checklist

❑ The normal anatomical position refers to the human body standing upright, facing forward with arms at the side and palms of the hands turned forward.

❑ Directional terms are based on the imaginary vertical line drawn through the middle of the body called the midline.

❑ Anterior is toward the front of the body. Posterior is toward the back of the body. Lateral is away from the midline, and medial is toward the midline. Superior is toward the head of the body, and inferior is toward the feet. Proximal is toward the trunk of the body, and distal is away from the trunk of the body.

❑ Body areas include the cranium, thorax, abdomen, pelvis, and extremities.

❑ The respiratory system is responsible for taking in oxygen and delivering it to the blood, speech, and the movements of ventilation.

❑ The respiratory system includes the following structures: oropharynx, nasopharynx, epiglottis, trachea, larynx, lungs, bronchi, and alveoli.

❑ The circulatory system is the transportation pipeline to move blood throughout the body. Blood carries oxygen and nutrients to the cells and carries carbon dioxide and other wastes away from the cells.

❑ The circulatory system includes the following structures: arteries, veins, capillaries, and the heart.

❑ The nervous system controls the voluntary and involuntary activities of the body and provides higher mental functions such as thought, emotion, and memory.

❑ The nervous system includes the following structures: brain, spinal cord, motor nerves, and sensory nerves.

❑ The musculoskeletal system consists of the bones, joints, connective tissues, and muscles that work together to give the body form and allow it to move.

❑ The skeletal system includes the following structures: skull, facial bones, vertebrae, thorax, ribs, bones in the extremities, and pelvis.

❑ The muscular system involves voluntary, involuntary, and cardiac muscle.

❑ The integumentary system is the skin, which protects the body from the environment and harmful substances, helps regulate body temperature, and provides sensory input to the brain.

❑ The gastrointestinal system is responsible for processing food into nutrients. The urinary system is responsible for eliminating waste from the body in the form of urine.

❑ The reproductive systems of the male and female are closely associated with the urinary systems.

❑ Endocrine glands secrete hormones and include the pituitary, thyroid, parathyroid, and adrenal glands and the ovaries, testes, and pancreas.

❑ The lymphatic system links the digestive and circulatory systems by transporting vitamins and nutrients from the digestive tract into the blood. It also carries waste and fluid back from the tissues to the circulatory system and participates in the immune response of the body.

Key Terms

Abdomen The part of the body between the hips and the chest.

Anatomy The structure of the body.

Anterior Toward the front of the body.

Arteries Blood vessels that carry blood away from the heart.

Diaphragm The dome-shaped muscle that is largely responsible for ventilation.

Distal Away from the trunk of the body.

Inferior Toward the feet or bottom of the body.

Lateral Away from the midline of the body.

Medial Toward the midline of the body.

Midline An imaginary vertical line drawn through the middle of the body.

Normal anatomical position The position of a human body standing upright, facing forward, with arms at the side and the palms turned forward.

Pelvis The lower part of the trunk of the body.

Physiology The function of the body.

Posterior Toward the back of the body.

Proximal Toward the trunk of the body.

Superior Toward the head or top of the body.

Thorax The chest.

Veins Blood vessels that carry blood toward the heart.

Ventilation The mechanical process of moving air in and out of the lungs.

Xiphoid process The lowest part of the base. It is to be avoided during chest compression of the sternum.

First Responder NSC Objectives

COGNITIVE OBJECTIVES

- ❑ Describe the anatomy and function of the respiratory system.
- ❑ Describe the anatomy and function of the circulatory system.
- ❑ Describe the anatomy and function of the musculoskeletal system.
- ❑ Describe the components and function of the nervous system.

Check your understanding

Please refer to p. 439 for the answers to these questions.

1. Matching: Place the letter of the phrase in the right column next to the term it describes.

_____ Anterior   A. Toward the head

_____ Posterior   B. Toward the trunk
                          (torso)

_____ Lateral   C. Front of the body

_____ Medial   D. Away from the midline
                          of the body

_____ Superior   E. Back of the body

_____ Inferior   F. Away from the trunk
                          (torso)

_____ Proximal   G. Toward the feet

_____ Distal   H. Toward the midline of
                          the body

2. For each abdominal organ below, place the abbreviation for the quadrant in which it is located in the blank space.

_____ Stomach   RUQ (right upper
                          quadrant)

_____ Liver   LUQ (left upper
                          quadrant)

_____ Spleen   RLQ (right lower
                          quadrant)

_____ Gallbladder   LLQ (left lower
                          quadrant)

_____ Appendix

3. Label the following bones:

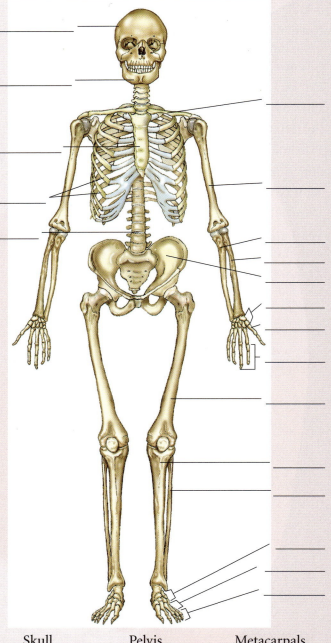

Skull	Pelvis	Metacarpals
Mandible	Humerus	Carpals
Vertebral	Radius	Tarsals
column	Ulna	Metatarsals
Sternum	Tibia	Phalanges
Ribs	Fibula	Clavicle
Femur		

4. The flap of tissue that closes over the trachea to protect the lower airway when a person swallows is the _____.

5. The voice box is also known as the _____.

6. The muscle that separates the organs in the chest from the organs in the abdomen is the _____.

7. The blood vessels in the neck that transport blood from the heart to the brain and head are the _____.

8. Blood that is rich in oxygen is transported from the lungs by the pulmonary vein, which empties into the _____ side of the heart.

9. The heart muscle receives its own supply of oxygenated blood from the _____ arteries.

10. The major artery of the upper extremity (arm) is the _____ artery.

11. The major artery of the lower extremity (leg) is the _____ artery.

12. The tiny, thin-walled blood vessels where the exchange of oxygen, wastes, and nutrients between the body and the environment occurs are called _____.

13. The largest, strongest chamber of the heart, which pumps blood to the body, is the _____.

14. The chamber of the heart that pumps blood to the lungs so that it can be oxygenated is the _____.

15. The two structures that make up the central nervous system are the _____ and the _____.

16. The network of nerves that are outside of the central nervous system and that carry messages between the brain and the body is the _____ nervous system.

17. The nerves that tell you that you are feeling something hot are called _____ nerves, while the nerves that tell your hand to let go of the hot object (make you move your hand) are called _____ nerves.

18. The type of muscle found in organs such as blood vessels is called smooth or _____ muscle, while the type of muscle attached to the bones is called skeletal or _____ muscle.

19. The heart is made up of muscle tissue with special properties. This type of muscle is called _____ muscle.

20. The hair, nails, and skin are the structures that make up the _____ system.

21. Which of the following is the uppermost layer of the skin?
A. Dermis
B. Subcutaneous layer
C. Epidermis
D. Basement membrane

22. Which of the following organs is part of the endocrine system?
A. Kidney
B. Lymph glands
C. Gallbladder
D. Pancreas

23. Which of the following is the term for the tiny air sacs in the lungs?
A. Bronchi
B. Alveoli
C. Pharynx
D. Bronchioles

24. You have assessed a patient and found that he has an injury to the back of his arm about 2 inches above his elbow. In giving your hand-off report, which of the following would you use to correctly describe the location of the patient's injury?
A. On the anterior side, distal to the elbow
B. On the posterior side, distal to the elbow
C. On the anterior side, proximal to the elbow
D. On the posterior side, proximal to the elbow

Checkyour understanding–continued

25. You are caring for a patient who was involved in a skateboarding crash. He tells you he has severe lower right arm pain, which is confirmed by significant deformity and swelling. Which of the following are most likely injured?
   A. Tibia and fibula
   B. Tarsals and radius
   C. Humerus and scapula
   D. Radius and ulna

26. You are responding to a motor vehicle collision, when dispatch notifies you that it is a two-car collision with a T-bone impact on the driver's door of one vehicle. You expect to find which of the following injuries on the impacted driver?
   A. Right upper arm
   B. Spleen
   C. Frontal bone
   D. Gallbladder

Chapter 6

Lifting and Moving Patients

LESSON GOAL

This chapter discusses proper techniques for lifting and moving patients in a variety of conditions and locations, and the equipment used to safely move patients.

OBJECTIVES

1. Define body mechanics.
2. Discuss the guidelines and safety precautions that need to be followed when lifting a patient.
3. Describe the indications for an emergency move.
4. Describe the indications for assisting in nonemergency moves.
5. Discuss the various devices associated with moving patients in the prehospital environment.
6. Demonstrate an emergency move.
7. Demonstrate a nonemergency move.
8. Demonstrate the application of equipment used to move patients in the prehospital environment.

In the Real World

You and your partner are the first to arrive at the scene of a single-vehicle rollover on a country gravel road. As you are parking your truck at the edge of the road, you are told by dispatch that the ambulance will be on scene in approximately 6 minutes. You grab your first-response bag and head toward the vehicle. The vehicle is a small pick-up truck that is now lying on its top in the ditch; thick black smoke is coming from under the hood of the vehicle. As you continue to make your way toward the truck, you see a male patient lying on his back and hanging partially out of the driver's side window. The patient is unconscious and does not respond to your voice. His respirations are fast and shallow and you do not see any signs of bleeding. Your immediate concern is moving the patient to a safer environment before continuing with your assessment and treatment. How can you safely and rapidly move this patient without any immobilization equipment?

Role of the Emergency First Responder

As an emergency first responder, you will often be the first medically trained individual to arrive on the scene of an incident. If the scene is unsafe for you or the patient, or if the patient's condition is critical, your role may include moving the patient to a safer location. In this chapter you will learn how to perform emergency moves in a way that minimizes the risk of further injury to you or the patient.

If individuals with a higher level of training are present, your role is to help them lift and move the patient. To respond competently in situations such as the opening scenario, you must understand and be confident in your role. You should also be familiar with equipment used by other health care providers.

Body Mechanics

One of the primary responsibilities of an emergency first responder is his or her own personal safety. Back injuries can result from using poor **body mechanics** when lifting and moving patients or equipment. Proper body mechanics refers to the safest and most effective way to use your body as an advantage when lifting and moving something. To determine how much help you may need you should consider the following issues before attempting to move any patient:

- The weight of the patient
- Access to the patient
- Your own abilities and physical limitations
- The terrain and distance you need to carry the patient

Other considerations to help prevent injury include attention to your own body mechanics as well as those of your partner when reaching for something or across something. Avoid reaching out more than 20 inches in front of you and avoid reaching for an extended time. Twisting your upper body while stretching out to reach for something is a common action that can increase the chances of back injuries.

Lifting Techniques

In general you should lift items with your leg muscles and not just with your arm and back muscles. You should also keep the weight of what you are lifting as close to your body as possible (Fig. 6-1). Your body should move as a single unit, not in separate pieces. Moving, for example, only your upper body without moving your hips and your lower body can create strain in your lower back and potentially cause an injury. The proper technique for lifting something includes the following:

- *Feet are spread comfortably,* approximately shoulder-width apart.
- *Knees are bent* so you are almost in a semisitting position. This position allows your center of gravity to be closer to the object.
- *If more than one person is lifting, the lift should be simultaneous.* Communication is important so that lifting can occur at the same time. Identify who is going to be the "Lead" person for the lift (usually the person at the head of the patient). The Lead person now communicates clearly and frequently with all the lifting partners as well as with the patient.
- *The back is not twisted.* Your back should remain straight and you should tighten the muscles of both

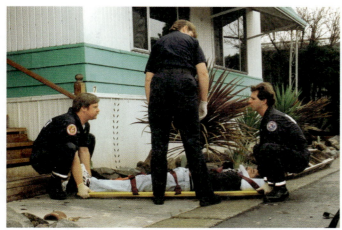

Fig. 6-1 Proper body mechanics. (From Shade B et al: *Mosby's EMT-intermediate textbook for the 1999 NSC*, ed 3, St Louis, 2007, Mosby.)

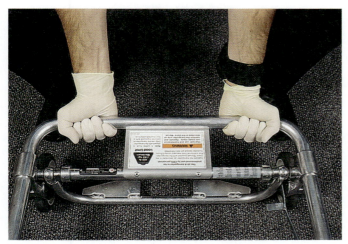

Fig. 6-2 Power grip. (From McSwain N, Paturas J: *The basic EMT: comprehensive prehospital patient care*, ed 2, St Louis, 2003, Mosby.)

your back and your abdomen to focus on lifting as a single unit.

- *Leg muscles are used.* The power of the lift should come from your legs and hips and not the weaker muscles in the back.
- *Weight is kept close to the body.* When reaching to lift something, you should ensure that you are as close to the object as possible because muscle strain can occur when reaching and lifting.

Power Grip

Hand positioning is important when lifting an object. To lift something effectively, the power grip or underhand grip is used (Fig. 6-2). With this grip, the palms of your hands and your fingers should be in complete contact with the device you are lifting. Your fingers should circle around the device at the same angle and your hands should be a comfortable distance apart, approximately 10 inches. To lower a device you should place your hands in a reverse power grip position.

Power Lift

The **power lift** is a way to effectively lift a heavy object using proper body mechanics. It is important during the power lift to do the following:

- Keep your back locked in its normal curvature and tighten your abdominal muscles.
- Place your feet comfortably apart, usually shoulder-width apart.
- Bring the center of your body over the object you are lifting to keep the lift as vertical as possible.

Skill 6-1 illustrates the power lift technique to lift a wheeled stretcher. You should use proper body mechanics, coordinate your movements with other rescuers, and take precautions when lifting and moving. These guidelines will help protect you, other rescuers, and the patient from potential injury.

Principles of Moving Patients

A patient is usually moved by the Emergency Medical Services (EMS) crew when ready for transport. Occasionally, however, you may take responsibility for moving the patient. The two types of patient moves are emergency (urgent) moves and nonemergency (nonurgent) moves.

Emergency Moves

In general, a patient should be moved immediately (with an **emergency move**) only in the following situations:

- *There is an immediate danger to the patient if he or she is not moved.* Such instances would include the following:
  - Fire or danger of fire is present.
  - Explosives or a danger of explosion is present.
  - The patient cannot be protected from other hazards on the scene such as traffic, electrical or chemical hazards, or other dangers.
- *Life-saving care cannot be given because of the patient's location or position.* For example, a patient in cardiac arrest might be found sitting in a chair or lying on a bed. This patient would have to be moved to a supine position on a hard, flat surface.

Skill 6-1

Two-Person Power Lift

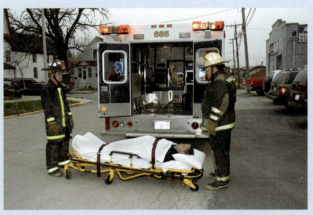

1. The two providers should stand at either end of the lowered wheeled stretcher. Feet are approximately shoulder-width apart.

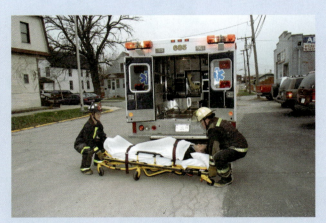

2. Bend the knees while keeping the back locked in its normal curvature and tighten the abdominal muscles. Use the **power grip** to grasp the stretcher. The center of the body should be over the stretcher.

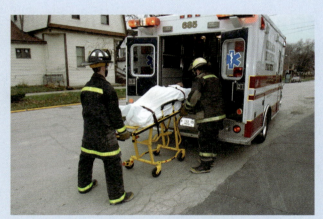

3. Upon command from the lead person, the two providers lift the stretcher simultaneously, maintaining communication and eye contact. Lift as vertically as possible, using the legs and not the back.

- *Access cannot be gained to other patients who need life-saving care.* This occurs usually with motor vehicle collisions.

Emergency moves are not guaranteed to protect the patient from injury or pain. Moving a patient even using an acceptable emergency move may actually cause pain and/or injury to the patient. It is important for you to remember that you are moving the patient because it is an *emergency*. The patient's life depends on you moving him or her to a safer location or into a more effective position. It is impossible to move a patient quickly and at the same time provide ultimate protection against further injury or pain.

Before moving a patient you need to ask the following question: "Does the benefit of moving the patient outweigh the risks associated with moving the patient?" Only if the answer is clearly "yes" should you consider moving the patient using an emergency move technique.

The greatest danger in moving a patient with an emergency move is the risk of worsening a spinal injury the patient may have. In an emergency move, you should make every effort to pull the patient in the direction of the long axis (the length) of the body to protect the spine. Every effort should be made not to move the patient's head away from the inline position formed between the head, neck, and shoulders.

Drags

There are several different drags that can be used as emergency moves such as the cloth drag, upper extremity drag, blanket drag, and incline drag. These drags can be used to move a supine patient out of danger. With any drag you should stabilize the patient's head and neck as much as possible and move the patient as a single unit in the direction of the long axis (the length) of the body. Skill 6-2 illustrates a variety of drags that can be used by a single provider in an emergency.

Carries

A patient can also be carried out of an emergency situation by either one or two providers. Ideally you should work with someone who is of similar build, height, and strength to ensure a balance when lifting and carrying a patient, although this is not possible at all times. Skill 6-3 illustrates a variety of one- and two-person carries. Rapid extrication of a patient out of a vehicle is an emergency move involving at least three providers. Rapid extrication is discussed further in the Team Work section of this chapter.

Nonemergency Moves

Nonemergency moves are performed when there is no immediate threat to the patient's life. Usually these types of moves are performed with other responders and should be carefully coordinated through frequent use of clear and effective communication. Practicing nonemergency moves with other potential emergency first responder partners will add confidence and coordination that will be beneficial when assisting with a patient move. At a minimum, you should know two nonemergency moves, the direct ground lift and the extremity lift. The direct ground lift should only be used with lighter patients who do not have a suspected spine injury. This lift should be used by a minimum of three providers. Skill 6-4 illustrates the direct ground lift.

The extremity lift should not be done if there are suspected injuries to any of the extremities or the head or neck. To perform an extremity lift, see Skill 6-5.

CAUTION!

Never pull a patient in any direction that does not follow the long axis of the body unless you have no other choice. Pulling a patient against the long axis of the body will potentially injure the spine.

CAUTION!

You will be called upon to make decisions about whether or not it is appropriate to move a patient. While in most cases you should not move your patient from the position in which he or she presents, emergency situations may arise where it is more dangerous not to move the patient. If moving the patient is required, use an emergency move that provides the most protection to the patient from further pain or injury.

Skill 6-2

Emergency Drags

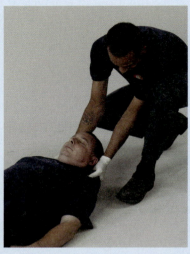

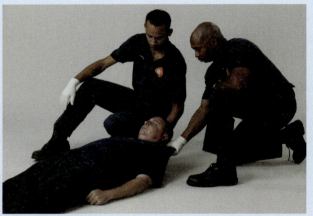

1. One-person clothing drag. Ensure you have a firm grasp on the patient's clothing and cradle the patient's head in your arms. (From Chapleau W, Pons P: *Emergency medical technician, making the difference,* St Louis, 2007, Mosby.)

2. Two-person clothing drag. (From Chapleau W, Pons P: *Emergency medical technician, making the difference,* St Louis, 2007, Mosby.)

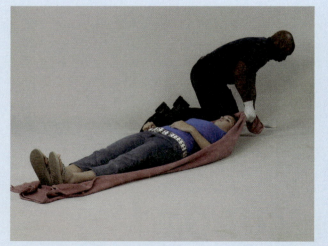

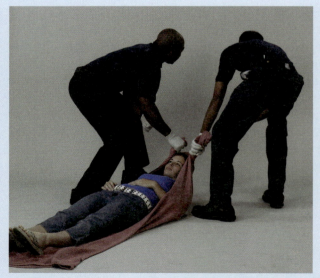

3. One-person blanket drag. You can place a blanket under the patient by placing the blanket next to him or her, rolling the patient toward you to place the blanket underneath him or her, and then rolling the patient back onto the blanket. Pull the blanket through to the other side. (From Chapleau W, Pons P: *Emergency medical technician, making the difference,* St Louis, 2007, Mosby.)

4. Two-person blanket drag. (From Chapleau W, Pons P: *Emergency medical technician, making the difference,* St Louis, 2007, Mosby.)

Skill 6-2

Emergency Drags—cont'd

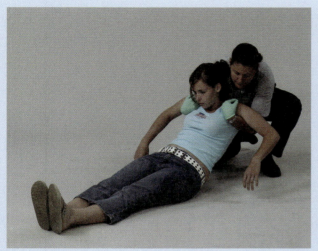

5. **One-person upper extremity drag.** Also called a shoulder drag. (From Chapleau W, Pons P: *Emergency medical technician, making the difference,* St Louis, 2007, Mosby.)

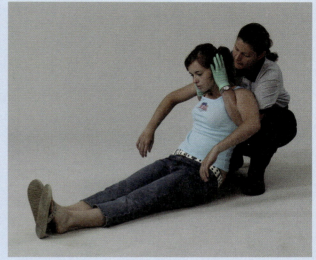

6. **One-person modified upper extremity drag for rapid extrication.** This move can be used to drag a person from a vehicle in an *emergency* situation if there is only one provider and the patient must be moved. (From Chapleau W, Pons P: *Emergency medical technician, making the difference,* St Louis, 2007, Mosby.)

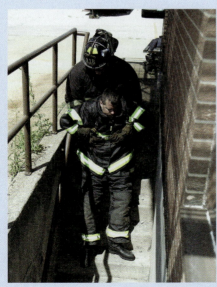

7. **Incline drag.** Use a modified upper extremity drag to move a person down stairs. The patient should be dragged in a head-first position. (From Chapleau W, Pons P: *Emergency medical technician, making the difference,* St Louis, 2007, Mosby.)

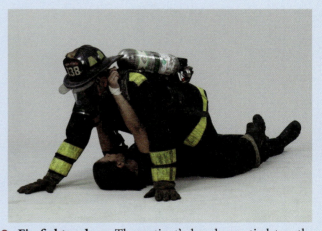

8. **Firefighter drag.** The patient's hands are tied together and passed over the provider's head. The provider crawls on hands and knees, keeping the patient's head as low as possible. This drag is used to drag patients out of a smoke-filled area. (From Chapleau W, Pons P: *Emergency medical technician, making the difference,* St Louis, 2007, Mosby.)

Skill 6-3

Emergency Carries

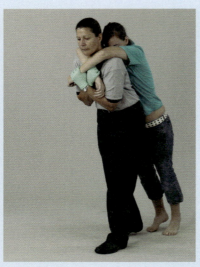

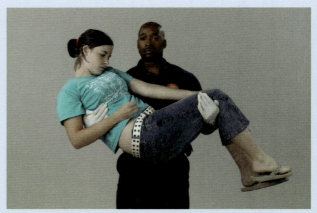

2. One-person cradle carry. This type of carry is generally only recommended for lighter patients. (From Chapleau W, Pons P: *Emergency medical technician, making the difference,* St Louis, 2007, Mosby.)

1. Pack strap carry. The provider firmly grasps the patient's arms around his or her neck and leans slightly forward to pull the patient onto his or her back. (From Chapleau W, Pons P: *Emergency medical technician, making the difference,* St Louis, 2007, Mosby.)

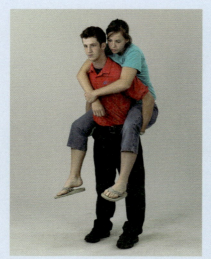

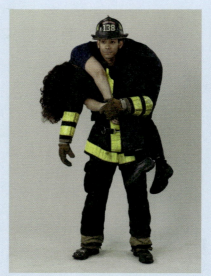

3. Piggyback carry. (From Chapleau W, Pons P: *Emergency medical technician, making the difference,* St Louis, 2007, Mosby.)

4. Firefighter carry. (From Chapleau W, Pons P: *Emergency medical technician, making the difference,* St Louis, 2007, Mosby.)

Skill 6-3

Emergency Carries—cont'd

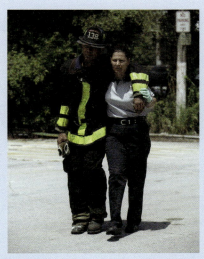

5. One-person assist. Also called one-person crutch. The patient's arms are grasped and placed around the provider's neck. The provider holds the patient's hand with one hand and the other is placed around the patient's waist. (From Chapleau W, Pons P: *Emergency medical technician, making the difference,* St Louis, 2007, Mosby.)

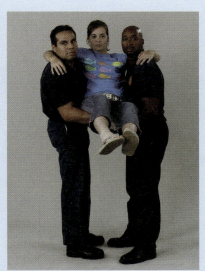

6. Two-person cradle carry. Two providers can cradle a patient between them to carry a patient to safety. (From Chapleau W, Pons P: *Emergency medical technician, making the difference,* St Louis, 2007, Mosby.)

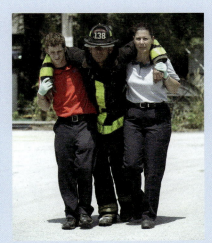

7. Two-person assist. Also called two-person crutch. The providers should ensure they are each gripping the patient's wrists. (From Chapleau W, Pons P: *Emergency medical technician, making the difference,* St Louis, 2007, Mosby.)

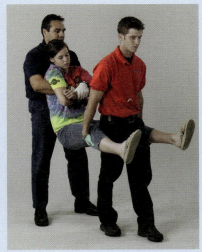

8. Two-person extremity carry. Carry a patient down a flight of stairs feet first. (From Chapleau W, Pons P: *Emergency medical technician, making the difference,* St Louis, 2007, Mosby.)

Skill 6-4

Direct Ground Lift

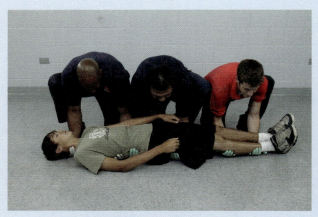

1. Two or three providers line up on one side of the patient. Providers kneel on one knee (preferably the same for all providers). (From Chapleau W, Pons P: *Emergency medical technician, making the difference*, St Louis, 2007, Mosby.)

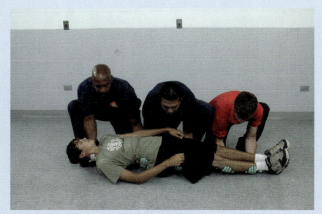

2. The provider at the head places one arm under the patient's neck and shoulder and cradles the patient's head while the other arm is placed under the patient's lower back. The second provider places one arm under the patient's knees and the other under the patient's lower legs. The third provider places arms above and below the waist. (From Chapleau W, Pons P: *Emergency medical technician, making the difference*, St Louis, 2007, Mosby.)

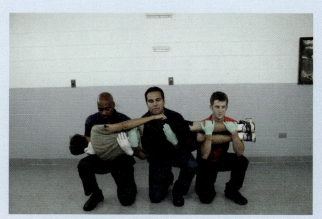

3. On signal, the rescuers lift the patient to their knees and roll the patient in toward their chests. (From Chapleau W, Pons P: *Emergency medical technician, making the difference*, St Louis, 2007, Mosby.)

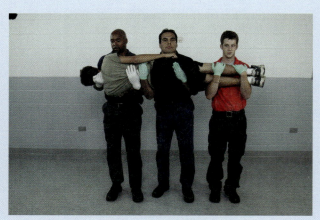

4. On signal, the rescuers stand and move the patient. To lower the patient, the steps are reversed. (From Chapleau W, Pons P: *Emergency medical technician, making the difference*, St Louis, 2007, Mosby.)

Skill 6-5

Extremity Lift

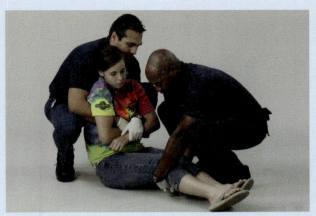

1. One provider kneels at the patient's head and another kneels at the patient's side by the knees. The provider at the head places one hand under each of the patient's shoulders and grasps the patient's wrists. The provider at the foot slips his or her hands under the patient's knees. Both providers move up to a crouching position. (From Chapleau W, Pons P: *Emergency medical technician, making the difference*, St Louis, 2007, Mosby.)

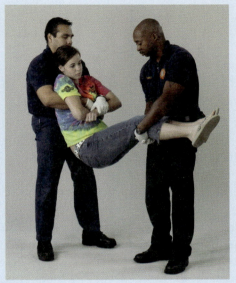

2. The providers stand up simultaneously and move with the patient. (From Chapleau W, Pons P: *Emergency medical technician, making the difference*, St Louis, 2007, Mosby.)

In the Real World—continued

After a brief discussion with your partner, you kneel above the patient's head. You place a forearm on either side of the patient's head, cradling his head and neck in your forearms. You then gather the patient's shirt in your hands. With slow, deliberate movements you pull the patient out of the vehicle while maintaining as much stabilization as possible. After the patient is free of the vehicle, your partner takes control of the patient's pelvis and legs. The two of you now move the patient out of the ditch and onto the protected shoulder of the roadway where you continue the assessment and treatment while waiting for the ambulance to arrive.

Transfer of a Supine Patient from Bed to Stretcher

You may be called on to help move a patient from a bed to a stretcher for transportation by an EMS crew. First be sure you understand why the patient is in bed. Is it an acute injury or illness such as a sudden onset of chest pain? Is the patient permanently bedridden such as a stroke patient? Is the patient recovering from a recent surgery or experiencing pain that led to the emergency call? If you understand the reason why the patient is in bed, you can choose the best method of transfer, either the direct carry or the draw sheet method. If the patient is experiencing pain, the direct carry is the most effective method. This method keeps the patient close to you and allows a better grip. The following steps indicate how to do a direct carry:

1. The wheeled stretcher is positioned perpendicular to the bed with the head end of the stretcher at the foot of the bed.
2. The height of the stretcher should be positioned as high as possible to allow placement of the patient without having the providers bend at the waist any more than necessary.
3. The straps are unbuckled and other items removed from the stretcher.
4. Both providers stand between the bed and the stretcher and face the patient.
5. The first provider slides an arm under the patient's neck and cups the patient's shoulder.
6. The second provider slides a hand under the patient's hips and lifts slightly.
7. The first provider slides his or her other arm under the patient's back.
8. The second provider places his or her arms under the patient's hips and calves.
9. The providers slide the patient to the edge of the bed.
10. The patient is lifted or curled toward the providers' chests.
11. The providers rotate and place the patient gently onto the wheeled stretcher.

If a quicker move is needed and the patient can tolerate movement, you should use the draw sheet method (Skill 6-6).

Patient Positioning

Proper patient positioning is as important as moving the patient. You should not reposition a trauma patient from the position they are found in unless it is absolutely necessary to treat immediate life-threatening injuries such as a compromised airway or significant hemorrhage. Repositioning a trauma patient may cause further injury to the patient's spine.

Most patients will best be served when they are placed in a supine position. The supine position is when the patient is lying on his or her back, looking skyward. This position allows the rescuer to have access to the patient's airway, observe the patient's respirations, and stay in the patient's field of vision.

The appropriate patient position depends on the patient's clinical presentation. An unresponsive, breathing, nontrauma patient should be placed in the **recovery position** (Fig. 6-3). The recovery position is the preferred position for an unconscious patient as it helps to keep the airway open and allows for easy access to the airway if it becomes obstructed or if the patient begins to vomit.

A patient who is experiencing difficulty breathing or chest pain should be allowed to rest in a position of comfort as long as there are no indications of a spinal injury. This is usually a sitting position with the patient leaning forward, with the hands on the legs, in an attempt to breathe more easily. You should allow the patient to stay in this position through your evaluation and treatment if the patient is responsive. You should also allow a nauseous or vomiting patient to remain in a position of comfort, positioning yourself appropriately to manage the airway. Remember that if the patient is comfortable, regardless of the nature of the call, it will be easier for both you and the patient to handle the emergency.

Skill 6-6

Draw Sheet Transfer

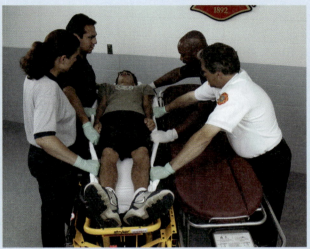

1. Providers should be on either side of the patient. Roll the edges of the sheet. (From Chapleau W, Pons P: *Emergency medical technician, making the difference,* St Louis, 2007, Mosby.)

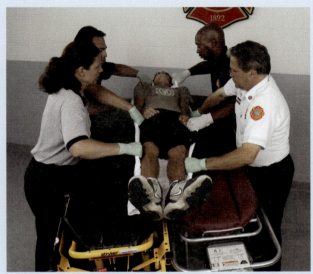

2. Lifting together on the count of three, providers lift and move the patient to the adjacent bed or stretcher. (From Chapleau W, Pons P: *Emergency medical technician, making the difference,* St Louis, 2007, Mosby.)

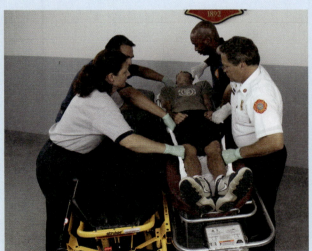

3. The patient is moved from the bed to the stretcher by pulling on the rolled-up sheet. (From Chapleau W, Pons P: *Emergency medical technician, making the difference,* St Louis, 2007, Mosby.)

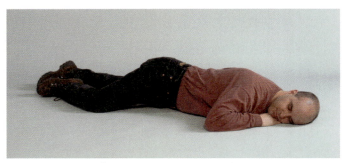

Fig. 6-3 Recovery position.

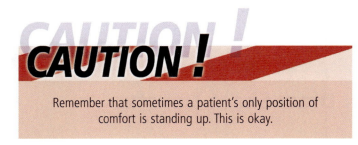

CAUTION!

Remember that sometimes a patient's only position of comfort is standing up. This is okay.

Log Roll

When a patient is in the prone (face down) position, he or she must usually be moved to a supine (face up) position so that a thorough patient assessment can be done.

Skill 6-7 illustrates the **log roll** of a patient who has no suspected spinal injury to check the front of the body. Skill 6-8 illustrates the log roll of a patient who has a suspected spine injury. Moving the patient's body as a single unit will help minimize the risk of further spinal injury. A minimum of three providers should be used for a log roll.

Skill 6-7

Log Roll with No Suspected Spine Injury

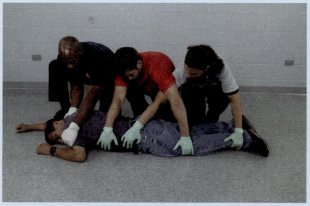

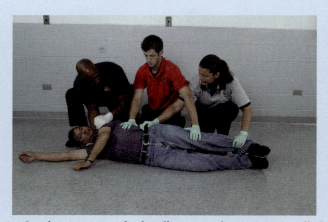

1. The three providers line up on the same side of the patient and are down on one or two knees. The provider at the head grasps the patient's arms and shoulders. The middle provider grasps the patient's torso and upper leg while the provider at the feet grasps the patient's feet and hips. (From Chapleau W, Pons P: *Emergency medical technician, making the difference*, St Louis, 2007, Mosby.)

2. On the person at the head's count, the patient is rolled as a single unit toward the providers. From this position the patient's anterior can be assessed or the patient can be rolled completely over to a supine position. (From Chapleau W, Pons P: *Emergency medical technician, making the difference*, St Louis, 2007, Mosby.)

Skill 6-8

Log Roll with Suspected Spine Injury from a Prone Position

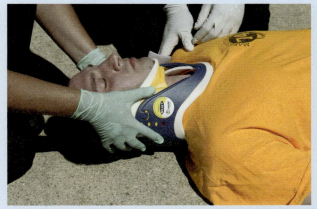

1. While one provider holds manual inline stabilization of the head and neck, a second provider applies a cervical collar. (From NAEMT: *PHTLS: basic and advanced prehospital trauma life support*, ed 5, St Louis, 2003, Mosby.)

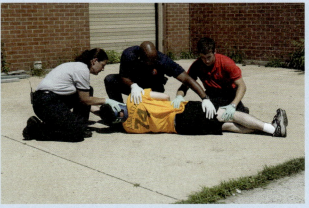

2. While the first provider continues to stabilize the head and neck, the second and third providers position themselves on the patient's side, placing their hands in positions to evenly distribute the patient's weight. With the first provider stabilizing the head and neck and the second and third providers in position at the patient's side, the patient is rolled onto the side on a 3-count. (From NAEMT: *PHTLS: basic and advanced prehospital trauma life support*, ed 5, St Louis, 2003, Mosby.)

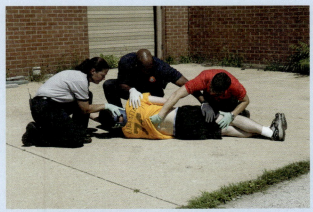

3. While the patient is in this position, a provider should examine the patient's back. (From NAEMT: *PHTLS: basic and advanced prehospital trauma life support*, ed 5, St Louis, 2003, Mosby.)

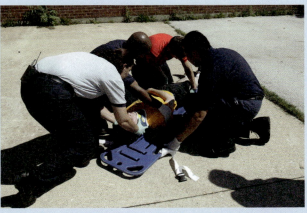

4. A fourth provider moves a backboard into position, and the patient is lowered onto the board on a 3-count. (From NAEMT: *PHTLS: basic and advanced prehospital trauma life support*, ed 5, St Louis, 2003, Mosby.)

Team Work

As an emergency first responder, you will often be asked to assist with the emergency medical technician (EMT) team to package and move the patient into the ambulance for transport to the hospital. You should become familiar with all the transportation equipment used by your local EMS agency and the skills used to move patients.

TRANSPORTING EQUIPMENT

Equipment used to transport patients or to get patients prepared for transport includes the following:

- *Stretchers and cots.* The **wheeled stretcher** (or wheeled cot) is the transporting device most commonly found in ambulances (Fig. 6-4). There are many varieties of wheeled stretchers and most allow the head to be raised and lowered. The **portable stretcher** can be made of canvas or heavy plastic and can be folded or collapsed when not in use (Fig. 6-5). The **scoop** stretcher splits into two pieces. Each piece can be placed on either side of the patient and then reconnected to "scoop" up the patient (Fig. 6-6). The **basket stretcher** can be used to lift patients out of difficult terrain or to a different level (Fig. 6-7).

- *Stair chair.* The **stair chair** is the preferred method of transporting a patient down a flight of stairs (Fig. 6-8).

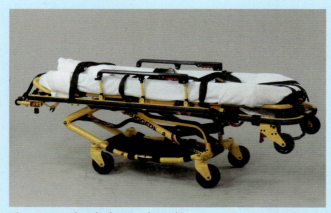

Fig. 6-4 Wheeled stretcher. (From McSwain N, Paturas J: *The basic EMT: comprehensive prehospital patient care,* 2003 ed 2, St Louis, 2003, Mosby.)

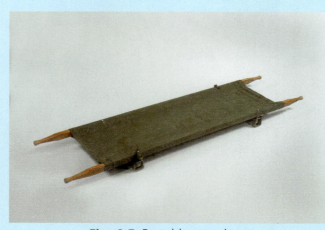

Fig. 6-5 Portable stretcher.

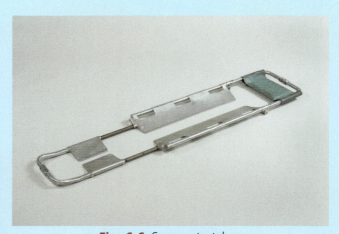

Fig. 6-6 Scoop stretcher.

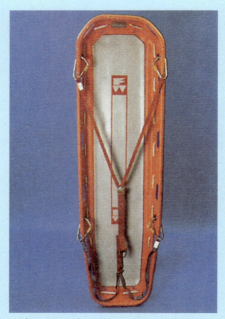

Fig. 6-7 Basket stretcher. (From Stoy W et al and Center for Emergency Medicine: *Mosby's EMT-basic textbook,* revised ed 2, St Louis, 2007, Mosby Lifeline.)

Team Work—cont'd

- *Backboards*. There are two types of backboards, the **long backboard** (or long spine board) and the short backboard (or short spine board). The long backboard is used for patients who are lying down or standing up and for those who must be fully immobilized to prevent worsening a potential spinal injury (see Chapter 12) (Fig. 6-9). The **short backboard** is usually used to remove patients in a sitting position from a vehicle. A **vest-type device** can also be used in place of a short backboard (Fig. 6-10).

You should practice with your local agency to learn the use of each piece of equipment so that you are able to assist in moving patients.

IMMOBILIZATION AND TRAUMA PATIENTS

The primary objective of any health care provider with any level of training should be to provide good patient care. You can increase your abilities to provide care by knowing how to interact with other caregivers. This chapter covers lifting and moving patients with minimal equipment and expertise, but in many situations more equipment and assistance may be needed.

With trauma victims, there is a great potential for spinal injury and extreme caution must be used to prevent further injury. This is accomplished through **spinal immobilization**. The techniques of spinal immobilization are discussed in Chapter 12. It is important to note that a spinal injury can be ruled out *only* by radiography studies such as an x-ray film, magnetic resonance image (MRI), or computed tomography (CT) scan. Therefore *any* trauma patient who has experienced a significant impact against the body should be immobilized.

A trauma patient who is found in a vehicle should be moved in a safe manner to avoid further injury. The method of moving this patient depends on the severity of the patient's condition based on the initial assessment. If the patient's condition is not critical and time can be taken to

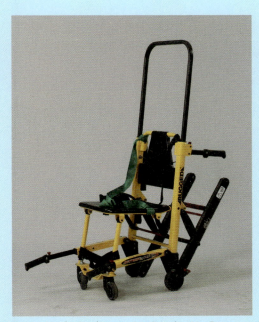

Fig. 6-8 Stair chair. (From McSwain N, Paturas J: *The basic EMT: comprehensive prehospital patient care,* 2003 ed 2, St Louis, 2003, Mosby.)

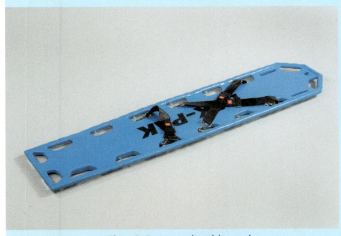

Fig. 6-9 Long backboard.

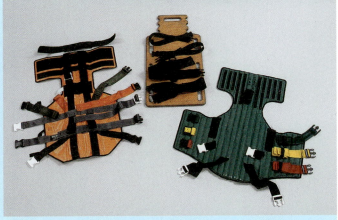

Fig. 6-10 Short backboard and vest-type devices.

Team Work—cont'd

securely package the patient before removal from the vehicle, the vest-type device or a short backboard should be used. Because both of these devices take several minutes to apply, they should not be used with a critical patient.

With a critical patient or a situation where time is of the essence, a patient can be removed from a vehicle using the **rapid extraction** technique. Skill 6-9 shows how four trained providers can remove a patient from a vehicle safely and effectively with this method.

If you learn these skills, you can increase your ability to provide patient care. Practice these and other skills regularly to stay sharp and mentally prepared to assist. Such practice also gives you the opportunity to work as a team with members of your EMS system.

In the Real World—Conclusion

After the ambulance arrives you give the EMTs a detailed description of the patient's current assessment and treatment, including your movement technique. After turning care of the patient over to the EMTs you and your partner now turn your attention to the vehicle fire and assisting the other agencies on the scene.

Skill 6-9

Rapid Extrication

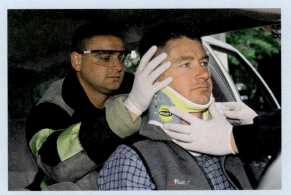

1. One provider holds manual inline stabilization of the head and neck while another applies a cervical collar.

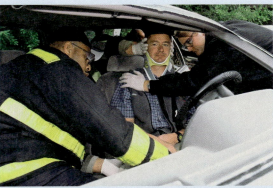

2. While manual stabilization is maintained, the patient's upper torso, lower torso, and legs are rotated in a series of short, controlled movements until the patient is in such a position that manual stabilization can no longer be maintained.

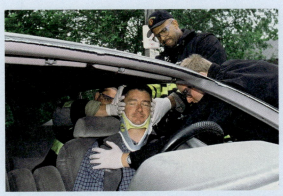

3. The person at the patient's legs comes around the outside of the vehicle to take over manual stabilization. The person previously holding manual stabilization moves to control the patient's lower torso and legs.

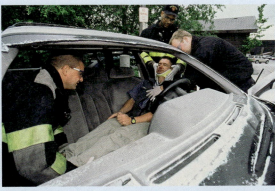

4. The patient is rotated until he or she can be lowered out of the vehicle door opening and onto a long backboard.

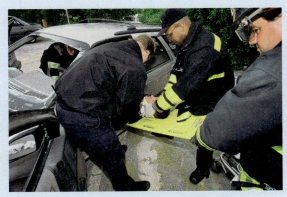

5. The patient is moved onto the long backboard.

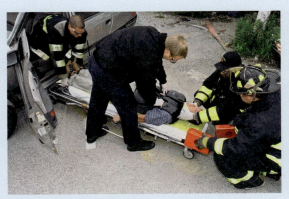

6. The patient is secured to the long backboard.

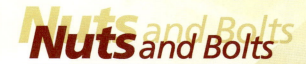

Nuts and Bolts

Critical Points

Ask yourself several questions before moving a patient. Do I need to move this patient? Is there a danger to the patient or me if I do not move this patient? If I have to move this patient, what is the best method? Is there enough help available to move this patient? You should be able to answer these questions in all situations. Patients should be moved only in emergency situations. Remember, your first priority is your safety and the safety of others in your crew. Your next concern is the patient's safety. If possible, do not move the patient until EMS personnel complete an evaluation. If this is not possible, choose the best method to move your patient. Always use correct body mechanics to avoid injuring yourself and causing further injury to your patient. Plan ahead and stay safe.

Learning Checklist

❑ As an emergency first responder, your role may include moving a patient if the scene is unsafe for either you or the patient or if the patient's condition is critical.

❑ Proper body mechanics refers to the safest and most effective way to use your body as an advantage when lifting and moving something.

❑ Before moving any patient, you should consider the weight of the patient, your own abilities and physical limitations, and the terrain and distance you will need to carry the patient.

❑ General lifting techniques include using your legs and not your back, keeping the weight of the object as close to your body as possible, and moving your body as a single unit.

❑ The power grip is used to maximize the effectiveness of the lift. The palms of your hands and your fingers should be in complete contact with the object you are lifting. Your fingers should be at the same angle and your hands approximately 10 inches apart.

❑ The power lift is effective to lift a heavy object. You should keep your back locked, your abdominal muscles contracted, your feet approximately shoulder-width apart, and your body over the object. The lift should be as vertical as possible.

❑ An emergency move should be used only if there is an immediate danger to the patient if he or she is not moved, if life-saving care cannot be given because of the patient's location or position, or if access cannot be gained to other patients who need life-saving care.

❑ When performing an emergency move, you should always move the patient in the direction of the long axis of the body.

❑ Nonemergency moves are performed when there is no immediate threat to the patient's life and are usually performed with other providers.

❑ The direct ground lift and the extremity lift are examples of nonemergency moves.

❑ To move a supine patient from a bed to a wheeled stretcher, you can use the direct carry or the draw sheet method.

❑ A patient should not be repositioned unless necessary.

❑ An unresponsive, breathing, nontrauma patient should be placed in the recovery position.

❑ A patient who is having difficulty breathing or who has chest pain should be allowed to remain in a position of comfort. Nauseous or vomiting patients should also remain in a position of comfort.

❑ Log rolling is a technique to move a patient from a prone position to a supine position.

❑ Transporting agencies may require your help with transporting equipment, which might include wheeled stretchers, portable stretchers, scoop stretchers, basket stretchers, stair chairs, long backboards, short backboards, and vest-type devices.

❑ Rapid extrication is a technique used to remove a critical patient from a vehicle when time is of the essence. This will generally require at least three if not four providers.

Key Terms

Basket stretcher A device that a patient can be placed into and then lifted over rough terrain or to different levels.

Body mechanics The movement and positioning required to make a physical movement. Using proper body mechanics can prevent injury.

Emergency move Any move that is initiated because there is an immediate danger to the patient and provider.

Log roll A technique for moving a patient by rolling him or her onto the side to insert a device underneath the patient or to move the patient from a prone position to a supine position.

Long backboard A device that is long enough for a person's entire body to be completely immobilized as a single unit.

Nonemergency move The type of move that is designed to provide the best care of the patient in a controlled, safe environment.

Portable stretcher A piece of equipment that can easily carry patients down stairs or over rough terrain.

Power grip A way to hold your hands on something that you are lifting to have the most effective lifting technique.

Power lift A lifting technique used to lift heavy objects; the positioning emphasizes proper body mechanics.

Rapid extrication The rapid removal of a critical patient out of a vehicle; requires at least three providers.

Recovery position Position that places a patient on his or her side, keeping the airway open and allowing easy access to the airway. Unresponsive, breathing, nontrauma patients are placed in this position.

Scoop stretcher A patient-lifting device that can be separated into two halves and placed under the patient and then reconnected.

Short backboard Device that allows immobilization of the spine of a patient who is in a sitting position.

Stair chair A device that facilitates moving a patient down stairs.

Vest-type device A device that can be strapped to a patient to immobilize the spine; fits like a vest around the patient.

Wheeled stretcher A device that allows a patient to recline while being transported; generally used in ambulances.

First Responder NSC Objectives
COGNITIVE OBJECTIVES

- Define body mechanics.
- Discuss the guidelines and safety precautions that need to be followed when lifting a patient.
- Describe the indications for an emergency move.
- Describe the indications for assisting in nonemergency moves.
- Discuss the various devices associated with moving a patient in the out-of-hospital arena.

AFFECTIVE OBJECTIVES

- Explain the rationale for properly lifting and moving patients.
- Explain the rationale for an emergency move.

PSYCHOMOTOR OBJECTIVES

- Demonstrate an emergency move.
- Demonstrate the use of equipment to move patients in the out-of-hospital arena.

Check your understanding

Please refer to p. 439 for the answers to these questions.

1. List four principles of good body mechanics used in lifting.
   A. _____
   B. _____
   C. _____
   D. _____

2. Give an example of when an emergency move should be used.

   _____

   _____

   _____

   _____

3. The greatest risk to an injured patient in performing an emergency move is _____.

4. An unresponsive patient who is breathing and who does not have any injuries should be placed in the _____ position, in which the patient is lying on his or her _____.

5. The device to which a trauma patient is secured for spinal immobilization is called a/an _____.

6. A device in which a patient can be carried in a sitting position is called a/an _____.

7. Patients who are conscious and do not have injuries should be placed in which of the following positions while awaiting arrival of additional personnel?
   A. Lying on his/her side
   B. Lying on his/her back
   C. Position of comfort for the patient
   D. Recovery position

8. Which of the following is NOT a consideration in determining how much help you may need in moving a patient?
   A. The patient's weight
   B. Your own physical abilities
   C. The terrain and distance over which the patient is to be moved
   D. Disturbing the sleep of those who would be called to help

9. Your patient is a 45-year-old female complaining that she became nauseated and started vomiting a few hours after dinner. She indicates that she has pain in the upper right quadrant of her abdomen. Her airway is clear and her vital signs are normal; she is alert and responds appropriately to all of your questions. Although it seems a bit unusual to you, the patient seems most comfortable on her knees with her head and arms resting on the sofa. This seems to upset her husband, who wants her to get up and lie down on the sofa. While waiting for the arrival of the ambulance, which of the following is the best course of action?
   A. Allow her to remain in that position, monitor her condition, and explain to her husband that it is important for his wife to be as comfortable as possible.
   B. Encourage the patient to get up off the floor and lie on the sofa, assisting her if necessary.
   C. Insist that the patient lie in the recovery position.
   D. Suggest to the patient that she should get up and walk around to take her mind off the pain.

Chapter 7

Airway Management and Ventilation

LESSON GOAL

A patient who is not breathing or does not have an open airway has no chance of survival. The emergency first responder must be prepared to inspect the airway, open and clear the airway, maintain an open airway, and provide appropriate ventilation as needed for adults, children, and infants.

OBJECTIVES

1. Identify the major structures of the respiratory system on a diagram.
2. List the signs of inadequate breathing.
3. Describe the steps in the head-tilt/chin-lift.
4. Relate the mechanism of injury to opening the airway.
5. Describe the steps in the jaw thrust.
6. Describe the importance of having a suction unit ready for immediate use when providing emergency medical care.
7. Describe the techniques of suctioning.
8. Describe how to ventilate a patient with a resuscitation mask or barrier device.
9. Differentiate between providing ventilation for an infant or a child and for an adult.
10. List the steps for providing mouth-to-mouth and mouth-to-stoma ventilation.
11. Describe how to measure and insert oropharyngeal and nasopharyngeal airways.
12. Describe how to clear a foreign body airway obstruction in a responsive adult.
13. Describe how to clear a foreign body airway obstruction in a responsive infant and child with complete obstruction or partial airway obstruction and poor air exchange.
14. Describe how to clear a foreign body airway obstruction in an unresponsive adult.
15. Describe how to clear a foreign body airway obstruction in an unresponsive infant and child.

In the Real World

You are a law enforcement officer with a local police department. You and your partner are patrolling the business district during the evening hours. Around 8:00 PM dispatch sends you to a restaurant in the downtown area for an ambulance assist. You arrive at the scene within 2 minutes from dispatch; you grab your first-response bag and enter the restaurant. One of the wait staff directs you toward the back of the seating area where a group of people are standing around a table. As you approach the table you see a man lying on the floor on his back with another person shaking the man's shoulders and yelling at him. One of the bystanders states that they were eating dinner when the man on the ground started laughing at something that was said. The man then grabbed his throat and started coughing and choking. Just before your arrival the patient slumped to the floor, unconscious. You put on a pair of gloves and kneel at the patient's side. You notice that the patient appears to be in his mid-fifties and is not breathing. You also notice that his face and nail beds are blue in color.

One of the most important actions an emergency first responder can perform is to open a patient's airway and keep it open. The body is an organism consisting of countless specialized cells that make up the muscle, bone, and tissues. Each of these cells needs oxygen and fuel to produce the energy required to perform their specific functions. The cells consume the oxygen and fuel and give off carbon dioxide and waste products. Oxygen enters the body through the respiratory system. The airway must be open to accomplish this essential task. The body normally maintains the airway automatically. However, when a person's level of consciousness decreases because of a traumatic event or medical condition, the body may no longer automatically maintain the airway. Brain cells that do not have an adequate supply of oxygen for 4 to 6 minutes will begin to die. Once enough brain cells die, the body will die. For this reason it is important for you to understand the structure and function of the airway and the respiratory system and relate that knowledge to airway management and ventilation.

The Respiratory System

Air normally enters the body though the nose (and the mouth if the mouth is open). The nose filters the air, warms it to body temperature, and humidifies it. The fine hairs within the nostrils filter out larger particles of dust or other contaminants. The air then passes over small structures that resemble fins on a radiator (turbinates) and that warm and humidify the air.

The pharynx (throat) lies behind the nose and the mouth. It is divided into two parts, the oropharynx and the nasopharynx. The nasopharynx extends from behind the nose to the oropharynx. The oropharynx extends from the rear of the mouth to the upper end of the esophagus (food tube). The epiglottis is a leaf-shaped structure that prevents food, liquids, and foreign matter from entering the trachea (windpipe) while swallowing. The larynx (voice box) contains the vocal cords. Air moving over the vocal cords creates vibrations. You turn these vibrations into words by controlling your vocal cords. The 9-inch-long trachea is made of flexible cartilage and looks like a corrugated pipe. It connects the upper airway to the lungs. The lungs are made up of a complex system of tubes that branch off and decrease in size until the air is delivered to the alveoli (air sacs). These alveoli are encircled by capillaries (blood vessels) that transport oxygen to the cells of the body. Transfer of oxygen and carbon dioxide between the air and the blood takes place where the alveoli and capillaries meet. This transfer of gases is termed respiration. This action should be differentiated from **ventilation,** which refers to the mechanical movement of inhalation and exhalation to move air in and out of the lungs. **Hypoxia** is the term used when the body's cells are not receiving adequate oxygen through the processes of ventilation and respiration. Fig. 7-1 gives an overview of the anatomy of the respiratory system.

The mechanics of breathing (ventilation) rely on pressure changes that occur within the chest. The brain receives signals from receptors in the blood that are sensitive to carbon dioxide and oxygen levels. An increase in carbon dioxide level or a decrease in oxygen level in the blood signals the brain to increase the respiratory rate (rate of breathing). When you run up a flight of stairs, for example, your muscles require more oxygen, and a signal is sent to increase your respiratory rate.

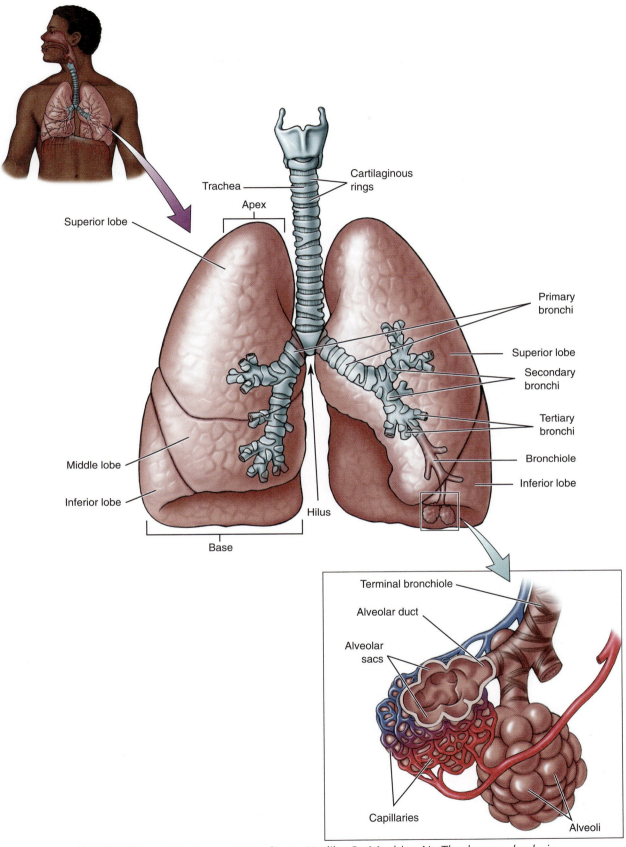

Fig. 7-1 The respiratory system. (From Herlihy B, Maebius N: *The human body in health and illness,* ed 2, Philadelphia, 2003, Saunders.)

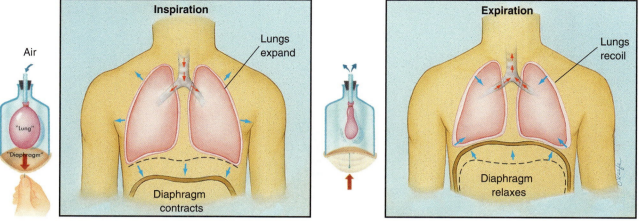

Fig. 7-2 The process of ventilation. (From Thibodeau G, Patton K: *Structure & function of the body,* ed 11, St Louis, 2000, Mosby.)

The lungs are protected within the semirigid structure created by the ribs and sternum. Between the chest and the abdomen lies a large muscle called the diaphragm. The diaphragm moves down and the chest moves out, causing the lungs to expand and creating a negative pressure in the chest. This causes inspiration and brings air into the lungs. Once the air reaches the alveoli, the oxygen is transferred to the red blood cells and carbon dioxide is passed back from the red blood cells to the alveoli. On expiration the diaphragm moves up, the chest moves inward, and air is exhaled. This cycle takes place approximately 18,000 times a day (Fig. 7-2).

A—Airway
Opening the Airway

When first approaching a patient, it is necessary to assess for responsiveness. You do this by asking the patient questions such as, "Are you okay?" If there is a verbal response, the patient has an open airway. If there is no response to your questions, you should gently tap the patient's shoulder. If there is still no response, you should assume that the patient is unconscious. One of the most important actions that you, as an emergency first responder, can perform is to open the airway of an unresponsive patient. When a patient becomes unconscious, the tongue may become flaccid (limp) and fall back into the airway (Fig. 7-3). If this is not corrected within a very short time, irreparable brain damage and death may occur. Simply opening the airway can alleviate this obstruction. Since the tongue is attached to the lower jaw, moving the jaw forward will move the tongue out of the airway.

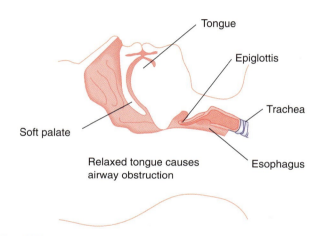

Fig. 7-3 In an unconscious patient, the tongue may fall into the back of the airway. (From McSwain N, Paturas J: *The basic EMT: comprehensive prehospital patient care,* ed 2, St Louis, 2003, Mosby.)

Head-Tilt/Chin-Lift

The best method for opening the airway in uninjured, unresponsive patients is the **head-tilt/chin-lift** method. Research has shown that this maneuver provides the most effective airway position. The head-tilt/chin-lift method should not, however, be used with trauma patients. If the cervical spine has been injured, moving the head back in a head-tilt/chin-lift could cause irreversible damage to the spinal cord.

To perform the head-tilt/chin-lift maneuver, you place one hand on the patient's forehead and apply enough pressure to tilt the head back. With your other hand you lift up and pull the patient's jaw forward with your fingers on the bony part of the chin (Fig. 7-4).

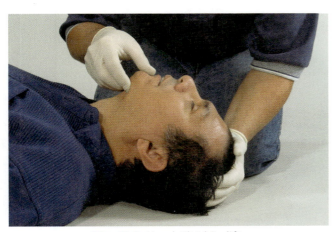

Fig. 7-4 Head-tilt/chin-lift.

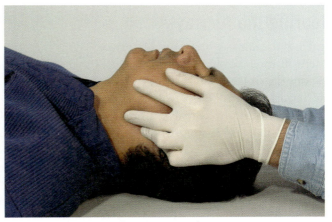

Fig. 7-5 Jaw thrust.

You should exercise the following precautions when using the head-tilt/chin-lift technique:

1. Avoid pressing your fingers deeply into the soft tissues of the chin because this can cause airway obstruction.
2. Avoid using your thumb to lift the chin. Instead you should use your fingers.
3. Keep the patient's mouth open.

Jaw Thrust

The **jaw thrust** without head tilt is an alternative method of opening the airway. This procedure works well but is tiring and technically more difficult than the head-tilt/chin-lift. The jaw thrust without head tilt is the safest technique for patients with suspected spinal injury and should be used as the initial method for establishing an open airway for all unresponsive trauma patients.

To perform a jaw thrust you position yourself behind the patient and place your fingers on the angles of the patient's lower jaw. You then lift with both hands to move the jaw forward. This action moves the tongue out of the way and opens the airway (Fig. 7-5).

Trauma Chin-Lift

A third alternative is the **trauma chin-lift** or the tongue-jaw lift. Like the other manual airway maneuvers, the trauma chin-lift will move the tongue out of the back of the airway. To perform the trauma chin-lift (tongue-jaw lift), you position yourself at the patient's side and grasp the patient's lower jaw with your thumb, placing your fingers beneath the patient's chin. You then pull up on the patient's chin to elevate the jaw and open the mouth (Fig. 7-6).

The disadvantages to this technique include the following:

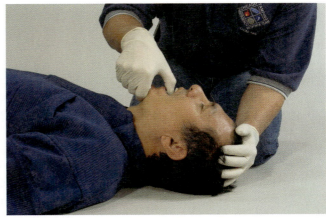

Fig. 7-6 Trauma chin-lift (also called the tongue-jaw lift).

- There is a risk of being bitten if the patient is partially responsive.
- The possibility of tearing a glove on a tooth causes risk to the rescuer.
- The patient's airway cannot be maintained and ventilated by a single provider; therefore two providers are required.

Inspecting the Airway

After the airway is opened, you should inspect the mouth to see if anything is blocking the airway. To perform an airway inspection, you open the patient's mouth with your gloved hand and look inside the mouth to see if it is clear (patent) or blocked by fluids (such as blood, mucus, or vomit), solids (such as food or other foreign objects), or teeth, including dentures. If you see something in the mouth, you should attempt to remove it. At the time of inspecting the airway, you may also note whether there is any air movement from the patient.

Clearing the Airway

Clearing the airway may be as simple as placing the patient in the recovery position, doing a finger sweep of the mouth, or suctioning the oropharynx. All foreign objects including blood, vomitus, teeth, or food should be cleared from the airway immediately, by whatever means possible and as often as needed, to prevent aspiration into the lungs.

The Recovery Position

The recovery position uses the force of gravity to allow fluids to drain from the mouth and helps to keep the airway clear (Fig. 7-7). This position also keeps the tongue from falling back and blocking the airway in an unconscious patient without suspected spinal injuries. To place a supine patient in the recovery position you would do the following:

1. Elevate the patient's left arm above his or her head or place it along the patient's left side with the palm facing his or her left hip. Cross the patient's right leg over his or her left leg.
2. While providing support to the head and neck, grasp the patient's right shoulder and roll the patient toward you. The patient's head should be as close to midline as possible. The head, torso, and shoulders should move simultaneously without excessive movement.
3. The patient should now be on his or her left side. Continue moving the patient off his or her left shoulder and onto the left anterior chest and abdomen area.
4. Bend the patient's right leg at the knee slightly, and place the right leg in front of the left leg for stabilization and comfort.

5. The patient's left arm can be placed at his or her side or left extended with the elbow bent to position the forearm at the top of the patient's head.
6. Place the patient's right hand under the chin and left cheek to help stabilize the head.

This position should be used as the first step to maintain an open airway in an unresponsive patient who is uninjured and breathing adequately.

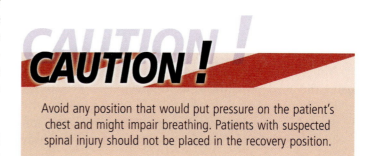

CAUTION!

Avoid any position that would put pressure on the patient's chest and might impair breathing. Patients with suspected spinal injury should not be placed in the recovery position.

Finger Sweeps

If upon inspection of the airway you see foreign material or vomit, it should be quickly removed. To do this, first roll the patient onto his or her side. Then, with a gloved hand, you can sweep out solid objects with one or two fingers. Liquid in the airway can be swept out using a cloth or gauze covering the fingers. Finger sweeps should be the initial method of choice for clearing a patient's mouth of objects. Blind finger sweeps should not be attempted. Blind finger sweeps may push the obstructing object further down into the patient's airway. Use a finger sweep for the infant, child, or adult victim only if the obstructing object can be directly visualized.

Suctioning

If placing a patient in the recovery position or doing a finger sweep is either ineffective or inappropriate (e.g., for a trauma patient), suction may be indicated. Your First Responder equipment and training may include some type of suction unit. If a patient's airway is obstructed by fluid or if the patient is making gurgling noises, you may use a portable suction unit to clear the mouth. Suction units can be manually or battery operated (Fig. 7-8). Suctioning uses negative pressure to keep the airway clear; therefore it is important to remember that while the suction is on, oxygen is not reaching the patient. Instead, oxygen is actually being removed or

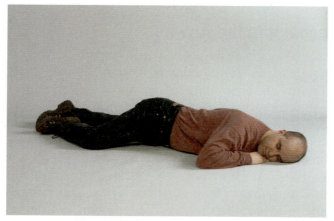

Fig. 7-7 The recovery position.

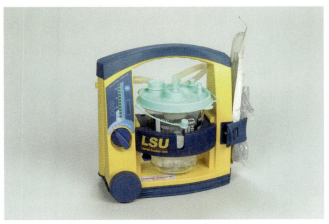

Fig. 7-8 Battery-powered suction unit.

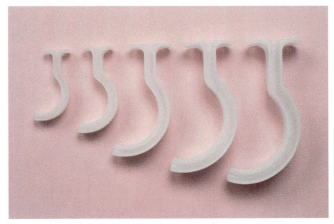

Fig. 7-10 Oropharyngeal airways.

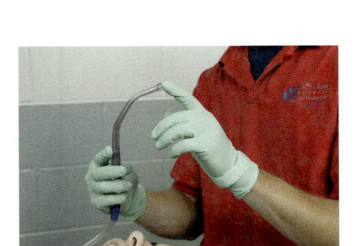

Fig. 7-9 Rigid tonsil-tip suction catheter. (From Chapleau W, Pons P: *Emergency medical technician, making the difference,* St Louis, 2007, Mosby.)

sucked out from the patient's airway at the same time as the obstructing fluids. If the patient has a totally obstructed airway full of blood or vomit, you should suction until the airway is cleared; otherwise, the patient will go too long without oxygen.

To suction the mouth of an unresponsive patient, a hard or rigid tonsil-tip suction catheter is preferred (Fig. 7-9). You should insert the suction catheter into the patient's mouth no deeper than to the base of the patient's tongue. You can measure this distance as the length between the corner of the patient's mouth and the tip of the patient's ear. Suction is applied only as you move the catheter out of the patient's mouth, not while inserting it into the mouth. Suction should never be applied for longer than 15 seconds at a time. After suctioning you should monitor the patient's breathing and pulse and provide ventilation if needed.

Mechanical suction units can be quickly overwhelmed by high volumes of fluid and are inadequate for removing solid objects such as teeth, foreign bodies, or food. To remove solid objects you should place the patient on his or her side and sweep out the mouth with a gloved hand. Then resume suctioning. Similarly, if a semiresponsive patient is actively vomiting but able to maintain his or her own airway, placing the patient in the recovery position will help.

Mechanical Airway Adjuncts

Once the patient's airway is open, it is necessary to maintain the open position. This can be accomplished by continuing to hold the patient's head in a head-tilt/chin-lift or jaw thrust position and by using mechanical airway adjuncts such as an **oropharyngeal airway (OPA)** or a **nasopharyngeal airway (NPA).** It is important to note that while a mechanical airway adjunct can help keep the patient's airway open, it should always be accompanied with a manual airway maneuver such as the head-tilt/chin-lift or the jaw thrust.

Oropharyngeal Airways

The OPA is a disposable device that is inserted into the oral cavity and positioned to move the tongue forward and keep the airway open. OPAs are made of hard plastic and come in many sizes to fit infants through adults (Fig. 7-10). They should be used only in unresponsive patients without a cough or **gag reflex** because patients with a gag reflex may vomit when the OPA is inserted, which could lead to further airway obstruction and other respiratory complications. Proper sizing is important because an OPA of the wrong size can actually *cause* an airway obstruction. An OPA that is too large may push past the oropharynx and cause an

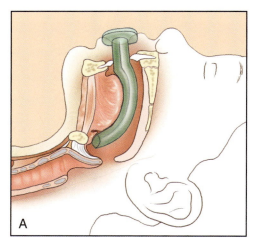

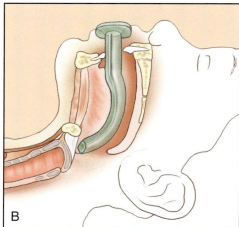

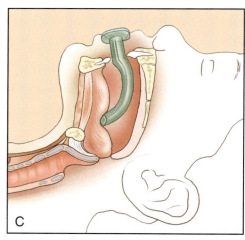

Fig. 7-11 A, A properly sized OPA keeps the tongue out of the airway and opens an effective air passage. **B,** An OPA that is too large may block the airway instead of opening it. **C,** An airway that is too small may not keep the tongue from blocking the airway. (From McSwain N, Paturas J: *The basic EMT: comprehensive prehospital patient care,* 2003 ed 2, St Louis, 2003, Mosby.)

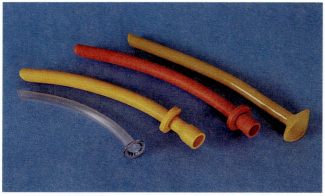

Fig. 7-12 Nasopharyngeal airways. (From McSwain N, Paturas J: *The basic EMT: comprehensive prehospital patient care,* ed 2, St Louis, 2003, Mosby.)

obstruction; one that is too small may push the tongue backward, obstructing the airway (Fig. 7-11). The proper size is selected by comparing the OPA to the distance between the corner of the patient's mouth and the bottom of the earlobe or angle of the jaw. The steps for sizing and inserting an OPA are listed and illustrated in Skill 7-1. If gagging is noted, the OPA should be removed immediately.

An alternative method for inserting an OPA uses a tongue blade. This is recommended for inserting an OPA into the airway of an infant or child. A tongue blade is used to press the tongue down and away. The airway is then gently inserted, with the patient in the upright (anatomical) position.

Nasopharyngeal Airways

An alternative to the OPA is the NPA (Fig. 7-12). This soft, rubbery device serves the same purpose as the OPA, but it bypasses some of the gag reflex nerves at the back of the tongue. Therefore the NPA is less likely to stimulate vomiting. This makes the NPA a good choice for responsive patients who need help keeping their tongue from obstructing the airway. Because your patient will be conscious, you should forewarn him or her that the NPA is lubricated but there may be some discomfort involved while inserting the NPA into the nostril. The technique for inserting an NPA is described and illustrated in Skill 7-2.

Because the NPA may slowly work its way out of the nostril after insertion, you should check for this movement on a regular basis and push it back into place when indicated. The NPA should never be forcefully inserted into the nostril if resistance is met since trauma to the nasal membranes may cause bleeding and further complicate airway management.

Skill 7-1

Inserting an Oropharyngeal Airway

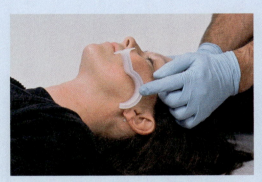

1. Put on appropriate PPE. The OPA should be sized appropriately so it fits between the angle of the patient's jaw, or from the tip of the earlobe to the corner of the patient's lips. (From NAEMT: *PHTLS: Basic and advanced prehospital trauma life support,* ed 6, St Louis, 2007, Mosby.)

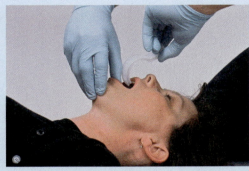

2. Open the patient's mouth by pulling down on the jaw. Insert the airway upside down with the tip facing toward the head. Gently run the tip along the roof of the mouth until it meets resistance. (From NAEMT: *PHTLS: Basic and advanced prehospital trauma life support,* ed 6, St Louis, 2007, Mosby.)

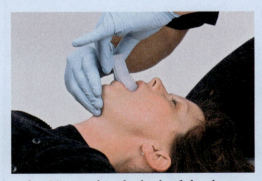

3. Once the OPA reaches the back of the throat, rotate it 180 degrees until the flange is on the teeth, level with the lips. (From NAEMT: *PHTLS: Basic and advanced prehospital trauma life support,* ed 6, St Louis, 2007, Mosby.)

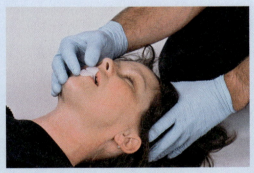

4. The OPA in its final position. If the patient begins to cough or gag at any time during the procedure or after the OPA is inserted, remove the OPA immediately. (From NAEMT: *PHTLS: Basic and advanced prehospital trauma life support,* ed 6, St Louis, 2007, Mosby.)

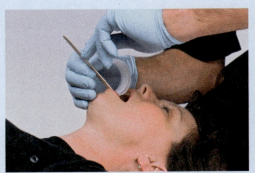

5. An alternative method for inserting an OPA uses a tongue blade and inserts the OPA in its normal anatomical position. (From NAEMT: *PHTLS: Basic and advanced prehospital trauma life support,* ed 6, St Louis, 2007, Mosby.)

Skill 7-2

Inserting a Nasopharyngeal Airway

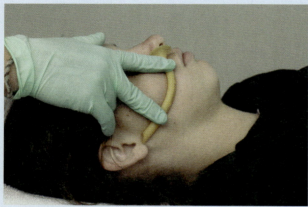

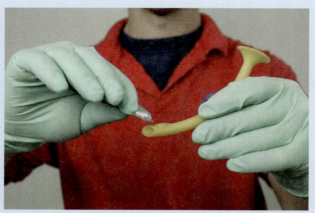

1. Put on appropriate PPE. Select the correct size NPA. Measure from the corner of the patient's jaw to the tip of the nose or from the tip of the patient's nose to the earlobe. Pick an NPA that is the same length. (From Chapleau W, Pons P: *Emergency medical technician, making the difference,* St Louis, 2007, Mosby.)

2. Inspect the nostrils for size and obstruction. Make sure the diameter of the NPA is not larger than the nostril. Use a water-soluble lubricant such as K-Y Jelly on the NPA; this will help it slide into a tight opening. Never use a petroleum-based lubricant like Vaseline. (From Chapleau W, Pons P: *Emergency medical technician, making the difference,* St Louis, 2007, Mosby.)

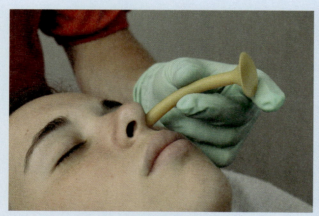

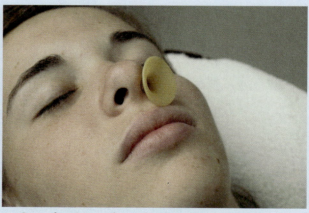

3. Insert the NPA into the right nostril first; the design generally makes insertion in this nostril easier. Insert the NPA posteriorly with the bevel toward the base of the nostril or the septum. Insert the NPA directly toward the back of the head. If you feel resistance, use slightly firmer forward and backward pressure while rotating the NPA slightly. Do not use excessive force. Stop the insertion and remove the NPA if the patient complains of pain versus discomfort. (From Chapleau W, Pons P: *Emergency medical technician, making the difference,* St Louis, 2007, Mosby.)

4. Once the airway clears the nostril, you will feel a decrease in resistance. Continue to insert the NPA until the flange of the NPA is touching the nostril. If the airway cannot be inserted into one nostril, try the other. (From Chapleau W, Pons P: *Emergency medical technician, making the difference,* St Louis, 2007, Mosby.)

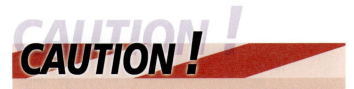

Be careful not to insert the airway in an upward movement toward the top of the patient's head.

B—Breathing

After ensuring that the airway is open, the next step is to look, listen, and feel for whether your patient is breathing. Look to see if the chest is rising and falling, listen for the sounds of breathing, and feel for any breaths against your cheek. By placing your ear next to the patient's nose and mouth and looking at the chest you can evaluate whether an unresponsive patient is breathing (Fig. 7-13).

Breathing is normally effortless. You do not walk into a room and nudge your partner and say, "Hey, did you notice that everyone is breathing in here?" Anything that draws your attention to the fact that someone is breathing is most probably a sign of distress. **Stridor,** a high-pitched whistling-type sound as a patient breathes in, indicates probable obstruction of the upper airways (between the pharynx and the vocal cords). **Wheezing** sounds, on the other hand, indicate obstruction (blood or other fluid) of the lower airways and are generally heard when a patient exhales. Other signs of distress include positioning (having to sit or stand) or the use of accessory muscles (neck and chest wall muscles). In other words, anything that indicates the patient is working harder to breathe is a sign of difficulty breathing (**dyspnea**). Respiratory arrest or the total lack of breathing is the most critical finding.

If a patient is able to speak and respond to your questions, you can assume he or she is breathing. However, as noted previously, it is also important to note the effort of breathing. If the patient seems out of breath or is only able to speak in short bursts of phrases, this is evidence of increased effort to breathe or respiratory distress (Box 7-1).

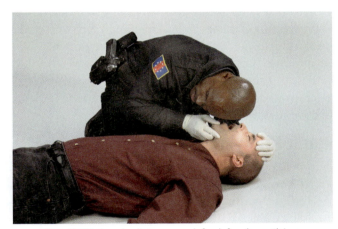

Fig. 7-13 Look, listen, and feel for breathing.

BOX 7-1   Signs of Respiratory Distress

- *Posture.* Patients will sit up or stand to breathe easier. It may be nearly impossible for them to breathe while lying down.
- *Speech.* Patients with significant respiratory distress will be unable to speak in complete sentences. They will only have enough breath to speak in short word bursts.
- *Muscle use.* Patients in respiratory distress will often use the muscles of the upper chest and neck when trying to catch their breath.
- *Changes in vital signs.* As the patient gets closer to respiratory failure, pulse and even respiratory rates will drop as the patient exhibits increasing fatigue brought on by the extra effort to breathe, and hypoxia. Skin color that is bluish can indicate hypoxia.

In the Real World—continued

You open the patient's airway with a head-tilt/chin-lift method and check for breathing. After confirming that the patient is not breathing, you use your pocket mask and attempt to ventilate. While you attempt ventilations, your partner contacts the responding ambulance and gives them an update on the patient. Your attempt to ventilate the patient is unsuccessful. You reposition the patient's head and again attempt to ventilate him, without success.

In unresponsive patients, you will need to examine the airway and check for breathing. A patient who is not breathing has only the oxygen that was already in his or her lungs and blood when breathing stopped. If the patient is not breathing, you must effectively breathe for them to prevent death. This is called **rescue breathing,** or ventilation, and refers to using your own exhaled air or other mechanical methods to give the patient's lungs oxygen. In the past, mouth-to-mouth ventilation was the first and only method of ventilation. Although this is still an effective emergency ventilation technique, the risk from contact with the patient's body fluids presents a potential health risk for the rescuer and should be avoided whenever possible as the only means of providing ventilations by a trained rescuer. A safer method is to use a **pocket mask** with a one-way valve or a **barrier device.** When treating patients as an emergency first responder, you should *always* practice body substance isolation (BSI) precautions. Barrier devices and masks serve the same purpose but the pocket mask with a one-way valve offers better protection to the rescuer and provides a more effective method of ventilation.

Mouth-to-Mask Ventilation

The pocket mask with a one-way valve provides a safe barrier between you and your patient. It is constructed of semirigid plastic with a soft, air-filled cuff. The mask should be transparent so you can watch for vomiting. The cuff should create a seal when you push it firmly against the patient's face. The mask has a one-way valve to divert the patient's exhalations. It may also have a supplemental oxygen inlet. Tubing that connects this inlet with an oxygen tank is used to provide a higher concentration of oxygen to the patient. Skill 7-3 lists and illustrates the steps for rescue breathing with a mouth-to-mask device.

Mouth-to-Barrier Ventilation

Barrier devices place a layer of thin film with a filter or valve between you and the patient. Barrier devices offer variable levels of protection based on their design. While the barrier device may prevent transmission of disease, it still requires very close contact with the patient. Barrier devices have no exhalation valve and air often leaks around the seal. A barrier device should present little resistance to your ventilation. The advantage of the barrier device is its compact size; some can even fit on a key ring (Fig. 7-14). As an emergency first responder, you should keep a clean pocket mask or barrier device readily available for any emergency. Skill 7-4 lists and illustrates the steps for rescue breathing with a mouth-to-barrier device.

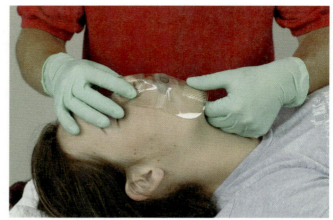

Fig. 7-14 Mouth-to-barrier device. (From Chapleau W, Pons P: *Emergency medical technician, making the difference,* St Louis, 2007, Mosby.)

TABLE 7-1   Rescue Breathing

	INFANT	CHILD	ADULT
Rate (breaths/ minute)	12-20	12-20	10-12
Time (seconds)	1	1	1

Mouth-to-Mouth Ventilation

Mouth-to-mouth ventilation is an effective method to deliver an adequate volume of air to a nonbreathing patient. Although it does not provide a high concentration of oxygen, the ease of obtaining an adequate seal and the overall quickness of getting into position, opening the airway, and breathing have shown it to be the most effective single-provider method for rescue breathing for a nonbreathing patient. However, to decrease the risk of exposure for the trained rescuer, this method is not recommended. The steps for rescue breathing with the mouth-to-mouth method are listed and illustrated in Skill 7-5. Table 7-1 summarizes the differences in rescue breathing between adults, children, and infants. If you are unable to provide mouth-to-mouth ventilation to a victim of cardiopulmonary arrest for any reason, give high-quality chest compressions without ventilations until more help arrives.

Foreign Body Airway Obstruction in Adults

Rescue breathing on a patient may not be successful. For example, if you did not see the chest rise and fall

Skill 7-3

Mouth-to-Mask Ventilation

1. Put on appropriate PPE. Position yourself at the patient's head and maintain an open airway through the use of manual or mechanical techniques.

2. Place the mask over the patient's nose and mouth. The pointed part of the mask should be over the nose with the wider part of the mask on the chin.

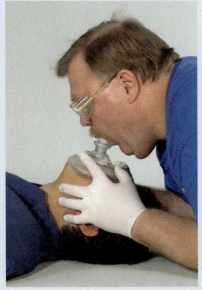

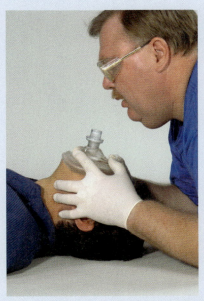

3. Place both of your hands on the mask while grasping the patient's jaw. Lift up slightly on the jaw while pressing on the mask to maintain a good seal between the mask and the patient's face.

4. Take in a normal breath, place your mouth over the mouthpiece, and breathe evenly into the patient's mouth for 1 second so you can visualize the rise of the chest.

5. Remove your mouth from the mouthpiece and allow the patient to exhale. Continue rescue breathing for the patient at a rate of 1 breath every 5 to 6 seconds (10 to 12 breaths per minute) for an adult or 1 breath every 3 to 5 seconds (12 to 20 breaths per minute) for an infant or child.

6. Continue to maintain an open airway and watch for any signs that the patient has vomited or has started breathing on his or her own.

Skill 7-4

Mouth-to-Barrier Ventilation

1. Put on appropriate PPE. Position yourself at the patient's head and maintain an open airway through the use of manual or mechanical techniques.

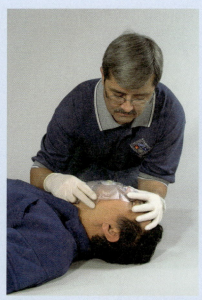

2. Place the barrier device over the patient's mouth.

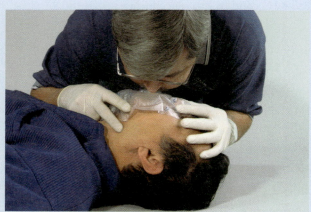

3. Place your mouth over the mouthpiece, pinch the nostrils, and breathe slowly into the patient's mouth over 1 second for an adult and 1 second for an infant or child. The delivery of your breath should cause the patient's chest to visibly rise.

4. Remove your mouth from the mouthpiece and release the patient's nose to allow the patient to exhale. Continue rescue breathing for the patient at a rate of 1 breath every 5 to 6 seconds for an adult or 1 breath every 3 to 5 seconds for an infant or child.

5. Continue to maintain an open airway and watch for any signs that the patient has vomited or has started breathing on his or her own.

Skill 7-5

Mouth-to-Mouth Ventilation

1. Put on appropriate PPE. Position yourself at the patient's head and maintain an open airway through the use of manual or mechanical techniques.

2. Place your mouth over the patient's mouth and pinch the patient's nose with your fingers.

3. Give each breath over 1 second for infant, child, or adult victims. The delivery of your breath should cause the patient's chest to visibly rise; avoid hyperventilation. For an infant, you may be able to place your mouth over both the infant's mouth and nose.

4. Remove your mouth and release the patient's nose to allow the patient to exhale. Continue rescue breathing for the patient at a rate of 1 breath every 5 to 6 seconds (10 to 12 breaths per minute) for an adult or 1 breath every 3 to 5 seconds (12 to 20 breaths per minute) for an infant or child.

5. Continue to maintain an open airway and watch for any signs that the patient has vomited or has started breathing on his or her own.

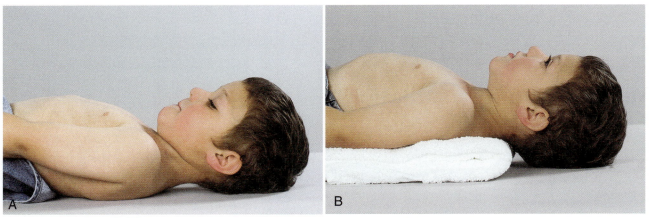

Fig. 7-15 A, Child without padding under shoulders. This position can block the airway. **B,** Child with padding under shoulders. This position opens up the airway.

with your rescue breath, or if you felt resistance against your breath entering the patient's airway, you can assume that the patient is not receiving the oxygen you are giving him or her. The patient may be choking on food or other foreign material or experiencing an airway obstruction caused by bleeding into the airway or vomiting. This is called a **foreign body airway obstruction (FBAO)**. If FBAO is not relieved quickly, it can result in cardiac arrest (see Chapter 9). Airway obstruction can be described as either partial or complete. Partial airway obstruction causes inadequate respirations that will not allow sufficient oxygen to reach the blood. With partial airway obstruction, the patient is coughing or gagging. This noise indicates that the patient is moving some air around the obstruction. Complete airway obstruction blocks any air from entering or exiting the lungs; therefore the patient cannot cough or speak.

Partial Airway Obstruction

If the patient is conscious, confirm that an airway obstruction exists. Ask the patient, "Are you choking?" or "Can you speak?" If the patient can respond verbally or can cough, the airway is partially obstructed. You should not intervene in this situation but should instead encourage the patient to continue coughing. The patient is still breathing around the obstruction and coughing will most likely expel the foreign object and relieve the obstruction. If the object is not expelled through coughing, you should ensure that the patient is transported to a medical facility for further treatment. You should also keep the patient within your sight. A patient with a partial airway obstruction can progress to a complete airway obstruction or become unconscious. In these situations, you must intervene.

Complete Airway Obstruction

If the patient is unable to speak and there is no air exchange, there is a complete airway obstruction. In this situation, abdominal thrusts are given to clear the obstruction. The steps to follow for performing abdominal thrusts are listed and illustrated in Skill 7-6. If the patient becomes unconscious, position the patient on his or her back and follow the steps listed in Skill 7-7.

Special Considerations
Infants and Children

The airways in infants and children are different from adult airways in that they are smaller and narrower. The tongue of an infant or a child is larger and takes up more space than in the adult airway. These anatomical differences make the airway of an infant or child more susceptible to obstruction. The less developed trachea is more flexible than an adult's, and the chest wall is more pliable. You must be aware of these differences when treating an infant or child. The primary cause of cardiac arrest in children is an uncorrected respiratory problem.

Infants and small children also have larger heads in proportion to their bodies. This can cause the neck to become hyperflexed and close off the airway. To prevent this problem, you should place a folded towel or your hand underneath the infant's or child's shoulders. This holds the airway in the correct position (Fig. 7-15). Another potential problem is hyperextension of the airway, crimping it off. To prevent this, carefully position the head in the sniffing position as shown in

Skill 7-6

Complete Foreign Body Obstruction (Conscious Adult)

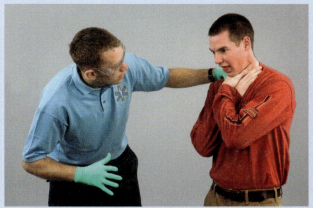

1. Ask the patient, "Are you choking?" or "Can you speak?" If there is no response, assume a complete airway obstruction. (From Henry M, Stapleton E: *EMT prehospital care,* ed 4, St Louis, 2000, Mosby.)

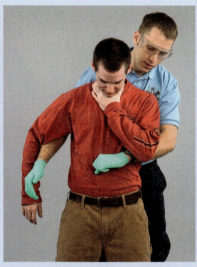

2. Position yourself behind the patient. Wrap your arms around the patient, placing the thumb side of one hand above the navel but below the patient's xiphoid process. (From Henry M, Stapleton E: *EMT prehospital care,* ed 4, St Louis, 2000, Mosby.)

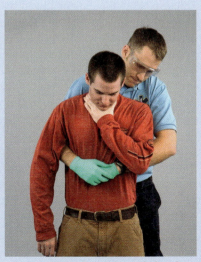

3. Place your second hand on top of the first and apply pressure in an inward and upward thrust. Repeat the thrusts until the object is expelled or the patient becomes unconscious. If the patient becomes unconscious, follow the steps of Skill 7-7. (From Henry M, Stapleton E: *EMT prehospital care,* ed 4, St Louis, 2000, Mosby.)

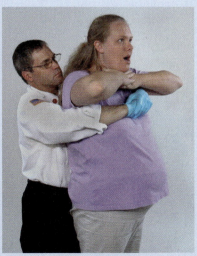

4. If the patient is obese or pregnant, you should use chest thrusts instead of abdominal thrusts. Place your arms around the patient's chest, under the patient's armpits. Give quick backward thrusts into the middle of the patient's sternum. Repeat the thrusts until the object is expelled or the patient becomes unconscious. (From Chapleau W: *Emergency first responder: making the difference,* St Louis, 2004, Mosby.)

Skill 7-7

Foreign Body Airway Obstruction (Unconscious Adult)

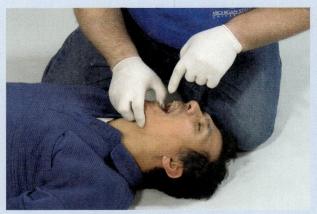

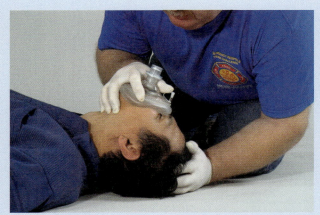

1. Open the patient's airway using either a head-tilt/chin-lift or trauma chin-lift; look for the foreign body airway obstruction. If you see the object, turn the victim's head to the side and gently remove the object using a finger sweep motion.

2. Open the airway and attempt to give a single ventilation. If you cannot ventilate after the first attempt, reposition the patient's head, open the airway, and try again to ventilate.

3. If your breaths do not go in, immediately begin chest compressions in the middle of the patient's chest, using the same technique as you would for CPR. Give 30 chest compressions before stopping to attempt ventilation again.

4. Following the 30 chest compressions, open the airway and look for the obstruction. If you are able to visualize the obstruction, turn the patient's head to the side and remove the object using a finger sweep motion. Attempt to ventilate the patient by giving two breaths. If you are able to ventilate the patient, assess for circulation by feeling for a carotid pulse. If the patient does not have a pulse, immediately begin CPR with 30 chest compressions. If the patient does have a pulse, support ventilations by giving rescue breaths until the patient begins to breathe spontaneously. Once the patient is breathing adequately, assist the patient into the recovery position and continue to monitor the patient's vital signs and assist as needed. If your service does not provide transport, stay with the patient until EMS arrives to take care of the patient.

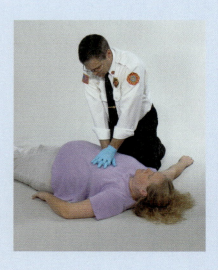

5. The sequence is the same for pregnant or obese patients.

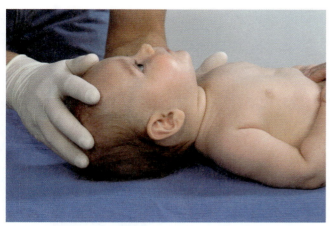

Fig. 7-16 Infant in the sniffing position.

Fig. 7-16. These potential problems are due to the flexibility of the immature trachea. See Chapter 14 for further discussion of the differences between pediatric and adult patients.

Foreign Body Airway Obstruction

For children older than age 1 year, the procedure for clearing a foreign body airway obstruction (FBAO) is the same as that for an adult but is performed with less force. In infants younger than 1 year of age, you should confirm that the airway is obstructed by observing for air movement and adequate breathing. A child's inability to cry can be a key indicator of a complete airway obstruction. If a complete obstruction is present and the child is conscious, position yourself behind the child and administer abdominal thrusts. Continue thrusts until the obstruction is dislodged or the child becomes unconscious. If the child becomes unconscious, open the airway using the head-tilt/chin-lift, and look into the mouth (Fig. 7-17). If you can see a foreign body, remove it using a finger sweep. If the obstruction is not visible, do not perform a finger sweep but attempt to ventilate. If this fails, reposition the head and attempt ventilation a second time. If you still cannot ventilate the child, immediately begin 5 cycles, or about 2 minutes, of cardiopulmonary resuscitation (CPR). CPR for the FBAO victim is performed in the same manner as regular CPR except open the victim's airway wide before each breath and look for the obstruction. If the obstruction is visible, remove it using a finger sweep and then attempt to ventilate the victim. Continue with CPR unless the child begins to breathe spontaneously. If the child still cannot breathe after 5 cycles of CPR, call Emergency Medical Services (EMS) and then continue CPR until EMS arrives.

In infants up to age 1 year you should confirm that the airway is obstructed by observing for air movement and an inability to cry. If an airway obstruction is present, sit or kneel with the infant in your lap to provide more stability. Place the baby face down, straddling your arm, and cradle

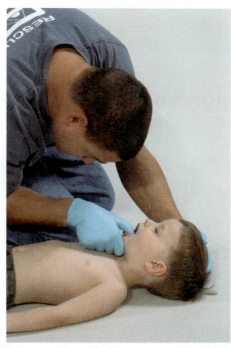

Fig. 7-17 Tongue-jaw lift (or trauma chin-lift) in a child.

the baby's face with your hand. The baby's head should be slightly lower than the chest, allowing gravity to help dislodge the obstruction. Using the heel of one hand, administer five back slaps between the infant's shoulder blades. Back slaps should be given with enough force to dislodge the foreign body but not so much force as to cause injury to the child. Immediately following the back slaps, sandwich the baby between your arms, roll the baby over, and administer five chest compressions. Chest compressions are performed in a similar manner to those required for cardiopulmonary resuscitation (see Chapter 9). Give the five compressions just below the nipple line, over about 1 second each, and with enough force to dislodge the foreign body. This sequence is repeated until the airway obstruction is relieved or the infant becomes unconscious.

If the infant becomes unresponsive, place the infant on a hard surface and begin CPR. First, open the airway and assess for breathing. Look in the infant's airway, and if the foreign body is visible remove it using a finger sweep. Never perform a blind finger sweep on any victim regardless of age. Once you have opened the airway, whether you were able or unable to remove the obstruction, assess for breathing and attempt to ventilate if the infant is not spontaneously breathing. Give two rescue breaths and watch for a rising chest. Next begin the steps of CPR, giving 30 continuous compressions and 2 breaths, except before the breaths look into the airway first for the obstruction and remove it if you see it. After 2 minutes or about 5 cycles of 30:2 CPR, activate Emergency Medical Services (EMS). Skill 7-8 lists and illustrates the steps to relieve an FBAO in an unconscious infant.

Skill 7-8

Foreign Body Airway Obstruction (Unconscious Infant)

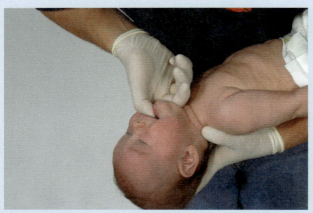

1. Position the infant on a firm, flat surface. Open the airway using a head-tilt/chin-lift or trauma chin-lift to inspect the mouth for a foreign object. If one is visible, use a finger sweep to clear it.

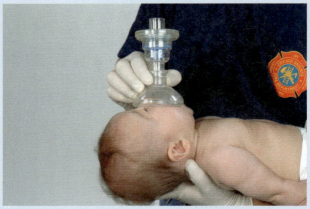

2. Open the airway and attempt to ventilate the infant. If the attempt fails, reposition the head and make another attempt to ventilate the infant.

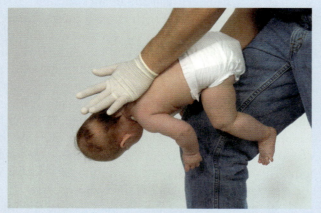

3. If ventilation is still unsuccessful, begin CPR by giving 30 compressions. After each cycle of 30 compressions, perform 1 extra step by opening the infant's airway and looking for the foreign body airway obstruction (FBAO). If you can visualize the object, remove it; if not, attempt to ventilate the infant again.

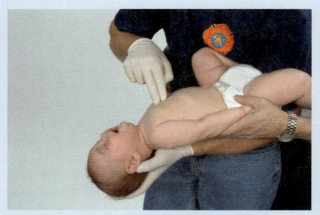

4. Repeat steps 2 and 3 until the object is removed.

5. Ensure that EMS has been activated. If you are alone, activate EMS after 5 cycles of CPR (about 2 minutes).

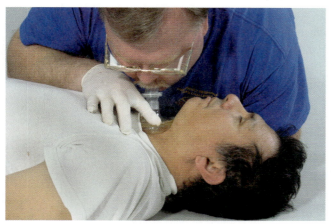

Fig. 7-18 Mouth-to-stoma breathing.

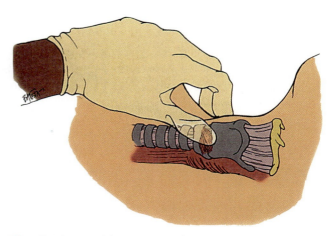

Fig. 7-19 Cricoid pressure. (From Sanders M: *Mosby's paramedic textbook,* revised ed 2, St Louis, 2001, Mosby.)

MOUTH-TO-STOMA VENTILATION

Because of illness or injury some patients may have had surgery to create an opening to their airway through the neck. A hole created in the neck that the patient breathes through is called a stoma. In order to breathe for these patients a seal must be maintained with the surface of the patient's neck around the stoma. Ventilations can be accomplished with these patients by placing a pediatric-sized mask or a barrier device over the stoma (Fig. 7-18). Rescue breathing is then accomplished using the same techniques as previously described except that the patient's nose is not pinched.

DENTURES

Dentures that are firmly held in place in the patient's mouth should be left intact. The dentures will actually help form the patient's mouth to create a better seal with a mask device. If, however, dentures or any other dental appliance are loose, they should be removed. Loose dentures or dental appliances could completely dislodge and obstruct the patient's airway. As an emergency first responder, you should continuously reassess the mouth of the patient who has dental appliances to ensure that the appliances have not come loose.

GASTRIC INFLATION/VOMITING

Although rescue breathing or assisting someone's ventilations can be necessary, it can also lead to air being pushed into the patient's stomach, causing it to bulge out. This is termed gastric inflation. Gastric inflation can cause the patient to vomit, which can lead to a further compromised airway. If you notice gastric inflation, you should do the following:

- Attempt to reposition the patient's head to allow air to flow more effectively into the lungs rather than the stomach.
- Make sure breaths are not being delivered too forcefully. Deliver breaths with only enough pressure to make the chest rise—no more. Rescue breathing with more pressure than it takes to make the chest rise will force air into the stomach, causing gastric inflation.
- Be prepared in case the patient vomits. You may need to roll the patient onto his or her side, perform a finger sweep, or suction the airway. If the patient vomits, the airway must be cleared before attempting to ventilate. Failure to do so can cause the material to be pushed into the lungs, causing further respiratory problems.
- You should never push on an inflated stomach to release the air as this may further harm the patient or cause the patient to vomit.

CRICOID PRESSURE

Cricoid pressure, or the Sellick maneuver, is a technique used to collapse the esophagus between the trachea and the cervical spine (Fig. 7-19). This maneuver prevents air from flowing into the stomach when rescue breaths or ventilations are given. Once cricoid pressure is applied it should not be released until the airway is secured with an advanced tube (see Team Work section). To apply cricoid pressure in a nonresponsive patient you should do the following:

1. Locate the patient's Adam's apple with your index finger.

2. Slide your finger down to the base of the Adam's apple.
3. Find the cricoid cartilage, which is the prominent horizontal ring at the base of the Adam's apple.
4. Use the tips of your index finger and thumb to apply firm backward pressure on the cricoid cartilage.

Cricoid pressure may be used when providing ventilations to a deeply unconscious patient and/or when an advanced airway is being inserted (see Team Work section). Applying and maintaining cricoid pressure will require additional help if one rescuer is ventilating and the other is performing chest compressions.

In the Real World—Conclusion

You suspect that the unresponsive patient has an occluded airway and position yourself to perform CPR. After 1 cycle of 30 chest compressions, a clump of food is dislodged from the patient's airway. After turning the patient on his side you use a finger sweep technique to clear the airway. You again attempt mouth-to-mask ventilations with success this time. After your initial ventilations you check for a pulse and find a strong, rapid carotid pulse. You continue to perform rescue ventilations with the pocket mask until the ambulance crew arrives a couple of minutes later.

The patient remains unresponsive and not breathing, so with the EMTs you assist with the placement of an oropharyngeal airway (OPA) and continue rescue ventilations with a bag-mask device and supplemental oxygen. The EMTs prepare to perform endotracheal intubation. After assembling their equipment, the EMT at the head of the patient asks you to stop ventilations while she attempts intubation. The intubation is successful, and you continue to ventilate the intubated patient once every 6 to 8 seconds while the EMTs check for tube placement, secure the tube, and prepare the patient for transport.

Team Work

First Responders may also be called upon to administer oxygen or assist other health care providers in providing oxygen or assisting with more advanced airway management. It is important to understand the principles behind these techniques to assist others more effectively.

OXYGEN ADMINISTRATION

Oxygen is necessary for life; a total lack of oxygen will cause certain death within a short time. Patients who have certain medical conditions or traumatic injuries may not have a total lack of oxygen but may not have sufficient oxygen circulating in their blood to support the body. Health care providers therefore often provide supplemental oxygen.

Oxygen Cylinders

Oxygen commonly comes in small portable tanks for use by emergency first responders. Larger tanks are mounted in ambulances to provide an adequate supply during transport. Smaller portable tanks that can be carried to the scene are made of steel or aluminum and are pressurized to approximately 2200 pounds per square inch (psi) when full. A gauge on the regulator attached to an oxygen tank gives the tank pressure (and therefore an indication of fullness) when the tank is turned on (Fig. 7-20). The sizes of tanks and the volumes they can hold are listed in Table 7-2.

The pressure in the tanks must be reduced before the oxygen can be administered to a patient. The regulator-flowmeter assembly reduces the pressure to 50 psi and provides a way to regulate the flow to the normal 2 to 15 liters per minute (LPM). Some special regulators can provide up to 25 LPM for use with a bag-mask device. Safety is a concern when using oxygen, and the following cautions should be observed:

1. Do not allow open flames anywhere near oxygen or oxygen equipment.
2. Do not allow grease or any other combustible material to touch the valves, fittings, or tanks.
3. Use only oxygen tanks, valves, or hoses. Do not use equipment made for other types of gas.
4. Always secure oxygen equipment to prevent it from becoming damaged.

Team Work—cont'd

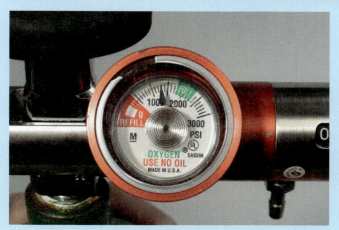

Fig. 7-20 The pressure gauge on an oxygen cylinder indicates the fullness of the cylinder. A full cylinder will read 2200 psi.

TABLE 7-2	Cylinder Sizes and Volumes
CYLINDER SIZE	**VOLUME CAPACITY (L)**
D cylinder	350
E cylinder	625
M cylinder	3000
G cylinder	3500
H cylinder	6900

5. Always make sure all fittings and hoses are securely fitted.

Skill 7-9 lists and illustrates how to prepare an oxygen cylinder.

Oxygen Delivery Devices

A common oxygen administration device used in prehospital settings is the **nonrebreather mask** (NRBM). This mask differs from a standard mask in its one-way valve and reservoir bag (Fig. 7-21). This reservoir bag accumulates oxygen while the patient exhales and allows 90% to 100% concentration to be delivered to the patient.

To apply the NRBM to a patient, do the following:

1. Attach it to the tank and turn on the tank.
2. Adjust the flowmeter to 12 to 15 LPM.

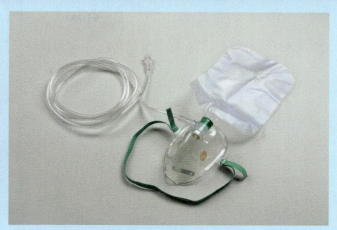

Fig. 7-21 Nonrebreather mask.

3. Place your finger over the one-way valve on the inside of the mask and inflate the reservoir bag fully.
4. With oxygen flowing, place the mask over the patient's mouth and nose. Adjust the elastic strap so a tight but comfortable fit is obtained.

To obtain near-100% concentration, the flow rate must be adjusted to keep the reservoir bag inflated during inspiration (Fig. 7-22).

A pediatric NRBM is used in much the same way except that the flow rate is decreased to keep the reservoir bag inflated only during inhalation.

The **nasal cannula** is another common device used in prehospital care. A nasal cannula is used for a patient who cannot tolerate having a mask over his or her face (Fig. 7-23). This claustrophobic feeling is common in patients who are having problems breathing, although your reassurance may help them overcome this feeling. The nasal cannula provides approximately 24% to 40% oxygen when administered at 2 to 6 LPM. Flow rates more than 6 LPM will cause discomfort to the patient and will not increase the oxygen concentration (Fig. 7-24). To apply the nasal cannula, do the following:

1. Attach the tubing to the oxygen tank and turn on the tank.
2. Adjust the flowmeter to the desired flow rate (2 to 6 LPM).
3. Place the prongs into the patient's nose and adjust the tubing for comfort.

Like the NRBM, the nasal cannula is available in pediatric sizes.

Skill 7-9

Preparing an Oxygen Cylinder

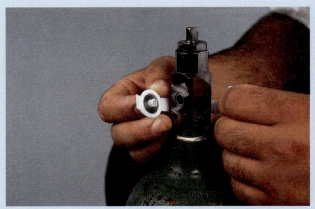

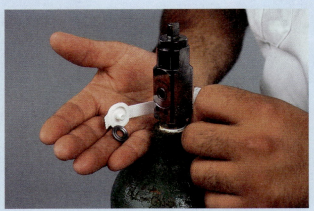

1. Select an oxygen tank (indicated by label or color of the tank—oxygen tanks are generally green). Remove the plastic cap from around the stem of the oxygen tank. (From McSwain N, Paturas J: *The basic EMT: comprehensive prehospital patient care*, 2003 ed 2, St Louis, 2003, Mosby.)

2. Be careful not to lose the O-ring inside the plastic cap. (From McSwain N, Paturas J: *The basic EMT: comprehensive prehospital patient care*, 2003 ed 2, St Louis, 2003, Mosby.)

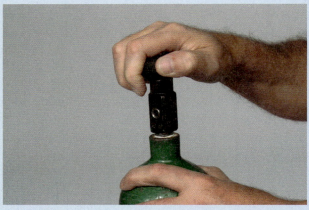

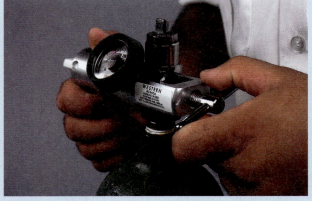

3. "Crack" the tank open for about 1 second to release any dust or debris and then close it. (From McSwain N, Paturas J: *The basic EMT: comprehensive prehospital patient care*, 2003 ed 2, St Louis, 2003, Mosby.)

4. Fit the oxygen regulator onto the tank. Align the pins on the regulator with the holes on the tank. Ensure that the O-ring is between the tank and the regulator. Tighten the regulator to the tank. (From McSwain N, Paturas J: *The basic EMT: comprehensive prehospital patient care*, 2003 ed 2, St Louis, 2003, Mosby.)

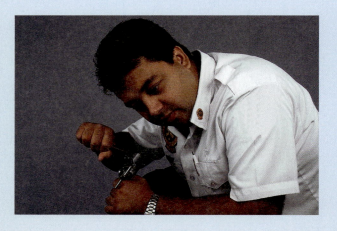

5. Turn the tank on by using the tank key and turning in a counterclockwise direction. Listen for any leaks and check the volume of the gauge to see how full the tank is. Attach oxygen tubing or oxygen delivery device. (From McSwain N, Paturas J: *The basic EMT: comprehensive prehospital patient care*, 2003 ed 2, St Louis, 2003, Mosby.)

Team Work—cont'd

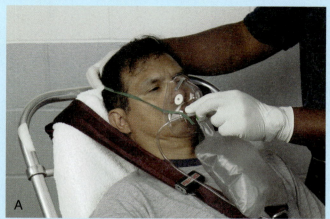

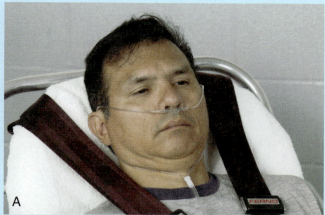

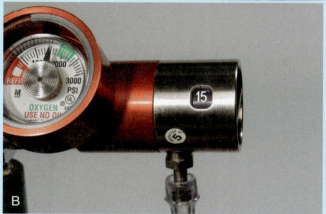

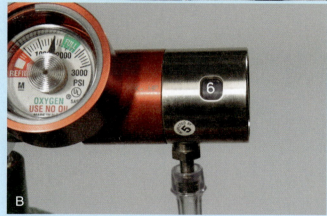

Fig. 7-22 A, Placement of a nonrebreather mask on a patient. **B,** Oxygen flow should be set at 12 to 15 LPM. (From Chapleau W, Pons P: *Emergency medical technician, making the difference,* St Louis, 2007, Mosby.)

Fig. 7-24 A, Placement of a nasal cannula on a patient. **B,** Oxygen flow should be set at 2 to 6 LPM. (From Chapleau W, Pons P: *Emergency medical technician, making the difference,* St Louis, 2007, Mosby.)

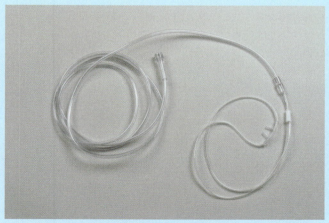

Fig. 7-23 Nasal cannula.

BAG-MASK VENTILATION

Bag-mask devices, sometimes referred to as self-inflating bags, are commonly used in both prehospital and hospital situations when ventilatory support (rescue breathing) is needed. The bag-mask has the following four major parts (Fig. 7-25):

1. The bag itself is a collapsible, soft plastic device. It is available in infant, pediatric, and adult sizes. The adult bag has a capacity of approximately 1800 mL of air, just short of the amount in a 2-L soda bottle. It provides considerably more than the required 800 mL of air an adult patient needs per ventilation, but it is nearly impossible to get all 1800 mL into the patient.
2. The bag-mask valve is a one-way valve. Many of the bag-mask devices contain a one-way value that diverts

Team Work—cont'd

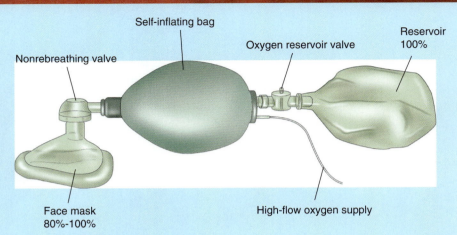

Fig. 7-25 The bag-mask device. (From McSwain N, Paturas J: *The basic EMT: comprehensive prehospital patient care*, ed 2, St Louis, 2003, Mosby.)

the patient's exhaled air out and prevents the exhaled air from returning into the bag.

3. The mask, like a pocket mask, is made of plastic, with an air-filled cuff.

4. The reservoir collects oxygen and allows a higher concentration of oxygen to be delivered to the patient.

The bag-mask device provides more efficient ventilation if two rescuers work together to ventilate the patient. One rescuer guarantees the mask's seal while the other squeezes the bag. As with a pocket mask, the ventilation rate should be 10 to 12 breaths per minute or 1 breath every 5 to 6 seconds. If you use the bag-mask device with oxygen attached, use a reservoir. The reservoir traps incoming oxygen and increases the oxygen concentration to near 100%. Advantages of the bag-mask include the following:

1. Can be used with or without oxygen
2. Close to 100% oxygen concentration when connected to an oxygen source and reservoir
3. Minimal risk of body fluid exposure
4. Disposable
5. Inexpensive

Disadvantages of the bag-mask device include its large size and the need for two rescuers to adequately ventilate the patient. To adequately ventilate a nonbreathing patient when using air without supplemental oxygen, 800 mL of air is needed. Only 600 mL is needed if 100% oxygen is used. While it may not seem hard to give 800 mL in a squeeze of the bag, a perfect mask seal is difficult to maintain. Facial hair, injuries, and loss of structure when dentures are

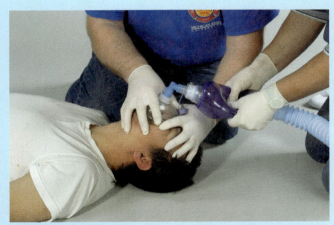

Fig. 7-26 The two-provider method of bag-mask ventilation is most effective.

removed make creating a tight seal challenging, even with two rescuers. Still you must ensure that the volume of each ventilation is sufficient to make the patient's chest visibly rise. If the chest does not rise, ventilation is not adequate. You should then check the seal between the patient's face and the mask and make sure the chest rises with each ventilation. You should practice regularly on a manikin to maintain this difficult but critical skill (Fig. 7-26).

ADVANCED AIRWAY MANAGEMENT

Advanced airway management is not typically a part of the emergency first responder's treatment protocols. However, emergency first responders, as members of a team of health care providers that may include EMT-Basics and/or Paramedics, may be called upon to assist in using these airway management devices.

Team Work—cont'd

Dual Lumen Airway

The **dual lumen airway** is an advanced airway that is inserted into either the trachea or the esophagus (Fig. 7-27). The dual lumen airway is generally considered only when a patient meets the following conditions:

1. Is unconscious
2. Is 16 years or older
3. Has an absent gag reflex
4. Is a minimum of 4 feet tall
5. Has apnea or a severely decreased respiratory rate

The dual lumen airway should not be used when the patient has an intact gag reflex, is younger than 16 years of age or shorter than 4 feet tall, has known esophageal disease, or has recently ingested caustic substances. The dual lumen airway has two sizes available. The smaller (37 French [37F]) is designed for use in patients 4 to 5.5 feet tall and the larger (41F) is designed for patients more than 5 feet tall.

To assist with the insertion of a dual lumen device, you should ensure that you have personal protective equipment (PPE) in place. This generally consists of gloves and goggles. You may be asked to provide ventilatory support as needed with a bag-mask or a pocket mask while the EMS providers prepare the equipment needed for the procedure. For at least 1 minute before insertion of the dual lumen device, 100% oxygen should be provided to the patient. You may also be asked to retrieve the equipment for the EMS providers. As an emergency first responder, you should be able to recognize a dual lumen airway device and understand when and why it is being used.

Endotracheal Tube

An **endotracheal tube** is a device inserted under direct visualization into the trachea and is considered the best method of airway management (Fig. 7-28). The procedure of inserting an endotracheal tube is commonly known as intubation. You may be asked to preoxygenate the patient with a bag-mask or other device or to retrieve the equipment. You may also be asked to apply cricoid pressure while the patient is being ventilated and intubated. It is important to remember not to let go of cricoid pressure until the endotracheal tube is in place. After the tube is inserted and secured you may be asked to ventilate the patient though the endotracheal tube. While this may seem easier than using a mask with a bag-mask device, it is important to remember that the tube cannot be allowed to change position. Excessive movement of the tube may displace it, leading to fatal complications. If you are unsure whether the tube has moved, tell EMS personnel immediately. It is important to recheck the tube's position. Never remain silent if you think the tube may have been accidentally displaced.

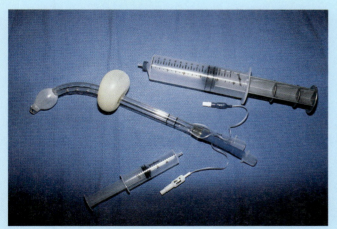

Fig. 7-27 Dual lumen airway device. (From McSwain N, Paturas J: *The basic EMT: comprehensive prehospital patient care*, ed 2, St Louis, 2003, Mosby.)

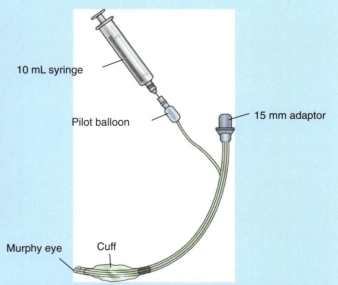

10 mL syringe

Pilot balloon

15 mm adaptor

Murphy eye   Cuff

Fig. 7-28 Endotracheal tube. (From McSwain N, Paturas J: *The basic EMT: comprehensive prehospital patient care*, ed 2, St Louis, 2003, Mosby.)

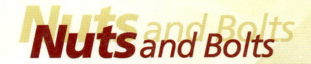

Critical Points

If there is any area in which the First Responder has the best opportunity to make the difference between life and death, it is in assessing, establishing, and maintaining the airway. Airway compromise may be the most preventable cause of death that a First Responder can face. Following the simple steps of checking for breathing and effort, examining the airway, opening and maintaining the airway, and supplementing breathing when it is inadequate or nonexistent will quite simply save lives. The First Responder should put the highest priority on establishing and maintaining a clear and open airway.

Learning Checklist

❑ The respiratory system consists of the nose, pharynx, oropharynx, nasopharynx, epiglottis, trachea, larynx, vocal cords, lungs, and alveoli.

❑ Inhalation occurs when the diaphragm moves down and the lungs expand.

❑ Exhalation occurs when the diaphragm moves up and the lungs get smaller.

❑ Hypoxia refers to the condition when the body's cells are not receiving adequate oxygen.

❑ Manual maneuvers to open the airway include the head-tilt/chin-lift, jaw thrust, and trauma chin-lift (or tongue-jaw lift). Manual maneuvers act to move the tongue and keep it from obstructing the airway.

❑ A head-tilt/chin-lift is performed by placing one hand on the patient's forehead and tilting it back while your other hand is used to pull the jaw forward by lifting up on the chin.

❑ A jaw thrust is performed by placing your fingers on the angle of the patient's jaw and lifting up with both hands to move the jaw forward.

❑ The airway can be cleared either by placing a patient in the recovery position and doing a finger sweep of the airway or by suctioning the patient's airway.

❑ Suction units can be manual or battery operated. Suctioning uses negative pressure to remove fluid or small objects out of the airway. You should never suction deeper than the base of the patient's tongue, only suction when moving the catheter out of the patient's mouth, and never suction for more than 15 seconds at one time.

❑ Mechanical airway adjuncts include the oropharyngeal airway and nasopharyngeal airway.

❑ The oropharyngeal airway should only be used in patients without a gag reflex; otherwise, it could induce vomiting. It is sized by measuring the distance between the corner of the patient's mouth and the tip of the ear.

❑ An oropharyngeal airway should be inserted into children and infants by using the tongue blade method.

❑ The nasopharyngeal airway can be used in patients with a gag reflex; it should be lubricated before insertion and is sized by measuring the distance between the patient's nose and the corner of the ear.

❑ Inadequate breathing can be indicated by a patient's posture, speech, muscle use, or changes in vital signs.

❑ Rescue breathing (or ventilation) can be accomplished through mouth-to-mask, mouth-to-barrier, or mouth-to-mouth ventilation.

❑ Rescue breaths for adults should be over 1 second and occur 10 to 12 times per minute (1 breath every 5 to 6 seconds).

❑ Rescue breaths for a child or infant should be over 1 second and occur 12 to 20 times per minute (1 breath every 3 to 5 seconds).

❑ A complete airway obstruction in an adult and child should be relieved by abdominal thrusts in a conscious patient. It should be relieved by a combination of inspecting and sweeping the airway, attempted ventilations, and chest compressions in the unconscious patient.

❑ You should never blindly finger sweep a victim's mouth. Only perform a finger sweep to remove a foreign object if the object is seen.

❑ A complete airway obstruction in an infant is relieved with back blows and chest thrusts if the infant is conscious. It is relieved with a combination of inspecting the airway, attempted ventilations, and chest compressions for the unconscious infant.

❑ If a patient has a stoma, ventilation can be performed by placing a pediatric-sized mask over the stoma and performing rescue breathing.

Key Terms

Bag-mask device Mechanical resuscitation device consisting of a self-inflating bag, one-way valve, reservoir, and a mask; squeezing the bag results in positive pressure (a breath) being delivered to the patient.

Barrier device A resuscitation device that places a layer of thin film with either a filter or a one-way valve between you and a patient.

Cricoid pressure A technique that collapses the esophagus between the trachea and cervical spine; used to prevent air from entering the stomach and the patient from vomiting during ventilation.

Dual lumen airway An advanced airway device that has two separate ports for the delivery of oxygen; can be inserted into either the trachea or the esophagus.

Dyspnea Difficulty in breathing.

Endotracheal tube An advanced airway device that is inserted directly into the trachea.

Foreign body airway obstruction (FBAO) An obstruction of the airway caused, for example, by choking on food or other foreign material or by bleeding into the airway or vomiting.

Gag reflex A response to stimulation of the posterior oropharynx causing gagging and vomiting in many people; generally, unconscious patients do not have a gag reflex.

Head-tilt/chin-lift A manual maneuver used to open someone's airway; the head is tilted back with one hand while the chin is lifted up with the other.

Hypoxia A condition where there is lack of oxygen to the cells of the body.

Jaw thrust A manual maneuver used to open the airway of a trauma patient; the patient's jaw is thrust forward without tilting the head back, which could potentially cause further injury to the spine.

Nasal cannula An oxygen delivery device that consists of two prongs that go into a patient's nose; delivers a low concentration of oxygen.

Nasopharyngeal airway (NPA) A mechanical device inserted into the nostril and used to prevent the tongue from obstructing the airway.

Nonrebreather mask Oxygen delivery device used to deliver higher concentrations of oxygen; consists of a mask, one-way valve, and a reservoir bag.

Oropharyngeal airway (OPA) A mechanical device inserted into the mouth and used to prevent the tongue from obstructing the airway.

Pocket mask A mask that can be used to deliver mouth-to-mask ventilation.

Rescue breathing Artificial ventilation provided to a patient who cannot breathe on his or her own.

Stridor A high-pitched, whistling sound that occurs when a patient breathes in if there is an obstruction (foreign body or tissue swelling) in the upper airway (between the pharynx and the vocal cords).

Trauma chin-lift Also called tongue-jaw lift. A manual maneuver used to open the airway and keep the tongue from obstructing the airway. Used to inspect the airway or to do finger sweeps of the airway.

Ventilation The mechanical movement of air being inhaled and exhaled; also refers to the artificial breathing given to a patient through a mask or your mouth.

Wheezing A high-pitched sound that occurs when air moves through narrowed airways; usually occurs on exhalation and generally indicates obstruction of the lower airways.

First Responder NSC Objectives
COGNITIVE OBJECTIVES

- Name and label the major structures of the respiratory system on a diagram.
- List the signs of inadequate breathing.
- Describe the steps in the head-tilt/chin-lift.
- Relate mechanism of injury to opening the airway.
- Describe the steps in the jaw thrust.
- State the importance of having a suction unit ready for immediate use when providing emergency medical care.
- Describe the technique of suctioning.
- Describe how to ventilate a patient with a resuscitation mask or barrier device.

Nuts and Bolts–continued

- Describe how ventilation of an infant or child is different from ventilation of an adult.
- List the steps in providing mouth-to-mouth and mouth-to-stoma breathing.
- Describe how to measure and insert an oropharyngeal (oral) airway.
- Describe how to measure and insert a nasopharyngeal (nasal) airway.
- Describe how to clear a foreign body airway obstruction in a responsive adult.
- Describe how to clear a foreign body airway obstruction in a responsive child who has complete or partial airway obstruction with poor air exchange.
- Describe how to clear a foreign body airway obstruction in a responsive infant who has complete or partial airway obstruction with poor air exchange.
- Describe how to clear a foreign body airway obstruction in an unresponsive adult.
- Describe how to clear a foreign body airway obstruction in an unresponsive infant.

AFFECTIVE OBJECTIVES

- Explain why basic life support ventilation and airway protective skills take priority over most other basic life support skills.
- Demonstrate a caring attitude toward patients with airway problems who request emergency medical services.
- Place the interest of the patient with airway problems as the foremost consideration when making any and all patient care decisions.
- Show empathy when communicating with patients who have airway problems and with their family members and friends.

PSYCHOMOTOR OBJECTIVES

- Demonstrate the steps in the head-tilt/chin-lift.
- Demonstrate the steps in the jaw thrust.
- Demonstrate the techniques of suctioning.
- Demonstrate the steps in mouth-to-mouth ventilation with body substance isolation (barrier shields).
- Demonstrate how to use a resuscitation mask to ventilate a patient.
- Demonstrate how to ventilate a patient with a stoma.
- Demonstrate how to measure and insert an oropharyngeal (oral) airway.
- Demonstrate how to measure and insert a nasopharyngeal (nasal) airway.
- Demonstrate how to ventilate infants and children.
- Demonstrate how to clear a foreign body airway obstruction in a responsive adult.
- Demonstrate how to clear a foreign body airway obstruction in a responsive child.
- Demonstrate how to clear a foreign body airway obstruction in a responsive infant.
- Demonstrate how to clear a foreign body airway obstruction in an unresponsive adult.
- Demonstrate how to clear a foreign body airway obstruction in an unresponsive child.
- Demonstrate how to clear a foreign body airway obstruction in an unresponsive infant.

Check *your understanding*

Please refer to p. 439 for the answers to these questions.

1. Which method is the most effective way to ensure your mouth-to-mask breaths are reaching the trachea?
   A. Chest rise/fall
   B. Abdominal rise/fall
   C. Pulse oximetry
   D. Patient becomes cyanotic.

2. The tube through which food passes from the mouth to the stomach is the _____.

3. The flap of tissue that protects the entrance to the trachea is the:
   A. Tragus
   B. Epiglottis
   C. Palate
   D. Pharynx

4. The tube through which air passes from the nose and mouth into the lungs (the windpipe) is called the _____.

5. The tiny air sacs in the lungs where oxygen and carbon dioxide are exchanged with the blood are called _____.

6. When the diaphragm moves down, creating negative pressure (a vacuum) inside the chest, air moves into the lungs. This process is known as _____.

7. Normally the respiratory rate increases when there is not enough _____ in the blood or when there is too much _____ in the blood.

8. When the muscles of an unresponsive person relax, this often causes the airway to be obstructed by the _____.

9. The best way to open the airway of an uninjured, unresponsive person is the:
   A. Head/neck lift
   B. Modified jaw thrust
   C. Tongue-jaw lift
   D. Head-tilt/chin-lift

10. You are eating at a local restaurant when a patron begins to cough and choke. You identify yourself and tell him you can help him. He now is not making any noise and is becoming cyanotic. What is your best course of action?
    A. Do not intervene, as he will get it out on his own.
    B. Begin chest compressions.
    C. Begin abdominal thrusts.
    D. Call 9-1-1 and wait for proper equipment.

11. A simple device placed into the mouth of an unresponsive patient without a gag reflex in order to help keep the tongue from obstructing the airway is a/an _____.

12. A patient who is responsive but who requires an adjunct to maintain his or her airway should have which type of airway adjunct placed?
    A. Oropharyngeal (OP)
    B. Nasopharyngeal (NP)
    C. Combitube
    D. Bite block

13. Which of the following usually indicates the patient has an upper airway obstruction?
    A. Wheezing
    B. Vomiting
    C. Stridor
    D. Grunting

14. The medical term for difficulty in breathing is _____.

15. Which of the following would indicate that a patient is not breathing at all?
    A. Apneic
    B. Tachycardic
    C. Hyperventilating
    D. Pulseless

Check your understanding–continued

16. You are caring for a patient who is not breathing. The most effective oxygen delivery device would be:
   A. Nasal cannula
   B. Nonrebreather mask
   C. Bag-mask
   D. Nebulizer mask

17. A person who is choking but is able to speak or cough has a/an _____ airway obstruction.

18. A conscious patient who is choking and cannot cough or speak requires the use of _____ to remove the obstruction.

19. When performing rescue breathing for an infant or small child, what should the emergency first responder do to make sure that the neck is not hyperflexed because of the large size of the head, since hyperflexing will close off the airway?

   _____

   _____

   _____

   _____

20. An emergency first responder may be asked to assist other EMS providers with more advanced airway adjuncts. One such device can be inserted blindly only in unresponsive patients who are over 16 years of age. This is called a/an _____.

21. A device that is squeezed by hand to ventilate a patient instead of using the rescuer's own breath is called a/an _____.

22. A device used to administer a high concentration of oxygen to a patient who is breathing on his or her own is called a/an _____ mask.

23. You are beginning rescue breathing on a 50-year-old male patient who has taken an overdose of a sedative medication. You place a pocket mask over his nose and mouth and obtain a good seal. As you exhale into the mask you find that air does not easily enter the patient's lungs. Which of the following actions should you take first?
   A. Exhale more forcefully into the mask.
   B. Begin giving a series of abdominal thrusts.
   C. Check that the head is in the proper position to open the airway.
   D. Remove the mask and give mouth-to-mouth ventilations.

Chapter 8

Patient Assessment

LESSON GOAL

This chapter will provide you with the knowledge you need to evaluate the scene for safety, to establish the number of patients, to assess the patient's mechanism of injury or nature of illness, and to determine the need for additional Emergency Medical Services (EMS) resources. The chapter focuses on the initial patient assessment, history, and physical examination.

OBJECTIVES

1. Discuss the components of scene size-up.
2. Describe common hazards found at the scene of trauma and medical patients.
3. Identify common mechanisms of injury and nature of illness.
4. Discuss the reason for identifying the total number of patients at the scene.
5. Summarize the reasons for forming a general impression of the patient.
6. Differentiate between assessing mental status in the adult, child, and infant patient.
7. Differentiate between patients with adequate and inadequate breathing.
8. Differentiate between assessing circulation in the adult, child, and infant patient.
9. Discuss the need for assessing the patient for external bleeding.
10. Identify reasons for prioritizing a patient for care and transport.
11. Demonstrate a focused history and physical examination.
12. Given a simulated patient, obtain a SAMPLE history.
13. Differentiate between the ongoing assessment of a critical patient and a noncritical patient.
14. Describe the information included in the emergency first responder "hand-off" report.
15. Provide a rationale for evaluating scene safety before entering a given scene.
16. Given a scenario, describe how patient situations can affect the evaluation of the mechanism of injury or nature of illness.
17. Give a rationale for the sequence of patient assessment.
18. Given a scenario, identify potential safety hazards and determine if the scene is safe to enter.
19. Given a simulated patient, assess the patient's mental status, airway, breathing, circulation, and disability.

In the Real World

You and another emergency first responder are called to the scene of a motor vehicle collision. Dispatch reports a two-vehicle collision with injuries and five people involved. On arrival, you see that one vehicle has apparently rear-ended another at a busy intersection. Bystanders report that an elderly male is in the front vehicle, and two adults and two children are in the rear vehicle. Police officers arrive and begin controlling traffic. You do not see any downed electrical wires or poles. You notice a green fluid leaking from the rear vehicle. Both vehicles are upright, resting on their four wheels. There is broken glass on the ground but all the windows are intact. No fire or smoke is present, the weather is good, and air temperature is not an issue. The bystanders are not violent or in the hazardous area.

Bystanders tell you that the vehicle in front slowed and the second vehicle ran into it, while traveling at a moderate speed. There were moderate damages to both vehicles, and the airbags were deployed in the rear vehicle. You suspect possible head, neck, facial, and eye injuries to the occupants held by airbags. You consider clavicle, chest, abdominal, and possible lumbar spine injuries in the occupants wearing restraints.

You identify one man in the front vehicle and a man, a woman, and two children in the second vehicle. You question bystanders and everyone states that only five people were involved in the collision. You notify the responding ambulance crew of the number of patients and the status of the scene.

Police are already on the scene, controlling traffic. The vehicles are not severely damaged so extrication is not required. There is no smoke or fire but an antifreeze leak is present. You contact the fire department to help with the spill and you begin to assist with the patients.

As an emergency first responder you must be able to rapidly assess the scene, size up potential hazards, and determine the need for additional resources. You must also be able to rapidly assess patients for life-threatening (critical) conditions and begin treatment. Assessment is learned as a series of separate skills, but in reality you will be doing many of these things at the same time. In the assessment process you rapidly take in information and sort it to make decisions. The only way to become proficient at assessment is to practice often and to learn from both the calls you handled well and those you did not handle as well.

Because as an emergency first responder you are the first to arrive on the scene and possibly the first to come in contact with the patient, your assessment skills may impact your safety, the safety of other care providers, the patient and his or her outcome, and bystanders at the scene. Assessment is the most important skill for emergency first responders. Assessment includes the following stages:

- Scene size-up
- Primary assessment
- Physical examination
- Patient history
- Ongoing assessment
- Hand-off report

Scene Size-up

Scene size-up is a quick determination of the entire scene and includes the safety of the scene, personal protection, and an assessment of the mechanism of injury or nature of illness before you actually contact the patient. Scene size-up begins the moment you receive the initial request for aid. The information provided by dispatch should give you an idea of what to expect when you arrive and what resources you may need to obtain. Dispatch should also inform you about the security of the scene. For example, you may have to stage (wait) a safe distance away from the scene until it has been made safe for you to enter by other agencies (such as the police department, the fire department, or the utility company) or until additional back-up has arrived. It is important to remember that communication with dispatch is two-way. You should ask questions as needed to prepare for your arrival and to ensure that proper additional resources are en route.

As you are traveling to the scene you should also be looking at the weather conditions. The weather can affect your ability to get to the scene safely and may also create an environmental concern for your patient such as exposure to cold or heat (see Chapter 16). Noting the time of day can alert you to potential traffic situations that will affect your access to the patient as well as the likely activities at the scene.

Personal Protection Equipment

When you respond to the scene of an emergency, your first concern is to use proper personal protection equipment (PPE) (see Chapter 2). You should put on gloves, eye protection, and a gown and mask, depending on the information from dispatch and from your size-up of the scene. Besides protecting yourself against all body substances, PPE can also include protective clothing specific to the environment. For example, in a motor vehicle collision (MVC) or fire situation, emergency first responders should wear full turn-out gear. Emergency first responders should also be clothed to protect themselves from extremes of weather. It is important to find out about any expected weather changes and to have appropriate clothing available. In the opening scenario, for example, the scene is an MVC. You should assume that blood is present, so put on gloves and consider whether additional body substance isolation (BSI) precautions are needed. In addition, if available and if appropriate you would put on full turn-out gear to protect yourself from any debris, glass, or fire at the scene.

A variety of specialized protective equipment and gear is available for use in very specific situations. Examples of special protective equipment would be biological and chemical suits. Biological and chemical protective suits come in different types and can provide added protection against hazardous materials and biological threats of varying degrees. A self-contained breathing apparatus (SCBA) can provide protection to the wearer from certain contaminated air. Only specially trained and properly fitted responders should wear or use specialized equipment.

Scene Safety

As an emergency first responder, you must ask yourself, "Is the scene safe?" whenever you arrive at the scene of an emergency. You must ensure that the scene is safe and remains safe from all preventable hazards. Table 8-1 outlines scene safety concerns at different scenes. When you arrive at an emergency scene, rapidly size up the scene and make scene management decisions (Fig. 8-1). In the scene size-up during the opening scenario, for example, you identify the traffic hazard and the fluid leak hazard. To evaluate the scene effectively, you must be aware of the whole environment and avoid having tunnel vision and focusing only on the patient. If a scene is unsafe and cannot be made safe, do not enter it. It is extremely important to know your limitations on determining scene safety. In some situations the safety of the scene may have to be determined by other responders who have received specialty training in areas such as tactical situa-

tions, fire, hazardous materials, vehicle extrication, or other types of special rescue. Once the scene is safe always take the appropriate precautions before entering the scene. Box 8-1 outlines some of these precautions.

Once the scene has been determined to be safe for you and your co-workers to enter, the safety of the patient

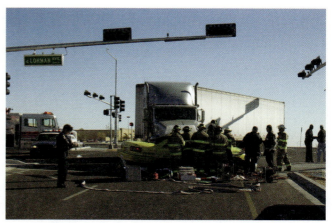

Fig. 8-1 When you arrive at an emergency scene, rapidly do a scene size-up. (From Chapleau W, Pons P: *Emergency medical technician, making the difference,* St Louis, 2007, Mosby.)

BOX 8-1   Precautions for Entering a Scene

- Never enter a scene that is potentially hazardous or unsafe; always wait for the scene to be made safe.
- Use caution and follow local protocols at suspected crime scenes and potentially violent scenes. Call for the police to make the scene safe before entering or leave if the situation suddenly becomes threatening.
- If possible, carry a portable two-way radio or cell phone to the scene so you can call for help if necessary.
- Realize your own limitations and do not exceed your abilities or training to manage a hazardous scene.
- Leave a scene if it becomes unsafe or you lose control.
- Always have an exit plan out of the scene and avoid blocking your route of retreat.

(Adapted from Dalton A, Limmer D, Mistovich J et al: *Advanced medical life support,* Upper Saddle River, NJ, 1999, Brady, Pearson Education, Inc.)

TABLE 8-1 Scene Safety Concerns

TYPE OF SCENE	QUESTIONS TO CONSIDER
Crash and rescue scenes	Is the traffic controlled? Are police on scene? Are downed electrical wires or poles present? Do you see any leaking fluids? Is the vehicle stable? Are broken glass and torn metal a hazard? Is fire or smoke present?
Confined spaces	How stable is the area? Could toxic substances be present? Is this a low-oxygen area?
Crime scenes	What is the potential for violence at this scene? Were weapons involved? Are police on scene?
Environmental concerns	Are the surfaces stable? Is water or ice present? Is the slope manageable? Is fog, snow, or lightning a hazard? Could extremes in heat or cold be a problem?
Violent conditions	Do you hear yelling and shouting? Is anyone making wild or aggressive gestures? Are weapons present or reported? Does this person have a known history of violence? Is the crowd controlled or in danger? Is there an animal on the scene?
Residence/building response	Is the area well lit or dark? Is someone present to help you gain access to the residence/building? Does the nature of the call suggest violence? Is gang graffiti present or any activity present that might indicate danger? Does the area have a history of violence? Is the building structurally stable? Is fire or smoke present? Are noxious fumes present?

(Adapted from Dalton A: *Advanced medical life support*, Upper Saddle River, New Jersey, 1999, Pearson Education, Inc.)

and the bystanders becomes your next priority while maintaining your own safety. You will need to keep the scene safe for yourself, other health care personnel, patients, and bystanders at all times. If the patient and/or bystanders cannot be protected from hazards at the scene, the patient and/or bystanders must be moved to a safer environment. It may be as simple as directing the bystanders to move from the traveled portion of a road or as complicated as having the patient decontaminated and moved from a hot zone.

Nature of the Event

During the scene size-up it is also important to determine whether a patient is a trauma patient or a medical patient. A trauma patient is one who has sustained an injury as the result of an external force. A medical patient is a patient who appears to have an illness or complains of symptoms of an illness. Once you make this determination, you determine the mechanism of injury (MOI) for a trauma patient and the nature of illness (NOI) for a medical patient. The assessment of the trauma patient may require more visual and hands-on assessment than the assessment of a medical patient. A medical assessment may require asking more questions to identify the nature of the illness.

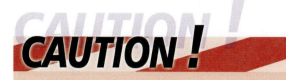

CAUTION!

Always assess the patient for possible trauma at a medical scene and for medical problems at a trauma scene. Do not assume the problem is only medical or only trauma. Often both can occur at the same time. Until proven otherwise, an unresponsive patient should be assumed to be a trauma patient.

Fig. 8-2 A frontal impact can cause potential injuries to the head, neck, chest, pelvis, and lower extremities. (From NAEMT: *PHTLS: basic and advanced prehospital trauma life support,* ed 5, St Louis, 2003, Mosby.)

Mechanism of Injury (MOI)

As you evaluate scene safety at a traumatic incident you should also look for clues to the MOI. To discover the mechanism of injury, or the cause of the injury, you need to consider the entire trauma scene and any physical forces that may have damaged the patient's body. For example, you can determine if a patient sustained a penetrating wound, such as a knife or gunshot wound, or was subjected to a blunt force that impacted the body, such as the steering column or windshield in an MVC. You can also determine whether the patient was injured by a blast injury, such as a propane tank blowing up when someone was lighting a barbecue grill. When possible, identifying certain characteristics of the instrument used to cause the trauma can be beneficial to the hospital treating the patient. If a knife was used, how long was the blade? If a gun was used, was it a hand gun or a rifle? Any information you can relay without delaying the patient's treatment or transport will be helpful.

You can also predict likely injuries to the patient by considering the impact site and tracing the destructive energy through the body. You cannot see the forces that occurred, but you can learn to look at a trauma incident, determine what force occurred and its path, and predict the most likely injuries. For example, injury patterns associated with MVCs are consistent with the type of impact involved. A frontal impact can cause the patient to move forward and upward in the vehicle, causing potential injuries to the head, neck, chest, and pelvis (Fig. 8-2).

Penetrating trauma can create both a permanent cavity and a temporary cavity. The permanent cavity is the path the projectile carves through the body, for example, the path a bullet takes through the body in a gunshot wound. The temporary cavity represents the energy that enters the body with the projectile, such as the bullet, and causes injuries away from the immediate path of the projectile. For example, the bullet may enter the leg and injure the muscle directly in its path (permanent cavity); it may also cause the tissues surrounding the path to be torn and compressed from the energy expanding out from the bullet path (temporary cavity) (Fig. 8-3).

In blunt trauma (trauma that does not actually puncture through the skin), the energy applied also creates a temporary cavity. Imagine hitting the side of a metal drum with a bat. With enough force, you would dent the side of the drum (permanent cavity). However, if you hit something more flexible, such as a piece of foam or a person, with a bat, the shape would return to normal, but inside a temporary cavity would be created by the force of the bat (Fig. 8-4).

To determine the mechanism of injury, it is important to look at the scene for clues as to what happened. You can also question bystanders, family members, and the patient to help determine the mechanism of injury. Table 8-2 describes various mechanisms of injury and their commonly associated injuries.

Nature of Illness (NOI)

With a medical emergency you will try to learn the NOI. You should talk directly with the patient whenever possible. If the patient is unable to answer your questions or you need further clarification, you may wish to speak with the patient's family members or bystanders about the scene and why you were called. For example, you can

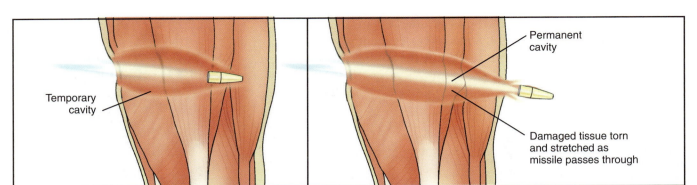

Fig. 8-3 Damage to the tissue is greater than the permanent cavity that remains. The faster and heavier the penetrating object, the larger the temporary cavity and the greater the zone of tissue damage. (From NAEMT: *PHTLS: basic and advanced prehospital trauma life support,* ed 5, St Louis, 2003, Mosby.)

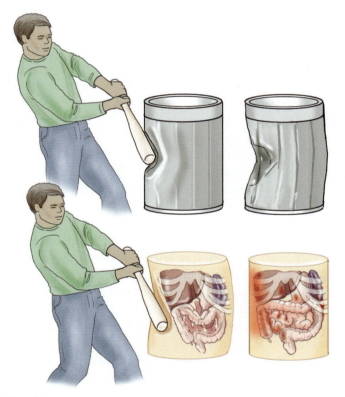

Fig. 8-4 A, Swinging a bat into a steel drum leaves a dent, or cavity, in its side. **B,** Swinging a bat into a piece of foam leaves no visible cavity. (From NAEMT: *PHTLS: basic and advanced prehospital trauma life support,* ed 6, St Louis, 2007, Mosby.)

ask the patient, family, or bystanders, "Why did you call for help?" Other important questions may include inquiring about the patient's past medical conditions, current medications, and other conditions leading up to the current event. The replies may help reveal the nature of the illness. Responses may include information such as the person has terrible stomach pain or difficulty breath-

ing. You can also look around the scene to uncover more clues about the nature of the illness, such as the following:

- An oxygen tank may indicate respiratory problems.
- Medication bottles may indicate specific illnesses.
- A patient curled up on his side holding his abdomen may have appendicitis or some other abdominal complaint.
- A patient outside on a cool, rainy night may have hypothermia.

Determining the nature of illness will help guide you in your assessment of the medical patient.

Number of Patients Involved

It is also important during the scene size-up to determine the number of patients at the scene and to decide whether additional resources are needed. Your call for additional resources should occur before contact with the patient because once you are involved in patient care you will have less of an opportunity to stop and call for help. You should thoroughly check the scene to be certain that you find everyone involved in the incident. Ask people at the scene if you have found everyone. If they cannot answer you definitively, continue your search. For example, look in a vehicle for children's things. Is a child missing? Could a child have wandered off or been ejected from the vehicle? In a situation of carbon monoxide poisoning inside a house, could another family member still be present inside? Continue questioning and investigating until you are confident that you have located all patients. Triage (the sorting and prioritizing of patients) should begin when you are confronted with multiple casualties (see Chapter 15).

TABLE 8-2 Common Mechanisms of Injury and Patterns of Injury

MECHANISM OF INJURY	PREDICTORS	ASSOCIATED PATTERNS OF INJURY
Motor vehicle crash (type of impact and damage to interior of car may help predict injuries)	Unrestrained	Multiple trauma, head and neck injuries, scalp and facial lacerations
	Airbag	Head and neck, facial, and eye injuries
	Restrained	Chest and abdominal injuries, cervical and lower-spine fractures, clavicle fractures
Motor vehicle/pedestrian crash (children are more commonly struck head-on, whereas adults are struck from side)	Low speed	Lower-extremity fractures
	High speed	Chest and abdominal injuries, head and neck injuries, extremity fractures
Fall from a height	Low height	Upper- or lower-extremity fractures
	Medium height	Head and neck injuries, upper- and lower-extremity fractures
	Great height (3 times the patient's height = critical injuries)	Chest and abdominal injuries, head and neck injuries, upper- and lower-extremity fractures
Fall from a bicycle	Without a helmet	Head and neck injuries, scalp and facial lacerations, upper-extremity fractures
	With a helmet	Upper-extremity fractures
	Hitting the handlebar	Internal abdominal injuries
Motorcycle crash	Low speed	Lower-extremity fractures and burns
	Medium speed	Head and neck injuries, upper- and lower-extremity fractures
	High speed	Chest and abdominal injuries, pelvic and femur fractures, head and neck injuries, upper- and lower-extremity fractures
Penetrating trauma	Low velocity (knives, ice picks, etc.)	Isolated to area of penetration, severe blood loss possible
	Medium velocity (handguns, .22s, shotguns, etc.)	Usually isolated to area of penetration, but a wider area of damage should be suspected; also may have ricocheting of bullet through body; severe injury more likely
	High velocity (high-powered rifles, assault weapons, etc.)	Area of damage much larger than area of penetration; critical life-threatening injuries more likely

(Adapted from Teaching Resource for Instructors in Prehospital Pediatrics [TRIPP], 1998, Version 2.0. Center for Pediatric Emergency Medicine [CPEM], New York.)

TABLE 8-3 Hazards and Available Resources

HAZARDS	RESOURCE
Electrical lines down	Fire service
	Electric utility company
Natural gas leak	Fire service
	Gas company
	Public utilities
Fire	Fire service
Hazardous materials (e.g., chemical spill, industrial incident)	Fire service
	Hazardous materials team
Rescue (such as water, confined space, high angle, trench, extrication)	Fire service
	Specialty rescue teams
Mass (or multiple) casualties	Law enforcement
	Fire service
	Local emergency management agency
Violent scene	Law enforcement
Loose animals on scene	Animal control

Additional Resources

When you arrive at an emergency scene, you should first confirm that additional personnel are en route to help manage the scene and the patient as needed. You may need police officers, firefighters, extrication specialists, a hazardous materials team, utility company workers, or a medical transport team (Table 8-3). Some teams may be dispatched automatically or you may be responsible for determining what resources are necessary. You may also need to communicate the number of patients and the severity of their injuries to help determine what type of medical resources are needed: a Basic Life Support (BLS) crew, an Advanced Life Support (ALS) crew, or helicopter service. You should follow your local guidelines to activate these services.

Once you have sized up the scene and determined that it is safe, your focus should be on patient assessment. However, you must remember that a scene can change and you should continue to monitor the situation and scene for safety and security concerns throughout the patient assessment.

Primary Assessment

A primary assessment, sometimes referred to as a primary survey or an initial assessment, is performed to determine whether a patient has any life-threatening problems and to manage those problems as they are found. The primary assessment has three main parts: forming a general impression of the patient; assessing the patient's responsiveness; and checking the patient's airway, breathing, circulation, and disability (ABCD). As you enter the scene look at the patient, think about what happened, and begin to evaluate the patient's condition. Notice the patient's responsiveness, level of anxiety, breathing, and skin. Is the patient awake, making sense, relatively calm, breathing adequately and without noisy breathing, and does the patient have good skin color? You should look for and observe these signs as you begin your initial assessment. Table 8-4 lists considerations for the primary assessment. It is important to note that while these steps are presented in a sequential manner, often times they will be performed simultaneously (Fig. 8-5). It is also important to note that not all steps may be completed in the primary assessment. If, for example, the patient has an obstructed airway and cannot breathe, the check for circulation must wait until the obstruction is relieved and rescue breaths can be given. The purpose of the primary assessment is to assess and treat life-threatening conditions as they are found.

General Impression

Your general impression of the patient and the patient's surrounding environment is formed before you have touched or started to assess the patient. The general impression helps you decide how to act and gauge the seriousness of the scene. To form a general impression of the emergency you need to quickly evaluate the scene and think about what is happening, what you have been told,

TABLE 8-4 Elements of the Primary Assessment

General impression	Medical or trauma (stabilize the spine) or unsure (treat as trauma)
	Environmental clues
	Age
	Gender
Assess responsiveness	Are patients awake when you get there?
	Do they respond when you talk to them?
	Do you need to touch them or use painful stimuli to get them to respond?
	How do they respond?
	Are they unresponsive to any stimuli?
Airway	Do you hear any noises (e.g., gurgling, snoring, stridor, or grunting)?
	If you open an airway or suction, does the noise improve?
Breathing	Are they breathing?
	Is the breathing fast or slow?
	Do you hear any wheezing or other noises?
	Are they using accessory muscles to breathe?
	How hard are they working to breathe?
	Can they speak? How many words between breaths?
	What is (are) their position(s)?
Circulation	Do they each have a pulse?
	Is it slow, fast, regular, or irregular?
	What are their skin colors and temperatures?
	Is there any major bleeding?
Disability	What are the patients' GCS* scores?
Priority	Are any of these critical patients?

*GCS, Glasgow Coma Scale.

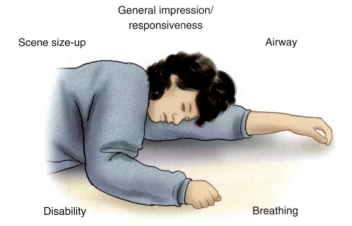

Fig. 8-5 While the steps in the primary assessment are presented in a sequential manner, often they can be performed simultaneously.

and what you observe. First you need to look at the scene and the patient to determine if the patient is a medical or a trauma patient. Does the patient appear to be injured? Are there signs of a mechanism of injury? Does the patient appear to be ill? Are there signs of a medical condition? If you are unsure, you should treat the scene as a trauma scene. You should consider the patient's approximate age, gender, presentation, and any other information you have been given. For example, if you first see a patient who is lying on the icy ground not moving and is very pale in color, you would assume that this is a more critical patient than someone that you see sitting up and alert in a chair inside a house.

Level of Consciousness

Once you have formed a general impression, the first thing to assess is the patient's level of consciousness or

In the Real World—continued

You have five patients: an elderly male in the first vehicle; and a male adult, a female adult, one preschool boy, and one infant girl in the second vehicle.

The elderly male in the first vehicle complains of chest pain, looks pale, and has wheezes when he breathes. He tells you the pain in his chest is bad and then stops talking. When your partner pinches his shoulder, he only moans. You check for a carotid pulse and find it weak and irregular. The patient's color is pale and his skin is cool to touch.

The two adults in the second vehicle are alert and talking and deny any injury. The man is bleeding slightly from his nose and the woman has no visual injuries. Both adults have regular radial pulses and good skin color.

The young boy is staring straight ahead. He glances at loud noises but does not stay focused on the noises. He answers quietly when you ask questions. He has a cough that sounds like a seal bark and has noisy breathing but continues to speak, expending significant energy to breathe; you can see his chest and neck muscles working. He speaks only one or two words at a time and his color is pale. He has a rapid radial pulse and his skin is pale in color and cool to the touch.

The infant girl is crying loudly and kicking but quiets down when her mother soothes her. Her color is pink and she is breathing adequately.

Your general impression is that the boy's condition is serious, that the elderly patient may have serious injuries, and the two adults and infant are stable at this time.

---

level of responsiveness. Assessing responsiveness involves the evaluation of how alert or awake the patient is and what kind of stimulus causes a response from the patient.

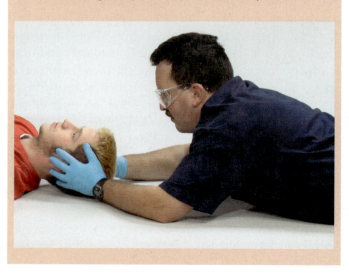

CAUTION!

If you think the patient's condition was caused by trauma, it is important to stabilize the spine at this point. Support the patient's head in line with the body. Further information on stabilizing the spine can be found in Chapter 12.

You should always begin your assessment by introducing yourself in a normal tone of voice, describing your training, and making it clear that you are there to help. This can be as simple as "Hello, my name is Jess. I'm an emergency first responder and I'm here to help you." For a medical patient, you can add, "Why did you call us?" or for a trauma patient, "Tell me where you hurt." If the patient is responsive and talking, you can identify the patient's chief complaint—the reason for calling for help. For example, if a patient tells you that she has "cramping abdominal pain," that is her chief complaint.

A patient who is awake and speaks to you spontaneously is considered to be alert (responsive). A patient who is not awake but wakes up or moves in some way when you speak is said to be responsive to verbal stimuli. If the patient does not respond when you enter the room or when you speak, you should try gently tapping the patient. If the patient still does not respond, try a more aggressive approach such as performing a sternal rub or placing a pen between the patient's fingers and gently squeezing the fingers together. A patient who responds to this technique is said to be responsive to painful stimuli. If the patient is not awake and does not respond to any stimuli, the patient is said to be unresponsive. This technique, called the AVPU (Alert, Verbal, Painful, Unresponsive) scale, is a quick way to determine a patient's level of responsiveness (Table 8-5).

For responsive patients you should also determine if the patient is oriented to the situation. Does the patient know who and where he or she is, what day it is, and what

TABLE 8-5   AVPU Scale

A—**A**lert	The patient is alert, awake, and talking to you. The patient knows his or her name, where he or she is, what day or time it is, and what happened.
V—Responds to **v**erbal stimuli	The patient responds to voice. The patient may not be alert or open the eyes spontaneously but he or she responds appropriately when you speak to him or her.
P—Responds to **p**ainful stimuli	The patient responds only to a painful stimulus such as a pinch of an earlobe or a sternal rub.
U—**U**nresponsive	The patient is not awake and is completely unresponsive to any type of stimuli.

happened? A patient can be awake and oriented or awake and disoriented. Disoriented patients may have a serious medical problem or a traumatic injury.

Airway

Chapter 7 covers airway obstructions and airway management in detail; this chapter focuses only on assessing the status of a patient's airway. Generally, a patient who is responsive and can speak has an open (or patent) airway. While this patient's airway may currently be functional, reassessment must be continuous as the airway may still be at risk. Noisy breathing indicates a partially obstructed airway. A patient who is trying to speak or cough but cannot make any noise has a completely obstructed airway. Partial or complete airway obstruction may be attributable to a foreign body, a narrowing airway caused by swelling, or trauma. Upon inspection, if there is anything visible blocking the airway of the child or adult, it should be removed immediately. Solid objects should be removed with your fingers while liquids such as blood or vomit should be removed either through positioning the patient in a recovery position or with suctioning. If the patient is unresponsive, you should assess the patient's airway and look, listen, and feel for breathing. You will need to open the patient's airway if breathing is noisy or if you do not hear breathing at all. Use the head-tilt/chin-lift maneuver to open the airway unless there is a possibility of trauma (Fig. 8-6). With trauma patients it is important to open the airway without moving the spine, to prevent further injury. This is best accomplished by having someone assist you and maintain head and spine stabilization while you use the modified jaw-thrust method without a head-tilt maneuver (Fig. 8-7). You must be sure the patient has a patent airway and that this open airway is maintained throughout the rest of your assessment and treatment.

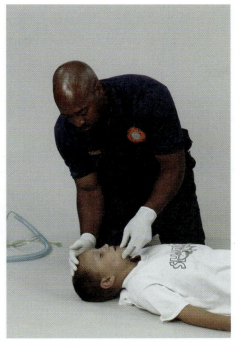

Fig. 8-6 Head-tilt/chin-lift. (From Chapleau W, Pons P: *Emergency medical technician, making the difference,* ed 1, St Louis, 2007, Mosby.)

Breathing and Ventilation

To assess breathing you should look at and listen to the patient as he or she breathes. If the patient is responsive and alert, you can ask yourself the following questions: Is the patient able to speak in full sentences without having to stop to take a breath? How hard is the patient working to breathe? Is the breathing adequate? Is the patient sitting upright? Patients who are having trouble breathing are usually sitting upright and leaning forward (sometimes called the tripod position) (Fig. 8-8). What is the patient's

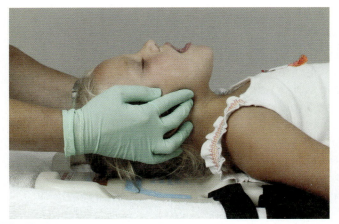

Fig. 8-7 Jaw thrust. (From Chapleau W, Pons P: *Emergency medical technician, making the difference,* ed 1, St Louis, 2007, Mosby.)

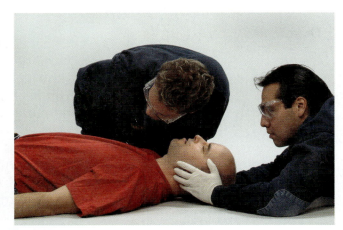

Fig. 8-9 If the patient is unresponsive, look, listen, and feel for breathing.

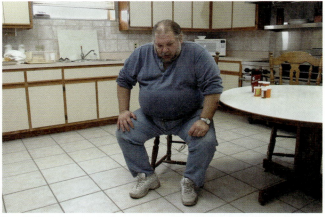

Fig. 8-8 Patients who are having difficulty breathing are usually sitting upright and leaning forward.

color? Is the patient showing signs of hypoxia such as cyanosis? How fast and how deep is the patient breathing? Remember, the quicker the breathing the shallower the breaths become, decreasing the amount of oxygen being delivered to the body. At this point in the primary assessment you should not take the time to count the actual breathing rate but you should quickly determine if breathing is adequate or inadequate. Is the patient using accessory muscles in the chest (between the ribs) or neck or abdominal muscles to breathe? The more energy the patient requires to breathe, the greater the distress of the patient. Can the patient speak and carry on a normal conversation? If so, breathing is adequate. If the patient's speech is interrupted by pauses to breathe, breathing is not adequate. Allow the patient to take the position that makes it easiest to breathe; this is usually sitting up.

If the patient is unresponsive, you should look, listen, and feel for breathing (Fig. 8-9). If the patient is breathing adequately, you can continue to reassess the patient. If the patient is not breathing adequately, open the airway and ventilate the patient using either a mouth-to-mask, a mouth-to-barrier, or a bag-mask device (see Chapter 7). Box 8-2 reviews the signs of inadequate breathing.

Supplemental oxygen should be given to any patient exhibiting signs of inadequate breathing and/or ventilation. Consider assisting breathing with a bag-mask and supplemental oxygen if the patient is breathing too fast (>20 breaths per minute) or too slow (<12 breaths per minute) or anytime there are signs of cyanosis. Some people are hesitant to assist the ventilations of a conscious patient with a bag-mask device. If the patient is showing signs and symptoms of inadequate ventilation and oxygenation, regardless of his or her level of consciousness, the patient should have ventilation assistance. If the patient has no respirations or very slow respirations, rescue breathing must be started (see Chapter 7).

Circulation

To determine the effectiveness of a patient's circulation, you should look for major bleeding, assess the pulse, and quickly assess the skin. As stated at the beginning of this section, it is important to remember that the components of assessment can be done in conjunction with each other. For instance, you can be looking at the patient's skin while observing that the patient is bleeding from the forehead and at the same time assessing the carotid pulse.

BOX 8-2   Inadequate Breathing

Look for:
- Restlessness, agitation, confusion
- Patient sitting upright
- Decreased level of consciousness
- Abnormal breathing rate and rhythm
- Pale, cyanotic, or flushed skin
- Use of additional muscles to breathe

Listen for:
- A patient who complains of not being able to breathe or pain with breathing
- A patient unable to speak or able to speak only a few words at a time
- Noisy breathing

Feel for:
- Abnormal chest movement
- Abnormal pulse

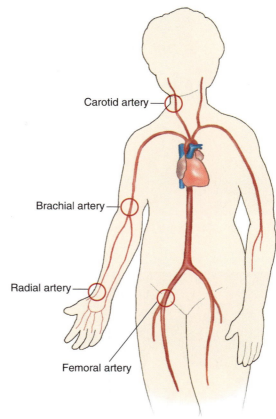

Fig. 8-10 Pulses may be assessed in the carotid, brachial, radial, or femoral arteries. (From McSwain N, Paturas J: *The basic EMT: comprehensive prehospital patient care*, ed 2, St Louis, 2003, Mosby.)

Assess the Pulse

Patients who are awake, breathing, and talking to you will have a circulating blood volume that can be confirmed by a pulse. However, if a patient is unresponsive you will need to check to see if he or she has a detectable pulse. A pulse can be felt anywhere an artery is located close to the skin surface, overlying a bony structure. The most common pulse sites that are palpated are shown in Fig. 8-10.

- **Carotid pulse.** A carotid pulse is the pulse felt over the carotid arteries in the patient's neck (Fig. 8-11). When you locate the carotid pulse in the patient's neck, you should keep the airway open, with one hand on the patient's forehead. You can use two or three fingers of your other hand to locate the larynx (Adam's apple) in the center of the patient's neck. Once this is located you can slide your fingers back toward yourself into the groove between the Adam's apple and the muscles on the side of the neck. You should gently feel for a pulse for at least 5 seconds but no more than 10 seconds. In an unresponsive, critical adult or child, you should immediately check the carotid pulse because this is considered a better check of circulation.
- **Brachial pulse.** A brachial pulse is felt in the fleshy part of the upper arm just under the bicep muscle

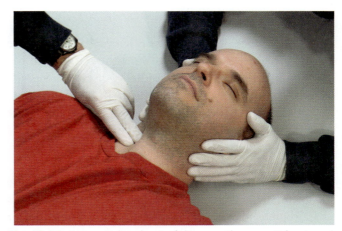

Fig. 8-11 A carotid pulse is felt over the carotid artery in the neck.

(Fig. 8-12). You should always assess the brachial pulse in an infant patient regardless of whether the patient is responsive or unresponsive because the brachial pulse is the easiest to locate and most reliable in an infant.

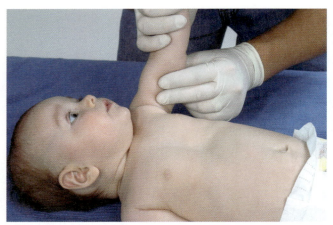

Fig. 8-12 A brachial pulse is felt over the brachial artery.

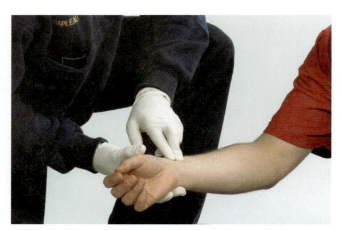

Fig. 8-13 A radial pulse is felt over the radial artery.

- **Radial pulse.** A radial pulse is felt on the thumb side of the wrist just lateral (toward the outside) to the tendon (Fig. 8-13). A radial pulse is generally checked on responsive adult patients, and if a radial pulse cannot be found the carotid pulse should be checked next. In responsive children you should assess the brachial or radial pulses first, followed by the carotid or femoral pulses.
- **Femoral pulse.** A femoral pulse can be found in the groin area. The femoral pulse can be used to assess circulation in responsive children if a brachial or radial pulse cannot be found. The carotid or femoral pulse should be assessed in an unresponsive child. In the newborn, assess the central pulse by palpating the base of the umbilical cord between your thumb and index finger.

Table 8-6 lists the best locations to check pulses in responsive and unresponsive adults, children, infants, and newborns. When you check a pulse you should assess if it is present or not present. Is the pulse slow or fast?

TABLE 8-6   Pulse Locations

PATIENT	PULSE LOCATION
Adult	
Responsive	Radial pulse
Unresponsive	Carotid pulse ≤10 seconds
Child	
Responsive	Brachial or radial pulse
Unresponsive	Carotid or femoral pulse
Infant	Brachial pulse
Newborn	Central pulse at base of umbilical cord

Normal pulse rates for an adult patient will be between 60 and 100 beats per minute and regular. Slow and fast pulses may indicate a significant problem. Is the pulse regular or irregular? An irregular pulse may indicate a cardiac problem. Is the pulse weak or strong? A weak pulse may be an indication of inadequate circulation. If the patient does not have a pulse, you should start cardiopulmonary resuscitation (CPR) immediately (see Chapter 9).

Major Bleeding

As part of the primary assessment you also need to assess the patient for major bleeding (hemorrhage). To do this you must look at both the patient and the scene. Does the patient have any visible active bleeding? Do you see a pool of blood anywhere at the scene? You should look to see if blood has collected in the patient's clothing or hair or is visible on the ground. It is also important to feel around the back of the patient to see if any blood has collected underneath the patient. If active hemorrhage is occurring, you must control it (see Chapter 11). You should also be aware of how much blood the patient has potentially lost. If a patient has lost a lot of blood, he or she may be in shock. Shock management is covered in Chapter 11. It is important to remember that although all bleeding can be potentially life-threatening, some bleeding can look more severe than it actually is. You should not let bleeding distract you from the priorities of assessing and maintaining the patient's airway, breathing, and circulation.

Assess the Skin

The patient's skin color and temperature can also be indications of the adequacy of circulation. Assessing the skin color of patients with natural dark-colored skin can best be accomplished by visually checking the palms of their hands or under their tongue, or by examining the inside lining (mucosal tissue) of the patient's lips or eyelids. Although a late sign, a bluish (cyanotic) discoloration indicates a lack of oxygen at the cellular level. Pale skin color may indicate a low body temperature, blood loss, or shock. If the patient's skin is flushed or red, the patient's temperature may be elevated. Cool skin may indicate a low body temperature or shock. Wet or sweaty skin may indicate physical exertion, severe pain, or shock. If the patient's color is pale, mottled, and cool to touch, the patient may be in shock. You should position a patient in shock on his or her back with the feet slightly elevated and cover the patient with a blanket (see Chapter 11).

Another circulation assessment that may be helpful when assessing infants and children 6 years of age or younger is checking the capillary refill time. Capillary refill time is checked by pressing on an area of the skin or thumb nail and releasing. Once released, color should return to the area within 2 seconds. If it takes longer than 2 seconds for the color to return to the area that was depressed, it may indicate decreased circulation. Delayed capillary refill by itself is not a reliable indicator.

Disability

An additional step in the initial assessment is sometimes designated as D for Disability. This step provides more of an assessment of a patient's brain (mental) function and is also called a neurological assessment. In this step the emergency first responder should assess the patient's mental function along with the patient's ability to move and control all extremities. Any sign of decreased or decreasing mental function can indicate a decrease in the amount of oxygen being delivered to the brain. One of the most complete ways to assess a patient's mental status (disability) is through the use of the Glasgow Coma Scale (GCS) score. The GCS score is used by other prehospital providers as well as in-hospital providers to assess the patient's mental function. The earlier the assessment can be done on a patient, the earlier a baseline value can be set so that subsequent evaluations can indicate whether a patient is improving, deteriorating, or staying the same.

The GCS score evaluates the patient's neurological functions based on three categories: eye opening, verbal response, and motor response. Each category identifies typical responses and has an assigned numerical value. The assessment is based on the patient's best response in each category and computation of the total score. The assessment should start at the top of each category with the best possible response (highest possible score)

TABLE 8-7 Glasgow Coma Scale

	POINTS
Eye Opening	
Spontaneous eye opening	4
Eye opening on command	3
Eye opening to painful stimulus	2
No eye opening	1
Best Verbal Response	
Answers appropriately (oriented)	5
Gives confused answers	4
Gives inappropriate response	3
Makes unintelligible noises	2
Makes no verbal response	1
Best Motor Response	
Follows command	6
Localizes painful stimuli	5
Withdraws to pain	4
Responds with flexion to painful stimuli	3
Responds with extension to painful stimuli	2
Gives no motor response	1
Highest possible score	15
Critical patient	≤13

and then move downward until a response is observed (Table 8-7).

Eye Opening (E)

The maximum number of points available for the patient's response to eye opening (E) is four points. If the patient readily opens his or her eyes without having to be asked, all four points are awarded. If, however, the patient only opens his or her eyes when asked, three points are awarded. If you must administer a painful stimulus to open the patient's eyes, two points are awarded, and only one point is awarded if the patient does not open the eyes to either a verbal or a painful stimulus.

Verbal Response (V)

After establishing the E response, you move on to assess the patient's best verbal (V) response. The maximum number of points available for verbal response is five. If the patient answers appropriately to a simple question such as "What happened?" or "Where do you hurt?" he or she would be awarded all five points. If the patient gives a confused response (such as "I don't know" or "I don't remember") to your questions, four points would be given. If the patient responds inappropriately (such as "The sky is blue") to your questions, only three points are given. If the patient simply makes unintelligible noise in response to your questions, he or she is awarded two points, and one point is awarded if a patient is unable to or does not give a verbal response.

Motor Response (M)

The final component of the GCS is the patient's motor response (M). The maximum number of points available for the motor response is six. If a patient is able to follow simple commands to move all extremities (such as "Show me two fingers" or "Push your foot against my hand"), all six points are awarded. If the patient does not respond to your request, you should apply a minor painful stimulus. If the patient tries to push away the painful stimulus (called localizing), he or she would receive five points. If instead the patient withdraws from the painful stimulus, four points are given. If the patient's response to the painful stimulus is to flex his or her extremities (move the arms and legs toward the body), three points are given. If the patient responds by extending his or her extremities away from the body, he or she is awarded two points, and one point is awarded if there is no response to the painful stimulus.

Reporting of the GCS Score

After assessing each component of the GCS (E, V, M) the points received for each component are added together to get a total GCS score. This score will range between a minimum of 3 and a maximum of 15 points. A total GCS score of 3 would mean that the patient is nonresponsive and without spontaneous eye opening, verbal response, or motor response. A GCS score of 15 means that the patient is conscious and alert. This patient is able to respond with spontaneous eye opening, verbal response, and motor response.

If the patient's GCS score is something other than 3 or 15, the score should be broken down by category and its awarded points. This type of reporting is necessary to identify the deficit in a category or categories. For example, if your patient opened her eyes when you administered a sternal rub or a pen-between-the-fingers squeeze (two points), gave inappropriate answers to your questions (three points), and withdrew her body away from a painful stimulus (four points), the total GCS score would be nine and would be reported as E-2, V-3, M-4.

Although this may seem confusing, with practice it can be accomplished quickly and efficiently and will be of great benefit to the receiving ambulance or hospital.

TABLE 8-8	Indicators of Critical Patients
General impression/ responsiveness	Unresponsive not moving, poor general impression
Airway	Obstructive sounds such as stridor, snoring, or gurgling (grunting in infants) Compromised airway
Breathing	Inadequate rate and quality of breathing Absence of breathing Difficulty breathing Accessory muscle use
Circulation	Uncontrolled bleeding Weak, absent, or irregular pulse Signs of cyanosis Cool, clammy skin (shock)
Disability	GCS ≤ 13 Confusion, disorientation Changing level of consciousness Pediatric—flaccid; glassy stare; does not acknowledge caregiver or emergency first responder

Prioritizing Patients

The primary assessment helps you separate or triage critical or serious patients from noncritical ones. Chapter 15 provides additional information on triage. With critical or serious patients you must continue to reassess the airway, breathing, and circulation and care for any life-threatening conditions until the patient is stable or more advanced care arrives. Table 8-8 shows a list of indicators that suggest a patient is likely to have serious or critical problems and should be prioritized for care and transport. Skills 8-1 and 8-2 illustrate the initial assessment of an unresponsive and a responsive patient, respectively.

Skill 8-1

Primary Assessment (Unresponsive Patient)

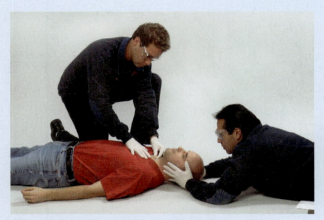

1. General impression. Assess responsiveness.

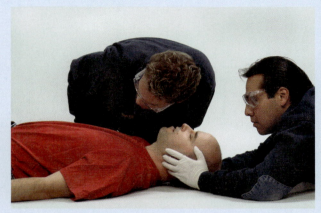

2. Assess airway and breathing.

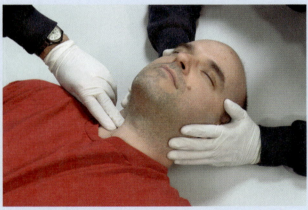

3. Assess for a pulse.

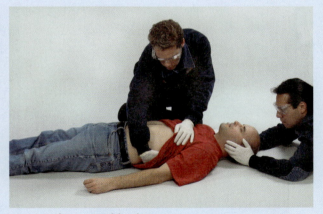

4. Assess for major bleeding.

6. Determine disability and assess priority.

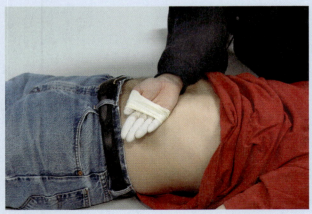

5. Assess the skin.

Skill 8-2

Primary Assessment (Responsive Patient)

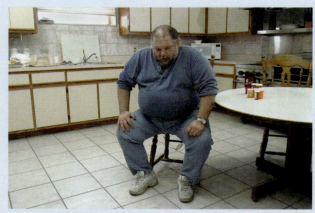

1. General impression.

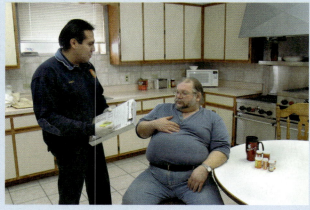

2. Assess responsiveness, airway, and breathing.

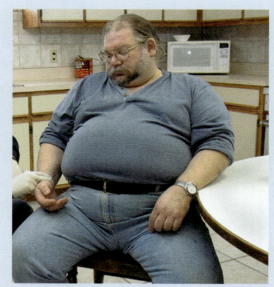

3. Assess circulation.

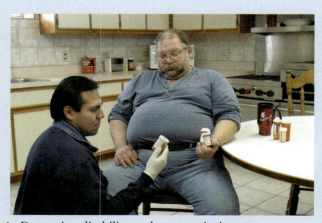

4. Determine disability and assess priority.

Communication

If you find an unresponsive patient during the initial assessment, you would call for additional help immediately. However, if the patient is responsive, you may wait until the initial assessment is complete before calling for additional help. Once you have prioritized the patient, you should update the responding EMS unit with a brief radio or cellular telephone report if possible.

The report should include the following patient information:

- Number of patients
- Age and gender of patient(s)
- Chief complaint
- Responsiveness
- Airway, breathing, circulation, and disability status

Secondary Assessment

After ensuring all life-threatening conditions have been identified and correctly managed during the primary assessment, you can now progress to the secondary assessment. The secondary assessment consists of obtaining a complete set of the patient's vital signs, performing a detailed physical examination based on the patient's presenting condition, and gathering a past medical history. A systematic and organized physical examination of the patient is performed to assist in identifying signs and symptoms of illness or injury and beginning appropriate treatment. A sign is defined as a finding that you can hear, see, feel, or measure during the physical examination, whereas a symptom is a problem or condition that a patient describes to you. The pneumonic OPQRST can be used for the evaluation of signs and symptoms and

pain (Table 8-9). After completing the physical examination the next step is to gather a past medical history. The exact nature of the history and physical examination depends on the patient's condition. For example, a patient with a sprained ankle may not require as full an examination as a patient of a motorcycle crash. This chapter describes the basic physical examination and the components of a past medical history that can be used on all patients. Later chapters provide additional information about patient assessment based on the patient's specific illness or injury. Although a head-to-toe format is used to present the information, it is important to realize that an assessment may not always be done in this way. Continuing with the example of a patient with a sprained ankle, the physical assessment would start with the injured ankle, and then spread out to other body parts as appropriate. This type of examination would be called a focused physical examination. Regardless of the type of assessment being performed, always keep the patient informed of what you are about to do and ask for his or her permission. Many patients view a physical examination with apprehension and anxiety; they feel vulnerable and exposed. Maintain a professional approach throughout the examination and display an appropriate compassion for the patient and the patient's situation.

Vital Signs

A set of vital signs consists of the patient's pulse rate, respiratory rate, and, if allowed, blood pressure. Vital signs provide a starting point for judging the effectiveness of prehospital care. As a "general rule," a set of vital signs should be taken every 15 minutes for noncritical patients and at least every 5 minutes for critical patients or whenever their condition changes.

TABLE 8-9 OPQRST Mnemonic for Evaluation of Pain or Signs and Symptoms

O	Onset	When did the problem start? What were you doing when the problem started?
P	Provocation	What, if anything, makes the problem worse? What, if anything, makes the problem better?
Q	Quality	How does the patient describe the problem? What does it feel like?
R	Radiation	Where is there pain? Does the pain spread anywhere else in the body?
S	Severity	On a scale of 1 to 10 (with 10 being the worst pain you have ever felt in your life), how bad is the problem?
T	Time	How long has the patient had the problem?

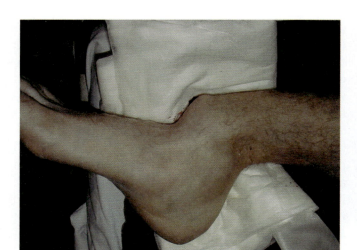

Fig. 8-14 Deformity of the right ankle. (From McSwain N, Paturas J: *The basic EMT: comprehensive prehospital patient care,* ed 2, St Louis, 2003, Mosby.)

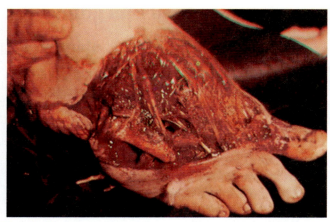

Fig. 8-15 Assess for any open injuries or wounds. This injury was caused when the foot was smashed over the footrest of a motorcycle. (From McSwain N, Paturas J: *The basic EMT: comprehensive prehospital patient care,* ed 2, St Louis, 2003, Mosby.)

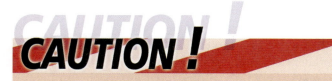

CAUTION!

The secondary assessment and physical examination may not be completed or even started if any life-threatening conditions are identified in the initial assessment.

Physical Examination

In the physical examination you should inspect (look) and palpate (feel) for signs of injury. The mnemonic DOTS (*Deformities, Open* wounds, *Tenderness, Swelling*) can be used throughout the physical examination. Each body part should be assessed for deformities. You may see this as an abnormal position of an extremity (Fig. 8-14) or a depression in the skull. You also assess for any open injuries or wounds (Fig. 8-15). It is important to note that if you find an object impaled in or sticking out from an open wound you should leave it in place and stabilize it. The management of an impaled object is discussed more thoroughly in Chapter 11. Patients may also report an area of tenderness or you may identify one as you palpate an area of the body. Palpation of the body should always be done gently but with purpose to avoid unnecessarily injuring the patient. The final thing to assess is swelling. You may be able to see swelling involving an uncovered body part, but you should also remember to palpate for swelling because you may not be able to see it through clothing. If you need to expose an area of the body while you are performing the physical examination, you should be gentle, consider the patient's privacy, and remember to keep the patient warm. Finally, you should always compare one side of the patient's body to the other to help identify abnormalities. For example, by comparing the left side of the chest to the right side you may see that the right side is swollen compared to the left.

The physical examination of a patient should be done in a systematic and orderly manner. You should practice your assessment skills often so you can quickly identify normal and abnormal findings. If a patient has a specific injury or complaint, you should generally start there; then expand the physical examination as needed. For example, if a patient has a sprained ankle you should focus first on the ankle and then expand the examination up the leg and to other body parts only as needed. The purpose of the physical examination is to identify other injuries not found in your initial assessment. In most cases you will just note where an injury is and move on with your assessment; however, in some instances immediate action must be taken. These immediate actions are listed below and on pp. 201-202 as they correspond to the appropriate body part. Skill 8-3 lists and illustrates a detailed physical examination of the entire body.

CAUTION!

If trauma is suspected, the patient's head and neck should have been stabilized in the initial assessment. As you proceed with the physical examination, you should not move the head any more than necessary as you look for injuries or abnormalities.

Text continued on p. 197

Skill 8-3

Secondary Assessment—Physical Examination

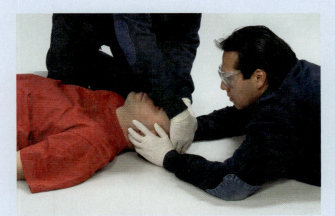

1. Inspect and palpate the scalp.

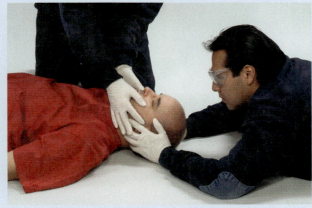

2. Inspect and palpate the face.

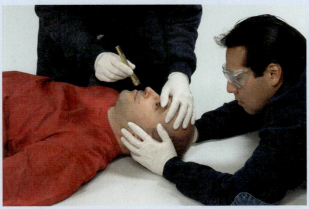

3. Look for eye injuries and pupil response. Do not palpate eye injuries.

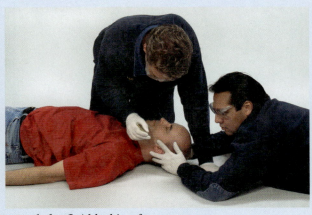

4. Look for fluid leaking from ears.

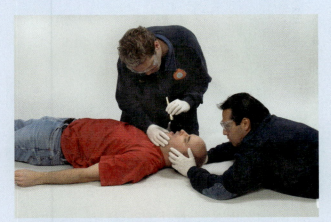

5. Check the mouth for any bleeding or injuries.

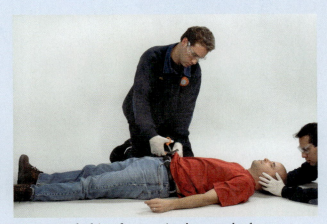

6. Remove clothing from patient's upper body.

Skill 8-3

Secondary Assessment—Physical Examination—cont'd

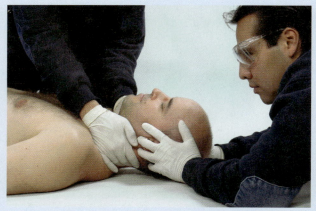

7. Inspect and palpate the front and the back of the neck.

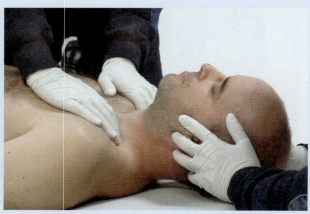

8. Inspect and palpate the chest.

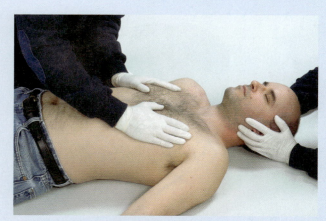

9. Compare both sides of the chest for any abnormality.

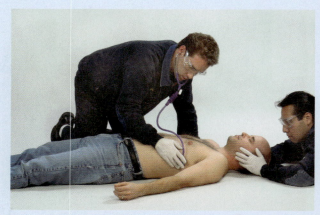

10. Auscultate the chest.

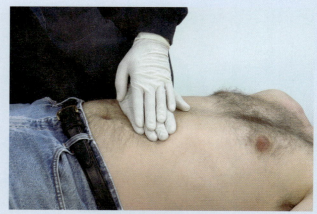

11. Inspect and palpate the abdomen.

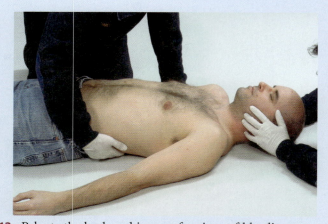

12. Palpate the back and inspect for signs of bleeding.

Skill 8-3

Secondary Assessment—Physical Examination—cont'd

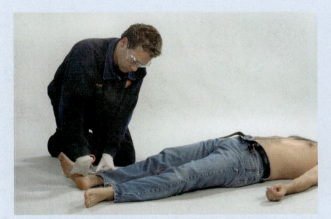

13. Remove clothing from patient's lower body.

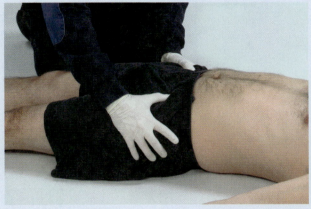

14. Palpate the pelvis.

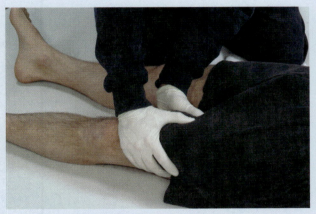

15. Inspect and palpate each upper leg.

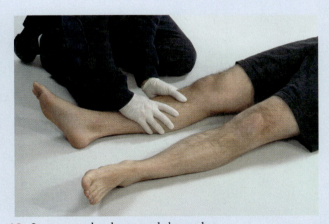

16. Inspect and palpate each lower leg.

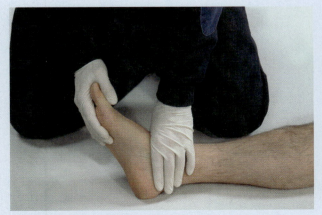

17. Assess movement and sensation in each foot.

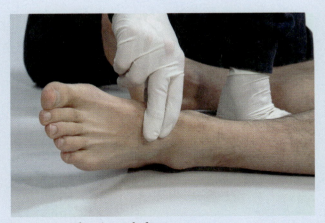

18. Assess pulses in each foot.

Skill 8-3

Secondary Assessment—Physical Examination—cont'd

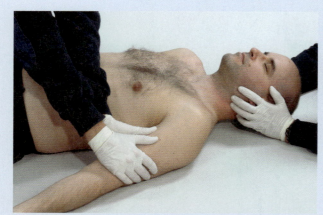

19. Inspect and palpate each upper arm.

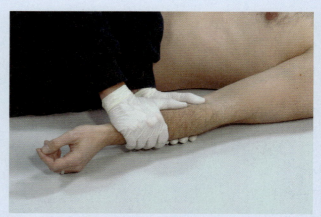

20. Inspect and palpate each lower arm.

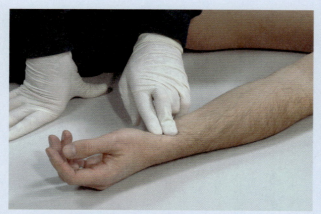

21. Assess radial pulse in each arm.

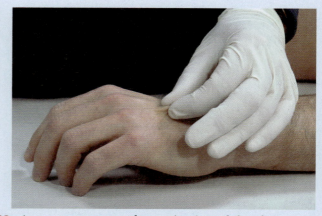

22. Assess movement and sensation in each hand.

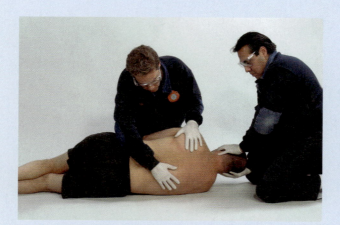

23. If possible, log roll patient and assess back.

Head

To examine the head you should run your fingers over the face and scalp to gently palpate for deformities or depressions in the bones of the face or skull. Remember to be gentle so that, in case of a skull fracture, you do not force pieces of bone down into the brain. You should run your fingers through the patient's hair to see if you can identify any injuries or tenderness. You should also look for open injuries or wounds anywhere on the face and scalp. You should not worry about finding the exact area of bleeding in the scalp because probing too much may actually increase the bleeding. Chapter 11 discusses management of open wounds to the head.

You should look for any fluid leaking from the nose or ears, which may indicate a skull fracture, and check the mouth for any bleeding or injuries. During the entire physical examination you should monitor the airway regularly because bleeding and clots can obstruct the airway or cause vomiting. You should not palpate eye injuries because this may cause additional injury to an already damaged eye. You should further note any complaints of tenderness and areas of swelling on the head and face.

Neck

If the patient is injured, you will need to keep the head and neck stabilized while you use gentle pressure to palpate for deformities. Specific areas of assessment include the position of the trachea (it should be midline in the neck and not shifted) and the presence of open wounds in the neck. Open wounds in the neck can be dangerous because the neck holds the trachea and has very large blood vessels; damage to these structures can be life-threatening. If air enters the open wounds, air bubbles can get into the blood vessels and cause blockage of the blood flow. If you discover an open wound during the physical examination, you should cover it completely with an airtight (occlusive) dressing (see Chapter 11). If the patient complains of tenderness when you palpate, there may be damage to the spine or the soft tissue that supports the neck. Because swelling can obstruct the airway, you will need to continually reassess the airway during the physical assessment. It is important to remember to inspect and palpate not only the front of the neck but also the vertebrae and skin on the back of the neck.

After you examine the neck, if you are trained to do so and have the equipment, a cervical collar should be placed on a trauma patient who requires one. More information on cervical collars is found in Chapter 12.

Chest

As you examine the chest you should remember the major organs that the thoracic cavity holds, such as the heart and lungs (Fig. 8-16). You should always compare the two sides of the chest to help identify any abnormali-

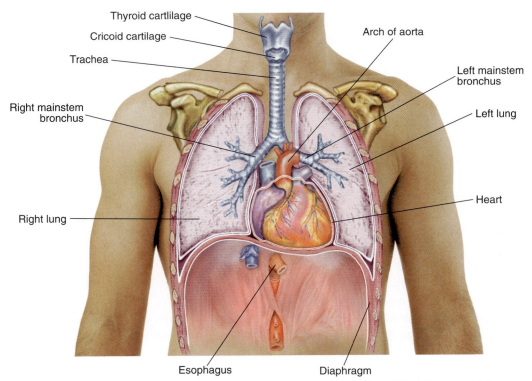

Fig. 8-16 Chest cavity and related anatomical structures. (Modified from Seidel H, Ball J, Dains J, Benedict G: *Mosby's guide to physical examination,* ed 6, St Louis, 2006, Mosby.)

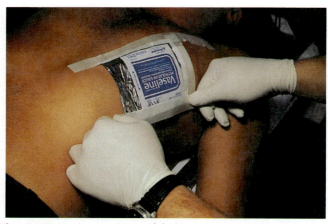

Fig. 8-17 Taping a piece of foil or plastic to the chest wall on three sides allows air to escape from the pleural space but not enter into it. (From NAEMT: *PHTLS: basic and advanced prehospital trauma life support,* ed 6, St Louis, 2007, Mosby.)

ties. You should inspect and palpate the chest for any deformity, which may indicate broken ribs. It is important to assess both the anterior (front) and the posterior (back) of the chest for open wounds. Open chest wounds, similar to open neck wounds, can let air flow into the chest and around the lungs, causing a potentially life-threatening injury. If you find an open chest wound, you should immediately apply direct pressure with a gloved hand and then apply an airtight (occlusive) dressing. Tape the dressing only on three sides, maintaining one open side for air to escape (Fig. 8-17). Inspect and palpate for tenderness and swelling, which may indicate a rib fracture and/or potential lung or heart damage.

Abdomen

You should gently palpate the abdomen for any injuries or tenderness. You may feel or see deformities in the abdomen. If you discover any open injuries to the skin and fatty tissue of the abdomen, you should cover them with an occlusive dressing such as plastic food wrap, again to keep air from entering the abdomen. If a wound is deep or if abdominal contents are visible or spilling out of the wound, you should cover the area with a sterile, moist dressing. It is important to note the location of any tenderness because it may provide a clue about underlying organ damage. The patient may tighten the muscles of an injured area (called "guarding") when you palpate the abdomen; you should watch out for this and avoid palpating obviously tender areas. You should report swelling or distention in the abdomen by quadrant location (see Chapter 5).

Back

If there are enough providers available when you are assessing a trauma patient, you should do a log roll (to protect the patient's spine from any potential injury) in order to inspect the patient's back (see Chapter 6). You should inspect and palpate the back for any obvious deformities, open wounds, tenderness, or swelling.

Pelvis

To assess the pelvis, apply gentle but firm pressure to the pelvic girdle to check for deformities. As you are palpating you may feel a crunching, or crepitus. Crepitus is the sound or a feeling of bone ends grating against one another or air trapped between tissue layers. It feels like bubble wrap popping. This feeling indicates a possible pelvic fracture. Injury in the pelvic area can cause extensive bleeding both internally and externally from the large blood vessels in this area. Tenderness and swelling may indicate a fracture or dislocation. If you have to move the patient, you should fully support the legs if you suspect an injury in the pelvic area.

Extremities

You should inspect and palpate each extremity for deformities of the bones, soft tissue, and joints. You should also look for open wounds and control any bleeding. Although injuries to extremities can be dramatic, you must not be distracted from assessing and managing the patient's life-threatening conditions. Tenderness or swelling in the extremities may result from a fracture, dislocation, or sprain. You should limit the movement of an injured extremity or support the area if the patient must be moved. To assess for numbness, ask the patient to identify the areas you touch. Ask the patient to move the arms and legs. If one arm or leg is weaker, the patient cannot move an extremity, or numbness is present, you should suspect a head or neck injury. Palpate the patient's radial pulses in the arms and pedal pulses in the legs to evaluate circulation. Remember to compare each extremity to the opposite extremity to help identify possible injuries and/or abnormalities.

History

It is important to collect the patient's complaint, past medical history, and event history as you assess the patient. The chief complaint is a very brief description of the reason for summoning assistance. In the best of circumstances, the patient will be able to answer all questions about his or her own medical history. In the event that the patient is unable to respond or cannot remember events leading up to the incident, you may need to seek

TABLE 8-10   SAMPLE Mnemonic for History Taking

S	Signs/symptoms	Sign—a condition you can see or measure
		Symptom—a problem a patient describes
A	Allergies	Allergies to medications, environment, or food
		Medical insignia tag
M	Medications	Prescription, over-the-counter, herbs, vitamins, "recreational" drugs
		Medical insignia
P	Pertinent past medical history	Recent medical, surgical, or trauma problems
		Seeing a doctor for problems
		Recent hospitalizations
		Medical insignia
L	Last oral intake	What was consumed?
		How much?
		How long ago?
E	Events leading to injury or illness	What were you doing when you became ill?
		What were you doing when you were hurt?
		Does anything else hurt or bother you?

other sources to assist in the gathering of a history. Consider checking with family members, friends, bystanders, law enforcement personnel, or others who may have answers to your history questions. Another source of medical information may be found by looking for medical identification jewelry or medical information on the patient's driver's license.

You can gather a patient's most relevant medical history by using the mnemonic SAMPLE (Table 8-10).

S—Signs and Symptoms

As you perform the physical examination and collect the patient's history, it is important to note the patient's signs and symptoms. A sign is a finding you can:

- *hear,* such as snoring
- *see,* such as a bruise
- *feel,* such as skin temperature
- *measure,* such as a fast pulse

A symptom is a problem a patient describes, such as a headache. Signs and symptoms give you clues about what is wrong with the patient. You should obtain additional information about the patient's signs and symptoms if you have time. Ask questions like the following:

- Can you describe the problem? (e.g., What color is the blood in your stool?)
- What kind of symptoms are you having? (e.g., Do you have any pain anywhere?)

- What makes the symptom worse or better? (e.g., Does it hurt more when you breathe?)
- When did the symptom start? (e.g., When did you first feel this pain? What were you doing when it started?)
- How long has the symptom been present? (e.g., How long have you had this problem or condition?)
- Has anything like this ever happened before? What happened the last time? (e.g., Has this ever happened to you before? Did you see a doctor about it?)

A—Allergies

It is important to determine if the patient is allergic to anything, such as medications, food, or things in the environment (e.g., grass, pollen, animals). Information about allergies is particularly important to communicate to other health care providers because certain allergies may have an effect on the treatment the patient receives or they may be the reason for the patient's condition. Patients with severe allergies may wear a medical insignia tag that indicates the allergy. It is important to ask the patient if he or she is allergic to anything and also to look for a medical insignia tag while performing a physical examination.

M—Medications

You should always ask patients what medications they are taking, including prescribed medications, over-the-counter medications, herbs, vitamins, and "recreational" drugs (e.g., cocaine, marijuana). You should also check whether patients have taken their prescribed medication as instructed. Have they taken it with any other medication or substance? How much did they take and when was it taken? This information should always be communicated because medications can help health care providers identify a patient's preexisting condition.

P—Past Medical History

Ask about the patient's pertinent past medical history to help you identify the present problem. A pertinent medical history would be anything that is relevant to the current condition. For example, knowing that a patient has diabetes can give you a clue that perhaps the patient's unresponsiveness is caused by a low blood sugar problem. You should ask questions such as the following to help you identify recent medical problems:

- Have you had any recent medical, surgical, or trauma problems?
- Are you seeing a doctor for any problems?
- Have you been in the hospital recently?

L—Last Oral Intake

You should find out when the patient last ate or drank anything. This is important in case, for example, the patient needs to undergo surgery. Knowing when a diabetic patient last ate may help you evaluate unresponsiveness. You can ask when and how much an infant ate and drank to evaluate potential dehydration.

E—Events Leading to the Injury or Illness

Information about events that occurred before the problem may provide clues about the patient's problem. For example, a patient may have inhaled gas in the garage before experiencing difficulty breathing; if you find this patient sitting on the couch in the house you need to ask what happened earlier to understand the problem. It is also important to determine the chronology of events that happened. For example, a patient may have been in a MVC. It is important to learn whether the patient had chest pain, was dizzy, or blacked out before the crash or if the patient was just trying to avoid a squirrel that ran into the street.

Reassessment

While caring for a patient you should perform a reassessment until additional EMS personnel arrive and take over care. You may or may not have time to complete this reassessment. With a critical patient you may focus entirely on the primary assessment and assessing and treating airway, breathing, or circulation problems. If the patient is not critical and the EMS response time is short,

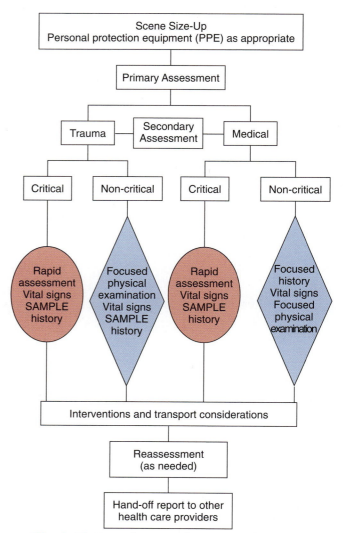

Fig. 8-18 Flow diagram of patient assessment.

you may have time to complete only an initial examination. If you have time, however, you should perform a primary assessment, complete a secondary assessment, and collect a SAMPLE history. The reassessment then repeats the primary assessment (ABCD) and vital signs at continuous intervals. It reassesses the patient's airway, breathing, circulation, and possible disability (mental status) to gauge the effectiveness of your treatment and to correct any identified problems. You should reassess the airway to ensure it is open and maintained. You should monitor the patient's breathing and pulse for rate and quality. You should recheck skin color, temperature, and condition and you should continually calm and reassure the patient as you wait for EMS to arrive. Any time a patient's condition changes, the patient should be reassessed. You should repeat the primary assessment frequently, at least every 5 minutes with a critical patient and at least every 15 minutes with a noncritical patient. **Fig. 8-18** illustrates the entire process of patient assessment.

Hand-Off Report

When the EMS responders arrive you should be ready to give a hand-off report. This report describes your assessments and interventions. With multiple patients you should start with the most critical patients so that they get immediate care and transport. The report should include the following patient information:

- Age and gender
- Chief complaint
- Responsiveness
- Airway and breathing status
- Circulation status
- Physical findings
- SAMPLE history
- Interventions provided
- Patient's current condition

Team Work

As part of the health care team it is beneficial for you, as an emergency first responder, to know how to take and report vital signs and how to accurately triage patients. This section of Team Work will focus on teaching you how to obtain vital signs and give you more information on triage.

VITAL SIGNS

You may be required to evaluate or help evaluate the patient's vital signs if time permits. The vital signs include the patient's breathing, pulse, skin, pupils, and blood pressure. As you assess a patient's vital signs the initial numbers you obtain will be important, but even more important will be the trends you identify as you reassess the vital signs. For example, if you assess a patient and find his or her pulse rate is high when you first arrive, but it slows to normal after you initiate treatment, then the patient is improving. On the other hand, if a patient's pulse rate is high and remains high or goes even higher, then the patient is not improving or may even be more unstable. As part of the ongoing assessment, vital signs are usually taken at a minimum of every 5 minutes in critical patients and every 15 minutes in noncritical patients.

Breathing

When evaluating breathing you should assess rate, quality, and, in some situations, breath sounds. To assess breathing you should observe the rise and fall of the patient's chest. You may find it easier to look at or feel the upper abdomen to count the respiratory rate. To measure the rate you should count the number of breaths in 30 seconds and multiply the number by 2. For example, if someone breathes 7 times in 30 seconds, the person's breathing rate would be 14 (7 × 2 = 14 breaths per minute). You can also count the number of breaths in 15 seconds and multiply by 4. You should usually not tell the patient you are assessing his or her rate

of breathing because patients may change their respiratory rate when they know someone is assessing their breathing. Normal breathing rates for adults, children, and infants are outlined in Table 8-11. A good tip is to take the patient's pulse rate first for 30 seconds and then, continuing to feel the pulse, observe the respiratory rate for another 30 seconds.

To assess the quality of breathing you need to evaluate how much energy the patient is using to breathe (i.e., the work of breathing), whether the patient is using accessory muscles to breathe, how deep the respirations are, and whether the breathing is noisy. As a general rule, until proven otherwise, breathing that is shallow, labored, or noisy is indicative of a patient with a serious problem (Table 8-12).

To assess breath sounds you may also auscultate or listen to the chest with a stethoscope (Fig. 8-19). When you assess breath sounds you should place the stethoscope in your ears with the earpieces facing forward and use the diaphragm of the stethoscope to listen from side to side on the chest. You are comparing the sounds and quality of respirations in each lung field in order to identify abnormalities. Some breathing sounds will be audible without a stethoscope. Abnormal breathing sounds are reviewed in Table 8-13. When possible it is best to auscultate multiple sites on each side of the chest and to auscultate the back of the chest as well (Fig. 8-20). Remember that abnormal breath sounds usually indicate a problem with the airway or lungs. Whenever abnormal breath sounds are present, you should monitor the patient closely for adequate oxygenation.

Pulse

The pulse is an indicator of the patient's circulatory function. When taking vital signs you should assess a radial

Team Work—cont'd

TABLE 8-11   Normal Respirations, Pulse, and Blood Pressure Measurements

	AGE	RESPIRATORY RATE (breaths/min)	PULSE RATE (beats/min)	BLOOD PRESSURE* (systolic/diastolic) (mmHg)
Newborn	Birth-6 wk	30-50	120-160	(74-100)/(50-68)
Infant	7 wk-1 yr	20-30	80-140	(84-106)/(56-70)
Toddler	1-2 yr	20-30	90-130	(98-106)/(50-70)
Preschool	2-6 yr	20-30	80-120	(98-112)/(64-70)
School age	6-13 yr	18-30	(60-80)-100	(104-124)/(64-80)
Adolescent	13-16 yr	(12-20)-30	60-100	(118-132)/(70-82)
Adult	>16 yr	12-20	60-100	(100-150)/(60-90)

*The normal systolic pressure in children aged 1 to 10 years can be calculated as 90 mm Hg + (child's age in years × 2) mm Hg. The lower systolic pressure in children aged 1 to 10 years can be calculated as 70 mm Hg + (child's age in years × 2) mm Hg.

TABLE 8-12   Categories for Quality of Breathing

QUALITY	EXAMPLE
Normal	No accessory muscle use, breathing is easy, average chest wall movement, regular respiratory pattern
Shallow	Limited or slight chest wall movement, may or may not use accessory muscles
Labored	Using more effort or work to breathe
	Using accessory muscles (neck, supraclavicular, intercostal, abdominal muscles)
	Nasal flaring
	Grunting (especially in infants), stridor, gasping
	Only able to say a few words before having to stop and breathe
	Bluish or cyanotic color
	Abnormal or irregular breathing patterns
Noisy	Increase in sound of breathing, such as snoring, wheezing, gurgling and crowing, stridor

pulse on both child and adult patients. A radial pulse should be measured with two or three fingers of your hand. You should not use your thumb to feel for a pulse because the thumb has its own pulse, which may be measured instead. If a radial pulse cannot be found, you should assess a carotid pulse on adults and a brachial pulse on children.

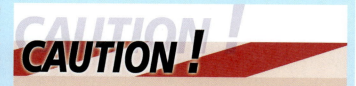

CAUTION!

Be cautious and use gentle pressure when you palpate a carotid pulse. You should never palpate a carotid pulse on both sides of the neck at one time.

Team Work—cont'd

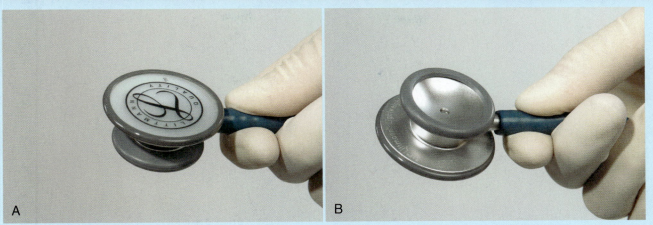

Fig. 8-19 Auscultation of the chest occurs with a stethoscope. **A,** Diaphragm of the stethoscope. **B,** Bell of the stethoscope.

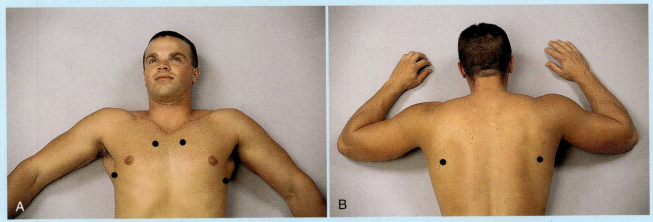

Fig. 8-20 A, Common anterior auscultation points. **B,** Common posterior auscultation points. (From American College of Emergency Physicians [Krohmer JR, editor]: *EMT-basic field care: a case-based approach,* St Louis, 1999, Mosby.)

TABLE 8-13 Abnormal Breathing Sounds

SOUND	CAUSE
Stridor	High-pitched noise from swelling or obstruction of upper airway
Wheezing	Whistling sound heard in lower airways because of obstruction or constriction of bronchioles
Grunting	Grunt usually heard on expiration in infant in respiratory distress
Absent breath sounds	Lack of breath sounds to an area attributable to lung being collapsed or not being ventilated

Team Work—cont'd

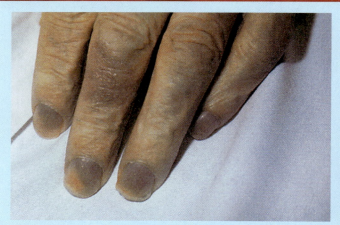

Fig. 8-21 To assess the skin you should look at the nail beds. Cyanosis indicates hypoxia. (From Henry M, Stapleton E: *EMT prehospital care*, ed 2, Philadelphia, 1997, W.B. Saunders.)

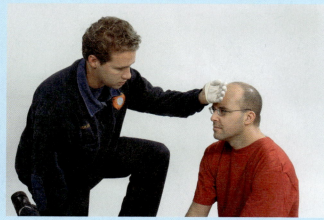

Fig. 8-22 Assess temperature by placing the back of your hand on the patient's skin. You may need to uncover the back portion of your hand to feel the change in skin temperature.

A brachial pulse should always be assessed on infants. Once you feel the pulse you should assess it for rate, regularity, and quality. To determine the pulse rate you should count the number of beats in 30 seconds and multiply by 2. Counting 43 beats in 30 seconds would equal a pulse rate of 86. You can also count the number of beats in 15 seconds and multiply by 4. Normal pulse rates for all age ranges are summarized in Table 8-11.

You should also evaluate the pulse for regularity. A normal pulse occurs at regular intervals. If the pulse is irregular, it may be a sign of cardiac problems. An irregular pulse should be measured for a full minute. When you assess the quality of the pulse, you are feeling to see if the pulse is weak or strong. If the pulse is rapid and weak, the patient may be in shock. If the pulse is rapid and bounding, it may indicate that the patient is anxious or has high blood pressure.

Skin Signs

Assessing the patient's skin can tell you a lot about a patient. Not only will you see injuries, but assessment will also give you clues about how well the heart and lungs are working. When evaluating the skin you should assess for color, temperature, condition, and (in children) capillary refill time. To assess color you should look at the patient's overall skin color, the mucous membranes of the mouth, the nail beds, and the conjunctiva of the eye (inner surface of the eyelid) (Fig. 8-21). You should expect these areas to be a pink color. In patients with dark skin color, the color of the nail beds, mucous membranes of the mouth, or conjunc-

tiva may be most useful. Abnormal skin colors may include the following:

- *Pale.* Pale skin indicates poor perfusion or impaired blood flow. This may be due to shock, emotional distress, or hypothermia.
- *Cyanotic.* A cyanotic or blue-gray color to the skin is usually due to lack of oxygen in the cells of the body and indicates respiratory problems. You will often see this color around the mouth and in the nail beds first.
- *Flushed.* Flushed or red skin may indicate exposure to heat, fever, high blood pressure, alcohol abuse, or the late stages of carbon monoxide poisoning.
- *Jaundiced.* A jaundiced or yellow color to the skin may be caused by liver diseases such as hepatitis.
- *Mottled.* A mottled or blotchy color to the skin may be caused by shock or hypothermia.

In addition to color you should assess the patient's skin temperature. You can assess the patient's temperature by placing the back of your ungloved hand on the patient's skin (Fig. 8-22). An ungloved hand is necessary so you can assess the true temperature of the patient's skin and determine the difference between your own temperature and the patient's temperature. Normal skin temperature is warm. Abnormal skin temperatures suggest decreased perfusion, infection, or heat and cold emergencies. Hot skin may be caused by fever, infection, poisoning, or exposure to heat. Cool skin is usually associated with poor perfusion or exposure to cold. Cold skin is usually caused by extreme exposure to cold.

Team Work—cont'd

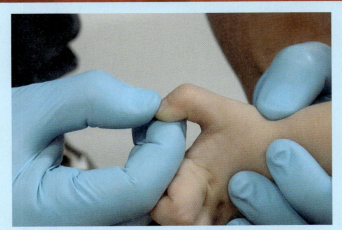

Fig. 8-23 Assessment of capillary refill time.

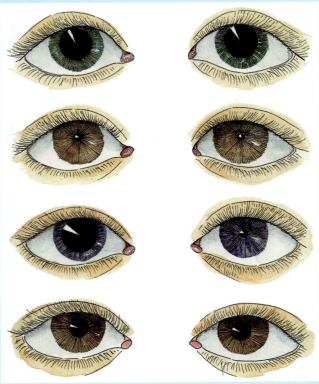

Fig. 8-24 **A,** Pupil dilation. **B,** Pupil constriction. **C,** Unequal pupils. **D,** Normal pupils.

When you assess the skin you should also assess the condition of the skin. The skin is normally dry. Wet, moist, or clammy skin may be associated with shock.

In infants and children 6 years of age or less you should also assess capillary refill time. Capillary refill time in conjunction with other findings is a reflection of how well the circulatory system is working. Capillary refill time can be delayed by decreased perfusion to an area. Capillary refill time is assessed by pressing on the patient's skin or fingernail until the skin underneath the depressed area turns white. Once the area turns white the pressure is released. You should note how long it takes for the color to return to the white area. This should occur in less than 2 seconds. If the capillary refill time is greater than 2 seconds, it is considered to be delayed. You should suspect shock or decreased blood flow to the area if capillary refill time is delayed (Fig. 8-23).

Pupils

The pupils of the eyes should be assessed for size, equality, and reaction to light. To assess the pupils, look at the pupils and then shine a light into them. Normally, pupils react by constricting equally to light. The pupils of both eyes are normally the same size and get smaller, or constrict, when light is shined on them. When it is dark the pupils get larger, or dilate. The size, equality, and reaction to light will give you clues about possible problems (Fig. 8-24).

- *Dilated.* Dilated or large pupils in the presence of bright light suggest drug exposure, poisoning, or decreased responsiveness. Death will also cause the pupils to dilate.
- *Constricted.* Constricted or small pupils in a darkened room or area suggest drug exposure, poisoning, or central nervous system (CNS) problems.
- *Unequal.* Unequal pupils are commonly associated with head injuries, stroke, or damage to the eye.
- *Nonreactive.* Pupils that do not react to light suggest the patient may have a head injury, stroke, or damage to the eye.

Blood Pressure

The blood pressure reflects the status of the heart and blood vessels. It is the pressure the blood exerts on the arteries as the blood flows through the vessels. To assess the blood pressure you will need a stethoscope and a properly fitting blood pressure cuff or sphygmomanometer. The blood pressure is represented by two numbers, the systolic and the diastolic blood pressures. The systolic blood pressure is the higher number and represents the pressure as the heart beats or pumps blood through the blood vessels. The diastolic blood pressure is the lower number and represents the pressure in the vascular system between heartbeats or when the heart relaxes.

Team Work—cont'd

Blood pressure values will vary depending on the age of the patient. Older patients tend to have higher blood pressures than younger patients. Normal blood pressures for the various age groups are outlined in Table 8-10. A high blood pressure can indicate hypertension (persistent high blood pressure) and may be associated with strokes or drug use. A low blood pressure can indicate hypotension (persistent low blood pressure) or decreased perfusion and may be due to shock or drug use. An extremely high or low blood pressure can be damaging to the organs of the body.

The blood pressure can be obtained by two methods, auscultation and palpation. When you auscultate the blood pressure, you will be using a stethoscope and listening for systolic and diastolic sounds. When you palpate a blood pressure, you will be feeling for the return of a pulse as the cuff is deflated. You will not obtain a diastolic pressure when you palpate. A palpated blood pressure is usually obtained when the environment is loud or you are unable to hear a blood pressure by auscultation.

To take a blood pressure the blood pressure cuff should be placed at least 1 inch above the crease of the elbow (antecubital fossa) and the bladder should be centered over the brachial artery. If you are taking a blood pressure by auscultation, you should then palpate the brachial artery before placing the diaphragm of the stethoscope over it. The diaphragm should not be placed under the blood pressure cuff. The valve on the bulb attached to the blood pressure cuff should be closed by turning it clockwise and the cuff should be inflated to approximately 200 mm Hg. If the air leaks out when you squeeze the bulb, the valve is not closed tightly enough. You then slowly loosen the valve to let air out of the cuff while listening for a tapping sound. You will need to look at the gauge to read the number where the tapping starts (systolic blood pressure number) and where it stops (diastolic blood pressure number). When the tapping stops you should rapidly release the rest of the air in the cuff. See Skill 8-4 for a demonstration of auscultating a blood pressure.

The blood pressure cuff should be placed in the same manner if you are palpating a blood pressure. However, instead of auscultating the brachial artery, you palpate the radial pulse before inflating the cuff. Be sure not to press too hard on the radial artery or you will stop the pulse. You should pump up the cuff in the same manner outlined in the previous paragraph. You will stop feeling a pulse when the cuff is pumped up. When you are slowly releasing the air from the cuff, feel the radial artery and look on the gauge

for when a radial pulse returns. The systolic pulse is the number at which the pulse returns. You will not get a diastolic pressure with this method because the pulse will not go away. Skill 8-5 demonstrates the palpation method for obtaining a blood pressure. Blood pressure should be documented with the systolic pressure over the diastolic pressure (e.g., 120/90) or with the systolic pressure palpated (e.g., 120 palpated).

There are many factors that can affect the accuracy of a blood pressure reading. When taking a blood pressure it is very important to choose the proper cuff size. The cuff should encircle the arm and should fasten securely. The cuff size should be equal to two thirds the length of the upper arm. A cuff that is too large or too loose will give a false low reading, while a cuff that is too small or too tight will give a false high reading. Other causes of false readings include letting the air out of the cuff too quickly, missing the first systolic sound, being unable to hear the sounds well, and positioning the cuff improperly.

In general, you should take a blood pressure reading in all patients who are 3 years old or older. In children who are under the age of 3, responsiveness, appearance, and respiratory status will be just as valuable in determining perfusion as the blood pressure measurement.

Vital signs will tell you how your patient is doing; they are most useful when assessed repeatedly for trends. If the vital signs do not match the patient's condition, you should question the patient about his or her normal vital signs to identify discrepancies. For example, if you obtain a high blood pressure reading you should ask the patient, if possible, if he or she has high blood pressure. When in doubt you should treat the patient and repeat the vital signs at regular intervals because they may be an indication of problems yet to come.

CAUTION!

You should not delay assessing or reassessing critical problems in adults or children in order to take a blood pressure. If you are going to take repeated blood pressures on a patient, leave the deflated cuff in place—it will save you time.

Skill 8-4

Auscultating a Blood Pressure

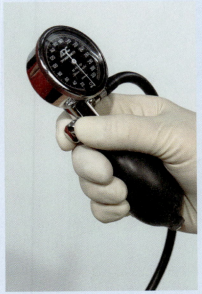

1. Place blood pressure cuff on patient and place stethoscope in your ears.

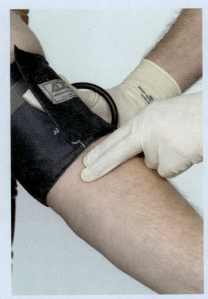

2. Palpate for the brachial artery.

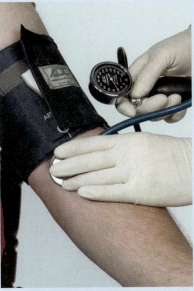

3. Place the diaphragm of the stethoscope over the brachial artery and hold it in place.

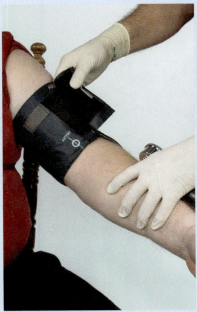

4. Tighten the valve on the bulb and inflate the cuff by squeezing on the bulb.

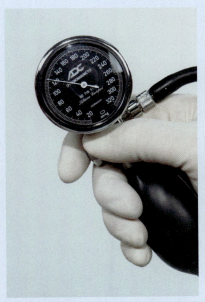

5. Slowly let the air out of the cuff and listen to the sounds. The first sound is the systolic pressure.

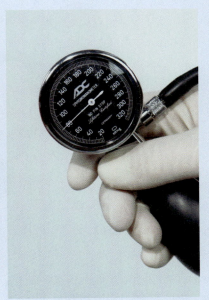

6. Where the sound stops is the diastolic pressure. Record the blood pressure as systolic/diastolic.

Skill 8-5

Palpating a Blood Pressure

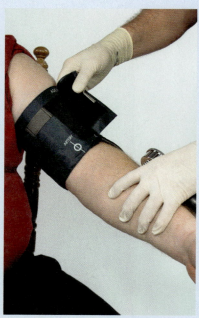

1. Place blood pressure cuff on patient.

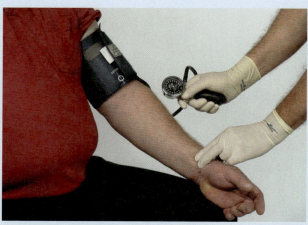

2. Place your index and middle fingers over the radial pulse.

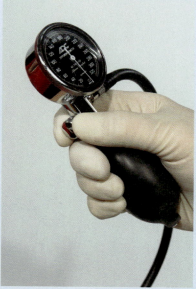

3. Tighten the valve on the bulb and inflate the cuff by squeezing on the bulb.

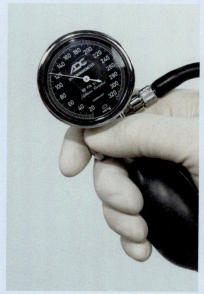

4. Slowly let the air out of the cuff and feel for a pulse. The systolic pressure is when a pulse can be felt. Record as "systolic/palp."

Team Work—cont'd

TRIAGE

Triage is the process of sorting patients. Triage is used when you have more patients than personnel or resources to care for them. You are sorting patients into categories for treatment. Many classification systems exist for triaging patients. The START Field Guide is an example of one of those systems and incorporates a 60-second assessment. During this 60-second assessment respiration, perfusion, and mental status are evaluated on the patients. Based on these findings patients are categorized as immediate, delayed, or nonsalvageable (or dead). Patients are placed in the immediate category if their injuries are critical and require few resources and personnel for management. Patients with severe bleeding who cannot respond to simple commands or who are breathing greater than 30 times a minute illustrate conditions that are placed in the immediate category. Patients who are not breathing and do not breathe when you open the airway are considered nonsalvageable. The remainder of the patients fit in the delayed category. Being aware of how to perform triage and the importance of triage is of vital importance to emergency first responders because they may be the first on the scene at a multicasualty incident. Triage is discussed in more detail in Chapter 15.

In the Real World—Conclusion

You perform a physical examination and collect a history for each patient in this incident. You prepare a hand-off report for the incoming EMS providers. Your report states the following:

"We have five patients who were involved in a moderate-speed, rear-end collision. Two are serious and three are stable. Our first serious patient is an elderly male who was conscious when we arrived and complaining of chest pain. As the chest pain became worse he became unconscious but he now continues to respond to painful stimuli. His breathing is regular and unlabored; his pulse is slow and irregular. His skin is cool and pale. He has no deformities, open wounds, tenderness, or swelling on his head, neck, chest, abdomen, pelvis, or extremities. We found a nitroglycerin patch on his chest when we palpated so we suspect he has a cardiac history. We manually stabilized his cervical spine and have maintained a jaw thrust.

"Our second serious patient was in the rear car. He is a 3-year-old boy with troubled breathing. His parents were taking him to the emergency department for breathing problems when the collision occurred. He is lethargic. He is oriented but does not stay focused on noises or conversations. His airway is clear and he has a seal-like cough. He is working hard to breathe, speaks only in one- or two-word sentences, and is using accessory muscles to breathe. His radial pulse is rapid. His skin is pale, cool, and dry. He denies any pain or tenderness. We did not find any deformities, open wounds, or swelling. He does not have any allergies. His parents gave him Dimetapp and Tylenol just before they left home 20 minutes ago. He has not had any recent medical problems. He drank a little juice with the medications. His parents report that he has been sick for a few days and is worse tonight. We kept him sitting in his car seat. His condition has remained the same.

"Our next patient. . . ."

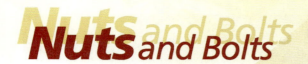

Critical Points

As a First Responder, you should know how to evaluate an emergency scene for safety, determine the number of patients, assess a patient's mechanism of injury or nature of illness, recognize the need for additional resources, and begin patient assessment and treatment.

Use the initial assessment to identify any life-threatening conditions. Treat any life-threatening conditions as they are identified. A complete physical examination may or may not be necessary depending on the injury.

You should always communicate your assessment and interventions to other health care providers.

Learning Checklist

❑ Assessment includes several stages: scene size-up, initial assessment, physical examination, patient history, ongoing assessment, and hand-off report.

❑ Scene size-up is a quick determination of the entire scene and includes the safety of the scene, personal protection, an assessment of the mechanism of injury or nature of illness, the number of patients involved, and the need for additional resources before you actually contact the patient. It includes information from dispatch, the weather, the traffic, and what you see at the actual scene.

❑ Scene safety is of utmost importance. If a scene is unsafe and cannot be made safe, do not enter it.

❑ A trauma patient is one who has sustained an injury as the result of an external force. A medical patient is a patient who appears to have an illness or complains of symptoms of an illness.

❑ The mechanism of injury refers to the physical forces involved in the injury.

❑ The nature of illness is the reason why you were called to help a medical patient.

❑ As part of the scene size-up you will need to determine the number of patients involved and whether additional resources are needed. Call for additional help before you initiate patient care.

❑ The primary assessment is performed to determine whether a patient has any life-threatening problems and to manage those problems as they are found. It is composed of forming a general impression, assessing responsiveness, and checking the patient's airway, breathing, circulation, and disability.

❑ The general impression is formed as you look at the scene and the patient, and it helps you to decide how to act and to gauge the seriousness of the scene. It considers the patient's age, gender, presentation, and any other information that you have been given.

❑ Use AVPU to assess a patient's responsiveness to determine if a patient is **a**lert, responsive to **v**erbal stimuli, responsive to **p**ainful stimuli, or **u**nresponsive.

❑ Assess airway and breathing; open the airway and begin rescue breathing if needed. If the patient is breathing spontaneously, assess the adequacy of breathing.

❑ To determine circulation, assess the pulse, look for major blood loss, and quickly assess the skin.

❑ To determine disability, assess the patient's mental status using the Glasgow Coma Scale (GCS) score.

❑ A systematic and organized secondary assessment includes a physical examination and focused history of the patient and is performed to identify signs and symptoms of illness or injury and begin appropriate treatment.

❑ The physical examination should involve inspection and palpation for signs of injury using the mnemonic DOTS (**d**eformities, **o**pen injuries, **t**enderness, and **s**welling). Each body part is assessed: head, neck, chest, abdomen, back, pelvis, and extremities.

❑ A patient's relevant medical history can be obtained using the SAMPLE mnemonic: S—signs and symptoms, A—allergies, M—medications, P—pertinent past history, L—last oral intake, and E—events leading to the injury or illness.

❑ The ongoing assessment is a repeat of the initial assessment at continuous intervals. You should reassess a critical patient at least every 5 minutes and a noncritical patient at least every 15 minutes.

❑ The hand-off report should include age and gender, chief complaint, responsiveness, airway and breathing status, circulation status, physical findings, SAMPLE history, interventions provided, and the patient's current condition.

❑ Vital signs include assessing the patient's breathing, pulse, skin, pupils, and blood pressure.

❑ The respiratory rate should be calculated by counting the number of breaths in 30 seconds and multiplying by 2. You should also assess the quality of breathing through observation of the work of breathing and auscultation of breath sounds.

- ❑ The pulse rate should be obtained by counting the number of beats in 30 seconds and multiplying by 2. The pulse should also be evaluated for regularity and quality.
- ❑ The skin should be assessed for color, temperature, condition, and capillary refill time (in children).
- ❑ The pupils should be assessed for size, equality, and reaction to light.
- ❑ Blood pressure can be measured through the auscultation method or the palpation method.
- ❑ Triage is the process of sorting patients when you have more patients than resources to care for them.

Key Terms

Auscultation The process of listening with a stethoscope.

AVPU The mnemonic for the scale used to determine a patient's level of response (A, alert; V, verbal; P, painful; U, unresponsive).

Blood pressure The pressure the blood exerts on the arteries as the blood flows through the vessels.

Capillary refill time The time it takes for color (blood) to return to the skin or nail bed after it has been squeezed to blanch the area; normal capillary refill time is less than 2 seconds.

Chief complaint The patient's initial or primary statement of the problem.

Circulation The movement of blood to allow for the exchange of nutrients and waste products through the body.

Crepitus A sound or a feeling of bone ends grating against one another or air trapped between tissue layers; feels like bubble wrap popping.

Diastolic blood pressure The pressure the blood exerts on the blood vessels when the heart is relaxed.

DOTS A mnemonic (Deformities, Open wounds, Tenderness, Swelling) for observations to make in the physical examination.

Focused history Information regarding the patient's medical problems, medications, and other information pertinent to the injury or illness.

General impression A quick evaluation of the scene to determine what has happened and the seriousness of the scene.

Hand-off report Verbally delivering information to another medical provider who is taking over the care of a patient.

Hemorrhage The loss of blood, or bleeding.

Mechanism of injury An impact or other cause of a patient's injury.

Medical patient A patient who appears to have an illness or complains of symptoms of an illness.

Nature of illness A determination of the patient's illness from findings.

Palpate To feel a part of the body to identify injury, pain, or tenderness.

Patent Open (e.g., a patent airway is an open and functioning airway).

Physical examination Assessing a patient to identify signs or symptoms of an illness or injury.

Primary assessment The first evaluation of the patient, to identify life-threatening problems.

Reassessment The reevaluation of the patient's initial assessment and problems.

Responsiveness The patient's neurological status, described by how and to what type of stimuli a patient reacts.

SAMPLE A mnemonic used to collect a patient history (Signs/symptoms, Allergies, Medications, Pertinent past medical history, Last oral intake, Events leading to the injury or illness).

Scene safety Evaluating the scene of an incident or illness for potential hazards to the emergency first responder, patient, crew, or bystanders.

Scene size-up The process of looking at the scene to determine safety factors and the mechanism of injury or nature of illness.

Sign A finding you can hear, see, feel, or measure during the physical examination.

Sphygmomanometer A device used to evaluate the blood pressure; also called a blood pressure cuff.

Stethoscope An instrument used to hear sounds within the body such as breath sounds or the blood pressure.

Nuts and Bolts–continued

Symptom A problem or condition that a patient describes.

Systolic blood pressure The pressure the blood exerts on the blood vessels when the heart is contracted.

Trauma patient A patient who has sustained an injury as a result of an external force.

Triage The process of sorting or categorizing patients into treatment and transport priorities in a multiple casualty situation.

Vital signs The patient's pulse rate, respiratory rate, skin signs, pupils, and blood pressure.

First Responder NSC Objectives
COGNITIVE OBJECTIVES

- Discuss the components of scene size-up.
- Describe common hazards found at the scenes of a trauma patient and a medical patient.
- Determine if the scene is safe to enter.
- Discuss common mechanisms of injury/nature of illness.
- Discuss the reason for identifying the total number of patients at the scene.
- Explain the reason for identifying the need for additional help or assistance.
- Summarize the reasons for forming a general impression of the patient.
- Discuss methods of assessing mental status.
- Differentiate between assessing mental status in the adult, child, and infant patient.
- Describe methods used for assessing if a patient is breathing.
- Differentiate between a patient with adequate and inadequate breathing.
- Describe the methods used to assess circulation.
- Differentiate between obtaining a pulse in an adult, child, and infant patient.
- Discuss the need for assessing the patient for external bleeding.
- Explain the reason for prioritizing a patient for care and transport.
- Discuss the components of the physical exam.

- State the areas of the body that are evaluated during the physical exam.
- Explain what additional questioning may be asked during the physical exam.
- Explain the components of the SAMPLE history.
- Discuss the components of the ongoing assessment.
- Describe the information included in the first responder "hand-off" report.

AFFECTIVE OBJECTIVES

- Explain the rationale for crew members to evaluate scene safety before entering the scene.
- Serve as a model for others by explaining how patient situations affect your evaluation of the mechanism of injury or illness.
- Demonstrate a caring attitude when performing patient assessments.
- Place the interests of the patient as the foremost consideration when making any and all patient care decisions during patient assessment.
- Communicate with empathy during patient assessment to patients as well as the family members and friends of the patient.
- Explain the rationale for the feelings patients might be experiencing.
- Explain the importance of forming a general impression of the patient.
- Explain the value of an initial assessment.
- Explain the value of questioning the patient and family.
- Explain the value of the physical exam.
- Explain the value of the ongoing assessment.

PSYCHOMOTOR OBJECTIVES

- Demonstrate the ability to differentiate various scenarios and identify potential hazards.
- Demonstrate the techniques for assessing mental status.
- Demonstrate the techniques for assessing the airway.
- Demonstrate the techniques for assessing if the patient is breathing.
- Demonstrate the techniques for assessing if the patient has a pulse.

- Demonstrate the techniques for assessing the patient for external bleeding.
- Demonstrate the techniques for assessing the patient's skin color, temperature, condition, and capillary refill time (infants and children only).

- Demonstrate questioning a patient to obtain a SAMPLE history.
- Demonstrate the skills involved in performing the physical exam.
- Demonstrate the ongoing assessment.

Check your understanding

Check your understanding

Please refer to p. 439 for the answers to these questions.

1. Looking for safety hazards and determining resource needs are two components of this assessment phase:
   A. Secondary survey
   B. Scene survey
   C. Primary exam
   D. Detailed exam

2. Classify each of the following situations as **S** (safe to enter) or **U** (unsafe, do not enter).
   An incident with downed power lines _____
   A call for an unconscious patient in an enclosed, confined space _____
   Police on scene motioning you into the house; you hear shouting in the house _____
   A local bar where a male is injured from a fight _____
   A home with the lights on and a family member motioning you for a chest pain call _____
   A semi-truck rollover, with a DOT HAZMAT placard and fluid leaking from the trailer _____

3. The way in which forces are applied to the body of a trauma patient producing injury is called the:
   A. Schematics
   B. Mechanism of injury
   C. Physical exam
   D. Primary survey

4. The purpose of the initial assessment is to determine if the patient has any:
   A. Medical history
   B. Life-threatening conditions
   C. Chronic disease
   D. Minor bleeding

5. Information that the patient or bystander tells you about his or her condition is called a/an:
   A. Sign
   B. Agreement
   C. Symptom
   D. Assessment

6. Describe what is meant by each of the letters in the mnemonic AVPU.
   A _____
   V _____
   P _____
   U _____

7. Match the letters of AVPU with the appropriate patient response.
   A. Complains of chest pain when you enter the room
   B. Does not move or make a noise even when you pinch her earlobe
   C. Moans when you pinch her shoulder
   D. Opens his eyes when you call his name

8. List four indications that a patient is not breathing adequately.
   1. _____
   2. _____
   3. _____
   4. _____

9. Classify each of the following patients as **A** (adequate breathing) or **I** (inadequate breathing).
   A 6-year-old with wheezing and use of neck, chest, and abdominal muscles _____
   A 70-year-old with snoring respirations _____
   A 10-year-old who has pink skin and who is talking in sentences _____
   A 50-year-old who tells you he has chest pain, and then takes several breaths before speaking again _____
   A 3-month-old who is grunting and whose color is pale with nail beds bluish in color _____
   A 14-month-old with pink color who is crying loudly _____

10. When assessing the patient's circulation, the First Responder should check which of the following?
    A. Lung sounds
    B. Vision
    C. Blood sugar level
    D. Pulse

11. How should the First Responder position a patient who has signs of inadequate circulation that may indicate shock?
    A. Seated
    B. Prone
    C. Supine with head elevated
    D. Supine with legs elevated

12. During the physical examination the First Responder will check for DOTS, which indicates:
    D _____
    O _____
    T _____
    S _____

13. The memory aid SAMPLE will assist the First Responder in remembering the information that should be obtained about the patient's history. What is the meaning of each letter in this mnemonic?
    S _____
    A _____
    M _____
    P _____
    L _____
    E _____

14. A noncritical patient should be reassessed every _____ minutes; a critical patient should be reassessed every _____ minutes.

15. In an adult, the normal rate of breathing is _____ times per minute.

16. In an adult, the normal pulse rate is _____ times per minute.

17. The radial pulse is found at the patient's _____, while the carotid pulse is found in the _____.

18. The patient who is not breathing should receive oxygen via which adjunct?
    A. Nonrebreather mask
    B. Bag-mask device
    C. Nasal cannula
    D. Simple face mask

19. Which of the following would help you in deciding whether your patient may be in shock?
    A. Ability to speak in full sentences
    B. Dry, pale mucous membranes
    C. Clear lung sounds
    D. Red, flushed, hot skin

20. When there are more patients at the scene of an emergency than there are personnel and resources to care for them, the First Responder will need to use a system to sort patients into categories for treatment. This process is known as _____.

21. You are the first to arrive on the scene. Your patient is a 19-year-old male who has been involved in a motorcycle crash during which he struck a guardrail at about 30 miles per hour. He is awake as you approach him but it seems unusual that he his shivering on such a warm day. He is pale and sweating despite the fact that he is shivering. He is breathing about 24 times a minute and his pulse is rapid and weak at the radial artery. The patient's left thigh is bent at an unusual angle and there is a piece of bone protruding through the skin. He has a large cut with profuse bleeding on his right upper arm. Which of the following is your priority in caring for this patient?
    A. Manually stabilize his cervical spine.
    B. Provide treatment for the wound to the patient's thigh.
    C. Take his blood pressure.
    D. Apply direct pressure to the bleeding arm wound.

Check your understanding–continued

22. You respond to a "man down" in a back alley where you find an elderly man prone on the gravel. The only response you receive is a grumble and squeal when you pinch his earlobe. His mental status according to the AVPU scale is:
   A. Alert
   B. Verbal
   C. Painful
   D. Unresponsive

23. It is your first shift and, of course, you get a call. Your partner asks you to get the vital signs. Which of the following measurements should you obtain?
   A. Lung sounds, pulse, blood pressure
   B. Pulse, respirations, blood pressure
   C. Pupil response, respirations, blood pressure
   D. AVPU, SAMPLE, DOTS

Chapter 9

Cardiopulmonary Resuscitation and AED

LESSON GOAL

Every day in the United States more than 1,000 adults die from sudden **cardiac arrest**; nearly half of these deaths occur outside the hospital. Sudden collapse is the first sign of cardiac disease in 50% of cases. Early **cardiopulmonary resuscitation** (CPR) is the single most important intervention to improve the patient's chances for long-term survival. This chapter describes how to assess an unresponsive victim and provide CPR if indicated.

OBJECTIVES

1. List the reasons the heart stops beating.
2. Define the components of cardiopulmonary resuscitation (CPR).
3. Describe each step (or link) in the sequence (or chain) of survival and how it relates to the emergency medical services (EMS) system.
4. List the steps of one- and two-rescuer adult CPR.
5. List the steps of infant and child CPR.
6. Describe the technique of external chest compressions on an adult, child, and infant.
7. List the circumstances when you can stop CPR.
8. Demonstrate the proper technique of chest compressions on an infant, a child, and an adult.
9. Demonstrate the steps of adult one- and two-rescuer CPR.
10. Demonstrate infant and child CPR.
11. Relate the concept of early defibrillation to the survival of a patient.
12. Demonstrate the application and operation of the automated external defibrillator (AED).

In the Real World

You are a firefighter and an emergency first responder assisting in fire suppression at a house fire when two other firefighters pull a man from the building. You quickly move to the man's side, removing your fire gear and putting on personal protection equipment (PPE). You attempt to arouse the man, but you get no response. Your partner comes to assist you. You open the man's airway and check for breathing. You place your cheek over the patient's face and, focusing on the man's chest, look for chest rise and feel for the man's breath against your cheek. The man is not breathing. You pull a pocket mask from your bag and give two breaths. Your partner checks for a pulse after you deliver the breaths and find that there is no pulse.

Studies have shown that early defibrillation saves lives. Other studies have shown that survival rates in cardiopulmonary arrest patients further improve if basic life support is given to the patient within 3 to 4 minutes and advanced life support within 8 minutes. The role of the emergency first responder is key to improving survival rates in these patients. Being the closest to these patients when they collapse puts these responders in the place to make the most important contribution toward their best outcome. Cardiopulmonary resuscitation and the use of automatic external defibrillators (AED) are extremely important skills for the emergency first responder.

Circulatory System

The circulatory system is responsible for transporting oxygen and other nutrients to all tissues of the body while also removing carbon dioxide and other waste products from the tissues. The basic components of the circulatory system are the "three Ps": the *pump* (the heart), the *pipes* (the blood vessels that link the system), and the *plasma* (the fluid portion of the blood). Recall from Chapter 5 that the heart is a fist-sized muscle with four chambers. The right and left upper chambers are called atria, and the right and left lower chambers are called ventricles (Fig. 9-1). The right atrium receives blood full of waste products and low on oxygen from the veins. The blood from the right atrium moves into the right ventricle through a one-way valve. The right ventricle then moves the blood to the lungs with each contraction. The exchange of fresh oxygen for carbon dioxide takes place in the lungs where tiny blood vessels (capillaries) surround each of the alveoli (air sacs) in the lungs. The walls of the microscopic capillaries are so thin and in such close contact with the alveoli that they create a membrane through which oxygen and carbon dioxide can easily

pass. Oxygen-rich blood is then returned to the left atrium. A valve opens to allow blood to flow from the left atrium into the left ventricle. Powerful contractions of the left ventricle move the oxygen-rich blood throughout the rest of the body. The one-way valves allow blood to flow between the atria and the ventricles while also preventing flow of blood from the ventricles back into the atria.

Arteries are the vessels that carry the oxygenated blood away from the heart. With each contraction, a pulse can be felt anywhere that an artery passes near the skin surface and over a bone. Strong arterial pulses can be felt on either side of the neck (carotid arteries), in the groin crease between the abdomen and thigh (femoral arteries), at the palm-side of the wrist near the thumb (radial arteries), and on the inner upper arm between the elbow and shoulder (brachial arteries; Fig. 9-2). The arteries continue to get smaller and smaller until they connect with arterioles and finally the capillaries. The exchange of oxygen for carbon dioxide occurs in the capillaries intertwined throughout the tissues in all parts of the body. Capillaries then dump deoxygenated blood into millions of very small veins. Veins are vessels that carry deoxygenated blood back to the heart. They gradually increase in diameter and decrease in number as they move the blood back to the right atrium so the entire process of circulation can begin again (Fig. 9-3).

Sudden cardiac arrest (SCA) is the term used when the heart stops beating and a pulse can no longer be felt. When blood stops flowing through the circulatory system, oxygen and nutrients cannot be delivered to the tissues and waste products cannot be removed. This can rapidly lead to tissue damage and major organ damage. The brain, for example, is the organ that is most sensitive to the lack of oxygen. Brain damage begins in just 4 to 6 minutes and becomes irreversible within 8 to 10 minutes without an adequate supply of oxygen. Some common reasons the heart stops beating are listed in Box 9-1.

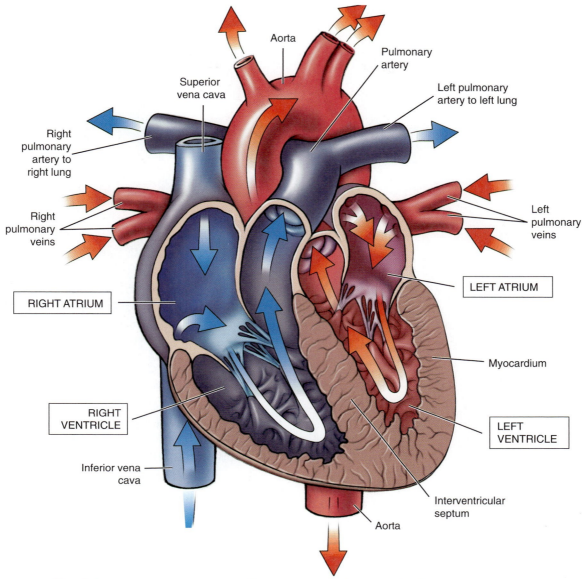

Aorta

Pulmonary artery

Superior vena cava

Left pulmonary artery to left lung

Right pulmonary artery to right lung

Right pulmonary veins

Left pulmonary veins

RIGHT ATRIUM

LEFT ATRIUM

Myocardium

RIGHT VENTRICLE

LEFT VENTRICLE

Inferior vena cava

Interventricular septum

Aorta

Fig. 9-1 Anatomy of the heart. (From Herlihy B, Maebius N: *The human body in health and illness,* Philadelphia, 2003, Saunders.)

Regardless of the cause of cardiac arrest, the treatment is always the same: ***Begin cardiopulmonary resuscitation immediately.***

Cardiopulmonary Resuscitation

Cardiopulmonary resuscitation (CPR) is a simple technique that is performed by emergency first responders on victims of cardiac arrest. The procedure combines rescue breathing and external chest compressions to oxygenate and circulate blood when the heart has stopped beating. Rescue breathing moves oxygen into the lungs where it can then move across thin tissue into the blood. External chest compressions move the oxygenated blood throughout the body. Even the best CPR produces less than one-third of the normal blood flow, however, and its effectiveness decreases over time. Most adult victims of cardiac arrest need an electrical shock to the heart called **defibrillation** to survive, and the goal of CPR is to maintain life until the defibrillator arrives. CPR by itself cannot sustain life indefinitely.

Sequence of Survival

The highest survival rates from cardiac arrest occur when a certain sequence of events is followed. This sequence has been called the **chain of survival,** or **sequence of survival.** The steps include recognizing an emergency and activating the emergency medical services (EMS)

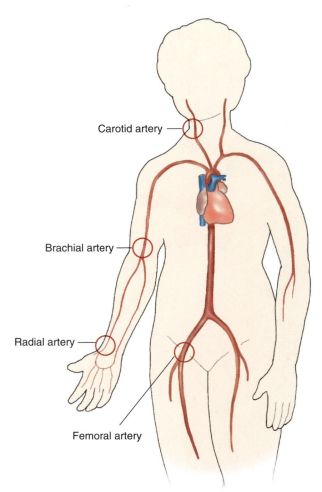

Fig. 9-2 Pulse sites. (From McSwain N, Paturas J: *The basic EMT: comprehensive prehospital patient care,* ed 3, St. Louis, 2003, Mosby.)

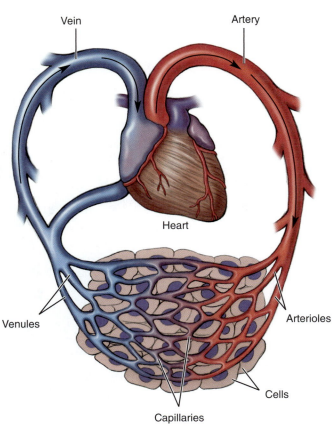

Fig. 9-3 Blood vessels and the circulatory system. (From Herlihy B, Maebius N: *The human body in health and illness,* Philadelphia, 2003, Saunders.)

BOX 9-1 Common Reasons the Heart Stops Beating

- Heart disease
- Respiratory arrest
- Stroke
- Seizures
- Diabetic reactions
- Poisoning
- Suffocation
- Drowning
- Trauma
- Bleeding
- Electric shock
- Severe allergic reactions
- Congenital abnormalities

---

system (i.e., calling 9-1-1); providing CPR, rescue breathing, or first aid; applying an automated external defibrillator (AED) and oxygen if available; and providing advanced care and hospital care as soon as possible (Fig. 9-4).

Recognition and Early Access

Rapid recognition of an emergency must occur. It is important for all communities to be educated to recognize the signs and symptoms of cardiopulmonary emergencies listed in Box 9-2 and to know how to contact the local EMS system. The goal is for everyone to be trained to provide basic rescue support and know to call for help. If more than one rescuer is at the scene, one rescuer should call for help and get an AED while the others begin CPR. In cases where the rescuer is alone, "phone first" should be the priority in order to activate 9-1-1 and obtain an AED. The rescuer should then perform 2 minutes or five cycles of CPR and then use the AED if it is available. This sequence should be used for all victims of sudden cardiac arrest, regardless of the victim's age. This means as soon as an emergency is recognized, the

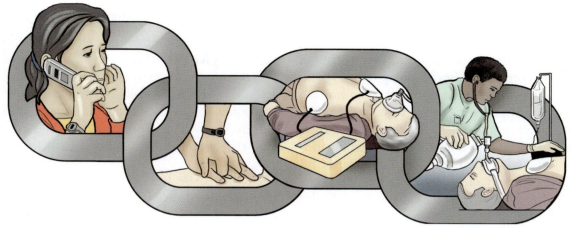

Fig. 9-4 The sequence of survival. (From Aehlert B: *ACLS quick review study guide,* ed 3, St. Louis, 2007, Mosby.)

BOX 9-2   Warning Signs and Symptoms of a Cardiac Emergency

- Dull, substernal chest discomfort, pain, pressure, or tightness
- Chest pain that radiates to left neck or jaw
- Shortness of breath
- A feeling of extra or skipped heartbeats
- A sensation that the heart is beating too hard, too fast, or too slow
- Nausea or vomiting
- Lightheadedness, dizziness, or fainting
- Sudden cold sweat
- Anxiety: A feeling of impending doom
- Denial that the symptoms may mean a cardiac emergency
- Sudden death

Not all warning signs and symptoms occur in every heart attack. Have the conscious patient stop all activity and activate EMS (if not already done) if the signs and symptoms last 5 minutes or longer.

---

first step is to call for help. If the collapse is witnessed and an AED is immediately available, the AED should be applied, interrupting the CPR.

"Phone fast" is the phrase used for unresponsive children and for victims of any age in cardiac arrest resulting from near-drowning, drug overdose, or an asphyxial arrest. In these instances, if you are alone, provide 2 minutes of CPR (five cycles) before leaving the victim to call for help and get the AED. If there is more than one rescuer at the scene, one person should immediately begin rescue efforts while the other goes for help. The reason is that in these instances respiratory arrest is more common than cardiac arrest. Providing rescue breathing immediately in these situations may prevent the patient from going into cardiac arrest.

Emergency medical dispatch (EMD) is another important component of early access. Specially trained dispatchers use priority medical dispatch protocols and give telephone instructions for managing a victim's airway problem, performing CPR, and operating an AED even to untrained individuals who are calling for help.

Early CPR

The best treatment for cardiac arrest before the arrival of the defibrillator and advanced cardiac care is CPR. Effective CPR helps preserve heart and brain function. To increase a patient's chances for survival, CPR must begin as soon as possible. Widespread community CPR training increases the odds of someone beginning CPR immediately on cardiac arrest victims before the arrival of medical help. Emergency first responders may, in addition to CPR, use airway management devices, supplemental oxygen, and defibrillation (using an AED).

To increase the public's willingness to perform CPR in a sudden cardiac arrest emergency, many communities are now teaching compression-only CPR to the lay public and having 9-1-1 dispatchers give compression-only CPR directions on 9-1-1 calls. Researchers have found some general themes that prevent the general public from providing CPR when needed. Some cite a concern for contracting an illness by coming into contact with body fluids when doing mouth-to-mouth breathing. Others stated that CPR is complicated and they have forgotten how to do it; still others cite fear of doing it wrong and hurting the patient as the main reason they do not act. Regardless of the reason, the goal of compression-only CPR is to encourage people to act when they find a cardiac arrest victim. Compression-only CPR has been demonstrated to be safe, and nearly as effective, as standard CPR in the first few minutes of a cardiac arrest. When the emergency first responder arrives at the scene and a lay rescuer is performing compression-only CPR, the emergency first responder should assume leadership for the CPR effort and begin ventilations, along with compressions, as soon as possible.

Defibrillation

Cardiac arrest usually results from an abnormal heart rhythm called **ventricular fibrillation (VF).** With VF, the electrical impulses of the heart suddenly become irregular and ineffective. This causes the heart to stop beating and prevents blood from flowing through the circulatory system, starving vital organs. Defibrillation is the only effective treatment for VF. The probability of survival decreases 7% to 10% for each minute that defibrillation is delayed. Most EMS systems encourage trained law enforcement, emergency first responders, the fire service, and even the lay public to use an **automated external defibrillator (AED)** (Fig. 9-5). The AED is a lightweight, safe, and accurate machine that gives the operator step-by-step voice prompts for AED operation. AEDs are covered in more detail later in this chapter. You should ask your instructor about the laws and practice guidelines for AED use in your area.

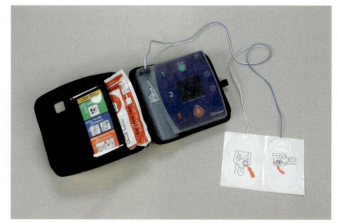

Fig. 9-5 Example of an automated external defibrillator (AED).

PUBLIC ACCESS DEFIBRILLATION

The goal of many communities is to promote public access defibrillation (PAD) because early defibrillation significantly improves survival in those who sustain a cardiac arrest. This is accomplished by training more people in CPR and AED use and placing AEDs in public places that are easily accessible. For example, AEDs are located in airports, shopping malls, and other such locations.

Early Advanced Care

Early **advanced care** is the final step in the sequence or chain. Advanced care refers to the sophisticated emergency equipment and treatment that can be used to help stabilize a patient before reaching the hospital. This can include endotracheal intubation to provide an airway and intravenous (IV) medications to help maintain a normal heartbeat and blood pressure after defibrillation.

The best chance for survival of a patient with sudden cardiac arrest occurs when all steps in the sequence are followed. Ideally, the first three steps in the sequence of survival involve the public. Citizens can recognize a cardiac arrest, call 9-1-1, begin CPR, and use an AED if available. Responsibility for patient care transfers to you, as an emergency first responder, upon your arrival. Often you and a layperson will work as a team until the patient's care is passed on to the ambulance personnel. You will then provide vital information to the ambulance staff about the scene and treatment of the patient before his or her arrival.

Techniques of CPR

The CPR principles of the **ABCs** (airway, breathing, and circulation) apply to patients in all age groups; however, some techniques vary depending on the age and size of the patient. To apply these different techniques, the following age definitions for health care providers should be used as a guideline:

- Infant: Birth to 1 year
- Child: Age 1 year to onset of adolescence or puberty (about 12 to 14 years of age)
- Adult: Adolescence age and older

CPR comprises a group of simple procedures performed in an orderly sequence. The first steps are similar to the initial assessment steps outlined in Chapter 7 and include assessing responsiveness, airway, breathing, and circulation (the ABCs). In all situations, it is necessary to continuously assess and provide care for ABC problems in that order: first the airway, then breathing, and finally circulation. You

BOX 9-3   Reasons Emergency First Responders Start, Stop, or Interrupt CPR

The emergency first responder must start CPR in the following situations:

- There are no signs of circulation (pulse, normal breathing, coughing, or movement).
- No clear DNAR (do not attempt resuscitation) order is available (see Chapter 3 for more information on DNAR orders).
- The emergency first responder should not start CPR in the following situations:

A person shows obvious clinical signs of irreversible death:

- Rigor mortis has set in. This temporary stiffening of the muscles occurs several hours after death.
- Dependent lividity is evident. This red or purple discoloration appears when blood seeps into the tissues on the part of body that is closest to the ground.
- Tissue decomposition is evident. Flesh decay is often accompanied by a distinctive foul odor.
- A valid DNAR order is presented.
- Attempts to perform CPR place the emergency first responder at risk of physical injury.

The emergency first responder can stop CPR in the following situations:

- Effective breathing and circulation have returned.
- Care is transferred to another health care professional with equal or higher certification.
- A qualified physician assumes responsibility.
- The emergency first responder is too exhausted to continue.
- The environment becomes dangerous to the emergency first responder or others.

Reasons to interrupt CPR include the following:

- If the scene is or becomes unsafe, you must move the patient without risking your own life.
- When moving a patient up or down stairs, interrupt CPR only as long as necessary to complete the move.
- When assisting with the transfer of the patient to the ambulance, you must try to provide effective chest compressions on the move.
- CPR must be interrupted for AED defibrillation as indicated.

should not move on to assess circulation until you have assessed and managed the airway and breathing.

CPR is begun only on patients who have no signs of circulation such as responsiveness to verbal or painful stimuli, movement, breathing, or a pulse. Box 9-3 lists reasons you might start, interrupt, or stop CPR. You also must learn your state's laws and follow local resuscitation protocols and standards of care. If there is a question whether to begin or stop CPR, you should always begin and continue resuscitation procedures. Unclear issues can be later clarified at the hospital.

Adult CPR
Assess Responsiveness, Summon EMS, and Position the Patient

Once you determine that the scene is safe and you have put on your personal protection equipment (PPE), you must first assess the person's responsiveness. You should

use the mnemonic AVPU (see Chapter 8) to assess responsiveness. First gently tap or squeeze the patient's shoulders and shout, "Are you all right?" If the patient is unresponsive and you are not a responding EMS member, you must make sure that EMS is called and that a defibrillator is on the way. Once you *know* that EMS is responding, you should position yourself and the patient.

Two or more rescuers should be used to roll a patient, if possible, and the patient must be positioned quickly, even if you are alone. The patient should be positioned on his or her back on a firm surface to ensure effective resuscitation. The patient's arms should be placed at his or her sides, and if the patient is lying on the side or face down, he or she should be carefully rolled as a single unit to prevent twisting the neck and back (see Chapter 6). Once the patient is supine and on a firm surface, you should position yourself beside the patient where you can comfortably provide both rescue breathing and chest compressions if needed.

A is for Airway

The tongue is the most common obstruction in unresponsive patients. In a conscious adult, food is the most likely cause of an obstructed airway. Once you have determined that a patient is unresponsive, the next thing to do is open the airway. This can be accomplished by the head tilt/chin-lift or the jaw thrust and the use of mechanical airway adjuncts such as the oropharyngeal and nasopharyngeal airways. If a foreign body obstruction is visualized, the airway will need to be cleared by a finger sweep of the mouth or by suctioning. Remember that the airway must be open and clear before you move on to check breathing. Refer to Chapter 7 for detailed information on airway management.

B is for Breathing

Once the airway (A) is open and clear, you need to determine if breathing (B) is present and adequate or if the patient needs assistance. To check breathing you should place your ear near the patient's mouth and nose while looking at the chest for chest rise and fall, *listen* for air movement, and *feel* for the flow of air on your cheek. You should look, listen, and feel for breathing for no longer than 10 seconds. If the chest does not visibly rise and fall and you do not hear or feel air movement, you must give two rescue breaths immediately. If the airway is obstructed, you should attempt to clear the airway through foreign body airway obstruction (FBAO) techniques.

The techniques of rescue breathing are discussed in Chapter 7. Mouth-to-mask, mouth-to-barrier device, and mouth-to-stoma methods are all quick, effective ways to provide rescue breathing. The most important principle of rescue breathing is to give each breath over 1 second until the chest begins to visibly rise. If the breaths are delivered with too much force or volume, air can enter the stomach causing gastric inflation and increasing the potential for vomiting. Vomiting in a cardiac arrest victim is a serious complication that can lead to long-term complications if the victim survives the immediate arrest. To decrease the risk of vomiting, deliver the breaths with only enough tidal volume and force to produce visual chest rise. If vomiting does occur, you should quickly roll the patient to one side to allow the airway to clear. Use your gloved fingers to sweep the mouth of any large objects or suction the airway before rolling the patient back and resuming resuscitation attempts. Cricoid pressure, described in Chapter 7, is a technique used during rescue breathing when multiple rescuers are available. This pressure obstructs the esophagus and reduces the risk of vomiting; it prevents the stomach contents from flowing into the mouth and lungs.

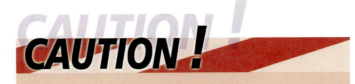

Some cardiac arrest patients have reflex gasping, respiratory efforts called **agonal breaths**. Sometimes called "dying breaths," these attempts are weak and not adequate to sustain life. If you are unsure whether the patient is breathing, begin rescue breathing.

C is for Circulation

When the patient's airway is open (A), breathing has been assessed, and two breaths have been given, if the patient is not breathing (B) the next step is to check for circulation (C). To assess circulation, feel for a carotid pulse while also looking for signs of normal breathing, coughing, or movement. It is important to keep the airway open by maintaining your hand on the patient's forehead while you feel for a carotid pulse. Feel for a pulse for 5 to 10 seconds as you continue to look for adequate breathing, coughing, or movement. If there is no breathing, coughing, or movement and no pulse, you must assume that the heart has stopped. Immediately begin to artificially circulate blood with chest compressions. If the patient has a pulse but is not breathing, you should give rescue breaths.

CHEST COMPRESSIONS

A chest compression is the application of external pressure on the lower portion of the sternum in a rhythmic manner. This pressure acts to artificially circulate the blood to major organs such as the brain and heart until defibrillation.

To properly perform chest compressions, do the following:

- Position yourself on your knees a couple of inches away from the patient's chest.
- Place the heel of your hand in the center of the patient's chest at the nipple line on the lower half of the sternum, avoiding the **xiphoid process**.
- Place your second hand on top of the first hand and interlace or extend your fingers so that only the heel of the hand remains on the sternum. If you have arthritic hands or wrists, you may wish to grasp the wrist of your hand that is on the patient's chest.
- Position yourself directly over the sternum and keep your elbows as straight as possible.
- Pivot downward from your hips to depress the sternum with enough force to move the chest 1½ to 2 inches in an adult of average size.

- Push hard and fast at a rate of 100 compressions/minute, allowing the chest to return fully to a normal position before the next compression. Minimize interruptions during compressions.
- Each compression cycle should be 50% depression and 50% relaxation. Avoid sharp, stabbing compressions, and keep your hands in contact with the patient's chest so that you will not lose your landmark.

COMPRESSION AND VENTILATION RATIOS

Emergency first responders should combine both ventilations (rescue breathing) and compressions when performing CPR to provide the patient with the best chance of survival. However, if the rescuer is unwilling or unable to provide rescue breaths, begin chest compressions without ventilations. For an adult patient, two rescue breaths are given after each set of 30 compressions. To provide the desired compression rate, of at least 100 compressions per minute, the chest must be compressed at more than one compression per second. To keep up the pace of compressions, it is recommended to count out loud: "1, 2, 3, . . . 30." After performing 2 minutes of CPR (approximately five cycles of the 30 compressions to two ventilations), you should stop CPR to recheck the patient's carotid pulse. If there is still no pulse, you should continue with CPR, stopping to recheck the carotid pulse every 2 to 5 minutes thereafter. Usually patients will not be revived with just CPR techniques; it will generally require defibrillation or other advanced techniques to regain a heartbeat. Remember, the purpose of CPR is to maintain blood flow to the vital organs (heart and brain) until an effective heartbeat can be restored. Chest compressions on pregnant or obese patients are performed in the same manner as outlined here, using both hands on the lower portion of the sternum in the middle of the chest at the nipple line (Fig. 9-6).

Once the advanced airway is in place (i.e., endotracheal tube), "cycles" of compressions and ventilations are eliminated. Continuous compressions are performed at a rate of 100/min with no interruptions. Ventilations are given over 1 second at 8 to 10 breaths/min. Emergency personnel should change the compressor role every 2 minutes in order to reduce fatigue and maintain high-quality CPR.

ONE- AND TWO-PERSON CPR

It is important as an emergency first responder to know how to perform CPR both as a sole rescuer and as part

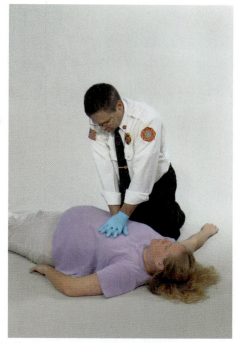

Fig. 9-6 Chest compression placement on a pregnant patient.

of a team. CPR is performed most efficiently by two or more persons. In two-person CPR, the rescuers can share the tasks of airway management, chest compressions, and cricoid pressure to avoid becoming fatigued. If you are performing CPR alone and a second person arrives, you can switch to two-person CPR or ask that the second person take over while you rest. As soon as a second rescuer is on the scene, you should also ensure that EMS has been called. A third person, if available, should apply cricoid pressure.

Additional helpers can bring equipment, shelter the patient and protect privacy, direct ambulance personnel to the patient, and ensure a clear exit for the ambulance. One- and two-person CPR procedures are listed and illustrated in Skills 9-1 and 9-2.

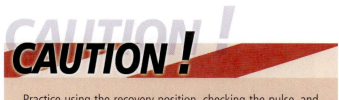

CAUTION!

Practice using the recovery position, checking the pulse, and feeling for landmarks for chest compressions and cricoid pressure on people of different ages, sizes, and shapes. Practice actual ventilations, compressions, cricoid pressure, and CPR *only* on resuscitation manikins.

Skill 9-1

One-Person Adult CPR

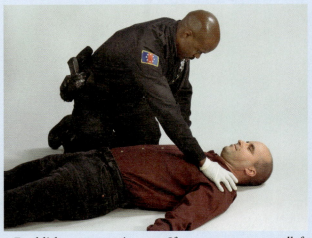

1. Establish unresponsiveness. If no response, go call for help and call 9-1-1.

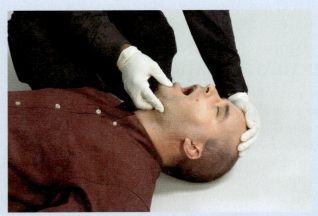

2. Open the airway with a head-tilt/chin-lift or jaw thrust.

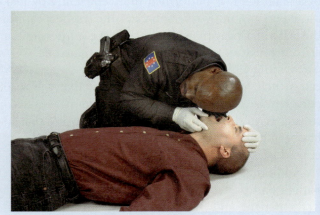

3. Look, listen, and feel for breathing.

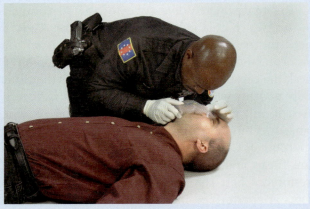

4. If no signs of breathing, provide two rescue breaths.

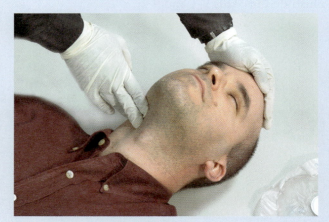

5. Check for a carotid pulse.

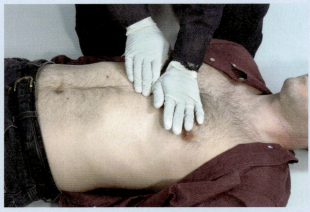

6. If there is no pulse, begin compressions on the lower portion of the sternum at the nipple line.

Skill 9-1

One-Person Adult CPR—cont'd

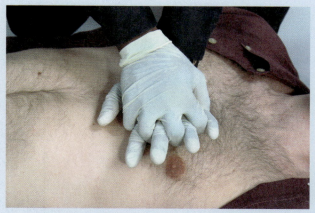

7. Place the heel of one hand in the appropriate spot, and place your other hand on top. Use the force from the heels of your hands only. Push hard and push fast, allowing the chest to recoil to normal position between compressions.

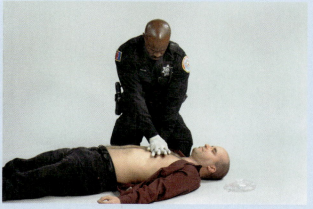

8. Position yourself directly over the patient's sternum, and keep your elbows as straight as possible to deliver 30 compressions.

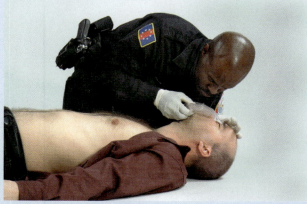

9. Provide two rescue breaths, each over 1 second in delivery, and observe for chest rise.

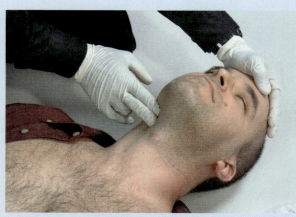

10. After approximately five cycles of 30 compressions and two ventilations, check again for breathing, movement, and a pulse. If a pulse or breathing is not present, resume CPR, and reassess the patient every few minutes. If there is a pulse but no signs of breathing, continue rescue breathing at a rate of one breath every 5 to 6 seconds.

Skill 9-2

Two-Person Adult CPR

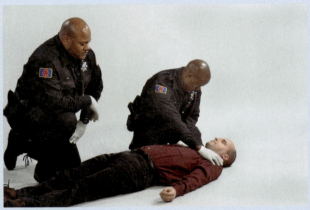

1. Establish unresponsiveness. If AED is available, the second rescue personnel should get AED and activate EMS. The first person should begin one-person CPR.

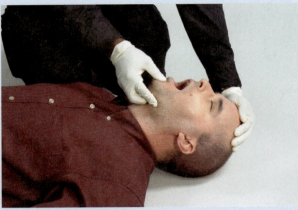

2. If patient is unresponsive, one rescuer should call for help while the other opens the patient's airway with a head-tilt/chin-lift or jaw thrust.

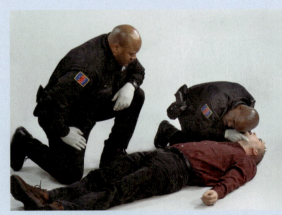

3. Look, listen, and feel for breathing.

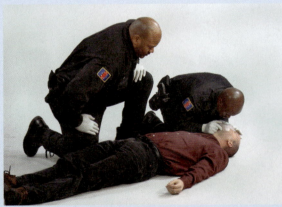

4. If there are no signs of breathing, provide two rescue breaths.

Skill 9-2

Two-Person Adult CPR—cont'd

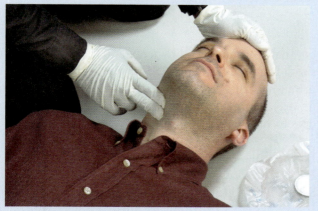

5. Check for a carotid pulse.

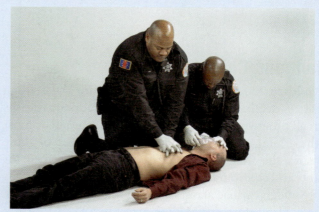

6. If the patient does not have a pulse, one person performs 30 chest compressions, followed by two ventilations given by the second person. Push hard and push fast, allowing the chest to recoil after each compression.

8. Rescuer personnel should switch between providing compressions and ventilations every five cycles of 30:2 CPR.

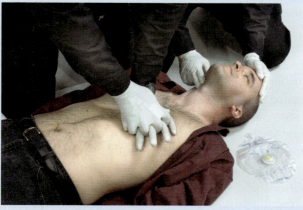

7. After five cycles of 30 compressions and two ventilations, the rescue personnel at the head should check for signs of circulation including breathing, coughing, movement, and a pulse. If no signs of circulation are present, resume CPR.

In the Real World—continued

You begin chest compressions while your partner goes to inform the ambulance crew that you are starting CPR. You have applied supplemental oxygen to the pocket mask to increase the amount of oxygen getting to the patient with each rescue breath. When your partner returns, you take over ventilations while your partner resumes chest compressions.

Infant and Child CPR

In children older than 1 year, injuries are the leading cause of death. Injuries cause more childhood deaths than all other causes combined, and unfortunately, most of these fatal injuries are preventable. Because of these statistics the first step in the sequence of survival for infants and children is modified to include injury prevention. Sudden cardiac arrest is rare in infants and children. Usually respiratory difficulty or arrest occurs first. Before 1 year of age, sudden infant death syndrome (SIDS), respiratory problems, foreign body airway obstruction (FBAO), and drowning are the most common causes of sudden death. To ensure the best chance for survival for infants and children in respiratory arrest, you should provide about 2 minutes of rescue intervention (basic life support [BLS]) before calling 9-1-1. This immediate support of the airway and breathing may prevent the infant or child from entering cardiac arrest. EMS activation is the third step and early advanced care is the final step. Defibrillation with an AED has been proven to be an effective intervention and is recommended for children 1 year of age and older. Currently, there is insufficient evidence to support AED use with infants younger than age 1. You should check your local protocols for providing infant and child CPR and defibrillation.

The overall sequence for BLS is the same for all ages. Assess scene safety, use PPE, check for unresponsiveness, position the patient, and care for the airway, breathing, and circulation. Correct any problems before moving to the next step. You should use the head-tilt/chin-lift, jaw thrust, cricoid pressure, and recovery position for patients of all ages. Because children and infants are anatomically different from adults, however, you must modify some of these assessments and procedures, as discussed later.

Airway

The infant's tongue is large for the size of the mouth, the airway is small, and the trachea is soft and collapsible. Proper head positioning may be the only rescue technique needed for an unconscious infant or child. Remember that you should not hyperextend the neck but instead should maintain the head in a neutral position. You can use a towel, diaper, or article of clothing folded to approximately 1-inch thick and placed under the infant's shoulders to maintain a patent airway.

Breathing

For unconscious infants and children, you should look, listen, and feel for breathing for *no more than 10 seconds*. If the patient's breathing is adequate and you do not suspect an injury from trauma, you should place the infant or child on his or her side in the recovery position; this position will promote airway drainage.

If the infant or child is not breathing, you need to give two rescue breaths. Each 1-second breath should be enough to make the chest rise while avoiding excessive volume. You should avoid fast or hard breaths because vomiting may occur if air fills the stomach; use the cricoid pressure maneuver if three rescuers are present. The smaller the child, the smaller the breaths that will be needed to make the patient's chest visibly rise. For infants, place your mouth over the nose and mouth and gently blow for 1 second for each breath. A rescuer with a small mouth may need to use the mouth-to-mouth method for larger infants. For children, slow mouth-to-mouth ventilations of 1 second work best. Inhale fresh air between rescue breaths. For unresponsive infants and children with signs of circulation but no breathing, give one breath that causes the chest to rise every 3 to 5 seconds, or 12 to 20 times a minute.

Barrier devices and bag-mask ventilation with supplemental oxygen are recommended for infants and children who are not breathing. You should review these procedures in Chapter 7 and practice using these techniques frequently to stay proficient.

Circulation

With infants, check the brachial pulse while looking for other signs of circulation such as normal breathing, coughing, or movement. The brachial pulse is checked because it is difficult to accurately assess a carotid pulse

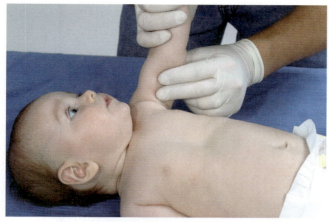

Fig. 9-7 Check the brachial pulse of an infant.

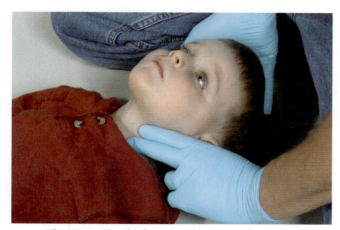

Fig. 9-8 Check the carotid pulse of a child.

on an infant's neck. To check the brachial pulse, you press your first and middle fingers gently on the brachial artery, located on the inside of the upper arm, for no more than 10 seconds (Fig. 9-7). With children, you should feel for a carotid pulse, similar to the technique used in an adult, for no more than 10 seconds (Fig. 9-8). If there is no pulse or if the heart rate is less than 60 beats per minute with signs of poor perfusion (pale, cool, mottled skin), you should immediately begin chest compressions.

CHEST COMPRESSIONS

Chest compressions for infants and children, as for adults, are applied to the lower half of the sternum between the nipples. For infants, the landmark is just below the nipple line. The chest should be compressed one-third to one-half its depth. As with the adult, you should avoid compressing the xiphoid process on the lower portion of the sternum. A second person should be able to feel a pulse with every compression you give. You should place

infants and children on a firm surface for CPR, as you would with an adult.

Infant: One-Person Technique. To properly perform chest compressions in an infant, you should do the following:

- Place your index finger on the sternum between the nipples to landmark.
- Lay your middle and ring fingers next to the index finger. Lift your index finger off of the chest or back and use only two fingers for compressions.
- Compress the chest one-third to one-half of the depth of the chest.
- Allow the sternum to return to its normal position following each compression without removing your fingers from the infant's chest.
- Provide smooth and rhythmic compressions with equal time for compression and relaxation. To compress the chest 100 times per minute, you will need to perform nearly two compressions per second.
- Give 30 compressions followed by two ventilations. After about 2 minutes, five cycles of 30:2 CPR, you should pause to check for signs of circulation. If signs of circulation are not present, you should continue CPR and stop to recheck circulation every minute afterward.

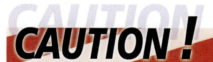

CAUTION!

If the chest does not rise with ventilations, you may need to use both hands to open the infant's airway and then visualize the position you had for compressions to deliver your next set of compressions on the infant's chest.

Infant: Two-Person Technique. If two or more emergency first responders are available, you can make the following modifications:

- Compress the infant's chest with the two-thumb-encircling-hands technique (Fig. 9-9).
- Place your thumbs side by side over the lower half of the sternum with your hands encircling the chest.
- Use both thumbs to compress the chest to one-third to one-half of the depth of the chest as you squeeze the thorax with your fingers.

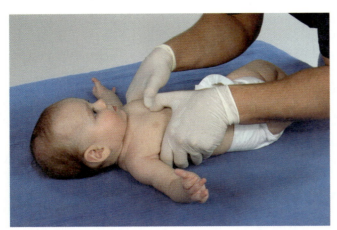

Fig. 9-9 Two-thumb-encircling-hands technique for infant chest compressions. Push hard and push fast, allowing the chest to recoil with each compression.

- Give smooth, rhythmic compressions and release the pressure between compressions to allow the chest to return to its normal position.
- Maintain the compression rate and ventilation: compression ratio the same as with the two-finger technique.
- After 15 compressions, pause briefly to allow the second rescuer to give two breaths.
- A third emergency first responder should apply cricoid pressure.

Skill 9-3 lists and illustrates one-person infant CPR.
Child: Single Person Technique. To properly perform chest compressions on a child, you should do the following:

- Place the child on his or her back on a firm surface.
- Position yourself vertically above the child's chest with your arm straight.
- Place the heel of one hand over the lower half of the sternum and avoid compressing the xiphoid process. Keep the fingers of your hand extended so that only the heel of your hand is compressing the child's chest (Fig. 9-10). If the child is larger and their chest can accommodate both hands, use the same compression technique as you would for an adult.
- Compress the sternum about one-third to one-half the depth of the chest.
- After each compression, you should allow the chest to return to its normal position. Compressions should be rhythmic and smooth with equal time for compression and relaxation.
- Provide compressions at a rate of approximately 100 per minute.

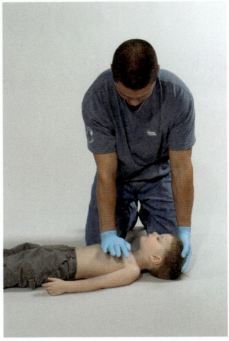

Fig. 9-10 Use the heel of one hand to provide chest compressions to a child. Push hard and push fast, allowing the chest to recoil with each compression.

- Maintain an open airway with one hand while compressing the chest with the other hand.
- After each set of 30 compressions, give two ventilations. You should pause to check for a pulse for no more than 10 seconds after the five cycles of CPR. If there is no pulse, or if the pulse rate is less than 60/minute with signs of poor perfusion, resume chest compressions and ventilations at a 30:2 ratio.

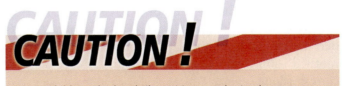

CAUTION!

In children, the head-tilt position may be inadequate to maintain an open airway. Between sets of 30 compressions, you may need to remove your hand from the chest to maintain the chin lift or jaw thrust to deliver a breath. After giving the breaths, you should visualize where your previous landmark was and provide compressions again.

Table 9-1 summarizes the differences between adult, child, and infant CPR techniques.

Skill 9-3

One-Person Infant CPR

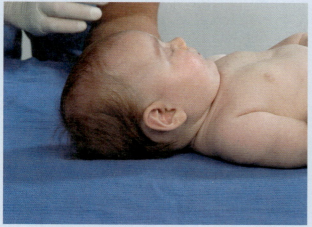

1. Establish unresponsiveness. If the infant is unresponsive, call for help or send someone to call 9-1-1.

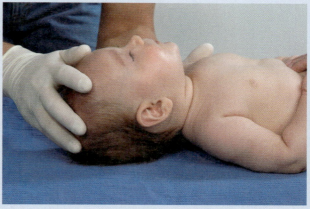

2. Open the airway using the head-tilt/chin-lift or jaw thrust, and look, listen, and feel for breathing for at least 5 seconds but no more than 10 seconds. If no breathing noted, provide two rescue breaths.

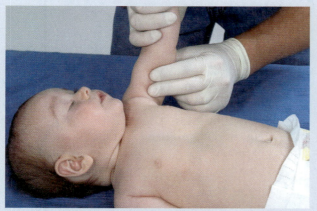

3. Check for a brachial pulse and other signs of circulation signs of normal breathing, coughing, or movement for at least 5 seconds but no more than 10 seconds.

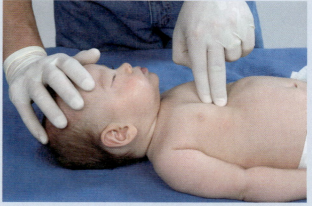

4. If there are no signs of circulation and the collapse of the infant is sudden and witnessed, immediately call for help then return to begin compressions. Sudden collapse is most likely caused by an arrhythmia. If the infant is unresponsive due to an "asphyxial" cause (i.e., drowning), the rescuer should provide five cycles of 30:2 compressions/ventilations (about 2 minutes) before leaving the victim to call for help.

TABLE 9-1   Summary of CPR Techniques

	ADULT (>12 YEARS)	CHILD (1 YEAR– PUBERTY)	INFANT (<1 YEAR OF AGE)
Rescue Breaths	1 second/breath	1 second/breath	1 second/breath
Pulse Check	Carotid pulse	Carotid pulse	Brachial pulse
Compression Method	Heel of one hand on bottom, heel of other hand on top	Heel of one hand, or for larger children, heel of one hand on bottom, heel of other hand on top (same as an adult)	Two fingers or two-thumb-encircling-hands technique
Compression Depth	1½-2 inches	⅓-½ depth of chest	⅓-½ depth of chest
Compression Rate	100/minute	100/minute	100/minute
Compression: Ventilation Ratio (Both One and Two Rescuers)	30:2 (one to two rescuers)	30:2 (one rescuer) 15:2 (two rescuers)	30:2 (one rescuer) 15:2 (two rescuers)

*With visible chest rise.

Child: Two-Person Technique. If two or more emergency first responders are available to give CPR to a child, you can make the following modifications:

- One person should manage the airway while the other does compressions. The person doing the compressions should pause after 15 compressions to allow the second person to give two breaths.
- A third person, if available, should apply cricoid pressure.
- At the end of 2 minutes, the rescuer managing the airway should assess of a pulse for no more than 10 seconds.
- At the end of five cycles, First Responders should change positions with minimal interruption if two or more rescuers are available. Emergency first responders will quickly become fatigued when doing CPR. Changing compressors every 2 minutes will ensure that high-quality chest compressions are given throughout the resuscitation effort.

CAUTION!

For larger children, the two-handed method of providing chest compressions is recommended.

Complications of CPR

Even when performed properly, the following complications can occur while giving CPR:

- *Gastric inflation.* To avoid gastric inflation, you should make sure the airway is open and ventilate just until the chest visibly rises. All ventilations should be provided smoothly and slowly to keep air out of the stomach. When enough emergency first responders are present, one rescuer should apply and maintain cricoid pressure.
- *Vomiting.* If vomiting occurs, you should immediately stop compressions, roll the patient to the side, and sweep the mouth with gloved fingers. Suction the airway if a suction device is immediately available. When the airway is clear, you can then reposition the patient and resume CPR.
- *Chest compressions.* In adults, broken ribs as a result of CPR are common. These broken bones can then cause other injuries inside the chest and abdomen. Correct hand position during chest compressions may help prevent broken bones, but it will not eliminate the risk. If you hear or feel bones break, you should verify that your hand position is on the lower half of the sternum and resume compressions. You should compress only with the heel of your hand and avoid compressions on the xiphoid process.

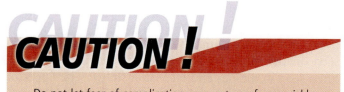

Do not let fear of complications prevent you from quickly and vigorously performing CPR. The alternative for the patient is death.

Family and Bystander Support

Most family members want to be close during the resuscitation of a loved one. You should let them be present as long as they do not interfere with the resuscitation process. If enough rescuers are present, one should talk to family, friends, and bystanders to gather a history of the event, explain procedures, and provide support. Those present will long remember your caring attitude and calm reassurance.

Effectiveness of CPR

CPR is an effective procedure that can help sustain life until a defibrillator and advanced care arrive. However, even perfectly performed CPR produces less than one-third of the heart's normal blood flow. A patient's chance for survival decreases within minutes, so it is important to quickly begin and aggressively perform CPR. Even with advanced EMS systems, cardiac arrest survival rates are low. You must understand that early CPR must be coupled with aggressive advanced care to keep a patient alive.

You may grieve, be disappointed, or have feelings of failure after an unsuccessful resuscitation attempt. These are common, normal emotional and physical aftershocks. These reactions do not mean that you are "weak" or "unstable," just that the event had a powerful impact on you. Methods you can use to reduce the stress of the event include the following:

- Attend a critical incident stress debriefing (CISD).
- Discuss the event with other rescuers.
- Try to maintain a normal routine.
- Eat a healthy diet and drink plenty of hydrating fluids.
- Get enough sleep.
- Avoid excess caffeine, alcohol, and nicotine.

Automated External Defibrillators

Early defibrillation is a key component to a cardiac arrest patient's survival. The time from the victim's collapse to defibrillation is the most important factor affecting whether the person survives the cardiac arrest. Survival rates of patients in cardiac arrest because of ventricular fibrillation drop 7% to 10% with each minute that defibrillation is delayed. To improve this situation, laws in many localities allow emergency first responders and trained lay public to use the automated external defibrillator (AED). Survival rates climbed from 3% to 19% in rural Iowa in the early 1980s when emergency medical technicians (EMTs) and emergency first responders were allowed to use defibrillators. Today AEDs are found in airplanes, stadiums, casinos, schools, and many workplaces. For example, the Las Vegas Casino AED Project has equipped security guards with AEDs, and their average time to defibrillation is 3 minutes. This study demonstrated a 59% survival rate to hospital discharge for patients whose initial rhythm was ventricular fibrillation (VF). With this type of data, it is important that EMS systems should strive to make early defibrillation (within 5 minutes) a high-priority goal.

The following section discusses the electrical system of the heart, defibrillator technology, and AED operation, maintenance, and quality assurance. Because many different models and brands of AEDs are available, only the universal principles of AED operation are presented here (Fig. 9-11). If you may operate an AED as an emergency first responder, you should know your state and local laws regarding AED use. You should also be familiar with the specific make and model of AED you will use. You should practice coordinating using an AED along with CPR and airway management skills. Practice sessions using realistic scenarios and protocols are most helpful.

The Heart's Electrical System

Electrical impulses trigger the heart's muscle to pump. Pacemakers inside the heart muscle stimulate an orderly contraction of the heart muscle. First the atria contract, then the ventricles follow. Heart disease can lead to blockages that disrupt the blood supply to the heart muscle and cause life-threatening electrical disturbances. As previously mentioned, the most common cause of cardiac arrest is a heart rhythm called ventricular fibrillation (VF). In VF the electrical impulses are so disorganized that the heart cannot pump blood. Circulation stops and the patient collapses. The only effective treatment for VF is applying an electrical current to the heart, a process called defibrillation. Defibrillation attempts to stop the

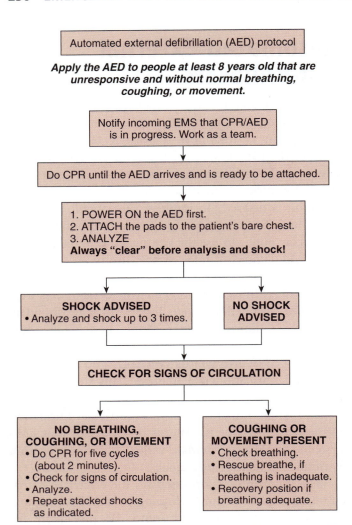

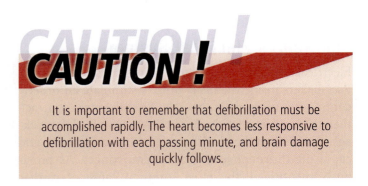

Fig. 9-11 Universal automated external defibrillation (AED) protocol.

chaotic activity in the heart so that the heart's normal pacemakers can resume an orderly rhythm that stimulates a heartbeat to pump blood.

CAUTION !

It is important to remember that defibrillation must be accomplished rapidly. The heart becomes less responsive to defibrillation with each passing minute, and brain damage quickly follows.

Defibrillation Technology

Defibrillation was first developed for use in hospitals. Physicians and then nurses were trained to interpret cardiac rhythms and hold paddles to the patient's chest to defibrillate. These early machines were large and heavy and required human interpretation of the rhythm seen on the monitor. This type of defibrillation is still often seen in movies and television shows. The operator dramatically rubs the paddles together and yells, "Clear!" and the patient nearly jumps off the stretcher. Portable manual defibrillators were developed in the 1970s, and several EMS systems trained their crews to use them. Although they saw an increase in survival rates in patients experiencing sudden death, the size, weight, and cost of the machines prohibited widespread use. The training was rigorous and time consuming. Early automatic defibrillators that interpreted the rhythm, charged automatically, and delivered the shock proved effective but dangerous because the machine shocked as it was programmed to do regardless of whether the area was clear.

Semiautomated defibrillators used today, however, are safe, accurate, lightweight, and easy to operate. These microprocessor-based machines accurately analyze the heart rhythm and provide directions to the operator. If a shock is indicated, it is delivered only when the operator pushes the SHOCK button. Many AEDs weigh less than 8 pounds and are programmed with both visual and audio prompts to follow predetermined protocols.

CAUTION !

The AED should be applied only to a patient who is unresponsive, not breathing and does not have a pulse. Do not apply the AED to a responsive patient even if you believe the patient may arrest. Keep the AED close by, and continue to monitor the patient's vital signs.

Special Considerations

Before using the AED you need to make sure that the scene is safe and then consider the following factors:

- *Children.* The AED is recommended for all children greater than 1 year of age. For children ages 1 through 8, a pediatric dose attenuator system (such as pediatric paddles) should be used if available. A rescuer should use a standard AED for pediatric victims of cardiac arrest if the adaptor system is not available.

- *Clothing.* The AED pads must be applied to the patient's dry, bare chest. All clothing (including a brassiere) must be removed.
- *Hairy chest.* If the patient has a hairy chest, the AED pads may not contact the skin. If the AED instructs you to "check electrode," excessive hair may be the problem. You can try firmly pushing on the pads first to see if that works. If there is still a problem, try quickly pulling off the pads, which might remove enough hair. If not, you may need to shave the area before applying a new set of pads.
- *Water.* Delivering shocks on a wet surface may cause burns to both the patient and rescuers. It may also cause the delivered electrical current to course around the patient's body but not through it. You should always move the patient from any standing water and dry the patient's chest before attaching the pads.
- *Transdermal medication patches.* Placing the pad over a medication patch may cause a burn or interfere with the shock. Carefully remove the patch and dry the chest before applying the pad. Dispose of the patch carefully so that no one is exposed to the medication.
- *Implanted defibrillators or pacemakers.* These devices are about the size of a deck of cards and can be felt under the skin. Placing a pad over these devices may interfere with the shock. Place the pad at least 1 inch to the side of an implanted defibrillator or pacemaker.
- *Metal surfaces.* Ensure that neither you nor the patient is in contact with a metal surface, to avoid injury.
- *Jewelry and glasses.* Placing an AED pad over a metal necklace may result in small burns and interfere with delivering the shock. Move the necklace out of the way or remove it. Glasses may also be removed, but don't let these tasks delay defibrillation. Keep the patient's belongings safe and later document their placement.

Universal Steps for AED Operation

It should be standard practice to bring your AED to every scene regardless of the information from dispatch or the situation you encounter. If you find a patient in cardiac arrest, one rescuer should provide CPR from one side of the chest while the AED operator is positioned on the other side of the chest. This position allows access to the AED controls and makes it easy to apply the pads without interfering with the compressor. You should assume this position whenever possible.

There are some variations among the different makes and models of AEDs, but the universal steps of AED operation are similar with all. You can train on one model and quickly learn another because of their simplicity. Skill 9-4 lists and illustrates the universal steps of AED operation.

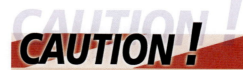

The rescuer operating the AED is in charge of the scene. This person is responsible for everyone's safety. No one should touch the patient during analysis, charging, or shocking. The AED operator must verbally and visually clear the area.

Remember the phrase *power-patient-analyze-shock.* These are the universal steps for AED operation and are described as follows:

1. Power

Press the AED power button. Allow the voice prompts to guide your actions.

2. Patient

Attach the pads to an unresponsive patient's bare, dry chest. If possible, do not stop CPR to apply the pads as this will cause an unnecessary delay. However, if a pause in CPR compressions is necessary to ensure correct pad placement, do your best to keep this delay to a minimum. Most pads already have the cable attached and a simple plug-in connector to the monitor. One model requires you to attach the wires to both the pad and AED, but the principles are the same. Remove the backing from the pad and apply it to the chest as directed on the pad. Place one pad on the upper right chest below the collarbone. Place the second pad on the left outer chest wall a few inches below the armpit (Fig. 9-12).

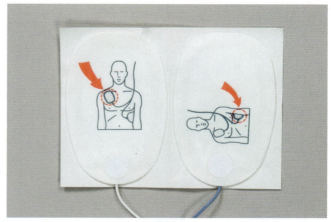

Fig. 9-12 AED pads contain diagrams for pad placement.

Skill 9-4

Universal AED Sequence

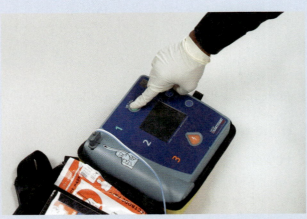

1. Place the AED next to the AED operator and turn on the AED.

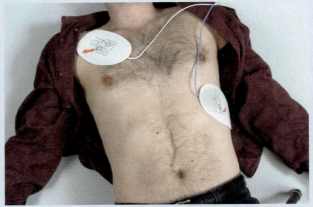

2. Attach the AED pads to the patient's chest as directed on the pads.

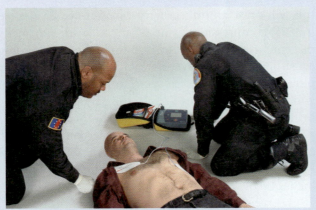

3. Allow the AED to analyze the patient's rhythm. Do not touch the patient.

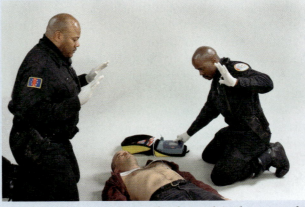

4. If the AED states that a shock is advised, ensure that everyone is clear of the patient.

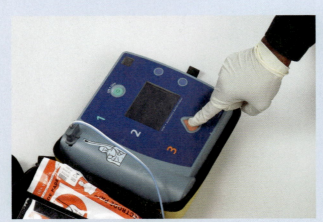

5. Press the SHOCK button.

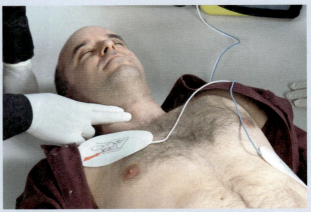

6. After the shock, immediately resume CPR for approximately 2 minutes (five cycles of 30:2).

3. Analyze

The machine may analyze automatically or prompt you to push the ANALYZE button. First clear the area. Plainly state, "Analyzing; do not touch the patient." Make a visual sweep of the area to double-check that the patient is clear. CPR and airway management stops. It may seem to take longer, but most machines analyze the rhythm within 15 seconds. If a shockable rhythm is present, the machine states, "Shock indicated," and will begin to charge.

4. Shock

Before pressing the SHOCK button, clear the area again. Loudly state that everyone should clear, such as by saying, "I'm clear, you're clear, everybody clear!" Visually sweep the area to be sure no one is touching the patient. Then push the SHOCK button. The delivered shock may cause the patient to "jump." You should deliver the first shock, if indicated, within 90 seconds of your arrival at the patient's side.

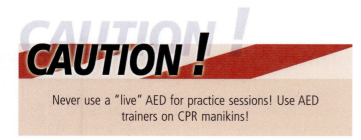

Never use a "live" AED for practice sessions! Use AED trainers on CPR manikins!

The AED is programmed to follow the universal protocol. The emergency first responder should follow the pattern of an AED shock followed by 2 minutes of CPR until the patient shows signs of circulation such as a pulse, breathing and movement, the AED states, "No shock advised," or EMS arrives. Check with your medical director for the maximum number of shocks allowed before the ambulance arrives. The following is a standard protocol:

1. Turn the AED on and attach it to the patient as soon as it is available. When indicated by the AED, shock once and then immediately start CPR without checking for a pulse.
2. Perform 2 minutes of CPR and then stop compressions. The machine then either automatically reanalyzes the patient's rhythm or prompts you to push the ANALYZE button.
3. If a "No shock advised" message occurs, immediately begin another cycle of CPR for 2 minutes.

4. If the patient begins to breathe or move, stop CPR and reassess the patient.
5. Provide rescue breathing if the patient's breathing is inadequate.
6. If breathing is adequate, place the patient in the recovery position.
7. Leave the AED attached until responding ambulance personnel ask you to remove it.
8. Continue to monitor the patient. Be prepared to use the AED again if indicated.

Lone Rescuer

You may be alone with an AED and a patient in cardiac arrest. Once you have established that the patient is unresponsive, you should immediately call for help. You should then open the airway and check for breathing. If the patient is not breathing, you should provide two rescue breaths and then check for a pulse. If the patient was found down for an undetermined about of time, you may give 2 minutes or five cycles of 30:2 CPR first. Many EMS response systems have adopted this protocol; check your local protocols to determine if you should attach the AED first or give CPR first. If CPR was initiated immediately when the victim collapsed, attach the AED as soon as it is available and follow the AED voice prompts. Shock the victim as soon as possible if you are instructed to do so by the AED voice prompts.

AED Maintenance

The AED operator must ensure the AED is ready and operational when needed. AED manufacturers provide specific recommendations for day-to-day and ongoing maintenance. These recommendations should be carefully followed. Many newer AEDs do daily self-tests but may require frequent inspection to make sure the "trouble indicator" is not on. An AED equipment checklist can help you become familiar with the device and identify any problems before you use the machine on a patient. You can ensure the machine is operational and materials are well stocked if you routinely complete an inventory checklist.

The following are suggested items to be carried with the AED:

- Three packages of AED pads (frequently check the expiration date)
- One pair of heavy-duty scissors
- A small towel
- Two to three disposable razors
- Several pairs of gloves
- Barrier devices

Event and System Quality Assurance

Your medical director or designee will do an in-depth case review every time CPR is given and the AED used. This review determines whether the patient was treated according to the protocol and the standards of practice. Also, data should be collected to help determine the strengths and challenges in your local EMS system. All steps in the sequence of survival should be monitored, and survival rates should be calculated.

Skill maintenance is a quality assurance issue. Emergency first responders who seldom respond to cardiac arrests need frequent practice drills to stay competent and comfortable with AED operation. As an emergency first responder, you should practice integrated airway maintenance, CPR, and AED operation in a variety of situations and scenarios. Skill reviews and practice ses-

sions are recommended at a minimum of every 6 months. You should check your local protocols for other recommendations and regulations.

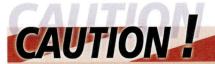

CAUTION !

CPR requires frequent scenario practice for an emergency first responder to remain proficient. CPR procedures are critical skills. Assess the basic ABCs on every patient you encounter. Cardiac arrest will be present in a very small percentage of your calls. Regular practice sessions will help you develop confidence and improve your CPR skills, thus increasing the chance of a successful resuscitation.

Team Work

One rescuer can adequately perform CPR, but it is best if additional helpers are available. The second rescuer should ensure that 9-1-1 has been called and rescuers are on their way. During two-rescuer CPR, the emergency first responder in charge of the airway can manage the airway aggressively by using supplemental oxygen, suction, and airway adjuncts (see Chapter 7). Chest compressions are more likely to result in good blood flow because there is less interruption. A third rescuer should apply and maintain cricoid pressure to avoid gastric inflation and vomiting. If other rescuers are available, they may question bystanders and the family to obtain the patient's history, bring equipment, ensure patient privacy, and lead ambulance personnel to the scene. Working as team in this manner benefits the patient and emergency first responders.

If advanced personnel have arrived on the scene and the patient has received an advanced airway such as an endo-

tracheal tube, you can still assist and be part of the resuscitation team by realizing that the protocols change slightly:

- *Adult patient.* Once an adult patient has been intubated, it is no longer necessary to pause during chest compressions to provide ventilations in the ratio of 30 compressions to two ventilations. Instead, ventilate the patient at a rate of 8 to 10 breaths per minute with a bag-mask device. The compressor role should be changed about every 2 minutes to prevent compressor fatigue.
- *Infant and child patient.* Once the infant or child patient has been intubated, it is no longer necessary to pause after a set of 15 chest compressions to provide a breath. Compressions should be delivered constantly at a rate 100 times per minute with 8 to 10 breaths per minute provided by a bag-mask device.

In the Real World—Conclusion

You and your partner continue to provide CPR as the ambulance crew arrives and begins to prepare the patient for defibrillation. The ambulance crew members secure the patient's airway with an endotracheal tube and begin to ventilate the patient with a bag-valve device and 100% oxygen. After a shock (defibrillation), the patient regains his pulse but is still not breathing. You assist the ambulance

crew to ready the patient and load him into the ambulance. You ride along in the ambulance. At the hospital, you contribute to the report the care you and your partner gave before the ambulance arrived. You return to the scene of the fire, which is now out. Together with your partner, you clean and restock your emergency first responder supplies and document an accurate account of the event.

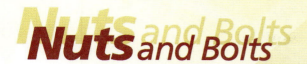

Critical Points

Constant circulation of oxygen-rich blood through the body is the foundation of life. When a patient's heart stops beating, death or disability is certain unless you act quickly and effectively to give CPR. The science of resuscitation shows that chances for surviving sudden cardiac death are best when a certain sequence of steps is followed. Emergency first responders therefore must work within the community to ensure early recognition and access to EMS, early CPR, early defibrillation, and early advanced care for all citizens. Early defibrillation is often called the most important step for survival of a cardiac arrest patient. As an emergency first responder, you are likely to arrive at the scene of a cardiac arrest first. You should be trained in CPR and AED use and that AED should be readily available. As an emergency first responder, commit yourself to frequent AED training that includes integrated CPR and AED skills. Practice your CPR skills frequently to remain proficient. Be proud of your CPR skills; as part of a well-trained EMS system, you can help save lives.

Learning Checklist

❑ The right atrium of the heart collects deoxygenated blood from the body. This blood moves through a one-way valve into the right ventricle. It then moves from the right ventricle to the lungs, where it picks up oxygen. The oxygenated blood then travels from the lungs to the left atrium. The blood then moves through another one-way valve into the left ventricle, where it is pumped to the rest of the body.

❑ Cardiac arrest occurs when the heart stops beating and a pulse can no longer be felt.

❑ The brain is the organ most sensitive to lack of oxygen. Brain damage begins within 4 to 6 minutes.

❑ Cardiopulmonary resuscitation (CPR) is an organized sequence of rescue breathing and external chest compressions.

❑ The chain of survival or sequence of survival includes recognizing an emergency and activating EMS; providing CPR, rescue breathing, or first aid; applying an AED and oxygen if available; and providing advanced care and hospital care as soon as possible.

❑ Cardiac arrest usually results from an abnormal heart rhythm called ventricular fibrillation (VF). Defibrillation is the most effective treatment of VF.

❑ CPR should be started when there are no signs of circulation and there is no clear do not attempt resuscitation (DNAR) order.

❑ CPR should not be started when a person is dead with obvious signs of irreversible death, when a valid DNAR order is present, or when attempts to perform CPR place the First Responder in physical danger.

❑ CPR can be stopped only when effective breathing and circulation have returned, care is transferred to someone of equal or higher medical certification, you are too exhausted to continue, or the environment becomes dangerous to the First Responder or others.

❑ Steps in adult CPR are as follows: assess responsiveness, summon EMS, and position the patient; open the airway; check for breathing; if there is no breathing, give two rescue breaths; check for a pulse and if there is not a pulse, begin chest compressions.

❑ Signs of circulation include feeling for a pulse while looking for signs of normal breathing, coughing, or movement.

❑ Compressions are performed on the lower half of the sternum, between the nipples in the adult. Use the heel of one hand and place your other hand on top. Depress the chest 1½ to 2 inches in a compression cycle of 50% compression and 50% relaxation. At least 100 chest compressions per minute should be performed. This is achieved with cycles of 30 compressions to two ventilations.

❑ If a second rescuer is available, two-rescuer CPR should be initiated with one person performing CPR and the other ventilations. The cycle of 30 compressions to two ventilations should be continued. If a third rescuer is available, he or she should provide cricoid pressure.

❑ Cardiac arrest is rare in infants and children. Usually respiratory arrest occurs first, which can then deteriorate into cardiac arrest if there is no intervention. For this reason, 2 minutes of basic life support (BLS) is performed before calling for help.

Nuts and Bolts–continued

- ❑ Defibrillation is currently a part of the pediatric sequence; it is recommended for children above the age of 1 year.
- ❑ Chest compressions for an infant (younger than 1 year of age) can be provided by placing two fingers just below the nipple line and then using two fingers to provide compressions. The chest should be compressed approximately one-third to one-half the depth of the chest at least 100 compressions per minute. Thirty chest compressions are provided followed by two ventilations. At the end of five cycles of compressions and ventilations, you should check for signs of circulation.
- ❑ Chest compressions for children between the ages of 1 and adolescence (usually age 12 to 14) are provided with the heel of one hand on the lower half of the sternum, between the nipples, avoiding the xiphoid process. The chest is compressed at one-third to one-half the depth of the chest, and the ratio of compressions to ventilations is 30:2 for single rescuers and 15:2 for two rescuers. At the end of 5 cycles of compressions and ventilations for a single rescuer or 10 cycles for two rescuers, you should check for signs of circulation. Resume CPR if there is no pulse or if the pulse is 60/minute or less with signs of poor perfusion.
- ❑ Complications of CPR include gastric inflation, vomiting, and broken ribs and other internal injuries.
- ❑ You should allow family members to be present during the resuscitation as long as they do not interfere with the process.
- ❑ CPR is effective to sustain life until a defibrillator and advanced care arrive.
- ❑ AED pads should be applied to the patient's dry, bare chest. If the patient has a hairy chest, it may need to be quickly shaved. Another option is to use one set of AED pads to remove as much of the chest hair as possible and then apply a new set to the area when the chest hair has been removed. Transdermal medication patches should be removed before using an AED. Place an AED pad at least 1 inch to the side of an implanted defibrillator or pacemaker. Remove jewelry and glasses from the patient and ensure that neither you nor the patient is on a metal surface.
- ❑ The universal steps for AED operation include turning the machine on, attaching the pads to the patient, pressing the ANALYZE button or allowing the machine to analyze the heart's electrical rhythm, and pressing the SHOCK button if a shock is advised by the machine. Following the shock, immediately resume CPR for 2 minutes.
- ❑ AED maintenance should be carried out in a systematic and regular way that follows the manufacturer's recommendations.
- ❑ Remember that CPR requires frequent scenario practice to remain proficient.

Key Terms

ABC The mnemonic used to help rescuers remember the sequence for the assessment and treatment of respiratory and cardiac emergencies. A is for airway, B is for breathing, and C is for circulation.

Advanced care (also called *advanced life support,* or *ALS*) The use of sophisticated emergency equipment including airway management and medications to help stabilize a patient.

Agonal breaths Often called "dying breaths." These breaths are weak, ineffective, gasping attempts that cannot sustain life. Rescue breathing is needed.

Automated external defibrillator (AED) A simple, lightweight, computerized device used to stop deadly heart rhythms.

Cardiac arrest When the heart stops beating and a pulse cannot be felt.

Cardiopulmonary resuscitation (CPR) The combination of artificial ventilation (rescue breathing) and chest compressions given to an unresponsive patient with no breathing or signs of circulation.

Chain of survival A term coined by the American Heart Association (AHA) to describe the sequence of interventions that increases survival rates from sudden cardiac death when performed rapidly. Early access, early CPR, early defibrillation, and early ACLS are the links in the adult chain of survival. The links of the pediatric chain of survival are prevention, early BLS rescue, early EMS access, and early ACLS.

Defibrillation The application of sufficient energy to the fibrillating heart muscle to stop all activity, with the hope that normal activity will return.

Ventricular fibrillation A lethal heart rhythm. Produces chaotic electrical activity in the heart, resulting in no blood flow out from the heart (cardiac arrest). Treated with defibrillation.

Xiphoid process The lowest part of the base of the sternum. It is to be avoided during chest compressions.

First Responder
NSC Objectives
COGNITIVE OBJECTIVES

- List the reasons for the heart to stop beating.
- Define the components of cardiopulmonary resuscitation (CPR).
- Describe each link in the chain of survival and how it relates to the EMS system.
- List the steps of one-rescuer adult CPR.
- Describe the technique of external chest compressions on an adult patient.
- Describe the technique of external chest compressions on an infant.
- Describe the technique of external chest compressions on a child.
- Explain when the First Responder is allowed to stop CPR.
- List the steps of infant CPR.
- List the steps of child CPR.

AFFECTIVE OBJECTIVES

- Respond to the feelings that the family of a patient may be having during a cardiac event.
- Demonstrate a caring attitude toward patients with cardiac events who request emergency medical services (EMS).
- Place the interests of the patient with a cardiac event as the foremost consideration when making any and all patient care decisions.
- Communicate showing empathy with family members and friends of the patient who has had a cardiac event.

PSYCHOMOTOR OBJECTIVES

- Demonstrate the proper technique of chest compressions on an adult.
- Demonstrate the proper technique of chest compressions on a child.
- Demonstrate the proper technique of chest compressions on an infant.
- Demonstrate the steps of adult one-rescuer CPR.
- Demonstrate the steps of adult two-rescuer CPR.
- Demonstrate child CPR.
- Demonstrate infant CPR.

Check your understanding

Check your understanding

Please refer to p. 439 for the answers to these questions.

1. The two upper chambers of the heart are called _____; and the two lower chambers of the heart are called _____.

2. The tiny blood vessels in the body tissues and around the air sacs in the lungs are called _____.

3. The blood vessels that carry blood away from the heart are called _____. whereas the blood vessels that carry blood back to the heart are called _____.

4. You are treating a patient who has stopped breathing and has no pulse. This condition is known as:
   A. Respiratory arrest
   B. Shock
   C. Cardiac arrest
   D. Defibrillation

5. The organ that is most sensitive to a lack of oxygen, which may suffer irreversible cell death after 8 minutes of apnea, is the _____.

6. The combination of rescue breathing and chest compressions is called _____.

7. The sequence of events in the chain of survival is _____, _____, _____, and _____.

8. Adults in cardiac arrest often need to have an electrical shock delivered to the heart. This procedure is called _____.

9. Which of the following will actually increase the amount of air delivered to the esophagus when using a bag-valve mask system?
   A. Squeezing too low and slowly
   B. Squeezing too quickly and forcefully
   C. Squeezing to half full
   D. Sellick maneuver (cricoid pressure)

10. As the amount of time between cardiac arrest and defibrillation increases, the likelihood that the patient will survive _____.

11. An AED is not recommended for use in children below the age of _____ years.

12. When an AED advises, "No shock indicated," the First Responder should check the patient's _____.

13. Often, cardiac arrest victims will exhibit reflexive, ineffective, gasping attempts to breathe. These are called _____ respirations and must not be mistaken for effective breathing.

14. Which of the following patients should have the AED applied?
    A. 67-year-old male with chest pain
    B. 10-month-old unresponsive female
    C. 37-year-old unresponsive diabetic female
    D. 52-year-old pulseless and apneic male

15. When assessing the circulation of an unresponsive adult patient, the First Responder should check which pulse?
    A. Radial
    B. Carotid
    C. Femoral
    D. Brachial

16. In an unresponsive infant, the First Responder should check the pulse located at which of the following locations?
    A. On the inside of the upper arm
    B. At the side of the neck
    C. At the patient's wrist
    D. In the groin

17. You are doing some last-minute holiday shopping at the mall. As you are waiting in line to pay for your purchases, the middle-aged man in front of you grabs his chest. He is ashen in color and has a distressed look on his face just before collapsing to the floor. Which of the following should be done first?
    A. Ask the cashier to page on the loudspeaker for any doctors in the store to come to the checkout.
    B. Start CPR.
    C. Make sure that someone is calling 9-1-1.
    D. Ask if anyone knows his medical history.

18. The landmark for chest compressions for all ages is which of the following?
    A. Middle of the sternum
    B. Xiphoid process
    C. Lower half of the sternum
    D. Nipple line

19. Looking for the signs of circulation include looking for which of the following?
    A. Pulse, breathing, movement
    B. Coughing, movement, breathing
    C. Pulse, normal breathing, coughing, movement
    D. Agonal respirations

20. You are a lone rescuer who arrives at the scene with an AED. A 45-year-old man is in cardiac arrest. Bystanders relay that he collapsed 4 to 5 minutes earlier, with no bystander CPR. You should first do which of the following?
    A. Wait for your partner
    B. Do CPR for 1 minute
    C. Attach the AED immediately
    D. Open his airway

21. While in the course of a cardiac arrest, your AED states "Shock advised." You charge the AED, and it is ready to deliver energy. What is the very next step you must take?
    A. Push the "SHOCK" button
    B. Resume CPR
    C. Put in an airway (oral/combitube)
    D. Make sure all are clear of the patient

Chapter 10

Medical Emergencies

LESSON GOAL

As an emergency first responder, you will encounter patients who present with various medical conditions and complaints. You may need to intervene with special skills in certain situations, but most often you will treat patients with common medical complaints. This chapter describes the appropriate care for the medical emergencies you are most likely to encounter.

OBJECTIVES

1. Identify the patient who presents with a general medical complaint.
2. Demonstrate the steps of emergency medical care for a patient with a general medical complaint.
3. Identify the patient who presents with a specific medical complaint of altered mental status.
4. Demonstrate the steps of emergency medical care for a patient with an altered mental status.
5. List some different causes of altered mental status.
6. Differentiate between hypoglycemia and hyperglycemia.
7. Identify the patient who presents with a specific medical complaint of seizures.
8. Demonstrate the steps of emergency medical care for a patient with seizures.
9. Identify the patient who presents with a behavioral emergency.
10. Demonstrate the steps of emergency medical care for a patient with a behavioral change.

In the Real World

You provide vital services in your emergency medical services (EMS) system as a community health representative and an emergency first responder. The nearest ambulance is at least 30 minutes away from your community on the Pine Ridge Indian Reservation. Early one morning, a young man knocks frantically at your door. "Jimmy is having a seizure! We need you right away!" You grab your radio and your emergency first responder kit. The two of you drive across the village to Jimmy's house. On the way, you radio for an ambulance.

As an emergency first responder, you may be called for patients with a variety of medical complaints. These complaints may result from long-term (chronic) disease processes that affect one or more body systems, or the complaint may be sudden (acute) in nature such as chest pain, difficulty breathing, a sudden change in mental status, abdominal pain, poisoning, insect stings or animal bites, exposure to extremes in heat or cold, or a behavioral emergency. Traumatic injuries may also mask medical emergencies. For example, a patient found unresponsive after a motor vehicle collision (MVC) may be unresponsive because of an injury from the collision or may have had a medical emergency, such as a heart attack, which then resulted in the collision.

Although there are many specific medical emergencies, the general assessment and management is the same for any patient. As an emergency first responder, this involves mainly supportive care and treating signs and symptoms. This chapter describes the care of a patient with a general medical complaint and provides specific information on some common medical emergencies that an emergency first responder may encounter.

General Medical Emergencies

With any patient assessment, you must begin with a scene size-up. This includes putting on personal protection equipment (PPE) as appropriate, ensuring the scene is safe, assessing the mechanism of injury or nature of illness, and determining the need for additional resources.

After the scene size-up, you form a general impression of the patient and then conduct a primary assessment. You should identify and treat any life-threatening conditions within the primary assessment and communicate the patient's condition to other health care providers as required.

After the primary assessment for a conscious patient, you should begin the secondary assessment by gathering the patient's SAMPLE history. It is important to ask conscious patients for their chief complaint or the reason they called for help. However, you should remember that this complaint may not be the patient's primary underlying problem. The chief complaint is what the patient *perceives* as the primary problem. After the SAMPLE history, you should take the patient's vital signs, if you have been trained to do so, and perform a physical examination as indicated. You should focus on the area of the chief complaint during your physical examination of conscious patients.

For unconscious patients or those without a specific chief complaint, you should perform a systematic hands-on physical examination and try to collect a general SAMPLE history from family, friends, or bystanders (Fig. 10-1).

The care of a medical emergency is based on the patient's signs and symptoms. Recall from Chapter 8 that signs are abnormalities that can be seen, felt, or heard in your assessment of the patient's body, such as bruises, cuts, bony deformities, or an irregular pulse. Symptoms are complaints or abnormal feelings that the patient describes to you such as nausea, difficulty breathing, dizziness, or pain. You should assume there is a medical emergency if the patient has unusual signs and symptoms or has vital signs outside of the normal ranges.

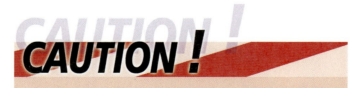

CAUTION!

Always look to see if a patient is wearing a medical alert tag. A medical alert tag can give information about certain allergies, medical conditions, or medications. It may be a necklace, bracelet, pin, or tag.

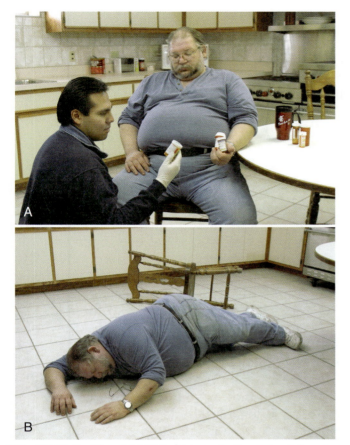

Fig. 10-1 **A,** The SAMPLE history is important in your assessment of the patient with a medical emergency. **B,** For an unconscious patient, or one without a specific chief complaint, perform a systematic physical examination.

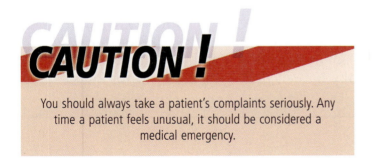

You should always take a patient's complaints seriously. Any time a patient feels unusual, it should be considered a medical emergency.

After completing your primary and secondary assessments and treating any signs and symptoms, you should perform ongoing assessments while you wait for additional health care providers to arrive. You should report any changes in the patient's condition to incoming units. It is important to continually comfort, calm, and reassure the patient while waiting for additional resources.

The steps for emergency care for a patient with a general medical complaint are detailed in Box 10-1.

BOX 10-1 Care for a General Medical Complaint

- Complete a scene size-up.
  - Establish a safe environment for rescuers, patient(s), and bystanders.
  - Request additional resources as needed (including EMS).
- Perform an initial (primary) assessment.
  - Identify and treat any life-threatening conditions.
- Obtain vital signs and SAMPLE history.
- Treat the patient's signs and symptoms as indicated.
- Perform a detailed physical examination (secondary assessment) as indicated.
- Maintain patient comfort.
- Calm and reassure patient as needed.
- Perform reassessment as indicated.
- Report any changes in the patient's condition.

Specific Medical Emergencies
Difficulty Breathing

A frequent and potentially life-threatening situation emergency first responders will be called to assist a patient with difficulty breathing. Respiratory emergencies involve some disruption in the patient's normally effortless act of breathing. For example, disease or foreign bodies may cause airway obstructions that make breathing difficult or ineffective. There are many reasons why a patient may have difficulty breathing. As an emergency first responder, you do not have to identify the cause of the respiratory emergency, but you must be able to distinguish adequate from inadequate breathing and perform general management steps.

As part of a SAMPLE history, a way to assess a patient's complaint of pain or difficulty is to use the OPQRST (*O*nset, *P*rovocation, *Q*uality, *R*adiation, *S*everity, *T*ime) mnemonic. Table 10-1 provides a SAMPLE history that incorporates OPQRST for a patient with difficulty breathing.

Common respiratory conditions that can lead to respiratory emergencies include **chronic obstructive**

TABLE 10-1 SAMPLE History for Difficulty Breathing

S   *Signs and symptoms* of respiratory distress include the following: obvious distress; signs of increased effort; fast, slow, or labored breathing; wheezing or other respiratory noises. For the complaint of breathing difficulty, use OPQRST:

Onset—Ask the patient when the problem started.

Provocation—Does anything make breathing better or worse (e.g., increased activity, sitting, standing, lying down)?

Quality—How does the patient describe the distress? Tightness in the chest or shortness of breath? Is there any associated pain? Where is the pain? Is the pain worse with breathing? Sharp pain or dull?

Radiation—Does the pain go anywhere else (e.g., the arm, neck, or jaw)?

Severity—On a scale of 0 to 10, with 10 being the most difficult it has ever been to breathe, how severe is the difficulty breathing? If this has happened before, how does this episode compare to other episodes?

Time—How long has the patient had difficulty breathing (e.g., it may have started a couple of days ago, but it has been getting much worse over the last half hour)?

A   *Allergies.* A history of allergies may give important clues for a patient with shortness of breath. For example, an acute episode of asthma is often triggered by allergies to such things as dust, pollen, or animal dander. An anaphylactic (severe allergic) reaction may be the result of a bee sting to which the patient is allergic.

M   *Medications.* The medications that a patient takes can indicate an underlying medical condition. For example, a patient may have an inhaler for asthma. If medications are readily available, you should have them gathered for the responding EMS team. Patients with chronic lung disease may have oxygen at home. Oxygen is considered a medication, and you should note the type of device and the dose (liters per minute).

P   *Pertinent past medical history.* Common conditions that are associated with breathing difficulty include asthma, emphysema, chronic bronchitis, congestive heart failure, or pulmonary edema.

L   *Last oral intake.* The last oral intake (solid or liquid) may be important for medical attention that is received at the hospital.

E   *Events leading to the illness.* What was the patient doing before he or she began to have difficulty breathing? Has it been getting worse over time? Has he or she received treatment for this type of problem before? When and what happened? Try to establish a brief time sequence (e.g., the patient had fever and chills for 2 days before the breathing difficulty started).

pulmonary disease (COPD), asthma, pulmonary edema, and hyperventilation.

Chronic Obstructive Pulmonary Disease (COPD)

COPD is a collection of diseases that cause obstruction of the airways and make breathing difficult. These diseases include chronic bronchitis and emphysema. The most common cause of COPD is cigarette smoking. **Chronic bronchitis** is an inflammation and irritation of the bronchi causing excessive production of mucus. Patients with this disease generally have a chronic cough,

and their skin may be dusky or pale. **Emphysema** is a lung disease that causes destruction of the alveoli, making it difficult to exchange oxygen and carbon dioxide in the lungs. These patients frequently also have chronic bronchitis and may have coughing and wheezing.

Asthma

Asthma is a disease that causes reversible narrowing and spasm of the bronchi and excessive mucus production. These patients will have distress, particularly on exhalation, and they often have an audible expiratory wheeze.

Asthma frequently occurs as an allergic response, although it can also be in response to exercise or an infection such as a cold or the flu.

Pulmonary Edema

Pulmonary edema is a condition in which fluid, for a variety of reasons, accumulates in the lungs. A late sign of acute pulmonary edema is frothy, pink sputum coming out of the patient's mouth.

Hyperventilation

Hyperventilation is a condition characterized by a persistent, increased rate of breathing that is often the result of emotional stress, but hyperventilation may also indicate a serious underlying medical condition (e.g., head injury, severe metabolic problem). The patient with stress-induced hyperventilation may appear nervous and agitated and may be calling for help in breathing or asking for oxygen. The patient may also complain of sharp chest pain and numbness and tingling in the extremities. The hyperventilating patient has rapid and shallow respirations that do not allow optimal gas exchange. The emergency first responder should coach this patient and try to get his or her breathing to be a more effective rate and depth. Getting the patient to breathe more deeply and slowly may cause the symptoms to subside and then disappear. If the patient appears cyanotic at any point, oxygen should be given; however, most hyperventilating patients will respond to the control of the rate and volume of breathing.

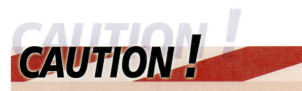

CAUTION!

It is important to remember that a rapid respiratory rate may have many medical causes. Always look first for a life-threatening condition.

> **BOX 10-2 Care for a Patient with a Respiratory Emergency**
>
> - Complete a scene size-up.
>   - Establish a safe environment for rescuers, patient(s), and bystanders.
>   - Request additional resources as needed.
> - Perform an initial (primary) assessment.
>   - Identify and treat any life-threatening conditions.
>   - Assist ventilations as required.
>   - Administer oxygen if appropriate.
>   - Obtain vital signs and SAMPLE history.
>   - Assess OPQRST.
> - Treat the patient's signs and symptoms as indicated.
>   - Some patients with a history of breathing difficulty may have prescribed inhalers for use—you may need to remind the patient to use the inhaler or assist the patient.
>   - Do not allow the patient to use an inhaler not prescribed to the patient.
> - Perform a detailed physical examination (secondary assessment) as indicated.
>   - Allow the patient to remain in a position of comfort.
>   - Patients with breathing difficulty may not tolerate being placed in a supine position. They may wish to be in a sitting position, leaning forward.
> - Calm and reassure the patient as needed.
> - Perform reassessment as indicated.
> - Report any changes in the patient's condition.

Any patient in respiratory distress should be taken seriously, however. Certain illness and injuries may cause hyperventilation. Regardless of the cause of the respiratory emergency, the management is the same for an emergency first responder. Box 10-2 lists the emergency care of a patient with a complaint of difficulty breathing.

Chest Pain

Chest pain is another common medical complaint that an emergency first responder will be called on to assist with. Chest pain can be caused by a number of reasons but, as an emergency first responder, you need to assume that any patient with chest pain has a life-threatening condition until proven otherwise. Typically, chest pain can indicate a problem with the heart, lungs, or the musculoskeletal system. Problems with the heart and lungs are discussed in the following sections. The musculoskeletal system is addressed in Chapter 12.

Heart

Acute coronary syndromes is a term used to describe a group of cardiac emergencies. These cardiac emergencies include **myocardial infarction, angina,** and abnormal heart rhythms (dysrhythmias).

MYOCARDIAL INFARCTION

A myocardial infarction (MI), or "heart attack," is caused by the blocking of an artery that provides the heart muscle's blood supply (a coronary artery). These patients generally describe a sudden onset of pressure-like pain in the chest that may radiate into the jaw, through to the back, or into the left arm. Older patients and diabetic patients may not experience or complain of pain, and changes in mental status may be the only clue.

ANGINA

Angina is also a condition caused by narrowing of the coronary arteries. These patients may have symptoms similar to an MI, but the pain passes with rest, nitroglycerin (a heart medication), or oxygen.

DYSRHYTHMIAS

Abnormal heart rhythms can cause less effective pumping of the heart and circulation of the blood. An automated external defibrillator (AED), for example, detects the presence of ventricular fibrillation (VF) and prepares to deliver an electric shock (see Chapter 9). Ventricular fibrillation is an example of a lethal dysrhythmia that can lead to sudden death.

The general signs and symptoms of acute coronary syndrome are listed in Box 10-3. Early recognition of these signs and symptoms is critical to ensure rapid intervention.

Lungs

Illness or injury in the lungs can also cause chest pain. Examples of conditions that occur in the lungs are pulmonary embolus (PE) and congestive heart failure (CHF).

PULMONARY EMBOLUS

A life-threatening cause of chest pain is a pulmonary embolus, or a blood clot, that has lodged in the lungs. These patients will complain of a sudden onset of sharp chest pain, which may become worse when they breathe deeply.

CONGESTIVE HEART FAILURE

Congestive heart failure (CHF) is a condition in which the heart is weakened by disease and is unable to pump efficiently. The result is a buildup of fluid in the lungs called pulmonary edema, which then leads to breathing difficulty. Patients with pulmonary edema will often have **crackles** or other noises that can be heard at the base of the lungs with a stethoscope. These noises may also be audible without a stethoscope in patients in severe distress. The signs and symptoms of CHF include difficulty breathing and swelling of the feet, ankles, or legs.

Similar to the assessment of a patient with difficulty breathing, if a patient complains of chest pain it is important to use the SAMPLE history with OPQRST to determine the extent and type of pain (Table 10-2). The management of chest pain is outlined in Box 10-4.

BOX 10-3   Signs and Symptoms of Acute Coronary Syndromes

- Pale, cool, clammy skin
- Cyanotic lips and nail beds
- Altered mental status
- Indigestion
- Vomiting and nausea
- Chest pain or discomfort (may radiate to other parts of body)
- Difficulty breathing
- Sense of impending doom (a feeling the patient has that he or she is going to die)
- Irregular pulse rate

CAUTION !

Patients with chest pain may be very anxious and feel as if they are going to die. Or they may deny that anything is wrong with them. You should always remain calm and professional, reassure patients, and try to get them to relax or rest.

Altered Mental Status

A sudden or gradual decrease in a patient's level of responsiveness or understanding is called an altered level of consciousness or **altered mental status.** This condition can range from disorientation to a complete lack of responsiveness. Altered mental status can result from

TABLE 10-2 SAMPLE History for Chest Pain

S   *Signs and symptoms* of cardiac emergencies include chest pain; difficulty breathing; swelling in the legs, ankles, or feet. For the complaint of chest pain, use OPQRST:

*O*nset—Ask the patient when the problem started.

*P*rovocation—Does anything make the pain better or worse (e.g., increased activity, sitting, standing, lying down, taking medication)?

*Q*uality—How does the patient describe the pain? Where is the pain? Can the patient point to it? Is there any associated pain? Is the pain worse with breathing? Sharp pain or dull?

*R*adiation—Does the pain go anywhere else (e.g., the arm, neck, or jaw)?

*S*everity—On a scale of 0-10, 10 being the worst pain ever experienced, how severe is the pain? If this has happened before, how does this episode compare to other episodes?

*T*ime—How long has the patient had the chest pain (e.g., it may have started a couple of days ago, but it has been getting much worse over the last half hour)?

A   *Allergies.* A history of allergies may be significant. Record any allergies the patient has.

M   *Medications.* The medications that a patient takes can indicate an underlying medical condition. For example, a patient may have nitroglycerin for angina that he or she takes periodically, or he or she may be on medication for congestive heart failure. It is important to try to gather any medications for the responding EMS team.

P   *Pertinent past medical history.* Common conditions that are associated with chest pain include heart disease, recent heart surgery, and chronic obstructive pulmonary disease.

L   *Last oral intake.* The last oral intake (solid or liquid) may be important for medical attention that the patient will receive at the hospital.

E   *Events leading to the illness.* What was the patient doing before he or she began to have chest pain? Has it been getting worse over time? Has he or she received treatment for this type of problem before? When and what happened? Try to establish a brief time sequence (e.g., the patient was mowing the lawn before the chest pain started).

BOX 10-4   Care for a Patient with Chest Pain

- Complete a scene size-up.
  - Establish a safe environment for rescuers, patient(s), and bystanders.
  - Request additional resources if needed.
- Perform an initial (primary) assessment.
  - Identify and treat any life-threatening conditions.
- Obtain vital signs and SAMPLE history.
  - Assess OPQRST.
- Treat the patient's signs and symptoms as indicated.
  - Administer oxygen as needed.
  - Some patients with a cardiac history may have prescribed medication for chest pain/discomfort—you may need to assist them or remind them to take the medication.
  - Do not allow the patient to take any medication not prescribed to the patient.
- Perform a detailed physical examination (secondary assessment) as indicated.
- Allow patient to remain in a position of comfort.
  - Do not allow patients with chest pain to exert energy because this may increase discomfort and pain.
- Calm and reassure the patient as needed.
- Perform reassessments as indicated.
- Report any changes in the patient's condition.

many causes including fever, infections, poisoning (including drugs and alcohol), low blood sugar, insulin reactions, head injury, decreased levels of oxygen in the brain, or a psychiatric condition.

As an emergency first responder, your focus should be supporting the patient and maintaining scene safety. Depending on the cause of the incident, the patient's mental status may rapidly return to normal, may deteriorate, or may stay altered indefinitely.

CAUTION !

Do not put anything in the patient's mouth or allow well-meaning bystanders to do so. Many people have a misunderstanding that patients may "swallow their tongue" and try to put a spoon or other object into the patient's mouth. Sometimes bystanders and family members, in their attempt to make the patient comfortable, place objects such as a pillow under his or her head. These types of actions could harm the patient by compromising the airway.

With unconscious patients, you will need to continually assess and ensure that the airway remains open and provide rescue breathing if indicated. You should have suction available if possible to keep the patient's airway clear. Airway adjuncts (i.e., an oropharyngeal or nasopharyngeal airway) can be used as needed to keep the patient's tongue from the back of the throat and keep the airway open. You should follow your EMS system's protocols for the use of airway adjuncts. Breathing patients should be placed in the recovery position unless you suspect a possible spine injury.

Your SAMPLE history is an important aspect of your assessment of a patient with an altered mental status. Remember that you may need to get a history from a family member or bystander if the patient is disoriented or not responding. Assessing mental status can be done using the AVPU scale and the Glasgow Coma Scale (GCS) (see Chapter 8).

The general steps for emergency care of a patient with altered mental status are detailed in Box 10-5.

Diabetes

One of the more common causes of an altered mental status without a history of injury is diabetes. The body's cells need metabolism to be taking place continuously. Metabolism is the process that creates energy. For metabolism to take place, the cells must receive oxygen and fuel and be able to dump off carbon dioxide and waste.

The cell's primary fuel source is **glucose** (sugar). Glucose cannot enter the cells unless it is accompanied by a hormone called **insulin.** Insulin is produced in the pancreas and, in most people, insulin is delivered into the blood to accompany glucose into the body's cells as needed. Diabetes is a disease in which the pancreas does not produce an adequate amount of insulin based on the body's demand. Diabetes may also be the result of the body not using insulin effectively.

Some patients can make up for insulin deficiencies through a special diet; however, others must take insulin doses in balance with their sugar intake. Because of the balance that is needed between insulin and glucose in the body, there are two types of diabetic emergencies: **hyperglycemia** and **hypoglycemia** (Fig. 10-2).

BOX 10-5   Care for a Patient with an Altered Mental Status

- Complete a scene size-up.
  - Establish a safe environment for rescuers, patient(s), and bystanders.
  - Request additional resources as needed.
- Perform an initial (primary) assessment.
  - Identify and treat any life-threatening conditions.
  - Ensure and maintain an open airway.
  - Ensure and maintain adequate respirations and oxygenation.
- Obtain vital signs and SAMPLE history as indicated.
  - Do not place anything in the mouth of an unconscious patient.
- Perform a detailed physical examination (secondary assessment) as indicated.
- Consider placing spontaneously breathing patients without potential spinal injury in the recovery position.
- Maintain patient comfort as needed.
- Calm and reassure the patient as needed.
- Perform reassessments as indicated.
- Report any changes in the patient's condition.

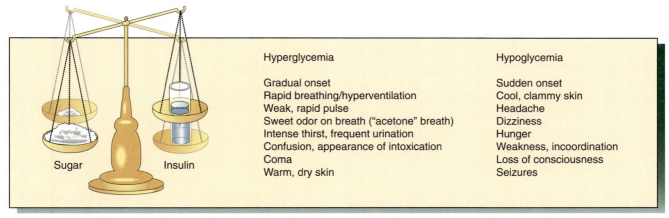

Hyperglycemia	Hypoglycemia
Gradual onset	Sudden onset
Rapid breathing/hyperventilation	Cool, clammy skin
Weak, rapid pulse	Headache
Sweet odor on breath ("acetone" breath)	Dizziness
Intense thirst, frequent urination	Hunger
Confusion, appearance of intoxication	Weakness, incoordination
Coma	Loss of consciousness
Warm, dry skin	Seizures

Sugar   Insulin

Fig. 10-2 Signs and symptoms of hypoglycemia and hyperglycemia. (From McSwain N, Paturas J: *The basic EMT: comprehensive prehospital patient care,* ed 3, St. Louis, 2003, Mosby.)

HYPERGLYCEMIA

Hyperglycemia, or high blood sugar, has a gradual onset and is caused when there is glucose available but not enough insulin to accompany the glucose into the cells to be metabolized. This can occur if the patient ingests too much sugar or does not take enough insulin. These patients may appear intoxicated or confused, but their vital signs and appearance may otherwise appear to be normal. While gradually progressing, this condition can deteriorate into a coma and ultimately death if not treated.

HYPOGLYCEMIA

Hypoglycemia, or low blood sugar, occurs when the patient has too much insulin and too little glucose. This can occur, for example, if the patient misses a meal, is exercising, or takes too much insulin. This condition has a rapid onset and the patient may appear to be in shock and become dizzy and weak. Ultimately the patient may lose consciousness and may have seizures. Another name for hypoglycemia is insulin shock.

The emergency management for a diabetic emergency is the same as the general management for altered mental status. You can find out if the patient is a known diabetic through your SAMPLE history and by looking for a medical alert insignia. Your SAMPLE history for altered mental status should always include questions such as the following:

- Do you have diabetes?
- Do you take insulin? If so, when did you last take it? How much did you take? What type of insulin?
- When did you last eat?

- What did you eat?
- Have you exercised recently?

Your local protocols may allow you to give *fully alert* patients with a diabetic emergency a form of sugar (such as orange juice or a piece of candy). You should watch the patient carefully and treat for any signs of airway compromise and shock (see Chapter 11).

Seizures

Another frequent cause of altered mental status is seizure activity. A **seizure** is a sudden attack that usually results from a nervous system malfunction. It is like a short circuit in the electrical activity of the brain. There are many causes of seizures, including chronic medical conditions, fever, infections, poisoning (including drugs and alcohol), low blood sugar, brain injury, decreased levels of oxygen, brain tumors, and complications of pregnancy. The cause of the seizure may also be unknown. Seizures are rarely life threatening but they can be extremely frightening to family members or bystanders. Any patient having a seizure should be seen by a physician as soon as possible.

Some seizures produce violent muscle contractions called **convulsions.** The patient's body may stiffen and then jerk violently. The patient may lose bowel and bladder control and may briefly stop breathing. Most patients become unresponsive during a seizure. The patient may vomit during seizures, which can compromise the airway, so you should be prepared to manage the patient's airway. Seizures may be brief, lasting less than 5 minutes, or may last a long time. Seizure activity may be continuous or it may stop and start without the patient ever regaining consciousness (status epilepticus). Prolonged seizures can be a life-threatening medical emergency that requires additional advanced medical care. Following a seizure, patients are usually confused, tired, and often fall sleep.

Remember that your role as an emergency first responder is to provide supportive care to a patient having seizures. It is important to protect the patient having a seizure from the surrounding environment. You should, for example, move dangerous objects away from the patient. You should try to protect the patient's privacy as much as possible and ask bystanders to keep a respectful distance. Never restrain the patient, because this could cause injury if the patient's muscles contract violently against the restraints. You should not put anything in the patient's mouth because it could cause significant oral trauma when the patient's jaw muscles contract. Seizure patients often bite their tongue or cheek, causing minor bleeding, and they may also have excessive saliva. Therefore, you should have suction available, if possible, to remove secretions as needed. You should continually ensure that the airway is open and provide rescue breathing if needed. If available, and if you are trained in its use, you should provide oxygen to the patient. If there is no indication of spinal injury, you should place the patient in the recovery position when the seizure has ended.

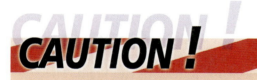

If the patient has obvious signs of inadequate breathing (i.e., appears bluish [cyanosis]), you should attempt to ventilate the patient while he or she is actively seizing.

You should give a detailed account of your observations of the seizure to the responding health care providers. As the emergency first responder, you may be the only witness to the seizure, and therefore your description of the patient's activity may be crucial for later determination of the cause of the seizure. The steps for emergency care for a seizure patient are detailed in Box 10-6.

Stroke

Another potentially life-threatening cause of altered mental status is a **stroke,** or **cerebral vascular accident (CVA).** These patients have narrowed arteries similar to

> ### BOX 10-6   Care for the Patient Having a Seizure
>
> - Complete a scene size-up.
>   - Establish a safe environment for rescuers, patient(s), and bystanders.
>   - Move objects that may injure the patient while he or she is seizing.
>   - Protect the patient's privacy.
>   - Do not restrain the patient.
>   - Do not place anything in the patient's mouth.
>   - Request additional resources as needed.
> - Perform an initial (primary) assessment.
>   - Identify and treat any life-threatening conditions.
>   - Ensure and maintain a patent airway.
>   - Suction/clear airway as needed.
>   - Ensure and maintain adequate respirations and oxygenation.
>   - If signs/symptoms of inadequate ventilation/respirations are present, attempt to ventilate the patient even while he or she is having a seizure.
> - Obtain vital signs and SAMPLE history as indicated.
> - Treat the patient's signs and symptoms as indicated.
> - Perform a detailed physical examination (secondary assessment) as indicated.
>   - Assess for local trauma that may have occurred during the seizure.
>   - Treat injuries as indicated.
> - Consider placing the spontaneously breathing patient with no suspicion of spinal injury in the recovery position.
> - Maintain patient comfort as needed.
> - Calm and reassure patient as needed.
> - Perform reassessments as indicated.
> - Report any changes in the patient's condition.

those that cause a heart attack; however, with stroke, rather than disrupting circulation to the heart muscle, blood flow to the brain is disrupted, causing death of brain tissue. Therefore, stroke has also been called a "brain attack."

A condition called transient ischemic attack (TIA) presents with signs and symptoms similar to stroke; however, a TIA is reversible (i.e., no permanent damage occurs). This is much like the way angina has signs and symptoms similar to a heart attack but is relieved with rest or nitroglycerin. The effects of a TIA typically last less than 1 hour.

Because it is difficult to differentiate between TIA and stroke, all patients with the signs and symptoms of stroke should be evaluated as soon as possible by a physician. Early detection of the signs and symptoms of stroke is critical to the patient's survival. Box 10-7 lists the signs and symptoms of stroke.

During your assessment of a patient suspected of having a stroke, you may use a screening test, such as the Cincinnati Prehospital Stroke Scale, which quickly assesses facial droop, arm drift, and speech pattern (Table 10-3).

While waiting for the arrival of EMS, you should provide supportive care to the patient suspected of having a stroke. This includes airway protection, rescue breathing, seizure precautions, and CPR if needed. You should also provide reassurance and comfort to the patient.

Acute Abdomen

Acute abdomen is a term used to describe a sudden onset of abdominal pain. The pain may be the result of a medical emergency (e.g., appendicitis) or trauma (e.g., blunt injury or internal bleeding). A patient with an acute abdomen may not experience pain just in the abdomen. The pain may be referred to different parts of the body such as the neck or back. A patient may also guard the abdomen. **Abdominal guarding** is a characteristic fetal-like position that someone with acute abdominal pain may take to help alleviate the pain (Fig.10-3).

BOX 10-7   Signs and Symptoms of Stroke

- Facial drooping/asymmetry
- One-sided paralysis
- Slurred speech
- Seizures
- Dilated pupil(s)
- Weakness, lack of coordination
- Nausea and vomiting
- Dizziness
- Blurred vision

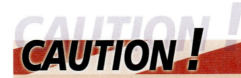

A patient with an acute abdomen may vomit. You should watch for vomiting and be ready to suction and clear the airway. In addition, you should save any vomitus to give to the responding EMTs. Analysis of the vomitus at the hospital may provide clues for the cause of the acute abdomen.

TABLE 10-3   Cincinnati Prehospital Stroke Scale*

Facial droop	Ask patient to show teeth or smile. Normal—equal symmetry Abnormal—unequal symmetry or no movement on one side
Arm drift	Ask patient to close eyes and hold out both arms for 10 seconds. Normal—equal or no movement Abnormal—one arm drifts lower than the other
Abnormal speech	Ask the patient to say, "You can't teach an old dog new tricks." Normal—patient uses correct words without slurring Abnormal—patient slurs words, uses wrong words, or is unable to speak

*Acute abnormality in any of these categories is strongly suggestive of stroke.

In the Real World—continued

Fortunately you know the patient and his medical history well. Jimmy has epileptic seizures that are usually well controlled by medication. Last week, however, Jimmy missed an appointment with his physician. When you arrive, you quickly size up the scene. You see that Jimmy is on the ground in his front yard with a small crowd of bystanders gathered around him. He is having a seizure. Seeing no hazards in the scene, you quickly move to protect him from harming himself by moving objects away from him. You ask bystanders to move out to the road to flag in the ambulance. This also helps to protect Jimmy's privacy. You note that Jimmy's eyes seem to be deviating to the left during the seizure. The seizure activity stops as you open Jimmy's airway and suction a small amount of blood and saliva from his mouth. You check for signs of trauma but see none. You roll Jimmy into the recovery position to help keep his airway clear.

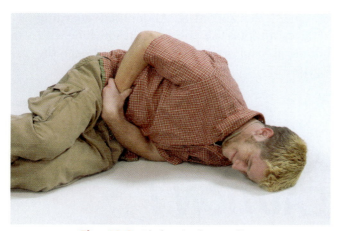

Fig. 10-3 Abdominal guarding.

As an emergency first responder, you should recognize that abdominal pain can have a life-threatening cause, and the patient should be seen by a physician as soon as possible. The signs and symptoms of an acute abdomen are listed in **Box 10-8**. Your SAMPLE history should use the OPQRST method of assessing any associated pain.

The emergency management of an acute abdomen for an emergency first responder is mainly supportive. You should maintain an open airway, provide rescue breathing if needed, and treat signs and symptoms of shock. You should also calmly reassure the patient until additional help arrives. If there are no signs or symptoms of shock, a conscious patient should be allowed to assume a position of comfort.

Behavioral Emergencies

Behavior is defined as the way a person acts or performs or a person's physical and mental activities. A **behavioral** emergency occurs when a patient exhibits behavior that is unacceptable or intolerable to the patient, family, or community. Such inappropriate behavior may be caused by extremes of emotion that lead to violence, or other causes. A behavioral emergency may also be caused by a psychological or physical condition such as the following:

- Situational stress
- Illness or injury
- Low blood sugar
- Lack of oxygen
- Inadequate blood flow to the brain
- Head trauma
- Excessive exposure to heat or cold
- Abuse of substances such as drugs or alcohol
- Psychological crises such as panic attacks or agitation, or bizarre thinking and behavior

Such behavior may threaten the patient's safety or lead to a suicide attempt. It may also pose a danger to others through threatening behavior or acts of violence.

BOX 10-8   Signs and Symptoms of an Acute Abdomen

- Abdominal pain
- Nausea and vomiting
- Abdominal guarding
- Distended or rigid abdomen
- Shock

As an emergency first responder, you may encounter patients with behavioral emergencies. It is important to do a thorough scene size-up and not enter a scene that is potentially unsafe unless you have undergone special training (e.g., as a law enforcement officer).

You should not leave patients having a behavioral emergency alone unless you are in danger. These patients may be at significant risk of injury to themselves if left alone. You should calmly reassure the patient and consider the need for (additional) law enforcement personnel if you or anyone on the scene may be at risk. If you think the patient may have overdosed on any substance, give any medications or drugs you find to EMS personnel when they arrive.

The following guidelines should be used while assessing patients with a behavioral emergency:

- Identify yourself, and let the person know you are there to help.
- Explain to the patient what you are doing.
- Do not make quick moves.
- Ask questions in a calm, reassuring voice.
- Ask the patient what happened, without being judgmental.
- Prove that you listen and understand by rephrasing or repeating parts of what the patient says.
- Acknowledge the patient's feelings.
- Respond with honest answers.
- Involve trusted family members or friends if needed.
- Assess the patient's mental status including appearance, activity, speech, and orientation for time, person, and place.

Box 10-9 summarizes the emergency management for a patient with a behavioral emergency. You should be prepared to stay on scene for a long time with a patient having a behavioral emergency. You should remain with the patient unless you are in danger.

Violent Situations

During the scene size-up, assess for potential violence situations. Ask family members and bystanders whether the patient has a known history of aggression or combativeness. Is the patient using threatening body language? Is the patient standing or sitting in a position that is threatening to himself or herself or others? Does the patient have clenched fists, tensed muscles, or weapons or other lethal objects? Is the patient yelling or verbally threatening harm to himself or herself or others? Assess the patient's physical activity. Is the patient moving

> **BOX 10-9   Care for a Patient with a Behavioral Emergency**
>
> - Complete a scene size-up.
>   - Establish a safe environment for rescuers, patient(s), and bystanders.
>   - Request additional resources as needed.
> - Perform an initial (primary) assessment.
>   - Identify and treat any life-threatening conditions.
> - Obtain vital signs and SAMPLE history.
>   - Maintain a comfortable distance from the patient.
>   - Maintain eye contact with the patient.
>   - Ask questions in a calm, reassuring voice.
>   - Encourage the patient to talk.
>   - Do not threaten, challenge, or argue with the patient.
>   - Tell the truth; never lie to the patient.
>   - Avoid unnecessary physical contact.
>   - Do not "play along" with visual or auditory disturbances of the patient.
>   - Involve trusted family members or friends.
> - Treat the patient's signs and symptoms as indicated.
> - Perform a detailed physical examination (secondary assessment) as indicated.
> - Maintain patient comfort.
> - Calm and reassure the patient as needed.
> - Perform reassessment as indicated.
> - Report any changes in the patient's condition.

toward you, holding any heavy or threatening objects, or making quick irregular movements?

Although helping people offers you a rewarding feeling as an emergency first responder, personal safety is your first responsibility. Being aware of potential situations where violence can occur and avoiding being placed in these situations will benefit you the most. Remember, you cannot perform your skills as an emergency first responder when you are injured or incapacitated. Always assess the environment for your safety before entering any situation. If you feel that your safety or the safety of others may be in jeopardy, you should wait to enter until the situation has been secured. This may involve waiting for properly trained individuals such as security or law enforcement.

Possible situations/environment that may escalate into violence include the following:

- Any incident in which guns or knives are involved
- Situations in which hostages are involved
- Situations in which physical assault has occurred
- Large gatherings of people such as a demonstration
- Situations in which your actions as an emergency first responder will disrupt an ongoing event such as a sporting event
- Environments in which drugs or alcohol are being consumed

Remember that the environment can change rapidly. A currently safe scene can change to violence without notice. You should always be aware of your current situation, and do not enter any environment that you are uncomfortable with.

After a period of combativeness and aggression, some seemingly calm patients may cause sudden and unexpected injury to themselves or others. You should make every effort to avoid acts of force that may injure the patient.

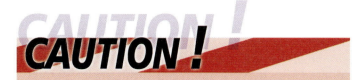

CAUTION!

When you recognize a violent or potentially unsafe scene, ensure that law enforcement has been called. If you are a police officer, additional units may need to be called. If you are an emergency first responder and the scene is not safe, *do not enter it.*

Restraints

Up until this point, this book has avoided the controversial subject of restraints. In general, because no patient should be treated or transported against his or her will, restraints are not recommended. *Restraints should be the responsibility of law enforcement officers.* Any patient requiring restraint should be considered a scene safety issue that can only be secured by involvement of law enforcement. Further direction may also come from medical directors.

There will be situations, however, in which restrained patients may require attention from emergency first responders. Special considerations with restrained patients include monitoring the patient's airway and ability to breathe and circulation distal to the restraints.

Team Work

In working with patients who have medical emergencies, you will encounter numerous medications. As part of the health care team, it is important that you recognize some of these medications, understand what they are used for, and, in some jurisdictions, know how to help administer them.

INHALERS

Many patients with chronic respiratory conditions such as asthma or COPD use inhaler medications called bronchodilators to relieve acute episodes of breathing difficulty. These inhalers come in a variety of brands such as Proventil, Ventolin, or Alupent; however, all of them work in the same way. They relax the smooth muscle in the bronchi of the lungs. This relaxation relieves the constricted airways and makes breathing easier.

The medication comes as a metered dose inhaler (MDI), which is a small device that gives a fixed dose of medication with each "puff" (Fig. 10-4). The patient inhales a puff of the medication into the lungs where it acts directly on the smooth muscle in the airways. A patient is prescribed a certain type of inhaler and a number of puffs to take when breathing is difficult. An inhaler may also be accompanied by a spacer device, which the patient uses to help trap more particles of the medication into the lungs. The emergency first responder should ask the patient if he or she has prescribed inhalers, whether they were used, and how often they were used. To assist a patient with an inhaler, you must ensure that the following conditions are met:

- The patient is in respiratory distress.
- The patient has a currently prescribed inhaler.
- There is a doctor's order to assist the patient with the inhaler. (Generally, only emergency medical technicians [EMTs] and paramedics assist with a patient's medications, but you should check your local protocols.)

Team Work—cont'd

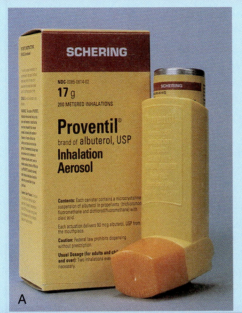

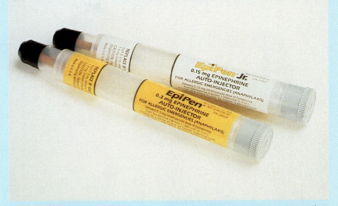

Fig. 10-5 Epi-Pen. (From McSwain N, Paturas J: *The basic EMT: comprehensive prehospital patient care,* ed 3, St. Louis, 2003, Mosby.)

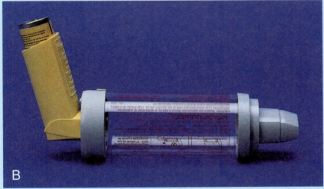

Fig. 10-4 **A,** An inhaler delivers a specific dose of medication to the lungs. **B,** A spacer device used with an inhaler increases the amount of medication going to the lungs. (From McSwain N, Paturas J: *The basic EMT: comprehensive prehospital patient care,* ed 3, St. Louis, 2003, Mosby.)

• The patient has not already taken the maximum number of puffs prescribed.

As an emergency first responder, you may also help the patient and the EMS team by retrieving the medication and reminding the patient that he or she should take it.

You should be aware that if a patient has taken this type of medication, he or she may have an increased heart rate, tremors, nervousness, or agitation. These are normal side effects of the medications and should be included in your report.

EPI-PEN

Patients with severe life-threatening allergies may be prescribed an Epi-Pen to carry with them. The Epi-Pen is an autoinjector that contains the drug epinephrine. Epinephrine acts to counter the effects of an anaphylactic reaction by constricting the blood vessels and opening up the airways.

The autoinjector is a device that contains a preloaded dose of epinephrine (Fig. 10-5). The injection is activated when it is forcefully plunged into the patient's shoulder or thigh. The device is inserted at a 90-degree angle to the skin and held in place for 10 seconds while the entire dose is released beneath the skin.

As an emergency first responder, you should ensure that the Epi-Pen is a currently prescribed medication of the patient. (Generally only EMTs and paramedics assist with a patient's medications, but you should check your local protocols.)

As an emergency first responder, you may also help the patient and the EMS team by retrieving the medication and reminding the patient that he or she should take it.

Only Epi-Pens that are designed and approved for pediatric use should be used with infants and children. Because of their smaller size, a different dose and length of needle may be required. Never use or encourage the use of an adult Epi-Pen on a pediatric patient.

NITROGLYCERIN

Nitroglycerin is a medication prescribed to patients with angina. It can come as either a spray or as a tablet

Team Work—cont'd

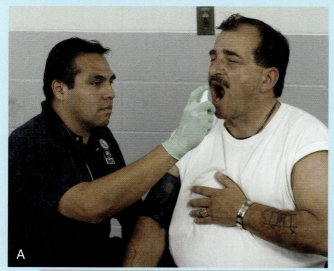

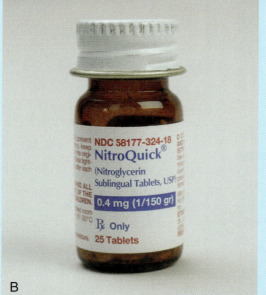

Fig. 10-6 Nitroglycerin. **A,** Spray. **B,** Tablet form. (From Chapleau W, Pons P: *Emergency medical technician: making the difference,* St. Louis, 2007, Mosby.)

(Fig. 10-6). Nitroglycerin acts to relax and open up the blood vessels and decrease the work the heart has to do. This decreases the need of the patient for additional oxygen and can relieve the symptom of chest pain.

Both the spray and tablet forms of the medication are delivered to the patient under the tongue. It is important to monitor the patient's vital signs before and after nitroglycerin administration. Because the medication dilates the blood vessels, nitroglycerin can cause the blood pressure to drop. For this reason, it should never be given to a patient with a systolic blood pressure of less than 100 mm Hg. Other side effects of the medication include headache and changes in the pulse rate.

Generally only EMTs and paramedics assist with a patient's medications, but you should check your local protocols. As an emergency first responder, you may assist in giving nitroglycerin by obtaining vital signs for the EMS team or by retrieving the medication and reminding the patient that they should take it.

OXYGEN

It is important to realize that oxygen is a type of medication. It may be prescribed to patients with COPD. For example, a patient may be prescribed to wear a nasal cannula and have the oxygen set at a flow rate of 2 liters per minute (LPM). Oxygen administration is discussed in Chapter 7.

In the Real World—Conclusion

After about 5 minutes, Jimmy starts recovering. He is still quite sleepy but able to answer questions appropriately. Jimmy admits to running out of his seizure medication 2 days ago. You contact the incoming ambulance and update the responding care providers on Jimmy's condition; you also receive an updated estimated time of arrival (ETA) for the ambulance.

You stay with Jimmy until the ambulance arrives. You give the EMTs a complete report as you help them prepare the patient for transport. When you return home, you complete your emergency first responder report and send it electronically to the receiving hospital. Your report arrives just as the ambulance pulls up at the hospital emergency department.

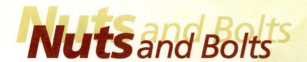
Nuts and Bolts

Critical Points

As a First Responder, you should perform a patient assessment when you arrive at any medical emergency. This standard approach helps ensure your safety and a standard of care. The standard assessment includes a scene size-up, initial assessment, physical examination, ongoing assessments, and providing comfort and reassurance to the patient while you wait for additional medical help to arrive.

Patients may have a reduced level of understanding or responsiveness. There are many reasons for an altered mental status. Your job as a First Responder is not to decide the cause but to provide safe, effective treatment to the patient.

Patients can be injured from exposure to heat or cold. After your patient assessment, it is important to try to maintain the patient's normal body temperature. Provide cooling or warmth as indicated.

A seizure is a sudden attack, usually related to a nervous system malfunction. Patients having isolated seizures are rarely in a life-threatening condition, but they should be monitored closely to prevent further injury. After your patient assessment, monitor the airway, remove dangerous items from the area, and carefully observe the patient.

A patient who is having a behavioral emergency exhibits behavior that is unacceptable to the family or community. You should perform a patient assessment and offer support and understanding to the patient.

Use good judgment to prevent injury to yourself, bystanders, and the patient when you encounter a violent scene. If a scene is not safe, do not enter it.

Learning Checklist

❑ The assessment of the medical emergency patient includes the scene size-up, initial assessment, SAMPLE history and vital signs, and a detailed physical examination as needed. You should calm and reassure the patient as needed and maintain patient comfort.

❑ You should focus on the area of the chief complaint during the physical examination of conscious patients.

❑ You should always look to see if a patient is wearing a medical insignia that indicates an allergy, medical condition, or medication.

❑ For unconscious patients or those without a specific chief complaint, you should perform a systematic physical examination and gather a SAMPLE history from family, friends, or bystanders.

❑ You should assume there is a medical emergency if a patient has unusual signs or symptoms or has vital signs outside of the normal ranges.

❑ Difficulty breathing can be assessed using the SAMPLE history and OPQRST mnemonic (Onset, Provocation, Quality, Radiation, Severity, Time).

❑ Common respiratory conditions that lead to respiratory emergencies include chronic obstructive pulmonary disease (COPD), asthma, pulmonary edema, and hyperventilation.

❑ Chest pain can be the result of a heart, lung, or musculoskeletal condition. Examples of heart conditions are myocardial infarction, angina, and dysrhythmias. Examples of lung conditions are pulmonary embolus and congestive heart failure (CHF).

❑ The OPQRST mnemonic should be used to assess chest pain.

❑ Altered mental status is a sudden or gradual decrease in a patient's level of responsiveness or understanding.

❑ Causes of altered mental status include fever, infections, poisonings (including drugs and alcohol), low blood sugar, insulin reactions, head injury, decreased levels of oxygen in the brain, or a psychiatric condition.

❑ Emergency medical management of a patient with an altered mental status includes ensuring the airway is open and providing rescue breathing and oxygen if appropriate.

❑ Diabetes is a common cause of altered mental status. The two types of diabetic emergencies are hypoglycemia and hyperglycemia.

❑ A seizure is a sudden attack that usually results from a nervous system malfunction.

❑ Causes of seizures include chronic medical conditions, fever, infections, poisoning (including drugs and alcohol), low blood sugar, head injury,

Nuts and Bolts—continued

decreased levels of oxygen, brain tumors, and complications of pregnancy.

❑ Prolonged seizures can be life threatening. Any patient who has a seizure should see a physician as soon as possible.

❑ Management of a seizing patient includes moving dangerous objects away from the patient, protecting the patient's privacy, not restraining the patient, ensuring the airway is open, and providing ventilations, if required.

❑ Stroke, or "brain attack," occurs when arteries leading to the brain are narrowed or blocked off preventing blood flow to the brain.

❑ The signs and symptoms of stroke include facial drooping, one-sided paralysis, slurred speech, seizures, dilated pupil(s), weakness, lack of coordination, nausea and vomiting, dizziness, and blurred vision.

❑ The Cincinnati Prehospital Stroke Scale is a method of quickly assessing for stroke. It includes assessing facial droop, arm drift, and speech pattern.

❑ You should give supportive care to a patient suspected of having a stroke. Provide airway protection, rescue breathing, and seizure precautions.

❑ An acute abdomen is a sudden onset of abdominal pain. Abdominal guarding is a characteristic position that someone with acute abdominal pain may take to alleviate the pain.

❑ Signs and symptoms of an acute abdomen include abdominal pain, nausea and vomiting, abdominal guarding, distended or rigid abdomen, and shock.

❑ A behavioral emergency may be caused by situational stress, illness or injury, low blood sugar, lack of oxygen, inadequate blood flow to the brain, head trauma, excessive exposure to heat or cold, abuse of drugs or alcohol, or psychological crisis.

❑ You should do the following with a behavioral emergency: maintain a comfortable distance from the patient, maintain eye contact with the patient, ask questions in a calm reassuring voice, encourage the patient to talk, tell the truth, do not threaten or argue, avoid unnecessary physical contact, and do not play along with auditory or visual disturbances.

❑ Scene safety is of utmost concern in a behavioral emergency. If the scene is not safe, do not enter it.

Key Terms

Abdominal guarding A characteristic fetal-like position that someone with acute abdominal pain may take to help alleviate the pain.

Altered mental status A sudden or gradual decrease in a patient's level of responsiveness or understanding.

Angina Chest pain caused by a lack of oxygen to the heart tissue.

Asthma A disease that causes reversible narrowing and spasm of the bronchi and excessive mucus production.

Behavior The way a person acts or performs, or a person's physical and mental activities.

Behavioral emergency A situation in which a patient exhibits behavior that is unacceptable or intolerable to the patient, family, or community.

Cerebral vascular accident (CVA) A disruption of blood flow to the brain caused by an occluded or ruptured artery. Also called a stroke.

Chronic bronchitis An inflammation and irritation of the bronchi causing excessive production of mucus.

Chronic obstructive pulmonary disease (COPD) A collection of diseases that cause obstruction of the airways and make breathing difficult.

Convulsions Severe, violent muscle contractions that can occur during a seizure.

Crackles Low-pitched bubbling sounds produced by fluid in the lower airways.

Emphysema A lung disease that causes destruction of the alveoli, making it difficult to exchange oxygen and carbon dioxide.

Glucose Sugar used by the cells for energy.

Hyperglycemia High blood sugar.

Hypoglycemia Low blood sugar.

Insulin Hormone produced by the pancreas that allows the cells to properly metabolize sugar.

Myocardial infarction (MI) Also called heart attack. A condition in which part of the heart muscle dies because of inadequate supply of oxygen.

Seizure A sudden attack that usually results from a nervous system malfunction resulting in varying levels of altered mental status.

Stroke A disruption of blood flow to the brain caused by an occluded or ruptured artery. Also called a cerebral vascular accident (CVA).

First Responder NSC Objectives
COGNITIVE OBJECTIVES

- Identify the patient who presents with a general medical complaint.
- Explain the steps in providing emergency medical care to a patient with a general medical complaint.
- Identify the patient who presents with a specific medical complaint of altered mental status.
- Explain the steps in providing emergency medical care to a patient with an altered mental status.
- Identify the patient who presents with a specific medical complaint of seizures.
- Explain the steps in providing emergency medical care to a patient with seizures.
- Identify the patient who presents with a specific medical complaint of behavioral change.
- Explain the steps in providing emergency medical care to a patient with a behavioral change.
- Identify the patient who presents with a specific complaint of a psychological crisis.
- Explain the steps in providing emergency medical care to a patient with a psychological crisis.

AFFECTIVE OBJECTIVES

- Attend to the feelings of the patient or family when dealing with the patient with a general medical complaint.
- Attend to the feelings of a patient or family when dealing with the patient with a specific medical complaint.
- Explain the rationale for modifying your behavior toward the patient with a behavioral emergency.

- Demonstrate a caring attitude toward patients with a general medical complaint who request emergency medical services (EMS).
- Place the interests of the patient with a general medical complaint as the foremost consideration when making any and all patient care decisions.
- Communicate empathy to patients with a general medical complaint and also to family members and friends of patients.
- Demonstrate a caring attitude toward patients with a specific medical complaint who request EMS.
- Place the interests of the patient with a specific medical complain as the foremost consideration when making any and all patient care decisions.
- Communicate empathy to patients with a specific medical complaint and to family members and friends of the patient.
- Demonstrate a caring attitude toward patients with a behavioral problem who request EMS.
- Place the interests of the patient with a behavioral problem as the foremost consideration when making any and all patient care decisions.
- Communicate empathy to patients with a behavioral problem, as well as with family members and friends of the patient.

PSYCHOMOTOR OBJECTIVES

- Demonstrate the steps in providing emergency medical care to a patient with a general medical complaint.
- Demonstrate the steps in providing emergency medical care to the patient with an altered mental status.
- Demonstrate the steps in providing emergency medical care to a patient with seizures.
- Demonstrate the steps in providing emergency medical care to a patient with a behavioral change.
- Demonstrate the steps in providing emergency medical care to a patient with a psychological crisis.

Check your understanding

Check your understanding

Please refer to p. 439 for the answers to these questions.

1. Which of the following is a sign of illness or injury that may be detected by the emergency first responder during his or her examination of the patient?
   A. Weakness
   B. Sweating
   C. Chest pain
   D. Nausea

2. An example of a symptom that your patient may relay is:
   A. Bruising
   B. Pale skin
   C. Chest pain
   D. Facial droop

3. The patient's level of awareness and responsiveness to the surrounding environment, which may be altered by drugs, injury, or illness, is known as their _____.

4. An unresponsive medical patient should be placed in the _____ position.

5. List the three findings evaluated in the Cincinnati Stroke Scale.
   _____

6. A true emergency caused by fluid accumulation in the lungs resulting in severe dyspnea and noisy, wet respirations is: _____.

7. Diabetic patients may experience hypoglycemia by which of the following:
   A. Eating too much
   B. Taking too much insulin
   C. Eating too much and taking their insulin as directed
   D. Forgetting to take their insulin

8. List three communication guidelines to be followed when assessing a patient with a behavioral emergency.
   1. _____   2. _____   3. _____

9. List four situations in which violence against an emergency first responder may occur.
   1. _____   3. _____
   2. _____   4. _____

10. If a scene is not safe and cannot be made safe, the emergency first responder should _____.

11. Which of the following may be indicative of a possible stroke (CVA)?
    A. Fever
    B. Hypotension
    C. Abdominal pain
    D. Inability to speak

12. Which of the following is appropriate when caring for a seizure patient?
    A. Move objects away from the patient
    B. Put a bite-stick or soft cloth in the mouth
    C. Restrain the arms and legs to prevent injury
    D. Place the patient on his back after the seizure

13. Which of the following is appropriate care of a patient with chest pain?
    A. Give nitroglycerin before vital signs
    B. Encourage vigorous physical activity
    C. Administer oxygen, obtain a history, call ALS
    D. Apply the AED patches and analyze the heart rhythm

14. Which of the following is the most important consideration for the patient with an altered mental status?
    A. Medical history
    B. Airway management
    C. Oxygen delivery
    D. Current medications

15. You respond to a community center where a patient has been found unresponsive. Bystanders tell you the patient was a bit confused a few minutes ago, and is now unresponsive. Your exam reveals a sweaty, cool patient with a MedicAlert bracelet that reads: "Diabetic." Which of the following is the most likely reason for the patient's condition?
    A. Asthma attack
    B. Hypoglycemia
    C. Psychiatric illness
    D. Myocardial Infarction

16. Your patient is an 80-year-old male who suddenly developed a fever, cough, and difficulty breathing and is now complaining of chills and body aches. Which of the following is the most appropriate question to ask in obtaining the patient's history?
    A. "What illnesses did you have as a child?"
    B. "What did your parents die of?"
    C. "Do you have any medical problems?"
    D. "Have you injured yourself recently?"

17. Which of the following is a common sign or symptom of a myocardial infarction?
    A. Sudden onset of a severe headache
    B. Pain that radiates down the arm
    C. Slurred speech
    D. Hives

18. OPQRST is a mnemonic that stands for:

    O _____   R _____
    P _____   S _____
    Q _____   T _____

19. You are treating a patient who is experiencing difficulty breathing, coughing, wheezing, and asking for his rescue inhaler. This patient should receive oxygen via which delivery method?
    A. Nasal cannula
    B. Mouth to mask ventilation
    C. Bag-valve mask ventilation
    D. Non-rebreather mask

20. Your patient is an 80-year-old male who suddenly developed difficulty speaking, vision problems, and difficulty grasping a glass with his right hand. Which of the following is the most likely cause of these symptoms?
    A. Stroke
    B. Heart attack
    C. Anaphylaxis
    D. Asthma

21. Match the terms in Column 1 with the correct definition in Column 2.

    Hypothermia   A. The manner in which a person acts

    Seizures   B. Low blood sugar

    Altered mental   C. Jerky, violent status muscle
    status   contractions

    Hypoglycemia   D. A sudden or gradual decrease
                            in responsiveness

    Behavior   E. A drop in body temperature

    Convulsions   F. Usually results from nervous
                            system disruptions

Chapter 11

Bleeding, Soft Tissue Wounds, and Shock Management

LESSON GOAL

As an emergency first responder, you must be able to appropriately assess and treat bleeding, soft tissue emergencies, and shock. This chapter presents information on procedures for the assessment and treatment of a variety of bleeding and soft tissue injuries. The emphasis is always on controlling bleeding, preventing further injury, and minimizing contamination. Early control of major bleeding can save lives. This chapter also emphasizes the importance of early identification of shock and shock management.

OBJECTIVES

1. Differentiate between arterial, venous, and capillary bleeding.
2. State the emergency medical care for external bleeding.
3. Given a scenario in which the patient is bleeding, select the appropriate personal protection equipment (PPE).
4. List the signs of internal bleeding.
5. List the steps in emergency medical care for a patient with the signs and symptoms of internal bleeding.
6. State the types of open soft tissue injuries.
7. Describe the emergency medical care for a patient with a soft tissue injury.
8. Discuss the emergency medical care considerations for a patient with a penetrating chest injury.
9. State the emergency medical care considerations for a patient with an open wound in the abdomen.
10. Describe the emergency medical care for a patient with an impaled object.
11. Describe the emergency medical care for a patient with an amputation.
12. Describe the emergency medical care for a patient with burns.
13. List the functions of dressing and bandaging.

In the Real World

You are called to assist an injured employee at a local steel fabrication plant. You are guided to the patient by coworkers. Assessing the safety of the scene as you go, you find a man holding a towel to his right forearm. As you pull on your gloves and put on your eye protection, you ask him to open the towel so that you can examine the wound. You see a 2-inch-long laceration with dark red blood flowing steadily from the wound.

Injuries to soft tissue and internal organs are potentially life threatening. The blood lost from these types of injuries can be significant and may result in shock and death. As an emergency first responder, your ability to identify and control bleeding may make the difference between life and death. In this chapter, you will learn about the different types of bleeding and how to control bleeding. You will also learn how to identify and treat signs and symptoms of shock and provide specific care for different types of soft tissue injuries.

Circulatory System

As explained in Chapter 9, the circulatory system is responsible for transporting oxygen and other nutrients to all tissues of the body while also removing carbon dioxide and other waste products. The basic components of the circulatory system are the heart, the blood vessels, and the blood. Chapter 9 discussed the anatomy and function of the heart. In this chapter, the blood vessels and blood are reviewed.

Blood Vessels

There are three main types of blood vessels: **arteries, veins,** and **capillaries** (Fig. 11-1).

Arteries

Arteries are the vessels that carry blood away from the heart. Typically arteries transport blood that contains high levels of oxygen compared to the blood transported by the veins. Arteries are composed of smooth muscles and are constantly changing in size to become either wider (as they dilate) or narrower (as they constrict) in response to the body's blood pressure needs. The pressure within the arterial system (the network of arteries) is usually higher than the pressure in the venous system. The largest artery in the body is the aorta.

Veins

Veins are the vessels that carry blood back toward the heart. Usually veins carry blood with low levels of oxygen and wastes, such as carbon dioxide, from the cells. Veins are not as muscular as arteries but still have some ability to dilate and constrict. The fluid in the venous system (the network of veins) is typically under lower pressure than the arterial system. The largest veins in the body are the superior and inferior vena cavae, which directs blood that is low in oxygen and high in waste back into the heart.

Capillaries

Capillaries are the smallest type of blood vessels. They connect arteries to veins and are the site of gas exchange in the lungs and other body tissues. It is here in the capillaries that the oxygen and nutrients being transported within the blood are exchanged for carbon dioxide and other wastes.

Blood

Blood is the fluid that is transported by the blood vessels. Blood consists of several elements including the following:

- *Red blood cells.* Red blood cells (RBC) are produced in the bone marrow and contain a molecule called **hemoglobin.** Oxygen binds to hemoglobin to be carried around in the blood to different parts of the body. In a sense, the hemoglobin acts as a "ferry" for oxygen.
- *White blood cells.* There are different types of white blood cells (WBC), but they all fight infection in the body.
- *Platelets.* Platelets are special cells that produce substances necessary for blood to clot. Clotting is one of the body's first defense mechanisms against bleeding.
- *Plasma.* Plasma is the straw-colored fluid that carries the cellular components (red blood cells, white blood cells, and platelets) of blood.

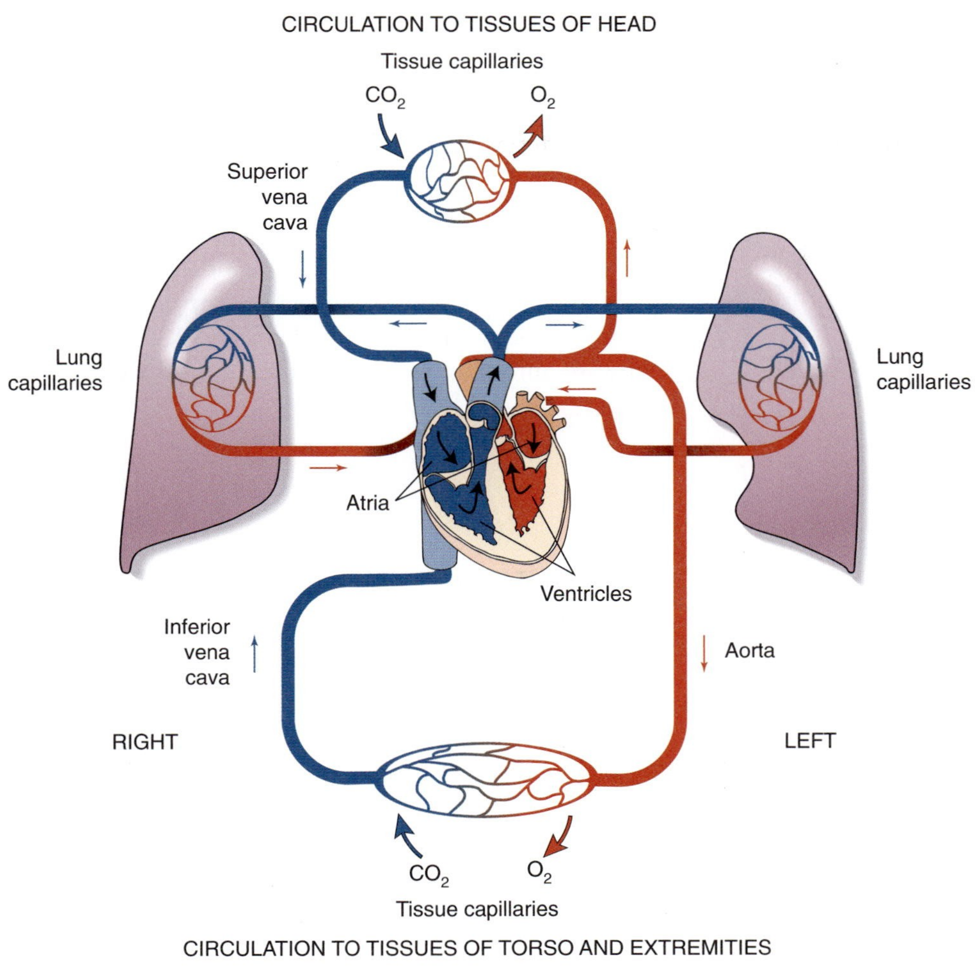

CIRCULATION TO TISSUES OF HEAD

Tissue capillaries

CO_2 O_2

Superior vena cava

Lung capillaries

Lung capillaries

Atria

Ventricles

Inferior vena cava

Aorta

RIGHT

LEFT

CO_2 O_2

Tissue capillaries

CIRCULATION TO TISSUES OF TORSO AND EXTREMITIES

Fig. 11-1 Blood flow through the circulatory system. (From McSwain N, Paturas J: *The basic EMT: comprehensive prehospital patient care,* ed 3, St. Louis, 2003, Mosby.)

Types of Bleeding

Bleeding refers to the loss of blood and is also called **hemorrhage.** The body naturally protects against blood loss in two main ways: producing blood clots and constricting (narrowing) blood vessels. A serious injury, however, may lead to bleeding that the body cannot control. If the damage or injury is too large for clotting to block the bleeding site, or if blood is being lost faster than the body can clot, the blood loss can become life threatening. Uncontrolled bleeding leads to shock (discussed later in this chapter) and possibly death. The goal with any type of bleeding is to stop or limit the amount of the patient's blood loss to prevent shock. If the patient is already exhibiting signs and symptoms of shock, the goal is to prevent further blood loss until the patient receives additional medical care.

Blood loss can occur outside the body (external) or inside the body (internal). Both types of hemorrhage can range in severity from minimal bleeding to life-threatening blood loss.

External Bleeding

Because external bleeding occurs outside of the body and can be seen, it can be easier to detect, identify the source, and control. There are three types of external bleeding based on the type of blood vessels involved: arterial, venous, and capillary bleeding (Fig. 11-2). As an emergency first responder, you should be able to recognize each type of external bleeding and understand its severity.

Arterial Bleeding

Arterial bleeding is the most severe type of hemorrhage and is most likely to quickly lead to overwhelming blood loss, shock, and death. Because arteries transport blood under higher pressure, arterial bleeding can be the most difficult to control. Blood will spurt from the open artery in a wound with each beat of the heart. Arterial blood is bright red because of the higher concentration of oxygen that it carries. Once the body has lost too much blood, the spurting stops—this is an ominous sign.

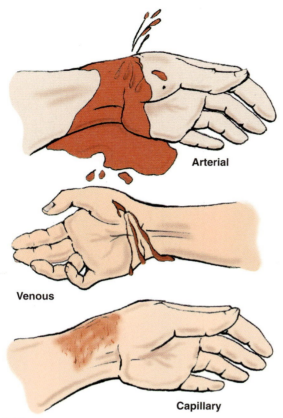

Fig. 11-2 Arterial, venous, and capillary bleeding. (From Stoy W et al: Center for Emergency Medicine: *Mosby's EMT-basic textbook,* revised ed 2, St Louis, 2007, Mosby.)

Venous Bleeding

Venous bleeding is blood that is escaping from the veins. This blood has already delivered oxygen to body tissues and therefore appears a darker red than arterial blood. Generally blood from the veins does not spurt out because it is under a lower pressure. Instead it flows steadily out of a wound. Bleeding from a vein can be heavy but in most cases it is easier to control than arterial bleeding because the pressure in the veins is lower.

Capillary Bleeding

Capillaries are microscopic blood vessels between arteries and veins. These vessels are so small that the blood merely oozes out. Capillary blood is darker red in color. **Capillary bleeding** is typically insignificant, clots spontaneously, and requires little intervention.

Based on the location, size, and severity of an injury, all three types of external hemorrhage may be occurring at the same time. Clearly identifying what type of external hemorrhage is involved will be difficult. Efforts should be focused on stopping the hemorrhage regardless of the type of external blood loss.

Assessment

When you arrive at any emergency scene, your own safety is your first priority. You should always perform a scene size-up before approaching the patient. As part of the scene size-up, it is important to protect yourself with the appropriate personal protection equipment (PPE). With bleeding patients, this requires the use of gloves at a minimum and possibly could require the use of a gown, eye protection, and a mask if there is risk of the blood spattering into the mucous membranes of the eyes, nose, or mouth.

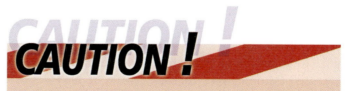

CAUTION !

Always use personal protection equipment (PPE) when treating patients who are bleeding to minimize the risk of infectious disease from contact with blood or other body fluids. Many communicable diseases are caused by bloodborne pathogens. Examples of pathogens to which you may be exposed include HIV and hepatitis B virus (see Chapter 2). A simple and effective way to protect yourself against disease is to use PPE.

After the scene size-up, you will form a general impression and establish the patient's level of consciousness. You will then perform an initial assessment of the patient. Part of the assessment for circulation during the initial assessment is to check for major bleeding. This can be accomplished by looking at the patient's body to see if there is any blood spurting out, by noticing pools of blood around the patient, or by quickly running your hands down the patient to see if there is any blood. Any obvious, significant external bleeding should be controlled at this time.

CAUTION !

Regardless of the need to control bleeding, your first priority is always to monitor and maintain the airway, breathing, and circulation.

After your initial assessment, you should look for other evidence of bleeding under the patient and within the patient's clothing during your more detailed physical examination. The amount of bleeding may be difficult to determine at first glance. Clothing can absorb and hide a great deal of blood and the patient's clothes should be removed as needed. You should ensure that you find and control all sources of external bleeding, if possible, during the physical examination. You should comfort, calm, and reassure the patient while waiting for additional help and continue your ongoing assessments as indicated. Remember that the patient may be scared and anxious. You should always explain what you are doing in a calm and professional manner. This will help the patient be more comfortable with the care you are providing. You should have the patient sit or lie down if he or she is bleeding or injured. This will make the patient more comfortable and potentially may lower his or her pulse rate, which may assist in slowing the bleeding of any wound.

Bleeding Control

There are four methods of controlling external bleeding. In order of preference, these are direct pressure, elevation, pressure points, and tourniquets.

DIRECT PRESSURE

The first step in controlling bleeding is to apply direct pressure on the wound. Direct pressure is applied by placing the flat pads of your gloved fingers and applying fingertip pressure directly on the point of bleeding. This pressure should be applied firmly and continuously until the bleeding stops. If possible, it is best to use some type of sterile dressing over the wound to cover it and to help prevent contamination. However, if blood is spurting out of a wound, direct pressure should be applied immediately during the initial assessment using only your gloved fingers or hand. When you put pressure on a bleeding wound, you must hold the pressure as long as the wound continues to bleed. The body needs time to allow the blood inside the injured vessel to begin forming a clot to initially decrease and then eventually stop the bleeding. Relieving the pressure too soon may let blood start flowing again and wash away incomplete clotting that had occurred. The body then has to start the clotting process all over again.

If fingertip pressure allows blood to ooze or flow freely from under the dressing, you should apply pressure with the palm of one or both of your hands. Remember that once you apply direct pressure, do not let up until the bleeding stops. If blood seeps out around a dressing, apply another dressing on top of the first dressing and continue with direct pressure. Do not remove a blood-soaked dressing, but continue to reinforce it with additional dressings. Each time you remove a dressing, you will interfere with the clotting process that has already begun.

A **pressure dressing** is a special type of dressing that can be used in some areas of the body where the blood vessels are closer to the body's surface such as the arms or legs. A pressure dressing involves placing one or more dressings over the wound while maintaining direct pressure. If hemorrhage continues, a bulkier type of dressing (such as a trauma dressing or a sanitary pad) is placed over the initial dressings and the dressings are then held in place with a **bandage.** Roller gauze, for example, can be used as a bandage for a pressure dressing. Once a pressure dressing is applied, it must be left in place. Direct pressure can be held over the top of the pressure dressing or additional dressings can be placed over blood-soaked ones if bleeding continues.

ELEVATION AND PRESSURE POINTS

Recent research has failed to show any patient benefit in using elevation or pressure points to control bleeding. Many protocols have been adjusted to remove them from use in bleeding control. If your protocol still includes their use, the description and rationales are included here.

Elevation. If direct pressure and pressure dressings do not control the bleeding in an extremity, and there is no evidence of musculoskeletal injury (see Chapter 12), you should elevate the extremity while maintaining direct pressure. Elevation of an extremity above the level of the heart can reduce the flow of blood to the wound and may help stop the bleeding.

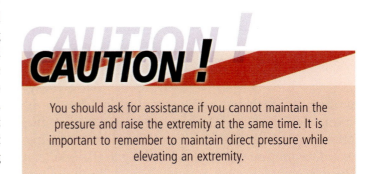

You should ask for assistance if you cannot maintain the pressure and raise the extremity at the same time. It is important to remember to maintain direct pressure while elevating an extremity.

Pressure Points. Pressure points are used as the next step to control bleeding if direct pressure, pressure dressings, and elevation do not work. Any place in the extremity where an artery can be compressed against a bony surface can be used as a pressure point **(Fig. 11-3)**. A

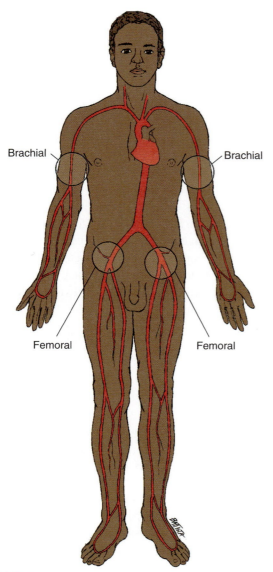

Fig. 11-3 Pressure on arteries proximal to the injury can be used to control bleeding in the extremities. (From Stoy W et al and Center for Emergency Medicine: *Mosby's EMT-basic textbook*, St Louis, 1996, Mosby Lifeline.)

pressure point should be located at a site between the trunk of the body and the bleeding wound. You can use pressure points in both the upper and lower extremities to reduce the amount of blood flowing to the wound. A pressure point is used in conjunction with direct pressure over the wound. As an emergency first responder, you will use the brachial artery as a pressure point for bleeding in the upper extremities and the femoral artery as the pressure point for bleeding in the lower extremities.

To use the brachial artery as a pressure point, you will need to locate the brachial artery in the injured upper arm. While holding the forearm in an elevated position

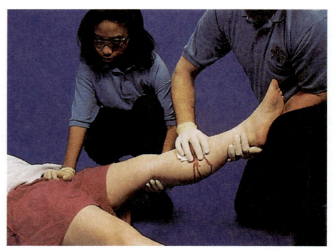

Fig. 11-4 Use the femoral artery for a pressure point and direct pressure with elevation to control bleeding in the lower extremity. (From Stoy W et al and Center for Emergency Medicine: *Mosby's EMT-basic textbook,* revised ed 2, St Louis, 2007, Mosby.)

and with direct pressure still placed on the wound, you should press the brachial artery against the humerus (bone of the upper arm) with your fingertips.

For bleeding to the lower extremities, the femoral artery is used as a pressure point. You should have the patient lie supine and then locate the femoral artery in the groin area between the genitalia and the pelvis with your fingers. You should then use the palm of your hand to compress the femoral artery against the pelvic bone (Fig. 11-4).

TOURNIQUETS

Recent research evaluating the use of tourniquets for bleeding control are describing significant patient benefit with limited risk, particularly in tactical or hazardous situations in which maintaining direct pressure is not possible. Tourniquets are used to control life-threatening bleeding not controlled by other measures such as direct pressure, pressure dressing, elevation, or pressure points. If a tourniquet must be used, its application is limited to control bleeding from the patient's arms and legs. In general, the use of tourniquets below the elbow or knee is not necessary unless circumstances do not allow application of direct pressure. General rules for applying a tourniquet include the following:

• Use as wide a piece of material as possible.
• Apply the material just above the injury.
• Wrap the material twice around the site.
• Tie a knot in the material.

In the Real World—continued

After applying pressure to the wound, you note that the patient has good pulses, movement, and sensation distal to the injury. There does not appear to be any deformity to the arm other than the laceration, and you surmise that the dark red flowing blood is venous in nature. You remove the towel, place clean gauze over the wound, and apply direct pressure. You continue to hold pressure to the wound and reassure the patient while you wait for the ambulance.

- Place a stick or other solid object on top of the knot.
- Try another knot over the placed object.
- Turn the object to tighten the material until the bleeding is controlled—you may not be able to completely stop the bleeding.
- Note the time the tourniquet was applied.
- Write TK on the patient's forehead along with the time the tourniquet was applied.
- Report the presence of the tourniquet to the arriving emergency medical services (EMS) crew.
- Never release a tourniquet once it has been placed.
- Once the bleeding is controlled, dress the wound to prevent further contamination
- Treat the patient for shock.
- Skill 11-1 illustrates the typical methods utilized to control external bleeding.

Internal Bleeding

Internal bleeding is blood loss that occurs inside the body. Because it occurs within the body, internal bleeding is much harder to identify and control. The causes of internal bleeding can range from tears in blood vessels to injured organs to musculoskeletal trauma. Similar to external bleeding, internal bleeding can range from minimal to life threatening depending on the amount of blood loss. Because internal bleeding is concealed from our visual assessment, even a minor case of hemorrhage can continue to bleed into an open cavity or into surrounding soft tissue long enough to create a life-threatening condition. For example, a fractured (broken) femur or pelvis can create enough internal bleeding to cause death. As an emergency first responder, you should know how to recognize and what to do in a situation of internal bleeding.

It is more difficult to assess internal bleeding than external bleeding. It is therefore important to be able to suspect internal bleeding based on mechanism of injury and the associated signs and symptoms. Internal bleeding should be suspected with any mechanism of injury involving blunt or penetrating trauma. For example, motor vehicle collisions, gunshot wounds, and explosions can all be causes of internal injury and bleeding. Also internal bleeding should be suspected in patients who have unexplained signs and symptoms of shock.

A painful, swollen abdomen or extremity may be a sign of serious internal blood loss. Other indicators of internal bleeding include discolored, tender, swollen, or hard tissues and the symptoms of shock, which are discussed later in this chapter. For example, a bruise indicates that there has been internal bleeding. Box 11-1 lists some of the signs and symptoms of internal bleeding. Box 11-2 summarizes the care for a patient with suspected internal bleeding. Because you cannot directly control internal bleeding (most internal bleeding can only be controlled through surgery), recognizing the signs and symptoms of internal bleeding and providing ongoing assessment of airway, breathing, circulation, and mental status is an emergency first responder's most important role.

Shock

Shock, or hypoperfusion, is a condition that results from a decreased volume of circulating blood. A decreased volume of blood in the blood vessels leads to a decreased supply of oxygen being delivered throughout the body. Cells that make up tissues and organs can function only if they receive an adequate supply of oxygen. If enough cells are deprived of an adequate amount of oxygen, the tissue becomes damaged; if enough tissue is damaged, whole organs cannot function properly and internal organs begins to fail. Organ failure can progress rapidly to failure of one or more of the body's systems. Eventually the entire body shuts down in response to system failure, and death quickly follows.

Shock can result from a failure of the heart's pumping ability (pump failure), from an abnormal dilation (widening) of the vessels (pipe failure) that prevents blood

Skill 11-1

Control of Bleeding

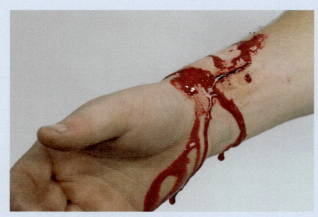

1. Identify source of external bleeding.

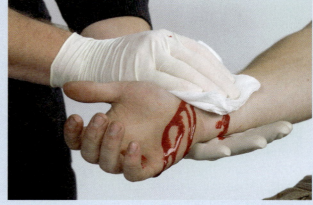

2. Apply direct pressure.

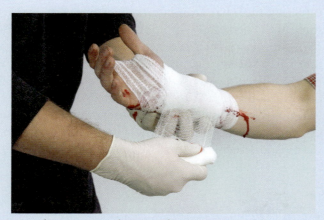

3. Apply a pressure dressing if appropriate.

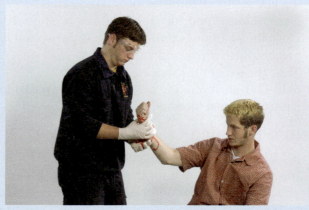

4. While maintaining direct pressure on the wound, elevate the extremity.

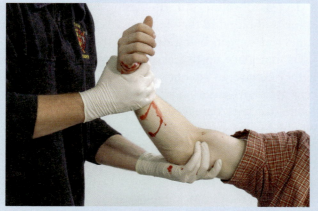

5. If bleeding is still not controlled, maintain direct pressure and elevation, and apply pressure to the appropriate pressure point.

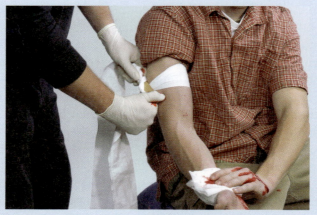

6. As a *last resort*, apply a tourniquet.

BOX 11-1   Signs and Symptoms of Internal Bleeding

- Signs and symptoms of shock
  - Increased pulse rate
  - Increase respiratory rate
  - Pale, cool, moist skin
  - Altered mental status
  - Nausea and vomiting
- Bleeding from any body orifice
- Blood-tinged vomit or feces
- "Coffee ground" vomit
- Dark, tarry stool
- Abdominal distention
- Abdominal rigidity or tenderness

BOX 11-2   Care for a Patient with Suspected Internal Bleeding

- Complete a scene size-up.
  - Establish a safe environment for rescuers, patient(s), and bystanders.
  - Request additional resources as needed (including EMS).
- Perform an initial (primary) assessment.
  - Identify and treat any life-threatening conditions.
- Obtain vital signs and SAMPLE history.
  - Identify signs and symptoms of internal bleeding.
  - If available and if you have been trained in its use, provide the patient with supplemental oxygen.
  - Watch for signs and symptoms of shock.
    - If shock develops, follow treatment for shock.
  - Keep the patient warm.
  - Do not give the patient any food or drink.
- Perform a detailed physical examination (secondary assessment) as indicated.
  - Provide care for other specific injuries as necessary.
  - Identify and manage any external bleeding and check for blood loss under clothing.
- Maintain patient comfort.
- Calm and reassure the patient as needed.
- Perform reassessment as indicated.
- Report any changes in the patient's condition.

from reaching all tissues, or from excessive fluid (blood) loss. All of these have the similar result of less blood and oxygen circulating around the body.

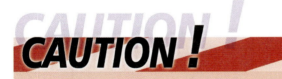

It is important to note that fluid loss can come from either external or internal bleeding (loss of blood) or from excessive vomiting or diarrhea (loss of body fluid). No matter what the cause of shock, the treatment you provide as an emergency first responder is the same.

It is important, as an emergency first responder, that you understand that shock is a condition that develops over time. How much time it takes for shock to develop depends on the extent and rate of circulatory failure. For example, a person who is spurting red arterial blood from his or her thigh is losing blood at a faster rate than if the person had venous bleeding from an injury to the arm. The faster blood is lost, the more quickly shock can develop. The body goes through different stages to attempt to stop shock from occurring. For example, if not enough blood is reaching the body tissues, the body will increase its heart rate in an attempt to push blood out of the heart faster while constricting the blood vessels to maintain blood pressure. This attempt by the body to stop shock from progressing is called **compensation.** However, if the source of the circulatory failure is not identified and treated, the body may eventually be unable to compensate any further and death will follow.

As an emergency first responder, you may not be able to identify and control the source or reason that shock is occurring. Your role, therefore, is to identify the signs and symptoms of shock and provide supportive care until more advanced medical care arrives.

Signs and Symptoms

The first signs and symptoms of shock reflect the body's attempt to compensate for the lack of circulating blood.

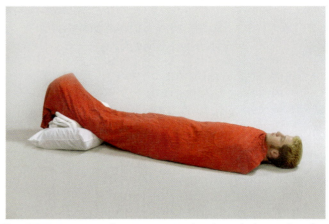

Fig. 11-5 Position the patient in shock with his or her feet slightly elevated and keep the patient warm.

These can include an increased pulse rate and respiratory rate while maintaining a normal blood pressure. A patient in shock may have an altered mental status or a decreased level of consciousness because of the decreased oxygen being delivered to the brain. The patient may be extremely restless and anxious or have trouble focusing. If the patient exhibits signs of an altered mental status such as agitation or being uncooperative and the injury or mechanism of injury suggests internal bleeding, you should always treat the patient for shock. When compensation begins to fail, the body can show changes in the skin condition, weakened pulses and more labored breathing, general weakness, nausea and vomiting, and a tremendous thirst. Ultimately the patient can become unconscious, have a large drop in blood pressure, and experience a further weakened pulse and breathing. Eventually the patient will die. Skill 11-2 illustrates the signs and symptoms of developing shock. Box 11-3 summarizes the signs and symptoms of shock.

Treatment

The general treatment of shock includes positioning the patient; maintaining the patient's airway, breathing, and circulation; keeping the patient warm; treating other injuries if appropriate; and calming and reassuring the patient.

Position the Patient

Generally, a patient in shock should be placed in a supine position. If the patient does not have any spinal or head injuries or fractured lower limbs that have not been splinted, you should elevate the person's feet no more than 12 inches off the ground (Fig. 11-5). This position may allow for some of the blood in the lower extremities to drain back into the circulatory system for use with the vital organs such as the brain, heart, and lungs. If the patient is conscious and is having difficulty breathing and does not have any spinal or head trauma, you may allow him or her to stay in a position of comfort either sitting

or semi-sitting if he or she is in the early stages of shock. Just because a patient is conscious does not mean that he or she cannot be in shock. Conscious patients who are suspected of being in shock or are candidates for shock should not be allowed to stand or wander around. They should be placed in either a sitting or lying position to conserve energy and decrease the workload of the heart.

Maintain Airway, Breathing, and Circulation

A person in shock is a critical, priority patient. Therefore, the initial assessment should be repeated at least every 5 minutes and should include at a minimum an assessment of the patient's pulse rate, respiratory rate, and mental status. Each set of the patient's vital signs should be compared to previous sets. Any change in the patient's vital signs may indicate a progression of shock. You should closely monitor the patient in case of vomiting and ensure that the airway is cleared and maintained in an open position. If available and if you are trained in its use, you should provide the patient with high flow supplemental oxygen through a nonrebreather mask. You should also ensure that any external bleeding is controlled and treat other additional injuries as needed.

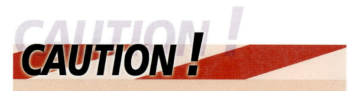

CAUTION!

You should never give a patient in shock anything by mouth. This includes food or drink. Even if the patient is tremendously thirsty, you must not give anything. Giving food or drink may cause the patient to vomit, which may compromise the airway. A patient in shock may need surgery and should therefore not have anything in the stomach.

Skill 11-2

Signs and Symptoms of Developing Shock

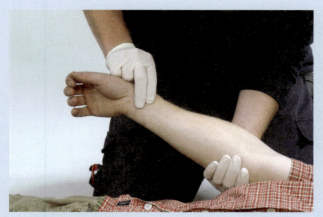

1. An increased pulse rate

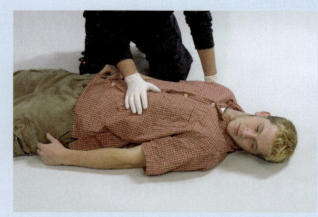

2. An increased respiratory rate

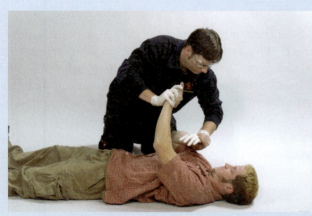

3. Anxiety, restlessness, or combativeness

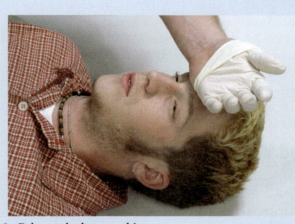

4. Pale, cool, clammy skin

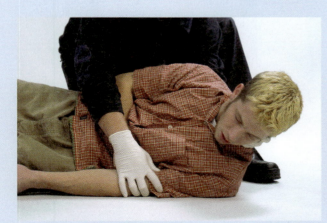

5. Nausea and vomiting

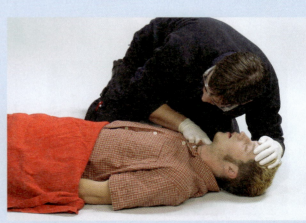

6. Weaker pulses and respirations; eventual loss of consciousness

Keep the Patient Warm

You should keep the patient dry and warm with blankets, jackets, or other pieces of clothing. It is important that something be kept under the patient as well as on top to ensure that body heat is not lost to the ground or the floor.

Provide Care for Specific Injuries

If appropriate or indicated, you should provide care for specific injuries, such as splinting musculoskeletal injuries (see Chapter 12).

Comfort, Calm, and Reassure the Patient

You should always act in a calm and professional manner and comfort, calm, and reassure the patient as indicated while you are waiting for additional EMS personnel.

Soft Tissue Wounds

A soft tissue wound can be defined as any interruption of the skin or underlying tissue (e.g., cuts, scrapes, or swelling). These types of injuries may create some of the most visually dramatic situations that an emergency first responder will encounter. As an emergency first responder, your priority is to control bleeding, prevent further injury, and reduce the chance of contamination or infection until a physician can see the patient.

A soft tissue wound can be classified as either closed or open.

Closed Wounds

A closed wound involves no break in the skin and no associated external bleeding. A **contusion** is a type of closed wound (Fig. 11-6). A contusion is more commonly known as a bruise. It is an injury in which tissue under the skin is damaged and blood vessels are torn. There is generally an area of discoloration because of blood leaking from the vessels into the soft tissue under the skin. Contusions are also associated with swelling and pain. The general management for a closed wound may be nothing at all if the wound is minimal. If the wound is larger, it can be treated with the application of ice and elevation of the body part, if possible, to reduce swelling and pain.

Open Wounds

An open soft tissue wound is one in which the skin has been broken and there is associated bleeding.

Abrasion

An **abrasion,** the most common open wound, is generally a superficial soft tissue injury (Fig. 11-7). An abrasion occurs when the outermost layer of skin is damaged by something scraping against it. For example, if a person falls off a bicycle, the bare skin of a hand or leg may scrape against the sidewalk, causing an abrasion. An abrasion is usually painful even though the injury is superficial and causes little or no oozing of blood.

Laceration

A **laceration** is a break in the skin of varying depth and length (Fig. 11-8). A laceration can occur by itself (e.g., when a finger is lacerated by a kitchen knife while slicing vegetables) or together with other lacerations or types of soft tissue injuries, such as can occur in a motor vehicle collision (MVC). The severity of lacerations can range from a paper cut to life-threatening wounds. Lacerations usually result from a forceful impact with a sharp object.

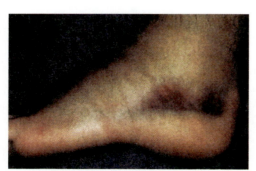

Fig. 11-6 A contusion. (From Stoy W et al and Center for Emergency Medicine: *Mosby's EMT-basic textbook,* revised ed 2, St Louis, 2007, Mosby Lifeline.)

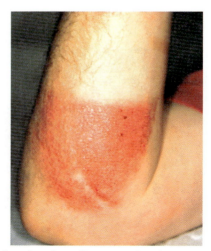

Fig. 11-7 An abrasion. (From McSwain N, Paturas J: *The basic EMT: comprehensive prehospital patient care,* ed 3, St Louis, 2003, Mosby.)

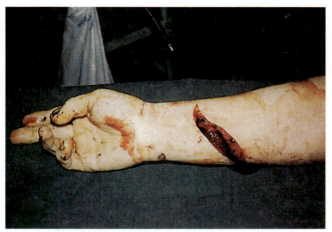

Fig. 11-8 A laceration. (From Stoy W et al and Center for Emergency Medicine: *Mosby's EMT-basic textbook,* revised ed 2, St Louis, 2007, Mosby Lifeline.)

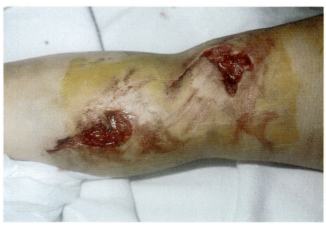

Fig. 11-10 An avulsion.

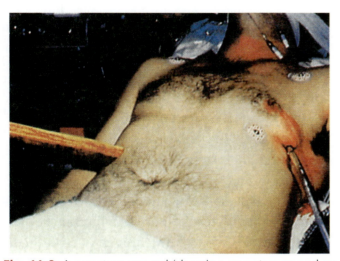

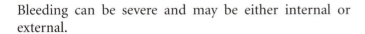

Fig. 11-9 A puncture wound (showing an entrance and an exit wound). (From London PS: *A colour atlas of diagnosis after recent injury,* London, 1990, Wolfe Medical.)

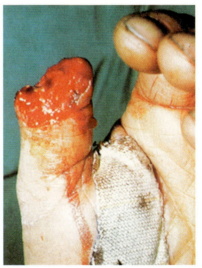

Fig. 11-11 Amputation of the tip of the thumb. (From McSwain N, Paturas J: *The basic EMT: comprehensive prehospital patient care,* ed 3, St Louis, 2003, Mosby.)

Bleeding can be severe and may be either internal or external.

Penetration or Puncture

A **penetration** or **puncture wound** is generally caused by a sharp, pointed object (Fig. 11-9). There may be little or no external bleeding, but internal bleeding may be severe. This bleeding may not be detected until the patient exhibits signs and symptoms of shock. An exit wound may also be present if the object had enough force to go through the body or body part. Gunshot and stab wounds, for example, may involve exit wounds. It is important to remember that both entrance and exit wounds need to have bleeding control. Bleeding control needs to be applied to all "holes" in the body.

Avulsion

An **avulsion** is a type of wound that occurs when a piece of skin or soft tissue is either partially torn loose or pulled completely off (Fig. 11-10). Avulsions can be found anywhere on the body and may be associated with other types of soft tissue wounds.

Amputation

An **amputation** is the separation of a body part from the rest of the body (Fig. 11-11). Amputations may involve a large amount of bleeding.

Management

When providing wound care, it is important to always protect yourself from exposure to body substances. As a

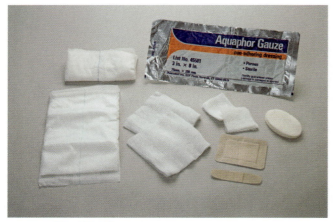

Fig. 11-12 Different types of dressings.

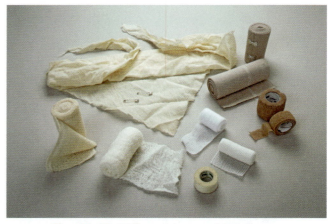

Fig. 11-13 Different types of bandages.

minimum you should always wear gloves when treating wounds. If there is a potential for any blood splatter eye protection, a face mask, and a gown should be worn in addition to the gloves. The steps for treating open soft tissue wounds begin with exposing the wound and controlling bleeding. If the bleeding is mild or stops, you should prevent the wound from further contamination by covering it with a sterile dressing and bandaging it securely in place.

Dressing and Bandaging

A **dressing** is a protective or supporting covering that is placed on an injured body part. A bandage holds a dressing in place. The functions of dressings and bandages are to help stop bleeding, prevent further damage to the wound, and reduce contamination and decrease the risk of infection. Dressings are available in many forms. Common dressings include 4 × 4-inch gauze pads, abdominal pads, and adhesive dressings (Fig. 11-12). Occlusive dressings are a special dressing made of nonporous material. This type of dressing is used for open chest wounds and neck wounds to prevent air from entering the wound and causing further damage. Bandages also are available in many forms, such as self-adherent (adhesive) bandages, gauze rolls, triangular bandages, and adhesive tape (Fig. 11-13). As an emergency first responder, you should be familiar with the types of dressings and bandages used in your system and that may be available to you. You should practice using dressings and bandages to better understand which are best for different types of injuries.

The general principles of dressing and bandaging include the following:

- Expose the injured area.
- Place a sterile dressing over the entire injury.

- Maintain direct pressure to control any bleeding.
- Use a bandage to secure the dressing with some pressure. Assess distal circulation and sensation to ensure the bandage is not too tight.
- If the dressing becomes saturated with blood, add another dressing and secure it in place with another bandage.
- Do not remove the bottom dressing in contact with the wound and remove the top layer only if the dressings get too thick to adequately apply pressure.

Skill 11-3 illustrates different dressing and bandaging techniques for different soft tissue injuries.

Special Considerations

Some kinds of soft tissue injuries require special considerations. Chest injuries, eviscerations, impaled objects, amputations, and foreign bodies in the eye are injuries that require special treatment.

Chest Injuries

A chest injury is any injury to the front, back, or side of the chest between the neck and upper abdomen. Chest injuries require special treatment because they can affect breathing. If the trauma goes deeper than the ribs and the muscles protecting the chest, the chest wall may be punctured. This can change the internal chest pressure, which in the normally sealed chest is needed for people to inhale and exhale effectively. If you hear air escaping from the wound or see bubbles in the blood outside the wound, this is called a **sucking chest wound.** Apply an **occlusive dressing** over the chest wounds. An occlusive dressing may include such things as a piece of Vaseline gauze, cellophane, foil, or flexible plastic. The dressing should be sealed, leaving a small opening such as one corner of the

Skill 11-3

Dressings and Bandages

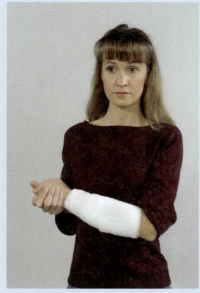

1. A wrist or forearm wound

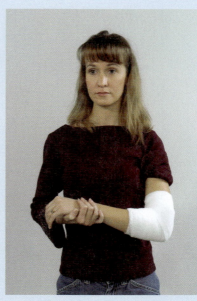

2. An elbow wound

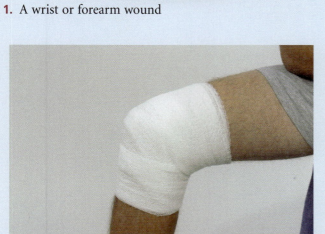

3. A knee wound

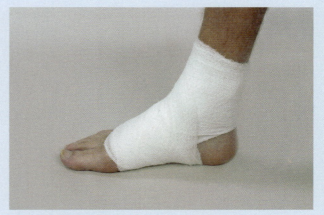

4. An ankle wound

Skill 11-3

Dressings and Bandages—cont'd

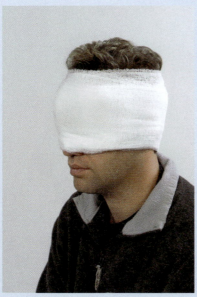

5. An eye injury (note that both eyes are covered for an eye injury to prevent further damage)

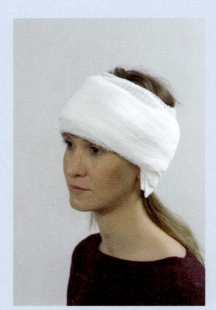

6. A head or ear injury

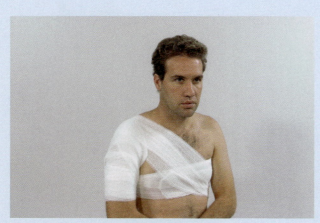

7. A shoulder or upper arm injury

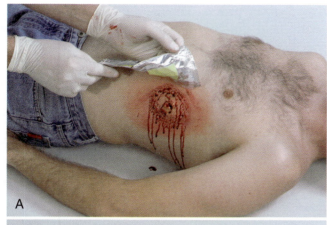

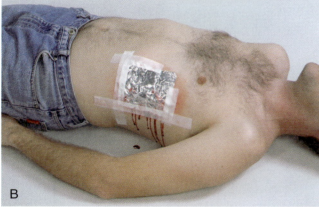

Fig. 11-14 A, Cover an open chest wound with an occlusive dressing. **B,** Tape the dressing, leaving a small opening to vent air.

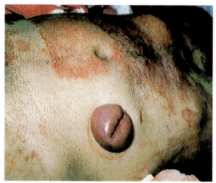

Fig. 11-15 An evisceration. (From McSwain N, Paturas J: *The basic EMT: comprehensive prehospital patient care,* ed 3, St Louis, 2003, Mosby.)

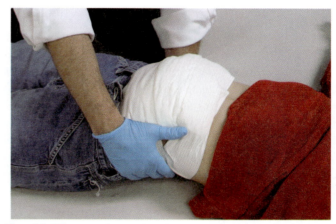

Fig. 11-16 An evisceration is covered with a thick, moist dressing and then covered with a dry, sterile dressing.

dressing left unsealed so that the bandage opens to allow air to escape on exhalation but closes to maintain the chest's pressure during inhalation. This allows the patient to breathe better and thereby maintain the body's oxygen level. You should place the patient on his or her injured side or in a semi-sitting position to allow the patient to breathe easier if you do not suspect a spinal injury. You should assess and treat the patient for any signs of shock (Fig. 11-14).

Eviscerations

An **evisceration** is a deep laceration through the abdominal muscle wall that allows internal organs to protrude from the abdomen (Fig. 11-15). Organs may protrude from an opening in the abdominal wall a small or large amount. The evisceration and the skin around it typically do not bleed. You should not attempt to replace the protruding organs inside the abdomen but should cover the wound with a thick, moist dressing so that the organs do not dry out. Cover the moist dressing with an additional dry, sterile dressing (Fig. 11-16). You should place the

patient in a position of comfort if spinal injury is not suspected and assess and treat the patient for any signs of shock.

Impaled Objects

Objects impaled in a wound present a challenging situation for you and other health care providers. Impaled objects can include such things as pencils, knives, tire irons, and even fence posts. There may be both an entry and exit wound, or just an entry wound. You should never remove an impaled object from a wound unless it is through the patient's cheek with uncontrolled bleeding and might interfere with airway management. You should leave the object in the wound and complete your assessment. You should also expose the wound area as much as possible without disturbing the object. Control bleeding, and manually secure the object to keep it from

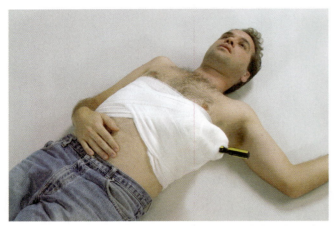

Fig. 11-17 An impaled object should be stabilized in place with bulky dressings.

water or to be placed directly on ice. It is important to reassure and comfort the patient. If the patient is not aware of the loss, it is a good idea to cover the stump with a blanket to protect the patient from psychological trauma. The patient will be better equipped to learn of the amputation later in a more stable environment.

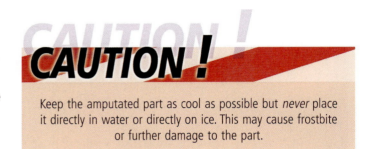

CAUTION!

Keep the amputated part as cool as possible but *never* place it directly in water or directly on ice. This may cause frostbite or further damage to the part.

moving and damaging surrounding structures. For example, a knife that is impaled in the abdomen but is not secured could lacerate internal organs or blood vessels and cause more damage each time it moves. Bulky dressings should be used to stabilize an impaled object, building them up to the top of the object or as far as possible to stabilize the object. If an object is too large to secure, you should keep the patient as still as possible, try to control bleeding, and reassure the patient while waiting for additional help. You should also assess and treat the patient for any signs of shock (Fig. 11-17).

Amputations

In the case of an amputated body part, the body may be able to control bleeding by clotting and contracting blood vessels. If the amputation site is bleeding, you should control the bleeding using direct pressure, pressure dressing, elevation, and pressure points as needed. Once the bleeding is controlled, apply dressings and bandages to help prevent further contamination.

As an emergency first responder, a priority is to care for the patient. This means that you should not abandon the patient or compromise patient care to attempt to find a severed part. If the amputated part can be located without compromising patient care, it should be preserved and sent with the patient to the hospital. The amputated part should be rinsed if necessary but not allowed to be saturated with water. Once cleaned of contaminates, the amputated part should be placed in a sealed plastic bag by itself. A second bag or container should then be filled with water and a few cubes of ice. The bag with the amputated part should be placed into the second bag or container holding the water and ice. Never allow the amputated body part to be submersed in

Nosebleeds

Nosebleeds are typically a result of trauma, an underlying medical condition such as high blood pressure, or just dryness of the air. Most nosebleeds can be easily controlled with simple techniques. If the patient is conscious and there are no indications of spinal injury, you can begin by having the patient sit upright and lean slightly forward. This position will help prevent blood from running into the back of the throat, potentially compromising the airway, plus it will decrease the amount of blood the patient swallows, helping to prevent vomiting. You should then pinch the nostrils together with a gloved hand. The patient may be able to pinch his or her own nostrils to stop the bleeding (Fig. 11-18). You should not allow the patient to sniffle or blow the nose, as this can lead to increased bleeding. You should not pack the nose with dressings or other such objects.

Ear Wounds

If there is a soft tissue wound to the external ear, you should apply dressings over the ear and not in the ear. You should then bandage the dressings in place as shown in Skill 11-3. Any bleeding from the ear should be considered a sign of head injury. Any fluid draining from the ear may be cerebrospinal fluid (see Chapter 12). Again, you should place a dressing over the ear (and not in the ear) and bandage the dressing in place.

Eye Wounds

An important consideration about eye wounds is that you will need to cover both of the patient's eyes even if only one eye is injured. This is because the eyes eye open with your fingers placed above and below the eyelids. Flush the eye for a minimum of 15 minutes with sterile water if possible. Never use any instruments to remove foreign objects from the patient's eye. If the object cannot be flushed out with water, bandage both eyes as described earlier.

Burns

Burns are classified according to the depth of the burn in skin and other tissue. The burn categories of first-, second-, and third-degree have generally been replaced by categories called superficial, partial-thickness, and full-thickness burns. They can also be classified by cause: thermal (caused by heat), chemical, and electrical.

Depth of the Burn

Sunburn is a typical **superficial burn.** It usually involves only the outer layer of skin. Superficial burns cause pain, reddening of the skin, and swelling. A **partial-thickness burn** involves the outer and middle layers of the skin. These burns cause deep, intense pain because the nerve endings are involved. The skin is reddened and usually has blisters. **Full-thickness burns** involve areas of charred or blackened skin, areas of redness, and blisters (Fig. 11-19). Full-thickness burns are pain free because the nerve endings in the layers of skin have been destroyed. However, full-thickness burns are generally associated with partial-thickness or superficial burns. In such cases, the patient will feel considerable pain.

Extent of the Burn

Burns are assessed by how much body surface area they cover. The **rule of nines** is an assessment tool that allows a quick calculation of the extent of a burn (Fig. 11-20). With the rule of nines, the body is divided up into segments that account for approximately 9% of the total body surface area. By combining the regions that are burned, an estimate of the extent of the burn can be reached. For example, if a person has burns to the right arm and the leg, 27% of his or her body surface area is burned.

Critical Burns

Burns are determined to be critical or noncritical depending on the type, extent, location, and depth of burn. Critical burns require immediate transport to a burn center and include the following:

- Any burns involving the respiratory system
- Partial-thickness burns over greater than 10% of the body
- Full-thickness burns

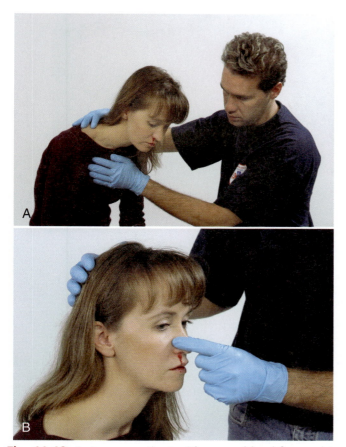

Fig. 11-18 A, Lean a patient with a nosebleed forward to prevent blood from draining into the airway. **B,** Pinch the nostrils together to stop the bleeding.

automatically move together. If one eye moves, it can automatically cause the other to move, which can further injure the wounded eye. By bandaging both eyes, you can prevent further injury. It is important to explain what is going on to the patient after you have bandaged his or her eyes because he or she will no longer be able to see.

FOREIGN BODY IN THE EYE

As an emergency first responder, you may be called upon to assist a patient with foreign matter in his or her eye. The causes of the foreign matter may be dirt, dust, chemicals, metal or wood shavings. The patient may complain of pain, increased tearing, blurred vision, or even loss of vision. Before treatment, ensure the environment is safe and you are utilizing appropriate personal protection equipment. If there are no indications of spinal injury, place the patient in a supine position with the head slightly lower if possible. Turn the patient's head toward the affected side so foreign matter cannot flow into the unaffected eye. Using your gloved hand, hold the affected

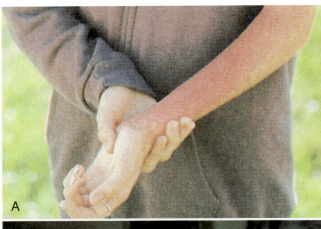

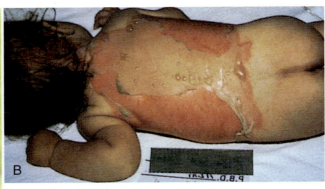

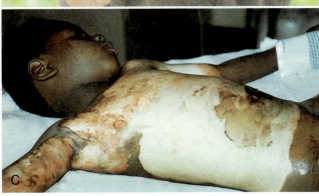

Fig. 11-19 A, Superficial burn. **B,** Partial-thickness burn. **C,** Full-thickness burn. (From McSwain N, Paturas J: *The basic EMT: comprehensive prehospital patient care,* ed 3, St Louis, 2003, Mosby.)

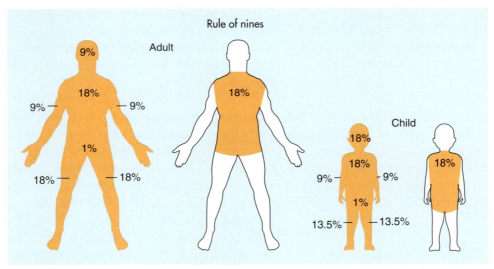

Fig. 11-20 The rule of nines. (From NAEMT: *PHTLS: Basic and advanced prehospital trauma life support,* ed 6, St Louis, 2007, Mosby.)

- Burns that involve the face, hands, feet, genitalia, or major joints
- Electrical burns
- Chemical burns

Thermal Burns

The initial treatment for burn patients is to *stop the burning process* by flushing the area with water or saline and to remove smoldering clothing and jewelry. It is important to note that some clothing may have melted to the skin. If you feel resistance when removing the clothing, you should leave it in place. Burn patients may have a compromised airway as a result of swelling of the airway caused by the heat. This can be a major complication. An inhalation injury may occur from breathing in hot, burning air or smoke at the scene, which can cause

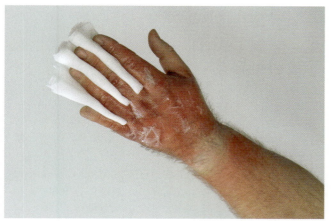

Fig. 11-21 With a burn to the hand or foot, separate the fingers and toes with dry dressings.

of water for at least 20 minutes. You should direct the flow of the water to the outer corner of the eye and cover both eyes with a dressing and bandage.

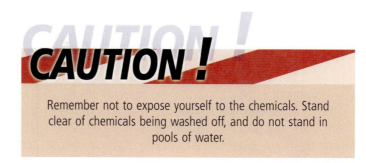

CAUTION !

Remember not to expose yourself to the chemicals. Stand clear of chemicals being washed off, and do not stand in pools of water.

so much swelling that the airway is closed off. You should continually monitor a burn patient's airway to ensure it remains open. Hoarseness, shortness of breath, or any trouble breathing may indicate a life-threatening injury.

To prevent further contamination of the burn wound, you should cover the burned area with a dry, sterile dressing. Do not put any type of ointment, lotion, antiseptic, or wet dressings on the burn. Do not break any blisters that form because this could cause contamination and later infection. If a hand or foot is burned, you should separate the fingers or toes with dressings (Fig. 11-21). You should ensure that the patient receives prompt transport to the hospital.

Chemical Burns

Chemical burns are a special situation. The chemical may be apparent, but some poisonous gases are colorless and odorless. You should consider all possible dangers when you arrive on a scene and ensure the safety of the scene before entering. It is also important to wear gloves and eye protection or other special clothing based on the chemical involved. You should immediately brush any dry powder from the patient to prevent further burns and then flush the area with large amounts of water for at least 10 minutes. You should then cover the burned area with a dry, sterile dressing.

Sometimes a burn is caused by a chemical that splashed on the patient. Splash injuries often involve the eyes. In such cases, flush the patient's eyes with copious amounts

Electrical Burns

Electrical burns are another dangerous situation. Again, it is important to ensure scene safety before approaching the patient. The electrical source should be turned off if possible before you enter the scene. You should never run to a patient, even one who is screaming for help. You should always assess the scene and ensure that it is safe to enter. You must not put yourself at risk for electrocution or electrical injury and become a patient yourself. When electricity enters the body, it travels the path of least resistance, usually through nerves and blood vessels. The patient's internal injuries are often much worse than the external injuries. With an electrical burn, you should anticipate an irregular heartbeat and monitor the patient closely for respiratory or cardiac arrest. If an AED is available, you should keep it close to the patient. You should check for an exit wound and an entry wound and ensure both are covered with dry, sterile dressings.

Infants and Children

The care of infants and children involves special considerations. They must be treated as pediatric patients, not as small adults. Pediatric patients have a greater surface area compared to their total body volume. This means that burns and other soft tissue injuries often result in greater fluid and heat loss. You should keep the environment warm when possible. Consider the possibility of child abuse when you are called to the scene of an injured child. If you find any evidence of possible abuse, give it to the responding EMS crew and privately share your suspicions. Do not be confrontational with any patient, family member, or bystander on the scene.

Team Work

USE OF PASG FOR PATIENTS

In your role as an emergency first responder, you may be asked to assist other health care providers with the PASG. The pneumatic antishock garment (PASG), also called military (or medical) antishock trousers (MAST), has been used for years in prehospital care. Your EMS system may use the PASG, and if so, you should be familiar with these devices. The trousers enclose the lower part of the body from the abdomen to the extremities. They have a pump to pump air into the trousers through a tube. The PASG can be used for suspected pelvic fractures and intraabdominal bleeding. As an emergency first responder, you may be asked to do the following:

- Retrieve the PASG.
- Assist in the application of the PASG under direct supervision.
- Prepare the patient, including removing the patient's clothing or lifting and moving the patient to a desired position.

The PASG should not be placed over clothes or shoes; remove the patient's lower clothing as needed. The abdomen and lower extremities should be assessed for wounds because these areas will not be accessible after the PASG is applied. The PASG has three separate regions that can be inflated or deflated: the abdomen, left leg, and right leg. One or both of the leg segments may be inflated without inflating the abdomen segment. The abdominal segment is not inflated without inflating both leg segments. Each segment also has its own stopcock that is opened to inflate or deflate that segment and closed to maintain pressure. The segments are secured with Velcro straps and the tubes for each segment are connected to the pump.

The PASG is usually applied in conjunction with a long backboard. The PASG is placed on the long backboard with the individual sections opened and the patient is then log rolled onto the board and into the PASG. This maneuver is usually performed at the time when the patient is placed on the long backboard for transport. The PASG is positioned on the long backboard in relation to the patient's ribcage. The top of the abdominal section of the PASG is placed just below the bottom rib. The PASG must not be placed over the rib cage because the pressure could hinder the patient's breathing. The PASG is inflated following medical direction.

The PASG can also be applied without using a long backboard. Grasp the PASG at the abdominal section, lift the patient's feet and calves, and maneuver the PASG up the body until the abdominal section is just below the rib cage. The PASG should not be applied if there is suspected injury to the neck. A patient whose condition is serious enough to require a PASG is usually placed on a long backboard, however, and it is easier to accomplish both at the same time.

In the Real World—Conclusion

You continue to monitor the bleeding under the gauze. When the gauze soaks through with blood, you reinforce it with additional dressings, continue to apply direct pressure, and elevate. The bleeding slows, and your patient is alert and breathing comfortably. You continually reassess and reassure the patient. When the EMS providers arrive, you have your hand-off report ready. You help them prepare your patient for transport. You are confident that you took the correct steps to quickly and effectively control the patient's bleeding and prevent possible shock.

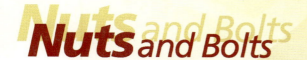

Nuts and Bolts

Critical Points

As a first responder, you will often treat bleeding and soft tissue injuries. Such injuries are not usually life threatening, but you must be prepared with the knowledge and equipment to quickly identify and effectively treat any problems. As a first responder, you must be able to identify and control bleeding. You should also be able to identify and treat a patient in shock. You must also be able to identify and care for other soft tissue injuries. Your role is essential for the patient's well-being.

Learning Checklist

❑ The circulatory system is composed of the "three Ps": the pump (the heart), the pipes (the blood vessels), and the plasma (the blood).

❑ There are three types of blood vessels: arteries, veins, and capillaries. Arteries carry blood away from the heart, veins carry blood toward the heart, and capillaries are the sites of gas exchange.

❑ Blood consists of red blood cells, white blood cells, platelets (which cause clotting), and plasma (the fluid).

❑ The types of external bleeding include arterial, venous, and capillary. Arterial bleeding is severe, has spurting blood from the wound with each heartbeat, and is bright red. Venous bleeding is darker red, flows steadily, and can be heavy. Capillary bleeding is oozing bleeding that is a darker red color. It is typically insignificant.

❑ Always wear the appropriate personal protection equipment (PPE) if a patient is bleeding (gloves for sure and eye protection, mask, and gown if there is risk of spatter).

❑ Bleeding control, in order of preference, is direct pressure (with or without pressure dressings), elevation, pressure points, and tourniquets (as a last resort).

❑ The brachial artery is used for a pressure point in upper extremity injury and the femoral artery is used for lower extremity injury.

❑ Signs and symptoms of internal bleeding include signs and symptoms of shock, bleeding from any orifice, blood-tinged vomit or feces, "coffee ground" vomit, dark tarry stool, abdominal distention, and abdominal rigidity or tenderness.

❑ Shock or hypoperfusion results from a decreased volume of circulating blood.

❑ Shock can result from a failure of the heart's pumping ability, from abnormal dilation of the vessels, or from excessive fluid loss.

❑ Signs and symptoms of shock include restlessness and anxiety, altered mental status, pale cool skin, increased respiratory rate, increased pulse rate, nausea and vomiting, and thirst.

❑ The treatment of shock includes positioning the patient; maintaining airway, breathing, and circulation; keeping the patient warm; providing care for specific injuries; and comforting, calming, and reassuring the patient.

❑ You should never give anything by mouth to a patient suspected of being in shock.

❑ A soft tissue wound is any interruption of the skin or underlying tissue.

❑ A closed soft tissue wound is a contusion.

❑ Open soft tissue wounds include abrasions, lacerations, penetrations or punctures, avulsions, and amputations.

❑ Soft tissue wounds are generally managed through the use of dressings and bandages.

❑ The general principles of dressings and bandages include exposing the injured area, placing a sterile dressing over the injury, maintaining direct pressure, securing the dressing with a bandage, and adding another dressing if the first becomes saturated with blood.

❑ Chest injuries should be managed with an occlusive dressing taped down with a small opening available to vent air.

❑ Eviscerations are managed by placing a thick, moist dressing over the abdominal organs and covering that dressing with a dry, sterile dressing.

❑ Impaled objects should be stabilized in place with bulky dressings.

❑ Your priority with an amputation is the patient. You should never abandon or compromise patient care to look for the body part.

Nuts and Bolts–continued

- ❑ Nosebleeds are controlled by having the patient sit forward and pinching the nostrils together. Do not pack dressings into the nose.
- ❑ Do not pack dressings into the ear. Loosely cover the ear with a dressing and hold it in place with a bandage.
- ❑ Cover both eyes with dressings and bandages if there is an eye injury to prevent further injury to the injured eye.
- ❑ The depth of the burn is classified as superficial, partial thickness, and full thickness.
- ❑ The rule of nines is a tool used to determine the extent of a burn.
- ❑ Burns can be critical. It is important to ensure the patient is transported promptly to a burn center.
- ❑ Treatment of burns includes stopping the burning, removing smoldering clothing and jewelry, continually monitoring the airway and breathing, and covering the burned area with a dry, sterile dressing. Do not put ointment, lotion, antiseptic, or wet dressings over a burn. Do not break any blisters. Separate fingers and toes with dry, sterile dressings.
- ❑ Treatment of chemical burns includes brushing any dry powder from the patient, flushing the area with copious amounts of water, and covering the burned area with a dry, sterile dressing.
- ❑ Always ensure the electric source is turned off before approaching a patient with an electrical injury.
- ❑ Infants and children have a greater surface area compared to their total blood volume. This translates into greater fluid and heat loss in pediatric burn patients.

Key Terms

Abrasion Injury from a scraping force involving the outermost layer of skin.

Amputation An extremity or other body part that is completely severed from the body.

Arterial bleeding Blood loss from the arteries.

Arteries Blood vessels that carry blood away from the heart.

Avulsion A type of wound that occurs when a piece of skin or soft tissue is either partially torn loose or pulled completely off.

Bandage An object that holds a dressing in place.

Capillaries Microscopic blood vessels that connect arteries to veins.

Capillary bleeding Blood loss from the capillaries.

Chemical burns Burns produced by chemical substances.

Compensation The body's response to try and stop shock from developing.

Contusion A bruise. A type of closed wound.

Dressing A protective or supporting covering that is placed over an injured site.

Electrical burns Burns produced by electricity.

Evisceration A laceration through the abdominal muscle wall that allows organs to protrude from the abdomen.

Full-thickness burn A burn involving all layers of the skin.

Hemoglobin A molecule that carries oxygen in the blood.

Hemorrhage The loss of blood, or bleeding.

Hypoperfusion Also called **shock**. A condition caused by decreased circulation of the blood.

Internal bleeding Blood loss inside the body.

Laceration A break in the skin of varying depth and damage.

Occlusive dressing A dressing that is airtight and nonporous.

Partial-thickness burn A burn involving the outer and middle layers of the skin.

Penetration/puncture wound A wound caused by a sharp, pointed object, with varying degrees of blood loss.

Pressure dressing A special dressing that places pressures over a wound site.

Rule of nines An assessment tool that allows a quick calculation of the extent of a burn.

Shock Also called **hypoperfusion.** A condition caused by decreased circulation of the blood.

Sucking chest wound A penetrating/puncture chest wound that is deep enough to penetrate the lungs, allowing air to escape the body through the wound.

Superficial burn A burn that involves only the outer layer of skin.

Veins Blood vessels that carry blood toward the heart.

Venous bleeding Blood loss from the veins.

First Responder NSC Objectives

COGNITIVE OBJECTIVES

- Differentiate between arterial, venous, and capillary bleeding.
- State the steps in emergency medical care for external bleeding.
- Establish the relationship between body substance isolation (BSI) and bleeding.
- List the signs of internal bleeding.
- List the steps in the emergency medical care of the patient with signs and symptoms of internal bleeding.
- Establish the relationship between BSI and soft tissue injuries.
- State the types of open soft tissue injuries.
- Describe the emergency medical care considerations for a patient with an open wound to the abdomen.
- Describe the emergency medical care for an impaled object.
- State the emergency medical care for an amputation.
- Describe the emergency medical care for burns.
- List the functions of dressing and bandaging.

AFFECTIVE OBJECTIVES

- Explain the rationale for BSI when dealing with bleeding and soft tissue injuries.

- Attend to the feelings of the patient with a soft tissue injury or bleeding.
- Demonstrate a caring attitude toward patients with a soft tissue injury or bleeding who request emergency medical services (EMS).
- Place the interests of the patient with a soft tissue injury or bleeding as the foremost consideration when making any and all patient care decisions.
- Communicate by showing empathy with patients who have a soft tissue injury or bleeding, as well as with family members and friends of the patient.

PSYCHOMOTOR OBJECTIVES

- Demonstrate direct pressure as a method of emergency medical care for external bleeding.
- Demonstrate the use of diffuse pressure as a method of emergency medical care for external bleeding.
- Demonstrate the use of pressure points as a method of emergency medical care for external bleeding.
- Demonstrate the care of the patient exhibiting signs and symptoms of internal bleeding.
- Demonstrate the steps in the emergency medical care of a patient with an open chest wound.
- Demonstrate the steps in the emergency medical care of a patient with open abdominal wounds.
- Demonstrate the steps in the emergency medical care of a patient with an impaled object.
- Demonstrate the steps in the emergency medical care of a patient with an amputation.
- Demonstrate the steps in the emergency medical care of an amputated part.

Check your understanding

Check your understanding

Please refer to p. 439 for the answers to these questions.

1. The medical term for bleeding is _____.

2. Uncontrolled bleeding may lead to a condition where there is not enough blood to carry oxygen to the tissues. This condition is known as _____.

3. You are caring for a victim who was ejected from a vehicle in a rollover incident who has multiple fractures. Which of the following fracture sites is most likely to lead to life-threatening bleeding?
   A. Radius
   B. Fibula
   C. Femur
   D. Humerus

4. Dark red, steady bleeding that may be heavy but is usually controllable is most likely from which of the following?
   A. Vein
   B. Artery
   C. Capillary
   D. Aorta

5. List, in order of use, the four methods an emergency first responder may use to control bleeding.
   A. _____
   B. _____
   C. _____
   D. _____

6. When a dressing over a bleeding wound becomes saturated with blood, the First Responder should _____.

7. List six signs or symptoms of shock.
   A. _____
   B. _____
   C. _____
   D. _____
   E. _____
   F. _____

8. An early indication of shock is an alteration in the patient's _____.

9. Which of the following would be considered appropriate initial burn care?
   A. Apply burn cream
   B. Break any blisters
   C. Cover with dry, sterile dressings
   D. Apply wet dressings

10. The most immediate concern for a patient who was pulled from a house fire that has soot in the nostrils and around the mouth is:
    A. Determining the percentage of body surface burned
    B. Applying burn cream
    C. Managing the airway
    D. Removing burned clothing.

11. Match the terms in the left column with the correct definitions in the right column.

_____ Abrasion

A. A cut caused by a sharp object such as a knife, piece of glass, or jagged metal

_____ Amputation

B. An open injury caused by a pointed object such as a nail

_____ Avulsion

C. An injury to the abdominal wall that allows the intestines to protrude through the opening

_____ Contusion

D. A body part such as (bruise) a finger, hand, or leg is completely severed from the body

_____ Evisceration

E. The surface of the skin is scraped away

_____ Laceration

F. The skin or an organ such as the ear is completely torn away from the body or may be left hanging from a flap

_____ Puncture

G. A discoloration of wound to the skin as a result of blood collecting under the skin when the skin is not broken but small blood vessels beneath it are crushed

12. While en route to a call for a construction worker who touched a high-voltage power line and is now unconscious, your primary concern should be:
    A. The patient remains electrified and is a danger to you even after the source of electricity is removed.
    B. The patient's heart may have stopped.
    C. There may be an exit wound where the electricity left the body, and it may be worse than the entry wound.
    D. The patient's injuries are often worse than they appear to be.

13. Appropriate care for a patient with a screwdriver sticking out of his chest would include which of the following?
    A. Removing the screwdriver and covering the wound
    B. Performing chest compressions
    C. Removing the screwdriver and applying oxygen
    D. Stabilizing the screwdriver in place

14. Your patient is a 36-year-old female who was thrown from and then stepped on by a horse. She responds to verbal stimuli, is pale and sweaty, and has a respiratory rate of 26 per minute. She is complaining of pain in her abdomen. There is an abrasion on her forehead, and her right forearm is deformed. She has a large bruise over the left upper quadrant of her abdomen. Her abdomen is very tender when it is palpated. Which of the following is the most beneficial treatment that a First Responder could provide before the arrival of the ambulance?
    A. Dressing and bandaging the wound on her forehead
    B. Manually stabilizing her forearm
    C. Giving her oxygen
    D. Making sure she has enough water to drink

Chapter 12

Musculoskeletal Injuries

LESSON GOAL

As an emergency first responder, you will encounter patients that have sustained an injury to either bone or muscle or both. Although these injuries may be painful and visually dramatic, rarely are they life threatening. Your ability to rapidly identify and effectively treat musculoskeletal injuries will reduce the patient's pain, prevent further injury, and minimize the risk of permanent injury.

OBJECTIVES

1. Describe the anatomy and function of the musculoskeletal system.
2. Demonstrate the assessment and management of a patient with a suspected musculoskeletal injury.
3. Differentiate between an open and closed musculoskeletal injury.
4. Perform manual stabilization of a suspected injury to the upper extremity, lower extremity, and spine.
5. Identify concerning mechanisms of injury for potential spinal injury.
6. Describe the signs and symptoms of a patient with a suspected spinal injury.
7. Demonstrate the assessment and management of a patient with a suspected head injury.
8. Describe the signs and symptoms of a patient with a suspected head injury.
9. Assess and treat a patient with a suspected spinal injury.

In the Real World

You are teaching a class of third-graders just before your scheduled recess. An overhead page summons you to the playground. As you exit the side door of the school, you see a crowd of teachers and students gathered around the jungle gym and you hear the crying of a child. As a trained emergency first responder for the school system, you start assessing the situation. You know that the school nurse is not scheduled to be at your school until the next morning. The vice principal sees you arriving and asks the others to step back so you can reach the patient. As the crowd parts, you see Heather, a student you had last year, sitting on the ground holding her left arm and crying. Ms. Tubbs is trying to calm Heather and asking her where she hurts. Ms. Tubbs tells you that Heather was playing on the jungle gym with the other students when she missed a bar and fell to the ground—a fall of about 5 feet. After falling, Heather immediately grabbed her left arm and started to cry. You ask the vice principal to make sure someone is contacting 9-1-1 and Heather's parents and also to pull her records and check for any medical history. You kneel down to Heather's level and make a quick scan of her. You notice that Heather's left arm is crooked just above the wrist area and that she has some abrasions to both her hands and her forehead but is not bleeding.

The musculoskeletal system involves all of the bones, muscles, and connective tissue of the human body. The musculoskeletal system gives the body shape, protects vital organs, and provides movement. Injuries to the musculoskeletal system can alter the normal structure and function of the body.

Musculoskeletal System

The adult body has more than 600 individual muscles (the muscular system) and 206 skeletal bones (the skeletal system). As you assess a patient suspected of having a musculoskeletal injury, you must rely on your knowledge of normal structure and function (Box 12-1). The musculoskeletal system also involves the body's intricate network of nerves and blood vessels. All bones are living tissue, and each bone has a blood and nerve supply.

When two or more bones of the skeletal system come together, their union creates a **joint.** The skeletal system joints allow the body to have movement. Movement is controlled by the coordinated efforts of the nervous system and muscles. Joints are held in place and stabilized by **ligaments.** Ligaments are tough fibrous bands of tissue placed at strategic angles that allow for twisting, flexion, extension, or rotation of that joint. Ligaments attach bone to bone. Muscles that control the movement of the skeletal system are attached to the bones by **tendons.** Tendons, too, are tough fibrous bands of tissue.

Skeletal System

The skeleton can be divided into two main sections: the **axial skeleton,** or the central part of the body, and the **appendicular skeleton,** or the extremities of the body (Fig. 12-1).

Axial Skeleton

The central part of the skeleton carries most of the weight of the body and comprises the bones that make up the skull, spinal column, and thorax. The skull comprises the cranium, which houses and protects the brain, and the facial bones. Facial bones include all the bones of the face including the mandible (jawbone), which is located to do airway maneuvers such as the jaw thrust.

The spinal column is made up of 33 individual bones. Each individual bone of the spinal column is called a vertebra. Between each vertebra is a fibrous disk that

---

BOX 12-1   Functions of the Musculoskeletal System

Skeletal System
- Support the body
- Protect vital organs (such as the brain, heart, and lungs)
- Assist with movement
- Make red blood cells

Muscular System
- Give the body shape
- Protect internal organs
- Assist with movement

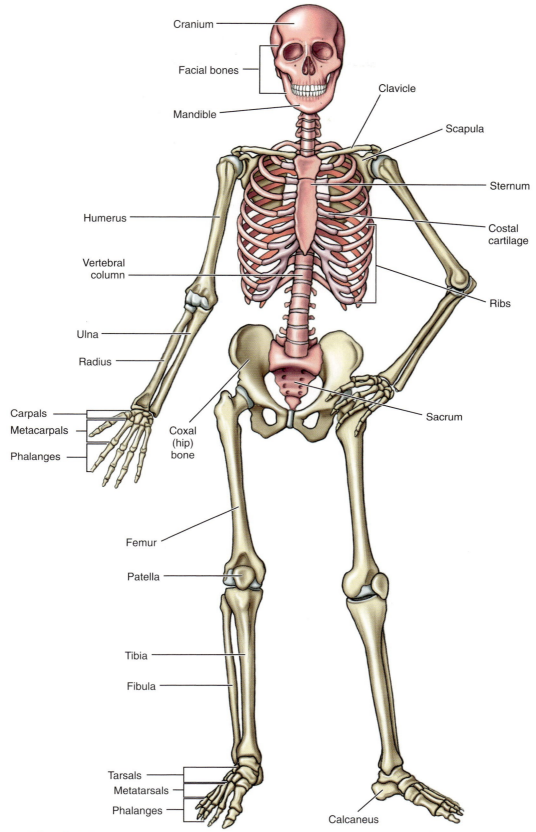

Fig. 12-1 The skeletal system. (From Herlihy B, Maebius N: *The human body in health and illness,* ed 2, Philadelphia, 2003, Saunders.)

allows for twisting and bending and also provides a cushion between the individual bones. The spinal column runs from the base of the skull to the bottom of the pelvis and houses and protects the spinal cord. The spinal cord is responsible for delivering and receiving messages to and from the central nervous system (CNS). The nerves of the spinal cord exit the spinal column between each vertebra and continue to each muscle and organ. In cases of injury to the spinal column, the patient may describe feelings such as "pins and needles," a sharp pain with movement, or a total lack of sensation or ability to move the extremities. A spinal injury may also cause paralysis of muscles.

The spinal column can be divided into five specific areas. The cervical area comprises the first seven vertebrae and is associated with the patient's neck. The next 12 vertebrae make up the back (posterior) of the chest and are referred to as the thoracic vertebrae. The lumbar portion of the spinal column is the patient's lower back and contains the next five individual vertebrae. The lumbar portion of the spinal column carries the most weight and has the largest-sized vertebrae. The sacral portion of the spinal column makes up the posterior portion of the pelvis and comprises five fused vertebrae called the sacrum. The final portion of the spinal column is identified as the coccyx (the tailbone) and comprises four fused vertebrae (Fig. 12-2).

The thorax (chest) comprises the clavicles (collarbones), the scapulas (shoulder blades), 12 pair of ribs, and the sternum (breastbone) (Fig. 12-3). The sternum can be further divided into three sections. The top is the manubrium, the center portion is the body, and the lower portion is the xiphoid. As described earlier, the thoracic portion of the spinal column makes up the posterior portion of the thorax. The main functions of the thorax are to add shape and form to the body while protecting the internal chest organs and to aid in the process of breathing (see Chapter 7).

Appendicular Skeleton

The appendicular skeleton comprises the pelvis and the upper and lower extremities. The pelvis is made up of two larger bones, which combine with the sacrum and coccyx to form the pelvic girdle. The bones of the lower extremities articulate (move) with the pelvis to form the hip joints. The pelvis protects the lower internal organs of the digestive and urinary systems and the internal female reproductive organs. The pelvis is a highly vascular (blood vessel–filled) area. Any injury to the pelvis can cause a significant loss of blood. Because the pelvis also forms an internal area where bleeding can be contained, bleeding from the pelvis may not be readily detectable.

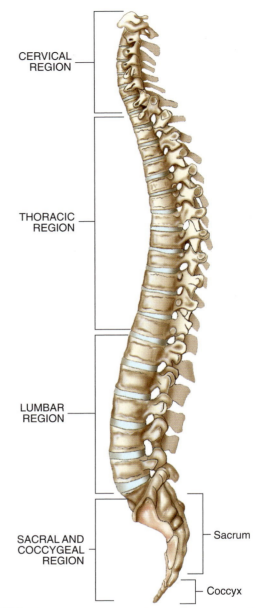

Fig. 12-2 The spinal column. (From McSwain N, Paturas J: *The basic EMT: comprehensive prehospital patient care*, ed 3, St. Louis, 2003, Mosby.)

The bones of the upper extremities (arms) include the humerus (upper arm), the radius (lateral side of the lower arm), the ulna (medial side of the lower arm), the carpals (wrist), and the metacarpals and phalanges (bones of the hand). The lower arm, consisting of the radius and ulna, is also called the forearm. The bones of the upper extremities articulate with the bones of the thorax at the shoulder joint, and the bones of the upper arm and forearm connect at the elbow joint. The bones of the forearm connect with the carpals to form the wrist joint.

The lower extremities (legs) consist of the femurs (thighs), the patellae (knee caps), the tibias (medial part

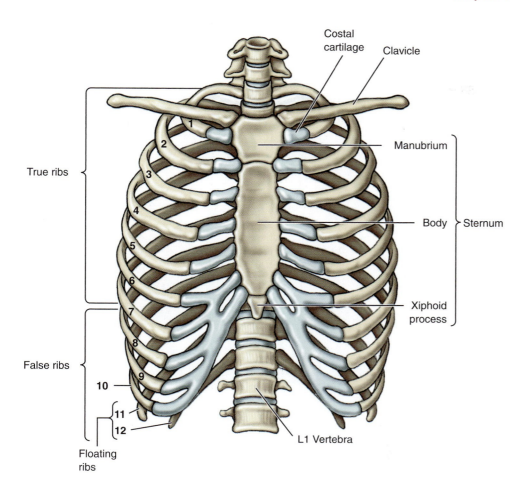

Costal cartilage
Clavicle
True ribs
1
2
3
4
5
6
7
Manubrium
Body
Xiphoid process
Sternum
False ribs
8
9
10
11
12
Floating ribs
L1 Vertebra

Fig. 12-3 The thorax. (From Herlihy B, Maebius N: *The human body in health and illness,* ed 2, Philadelphia, 2003, Saunders.)

of the lower leg), the fibulas (lateral part of the lower leg), the tarsals (ankles), and the metatarsals and phalanges of the feet. The femur articulates with the pelvis to form the hip joint. The lower portion of the femur articulates with the tibia and patella to form the knee joint. The bones of the lower leg (tibia and fibula) connect with the tarsals to form the ankle joint. The femur is a large bone that can cause significant bleeding if fractured (broken). Bleeding from an injured femur may be internal.

Muscular System

The muscular system is responsible for movement of the body and comprises three different types of muscles: skeletal, smooth, and cardiac. All muscles work by contracting and relaxing. This coordinated effort allows for such muscle activity as skeletal movement, movement of food through the digestive system, a beating heart, and many other tasks (Fig. 12-4).

Skeletal Muscle

Skeletal muscle is generally described as muscle that is connected to bone. Because it takes an active thought process to make these muscles contract and relax and

therefore move or stop moving, it is also called **voluntary muscle.** An example would be picking up a pencil to make a note during this section. At your will, you can pick up the pencil, make notes, and then put the pencil down through coordinated activities between your brain, nervous system, and selected muscles. Skeletal muscles also got you to class today, whether you drove a vehicle or walked. Any action of your body that you can start or stop uses skeletal muscle. Skeletal muscle also gives the body form and stabilizes joints. In addition, skeletal muscles generate heat and help maintain body temperature.

Smooth Muscle

The greatest difference between skeletal and **smooth muscle** is the ability to start or stop an action. Although the use of skeletal muscle generally requires a thought process, smooth muscle, or **involuntary muscle,** contracts or relaxes automatically. Involuntary muscles are found in areas such as the circulatory, digestive, urinary, and respiratory systems. For example, the walls of each blood vessel are made up of involuntary muscles. Your blood vessels will contract (become smaller) or dilate

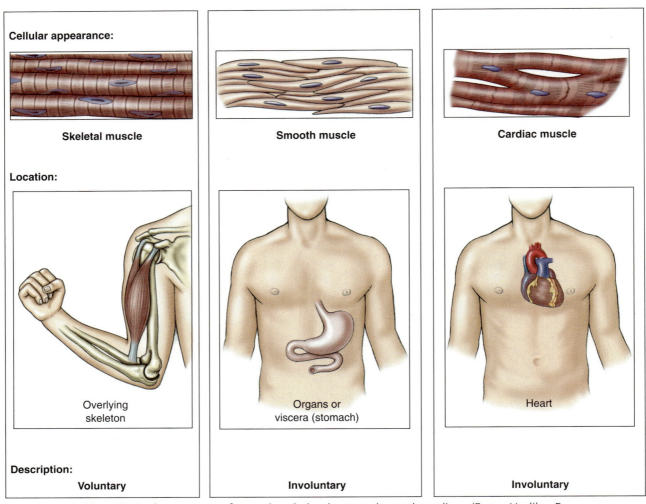

Cellular appearance:

Skeletal muscle

Smooth muscle

Cardiac muscle

Location:

Overlying skeleton

Organs or viscera (stomach)

Heart

Description:

Voluntary

Involuntary

Involuntary

Fig. 12-4 Three types of muscle: skeletal, smooth, and cardiac. (From Herlihy B, Maebius N: *The human body in health and illness*, ed 2, Philadelphia, 2003, Saunders.)

(become larger) without an active thought process. Although you may be able to initially interrupt the process of breathing, this is short lived. After a brief time period, the involuntary muscles of the respiratory system will take over and resume breathing.

Cardiac Muscle

A third type of muscle is **cardiac muscle.** Our hearts are composed of cardiac muscle. Cardiac muscle has the unique ability to generate its own electrical impulse independent of the nervous system and therefore cause its own contraction and relaxation. Cardiac muscle is not under voluntary control (e.g., you cannot consciously increase your heart rate) and is, therefore, a second type of involuntary muscle. Cardiac muscle is sensitive to any decrease in the oxygen or blood supply. Cardiac muscle can only tolerate an interruption of an adequate oxygen or blood supply for a short time period before suffering damage.

Mechanisms of Injury

Most musculoskeletal injuries are the result of some type of trauma. Trauma is the result of an outside force (direct, indirect, or twisting) that has a negative effect on the body (Fig. 12-5). A **direct injury** is a result of force applied directly to the injured part of the body. For example, a bat swung into a person's arm will injure the portion of the arm that is hit. An **indirect injury** is caused by a force applied to a different area of the body that is then transmitted to the injured part. For example, if the knees move into the dash as the result of a motor vehicle collision (MVC), that force could transmit back and injure the pelvis. A **twisting injury** results from an extremity being twisted or pulled.

When approaching the scene where a musculoskeletal injury may have occurred, you should pay attention to the surrounding environment and consider the forces involved. Certain injuries can be predicted based on the

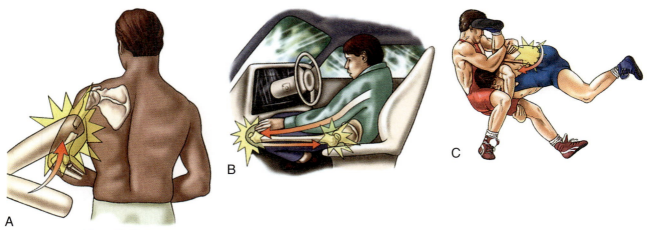

Fig. 12-5 A, A direct injury. **B,** An indirect injury. **C,** A twisting injury. (From Stoy W et al and Center for Emergency Medicine: *Mosby's first responder textbook,* revised ed 2, St. Louis, 2007, Mosby.)

mechanism of injury (MOI). This prediction can help identify potential injuries not just to the musculoskeletal system but also to soft tissue and internal organs lying underneath. Whenever possible, you should try to identify the MOI when trauma is involved and pass this information on to the receiving medical care system (Box 12-2).

Certain medical conditions or the process of aging may also have a role in musculoskeletal injuries. Bones become more fragile and brittle with age. Certain conditions, such as osteoporosis, can weaken bone structure. Under such conditions it takes a much smaller force to cause injury. Understanding how an injury has occurred will allow you to better assess and manage the patient.

Types of Musculoskeletal Injuries

Musculoskeletal injuries can be classified into many different types. The prehospital emergency care, however, is the same regardless of the type. As an emergency first responder, you are not responsible for distinguishing between the types of injury.

One way to classify a musculoskeletal injury is by defining it as open or closed. An injury in which the skin is broken is called an **open injury.** If the skin is not broken, it is referred to as a **closed injury.** Other classifications of musculoskeletal injuries include fractures, sprains, strains, and dislocations.

- *Fracture.* A **fracture** is another name for a broken bone. Fractures often involve injury to the nearby soft tissue, nerves, and blood vessels and result in bleeding and potential nerve damage (Fig. 12-6).
- *Sprain.* A **sprain** is an injury in which ligaments (which connect bone to bone) are stretched or torn (Fig. 12-7). A sprain does not involve injury to the actual bone but can produce significant pain and swelling.
- *Strain.* A **strain** is a muscle pull around a joint. Unlike a sprain, a strain does not involve the ligament and is characterized by pain with movement. There is little to no swelling of the joint (Fig. 12-8).
- *Dislocation.* A **dislocation** is the separation of a bone from its normal position in a joint. Dislocations damage blood vessels, nerves, soft tissue, and ligaments and can be very painful. Dislocations can also be associated with fractures.

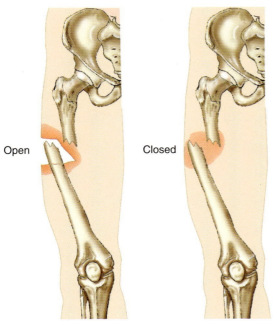

Fig. 12-6 Open versus closed fracture. (From NAEMT: *PHTLS: basic and advanced prehospital trauma life support,* ed 5, St. Louis, 2003, Mosby.)

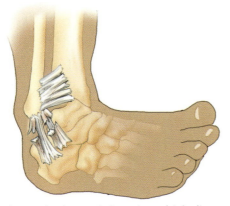

Fig. 12-7 A sprain is an injury in which ligaments are stretched or torn. (From McSwain N, Paturas J: *The basic EMT: comprehensive prehospital patient care Care,* ed 3, St. Louis, 2003, Mosby.)

In the prehospital environment, it is difficult to distinguish between these different types of injuries. *All musculoskeletal injuries are treated as potential fractures.*

General Assessment of Musculoskeletal Injuries

Before attempting a detailed assessment for injury to the musculoskeletal system, you must ensure that the scene

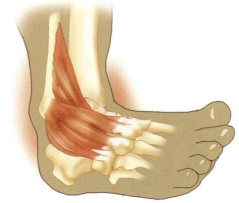

Fig. 12-8 A strain is a muscle pull. (From McSwain N, Paturas J: *The basic EMT: comprehensive prehospital patient care,* ed 3, St. Louis, 2003, Mosby.)

is safe and that all life-threatening conditions have been identified and treated. Musculoskeletal injuries are often painful and visually dramatic but rarely life threatening. Some patients may want you to focus on the obvious injury and will not understand that a greater threat to life may exist. You should not allow an obvious musculoskeletal injury to become a distracting injury. Remember to always complete your initial assessment ensuring an open airway, adequate breathing, circulation, and control of breathing before moving on to the detailed physical examination. Personal protection equipment (PPE) that is appropriate to the situation should be worn. This includes gloves at a minimum but may also include eye protection and a mask if there is a risk for blood spatter.

After the initial assessment and management of life-threatening conditions, a more detailed assessment of the injury can occur. It is important to always compare the injured side of the body to the uninjured side to assess the extent of the injury. You should completely expose the injured part of the body while you assess it further. As with any detailed assessment, you should assess for the following:

- *D*eformities
- *O*pen wounds
- *T*enderness
- *S*welling

During your SAMPLE history, you should evaluate the location and extent of the pain and determine the mechanism of injury. Some signs and symptoms of musculoskeletal injury are listed in Box 12-3. The three major signs and symptoms of injuries to muscles and bones include pain, deformity, and swelling.

BOX 12-3   Signs and Symptoms of Musculoskeletal Injury

- Patient holding an extremity (self-splinting)
- Swelling
- Deformity or angulation (abnormal appearance)
- Discoloration (bruising)
- An open wound
- Exposed bone ends
- Pain or tenderness over injury site
- A grinding or grating sound of bone ends rubbing over each other (crepitus)
- Loss of normal movement (paralysis)
- Limited or weakened movement of an extremity
- Pain with movement
- Inability to move joint; joint locked into position
- Loss of sensation or circulation distal to the injury site

Management of Musculoskeletal Injuries

The goal of managing any musculoskeletal injury, despite its type or cause, is to manage the patient's pain, prevent further injury, and minimize the risk of permanent injury. Depending on the situation, you may or may not have specialty equipment (such as commercial splints) to fully manage a musculoskeletal injury. However, there are general steps in managing any suspected musculoskeletal injury. The management steps include the following:

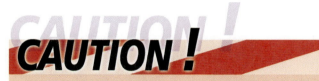

CAUTION !

With suspected spinal injuries, the patient's head and neck should be stabilized manually, and stabilization should continue until full spinal immobilization is completed. With a suspected injury to the upper leg, the patient's leg should be manually stabilized by holding the lower leg in place at the knee when possible.

Your assessment should also include checking the circulation, sensation, and movement in any injured extremity to identify any potential damage to blood vessels or nerves:

- *Circulation.* Assess the circulation of an extremity by feeling a pulse distal to the site of the injury. For example, if the injury is to the upper extremity, you should check a radial pulse. If the injury is to the lower extremity, check a pedal (foot) pulse. If there is no pulse, this means that blood is not flowing through the extremity and immediate treatment at the hospital is required.
- *Sensation.* Assess sensation by lightly touching the fingers or toes. If the patient can feel your touch, the nerve supply is probably intact.
- *Movement.* If the upper or lower extremity is injured (excluding the hand or foot), you should assess the movement of the hand or foot. Do this by asking the patient to squeeze your hand or to move his or her foot against your hand. Movement indicates that the nerves supplying the skeletal muscles are probably intact. Skill 12-1 demonstrates checking circulation, sensation, and movement in the hand and foot.

- *Manually stabilize the injury* (the patient may control this step). The injury should be gently stabilized with your hands or by the patient's hands at the joint above and the joint below the injury. If it is the joint that is injured, stabilization should occur at the bone above and below the injury. This will minimize the pain caused by excess movement. In addition to holding the joint or bone above and below the injury, you may also have to hold the sides or underneath the injured site. This will help prevent sagging of the injured site.
- Allow the patient to remain in a position of comfort if possible, but avoid moving the patient yourself.
- Control any bleeding unless it is coming from the patient's ears (see Chapter 11).
- Never attempt to straighten any musculoskeletal injury that is angled or misshapen, but attempt to stabilize it in the position found.
- Check and compare circulation, sensation, and movement both above and below the injury site and continue to monitor throughout your time with the patient. Any change in circulation, sensation, or movement should be reported immediately to the arriving medical care team.

Skill 12-1

Assessing Circulation, Sensation, and Movement

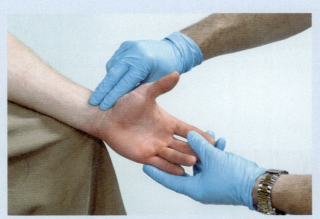

1. Assess the radial pulse for an upper extremity injury.

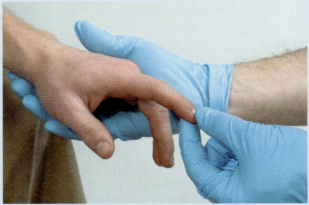

2. Assess sensation for an upper extremity injury by lightly pressing on a finger and asking the patient if he or she can feel it.

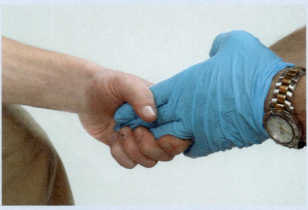

3. Assess movement for an upper extremity injury by asking the patient to move his or her hand or to grasp your hand.

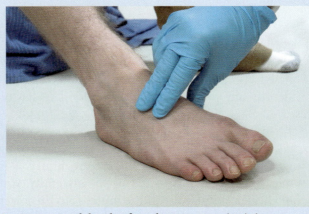

4. Assess a pedal pulse for a lower extremity injury.

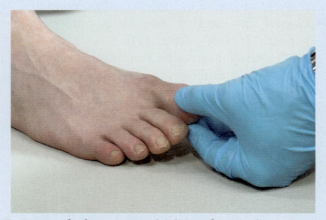

5. Assess of a lower extremity injury by pressing on a toe and asking the patient if he or she can feel it.

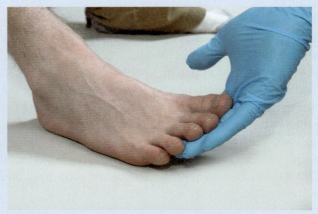

6. Assess movement for a lower extremity injury by asking the patient to point or flex the foot or move the foot against your hand.

- Dress any open wounds (see Chapter 11).
- Do not move the patient until the suspected musculoskeletal injury is appropriately splinted unless it is absolutely necessary.
- Consider the application of cold (such as an ice pack or a commercial cold pack) to the injury site to help control swelling and pain.
- If bone ends are visible, do not try to reposition or replace. You should instead cover the open wound to prevent further contamination.
- Calm, comfort, and reassure the patient.
- Splint the injury as required. As an emergency first responder, you may splint the injury yourself or you may assist other health care providers with splinting as required.

Splinting of a Musculoskeletal Injury

If possible, a musculoskeletal injury should be splinted. A **splint** is a device used to **immobilize**, or prevent movement of injured bones or joints, and to prevent further damage. **Box 12-4** outlines the reasons for splinting. The general principles for splinting a musculoskeletal injury are as follows:

1. Manually stabilize the injury as discussed in the general management section.
2. Remove or cut away clothing from injured site, and dress any open wounds.
3. Assess circulation, sensation, and movement distal to the injury.

---

4. Immobilize the joint above and the joint below the injured site with a splint. If it is a joint that is injured, splint the bone above and the bone below the joint.
5. Splint the injury in the position found. The hand or foot should be placed in a position of function.
6. After splinting, reassess circulation, sensation, and movement distal to the injury.
7. Pad the splint to prevent pressure points on the patient.

Skill 12-2 illustrates the general steps in splinting an extremity.

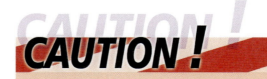

CAUTION!

If there are any deteriorating changes in circulation, sensation, or movement after a splint has been applied, you should maintain manual stabilization, loosen the splint, and contact medical control or the dispatched emergency medical services (EMS) unit if possible.

Splinting Equipment and Techniques

There are many types of equipment and techniques to perform splinting. Commercially made splints are available, although splints can also be improvised from such things as towels, pillows, rolled magazines, wood, or cardboard:

- *Rigid splint.* A rigid splint is made of firm, nonformable material that can be used to immobilize an injury.
- *Soft splint.* Soft splints are flexible, formable splints that provide gentle support of an injury. Air splints are a special type of commercially available soft splint. Once an air splint is applied over the injured site, it is inflated using only mouth air until a slight dent with your fingers can be made in the splint **(Fig. 12-9)**. **Skill 12-3** illustrates different types of splints used for different types of musculoskeletal injury.
- *Sling and swathe.* Injuries to the shoulder, clavicle, or humerus are best splinted using a sling and swathe technique **(Skill 12-4)**. Slings can be made out of any material such as a cravat or a commercial device. A swathe is a separate piece of material used to secure the extremity **(Fig. 12-10)**.

BOX 12-4   Reasons for Splinting

- Prevents movement of injured bones or joints
- Minimizes damage to muscles, nerves, and blood vessels
- Helps prevent a closed injury from becoming an open injury
- Minimizes restricting blood flow caused by bone ends compressing blood vessels
- Minimizes bleeding from associated tissue damage
- Minimizes pain by reducing movement of the bone and joint
  - If you are in doubt as to whether a musculoskeletal injury is present, you should apply a splint

Skill 12-2

Splinting an Upper Extremity Injury

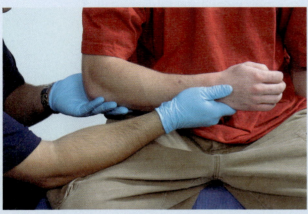

1. Provide manual stabilization of the joint above and the joint below the injury (the elbow and the wrist).

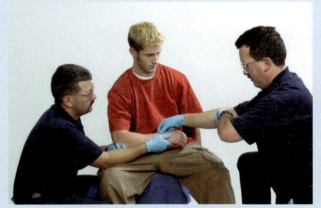

2. Assess circulation distal to the injury.

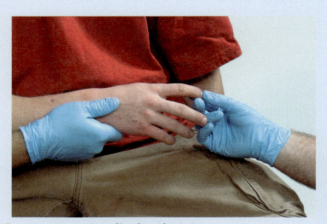

3. Assess sensation distal to the injury.

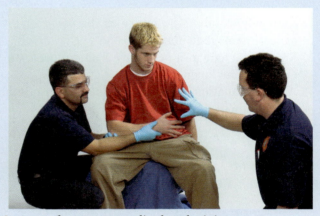

4. Assess for movement distal to the injury.

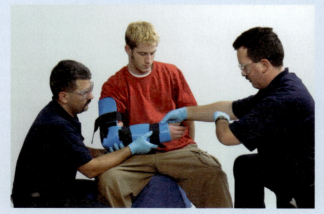

5. Apply a splint to immobilize the joint above and below the injury. Assess circulation distal to the injury after splinting.

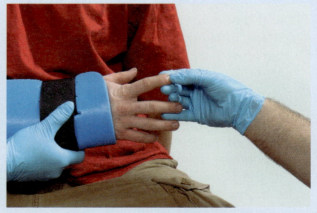

6. Assess sensation and movement distal to the injury after splinting.

In the Real World—continued

You assess Heather and find that she has no life-threatening injuries. As you continue to assess her, you get her to tell you what happened. She states that she was swinging on the jungle gym when she missed a bar and fell to the ground onto her outstretched arm. After some coaxing, she allows you to touch her left arm. You hold it under the injured site and feel a deformity at the distal forearm and wrist area.

You check for circulation and sensation both above and below the injury and find them to be the same; in addition, you find that Heather can move all of her fingers. You continue to hold Heather's left arm while directing Ms. Tubbs to clean her abrasions. You have Mr. Wheelock, another teacher, check to see that an ambulance has been called and to help direct the crew to Heather when they arrive.

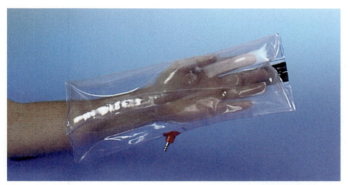

Fig. 12-9 An air splint. (From McSwain N, Paturas J: *The basic EMT: comprehensive prehospital patient care,* ed 3, St. Louis, 2003, Mosby.)

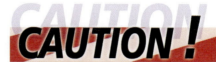

CAUTION!

It is important to remember that splinting generally requires two trained providers—one provider to maintain manual stabilization of the injured site and the other to apply the splint.

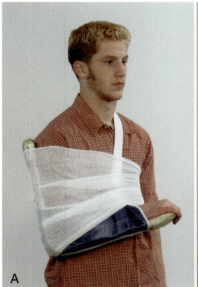
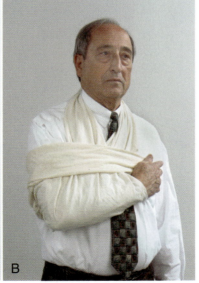

A   B

Fig. 12-10 **A,** Commercial sling and swathe of roller gauze. **B,** Sling and swathe with cravats.

Special Considerations

Any patient with a suspected spinal, head, or chest injury will require special considerations in assessment and management. Your initial assessment will always remain the same: identify and manage any life-threatening conditions.

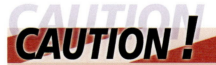

CAUTION!

A lack of pain in or around the spinal column does not rule out the possibility of a spinal injury.

Skill 12-3

Techniques of Splinting

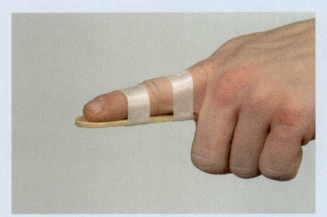

1. Splinting of an injury to a single finger.

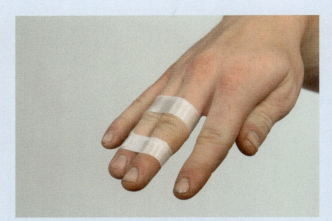

2. Splinting of an injury to two fingers.

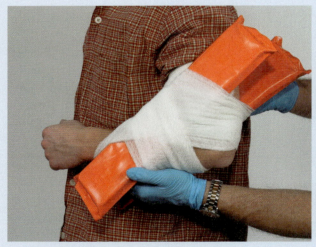

3. Rigid splint applied to an elbow injury.

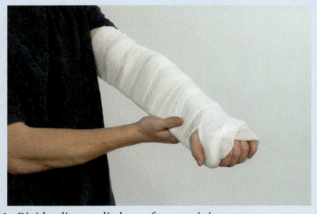

4. Rigid splint applied to a forearm injury.

Skill 12-3

Techniques of Splinting—cont'd

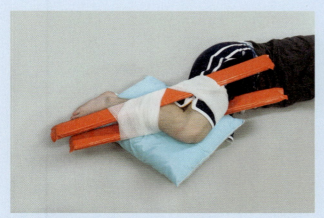

5. Rigid splint applied to a knee injury.

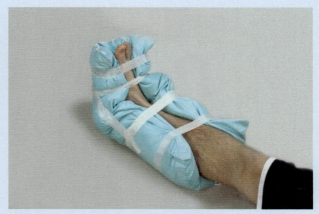

6. Soft splint applied to an ankle injury.

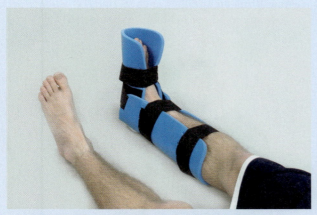

7. Semirigid splint applied to a lower leg injury.

Skill 12-4

Applying a Sling and Swathe

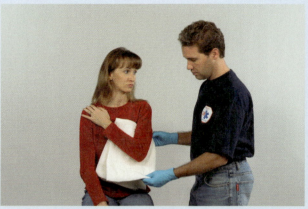

1. Check circulation, sensation, and movement distal to the injured site. Apply padding underneath the extremity on the side of the injury. Material for sling should be made into a triangle.

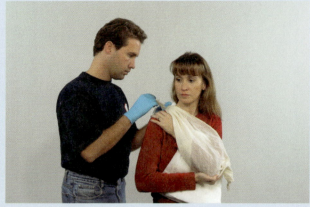

2. Apply a sling to support the weight of the extremity. The point of the triangle should be toward the patient's elbow. Bring the two long ends around the patient's neck and secure in a knot behind the shoulder.

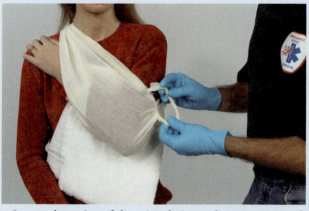

3. Secure the point of the triangle into a knot, or pin to the rest of the material to maintain support of the extremity.

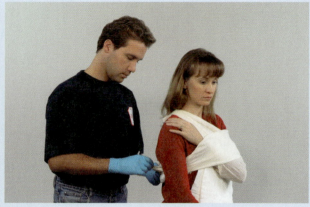

4. Apply a swathe to secure the extremity to the chest without restricting breathing. Recheck circulation, sensation, and movement.

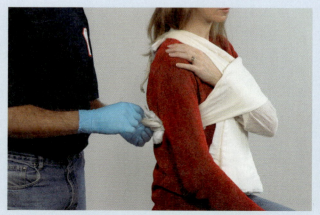

5. Pad behind both knots.

Suspected Spinal Injury

Any patient with a suspected spinal injury must be managed aggressively. Injuries to the spine can result in permanent paralysis if not recognized and treated. As an emergency first responder, you should be able to identify a suspected spinal injury and provide appropriate and rapid management.

Mechanism of Injury

A patient with a spinal injury can present with or without initial signs and symptoms. An important part of your assessment, therefore, is to assess the MOI. According to the Prehospital Trauma Life Support (PHTLS) committee, mechanisms of injury that should lead to the assumption of a spinal injury include the following:

- Any mechanism that produces a violent impact on the head, neck, torso, or pelvis (e.g., assault or entrapment in a structural collapse)
- Incidents that produce sudden forces to the neck or torso (e.g., a moderate- to high-speed MVC, a pedestrian struck by a vehicle, or involvement in an explosion)
- Any fall, especially in the elderly
- Ejection or fall from a motorized or otherwise powered transportation device (e.g., scooters, skateboards, bicycles, or motorcycles)
- Shallow-water diving incidents (e.g., diving or body surfing)

Assessment and Management

The initial assessment of the suspected spinal-injured patient is the same as with any other patient. You should wear appropriate PPE based on the situation, ensure the scene is safe, and identify and manage any life-threatening conditions. Special attention, however, should be given to controlling the airway. The jaw thrust without head tilt (see Chapter 7) should be used with all patients suspected of having a spinal injury. This maneuver is used to open and maintain the patient's airway while maintaining manual stabilization of the head and neck. The patient should not be moved until full spinal immobilization has been applied. If movement of the patient is necessary, for example, with an unresponsive trauma patient found in the prone position, do so with as much protection of the spine as possible. If an unresponsive patient is having difficulty breathing, assist his or her respirations. After the initial assessment, you should assess circulation, sensation, and movement in all four extremities when possible and complete a detailed assessment when needed.

BOX 12-5 Signs and Symptoms of Possible Spinal Injury

- Concerning mechanism of injury
- Altered mental status or unresponsive patient
- Pain associated with movement
- Pain independent of movement or palpation along the spinal column, upper extremities, or lower extremities
- Loss of sensation or movement in any extremity
- A sensation of "pins and needles" in an extremity
- Numbness, weakness, or tingling in the upper or lower extremities
- Pain or tenderness in or around the neck or back
- Soft tissue injuries associated with trauma to the head, neck, shoulders, back, or abdomen
- Loss of the use of the diaphragm muscle during breathing and increased use of the accessory muscles (patient has difficulty breathing)
- Loss of bowel or bladder control

The signs and symptoms of a possible spinal injury are listed in Box 12-5. Questions to ask a conscious patient suspected of having a spinal injury are highlighted in Box 12-6.

Manual Stabilization of the Head and Neck

Once you have recognized the potential for a spinal injury, your first step will be to manually stabilize the patient's head and neck in a neutral position. A neutral position can best be described as a position that maintains the normal curvature of the cervical spine, with the eyes facing forward and parallel with the ground if the patient is standing. This is best accomplished by placing your hands on the side of the patient's head and holding it still. You should not place your hands around the patient's neck because this might block his or her efforts to breathe. Manual stabilization of the head and neck can be provided for a patient lying on the ground, sitting upright, or found standing (Fig. 12-11). If the patient complains of increased pain or if you feel resistance while trying to position his or her head in a neutral position, you should *stop* immediately and maintain the patient's

BOX 12-6   Questions to Ask a Conscious Patient Suspected of Having a Spinal Injury

- Does your neck or back hurt?
- What happened?
- Where does it hurt?
- Can you feel me touching your fingers?
- Can you move your hands?
- Can you move your arms?
- Can you feel me touching your toes?
- Can you move your feet?
- Can you move your legs?

head and neck in the position it was found. Patients found lying face down (prone) should be log rolled onto their backs to maintain spinal stabilization whenever possible (see Chapter 6). Box 12-7 shows detailed steps to provide manual stabilization of the patient's head and neck.

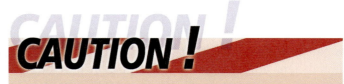

It is very important for manual stabilization of the patient's head and neck to be maintained until full spinal immobilization has been applied. Full immobilization requires the patient to be secured to a long backboard as discussed in the Team Work section.

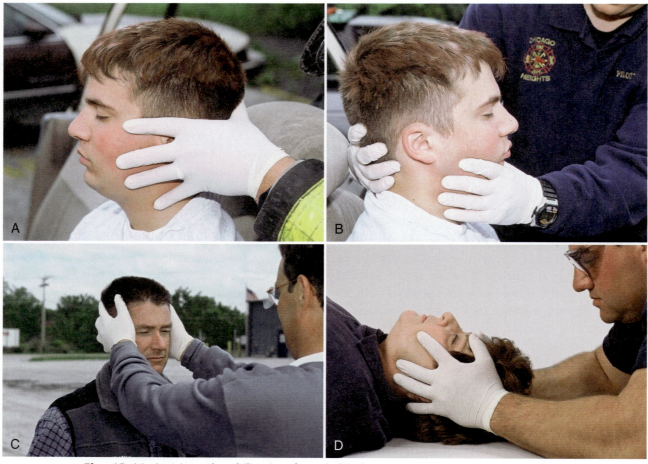

Fig. 12-11 A, Manual stabilization from behind a patient. **B,** Manual stabilization from the side of a patient. **C,** Manual stabilization from the front of a patient. **D,** Manual stabilization of a supine patient. (From NAEMT: *PHTLS: basic and advanced prehospital trauma life support,* ed 5, St. Louis, 2003, Mosby.)

BOX 12-7 Providing Manual Stabilization of the Patient's Head and Neck

1. Position yourself so you can place both hands on either side of the patient's head with your hands placed over the ears to hold and support the weight of the head.
2. Move the patient's head into a neutral position (eyes facing forward and level), maintaining the natural curvature of the cervical spine.
3. Place your forearms either on the floor or the patient's back or chest for support.
4. If the patient complains of pain or if you meet resistance during your movement of the head and neck into a neutral position, *stop* and maintain the head and neck in the position found.
5. Patients found prone (lying face down) should be log rolled to a supine (lying face up) position while maintaining manual stabilization.
6. Maintain manual stabilization until full immobilization has been secured.

BOX 12-8 Signs and Symptoms of Possible Head Injury

- Pain, swelling, deformity, or open wounds to the head
- Altered mental status or loss of consciousness following trauma
- Irregular breathing pattern
- Pupils that are unequal, slow, or nonreactive to light
- Loss of normal speech
- Weakness or paralysis of an extremity or both extremities on one side of the body
- Bleeding or fluid loss from the ears
- Exposed brain tissue
- Bruising or discoloration under or around both eyes
- Bruising or discoloration behind one or both ears

Suspected Head Injury

As with the suspected spinal injury patient, patients with a suspected head injury will need special attention and management. Injuries to the head can either be open or closed. Open injuries may involve bleeding. In particular, open wounds to the head and face will bleed profusely because of the large number of blood vessels in the area. A closed head injury may cause internal bleeding, swelling of the brain tissue, leading to minor or severe brain injury. Early recognition, management, and transportation of a patient with a suspected head injury to an appropriate facility are imperative.

Assessment and Management

Any patient who has an altered mental status or is unresponsive should be assumed to have a head injury and should be managed accordingly. During the initial assessment, in addition to identifying and managing any life-threatening conditions, it is also important to calculate a Glasgow Coma Scale (GCS) score and repeat this assessment in the ongoing assessment. When performing a physical examination of a suspected head injury patient, care should be used to avoid movement of the head and spine when palpating the skull. You should note any pain, swelling, or deformities of the skull, and do not probe open wounds or depressions in the skull. Signs and symptoms of a possible head injury are listed in Box 12-8.

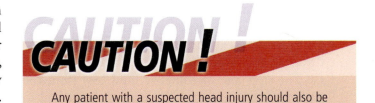

Any patient with a suspected head injury should also be considered to have a spinal injury.

In general, the management of a head injury patient includes the following:

- Do not move the patient unless it is absolutely necessary. If you have to move the patient, protect the spine as much as possible.
- Manually stabilize the patient's head and neck and maintain until the patient is secured to an immobilization device.

- Use the trauma jaw thrust to open and maintain the patient's airway.
- Assist the patient's ventilations if necessary.
- Apply supplemental oxygen if possible.
- Control minor external bleeding.
- Cover all open wounds.
- Do not stop any bleeding or fluid loss from the patient's ears. Cover with a sterile dressing to prevent contamination only (Box 12-9).
- Continue to monitor the patient's vital signs for changes (including his or her mental status).

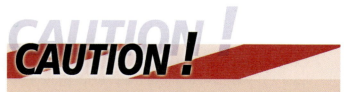

Do not tape or in any way constrict the patient's chest area because this may exacerbate breathing difficulty.

Suspected Chest Injury

Patients with chest trauma may have serious internal injuries. The most common chest injuries are rib fractures. These patients will almost always have chest pain and may experience significant difficulty with breathing. In these cases, you may need to assist their ventilations. Box 12-10 lists signs and symptoms that indicate possible chest injury.

Management

Management of a patient with suspected chest injury includes assisting ventilations as needed and providing supplemental oxygen to the patient if available. Traumatic injuries to the chest may also have caused spinal injuries. Patients with significant chest trauma should be managed and treated as if they have a spinal injury along with their chest injuries. A patient with chest injuries should be placed in a position of comfort, and you should allow the patient to self-splint the injured side if necessary. The management of chest injuries, such as an impaled object in the chest or an open chest wound, is discussed in Chapter 11.

Team Work

As an emergency first responder, you may be asked to assist in the further management of a patient with a suspected musculoskeletal injury. This assistance may include such things as applying a traction splint, helping to measure and apply a cervical collar, or performing spinal immobilization. Having a basic understanding of the procedures and common devices is essential to working effectively as part of the team.

CAUTION!

The following recommendations are meant to be general guidelines. Follow manufacturers' recommendations for the proper measurement and application of the splinting devices you will be using.

TRACTION SPLINT

A traction splint is a specialty commercial splint that is used to splint a fracture of the femur (thigh). As an emergency first responder, you may be asked to assist with the placement of a traction splint. It is important for you to be able to recognize the equipment and have an understanding of how the device is applied. Following is a list of general steps to take when applying a traction splint to a patient (Fig. 12-12):

1. Manually stabilize the joint above and below the injury site.
2. Remove or cut clothing away from the injury site.
3. Control any bleeding and apply dressings as needed.
4. Check circulation, sensation, and movement both above and below the injury site.
5. Attach ankle hitch and apply manual traction (pull firmly on the leg to keep it inline).
6. Place the traction device along the uninjured leg; lengthen the device to slightly longer than the uninjured leg.
7. If using a sling-type device, elevate the injured leg just enough to place the traction device under it.
8. If using a single pole device, place the device between the patient's legs.
9. Apply the proper straps as specified by the manufacturer and tighten.
10. Apply the securing device for the ankle.
11. Apply traction according to the manufacturer's recommendations.
12. Recheck circulation, sensation, and movement above and below the injury site.
13. Secure the patient to a long backboard.

CAUTION!

Several different types of traction splints are commercially available. You should find out the type used in your area and practice application of the device.

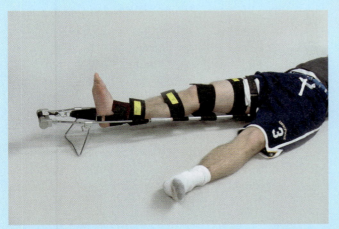

Fig. 12-12 A traction splint is used to immobilize a femur fracture.

CERVICAL COLLARS

Cervical collars are rigid devices that help support the head and neck and keep it from moving. The cervical collar on its own does not completely immobilize a patient's head and neck. As an emergency first responder, you may have to assist with the placement of a cervical collar on a patient with suspected spinal injury. Placement of a cervical collar requires two providers. One provider maintains manual stabilization of the head and neck, and the other sizes and places the cervical collar. Skill 12-5 illustrates the sizing and placement of a cervical collar.

Team Work—cont'd

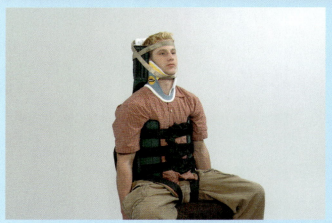

Fig. 12-13 A vest-type device can be used to immobilize someone sitting in an upright position.

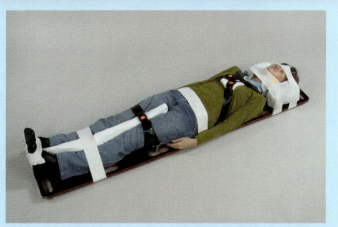

Fig. 12-14 Patient fully immobilized to a long backboard.

SPINAL IMMOBILIZATION

Any patient suspected of having a spinal injury should be fully immobilized. Full immobilization of the spine, just like immobilizing or splinting any other joint or bone, requires stabilization of the joint above and below the injured site. For spinal immobilization, the joint above is the head and the joint below is the pelvis. Full immobilization is generally done by moving a patient onto a long backboard. This may require log rolling the patient onto the board or, if the patient is sitting upright in a vehicle, the use of a short board or vest-type device (Fig. 12-13).

A short board or vest-type device is used to immobilize a patient sitting upright so that he or she can be turned and carried out of a vehicle without moving the spine. Once moved outside the vehicle, the patient is then immobilized to a long backboard.

As an emergency first responder, you will probably be asked to assist with immobilization of a patient with a suspected spinal injury because it requires at least three to four providers. It is important for you to recognize the need for spinal immobilization and to feel comfortable assisting other providers. The steps involved in immobilizing a patient to a long backboard include the following:

1. Apply and maintain manual stabilization of the patient's head and neck in a neutral inline position.
2. Measure and apply a cervical collar.
3. Place a long backboard along the side of the patient, with the foot end of the board at the patient's knees.
4. While maintaining manual stabilization, place two or three other providers on the side of the patient without the long backboard.
5. Providers at the side of the patient place their hands on the opposite side of the patient under the patient's shoulders and hips (and the lower legs if using three providers).
6. On the command of the provider maintaining manual stabilization of the head and neck, the patient is rolled just enough to slide the backboard under the patient.
7. The providers now place their hands between the patient's arms and chest and along the pelvis.
8. At the command of the provider maintaining manual stabilization of the head and neck, the patient is moved in a straight line upward and centered onto the backboard.
9. The patient can now be immobilized to the backboard with straps. The torso and legs are immobilized first with the head being immobilized last.
10. After the patient's head is secured to the board and full immobilization has been achieved, manual stabilization may be released.
11. Padding may be used to fill any voids or holes such as behind the patient's neck or between the patient's legs (Fig. 12-14).

Skill 12-5

Sizing and Placing a Cervical Collar

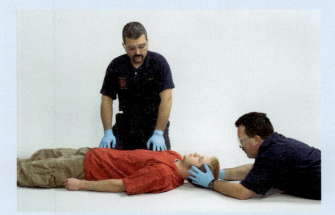

1. Apply and maintain manual stabilization of the head and neck in a neutral inline position.

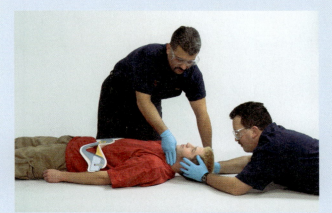

2. Using your fingers, measure the distance between the patient's lower jaw and shoulder (make sure your fingers are placed parallel to the patient's jaw).

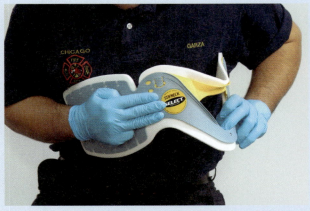

3. Find a cervical collar that matches the patient's measurements or adjust collar size to fit the measurement.

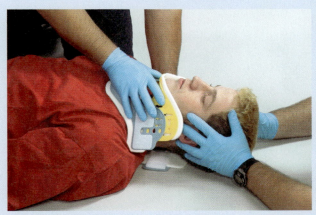

4. Apply the cervical collar and secure.

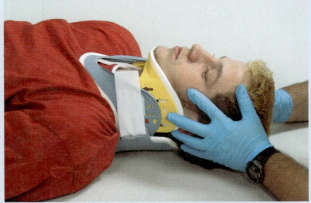

5. Maintain manual stabilization until the patient is fully immobilized to a long backboard.

In the Real World—Conclusion

When the ambulance arrives, you give the crew a report about Heather's injury and advise them that Heather's parents will meet them at the emergency department. You assist the crew with the splint for Heather's left forearm and wrist. Further assessment of Heather identifies no other injuries, so she is moved to the stretcher and transported to the hospital.

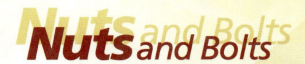

Critical Points

A First Responder requires an appreciation of the normal structure and function of the musculoskeletal system. A first responder must also understand that most musculoskeletal injuries are painful and visually disturbing but are rarely life threatening.

The initial method of stabilization for any musculoskeletal injury includes manual stabilization of the injury. Injured extremities on one side can be compared to the uninjured side. The First Responder should always check and compare circulation, sensation, and movement above and below any musculoskeletal injury site. Do not move a patient suspected of having a spinal or head injury unless absolutely necessary. If moving is necessary, do everything possible to protect the spinal column.

Learning Checklist

- ❑ The musculoskeletal system gives the body shape, protects vital organs, and provides movement.
- ❑ Musculoskeletal injuries can be painful and visually dramatic but are rarely life threatening. It is important to identify and manage life-threatening conditions first before treating musculoskeletal injuries.
- ❑ The skeleton is divided into the axial (central) skeleton and the appendicular (extremities) skeleton.
- ❑ The axial skeleton comprises the skull, spinal column, and thorax.
- ❑ The spinal column is divided into five areas: cervical, thoracic, lumbar, sacrum, and coccyx.
- ❑ The thorax comprises the clavicles, scapulas, ribs, and sternum.
- ❑ The appendicular skeleton comprises the pelvis and the upper and lower extremities.
- ❑ The pelvis is a highly vascular area and injury to the pelvis can cause significant loss of blood.
- ❑ There are three types of muscle: skeletal, smooth, and cardiac.
- ❑ Skeletal muscle (or voluntary muscle) is connected to bone and can be moved by conscious thought.
- ❑ Smooth muscle (involuntary muscle) contracts or relaxes automatically. An example is the muscle in the digestive system.

- ❑ Cardiac muscle (involuntary muscle) is unique because it can generate its own electrical impulse to contract.
- ❑ Musculoskeletal injuries result from a direct, indirect, or twisting-type force.
- ❑ An open injury is one in which the skin is open. A closed injury has the skin intact.
- ❑ With the detailed assessment, you should examine the patient for deformities, open wounds, tenderness, or swelling. It is important to compare the injured side of the body to the uninjured side to gauge the musculoskeletal injury.
- ❑ Assessment of musculoskeletal injuries should include checking circulation, sensation, and movement both above and below the injured site.
- ❑ Signs and symptoms of musculoskeletal injury include self-splinting, swelling, deformity, discoloration, open wounds, exposed bone ends, pain, crepitus, lack of or limited movement, and loss of sensation or circulation.
- ❑ The management of musculoskeletal injury includes manual stabilization of the injury; allowing the patient to remain in a position of comfort; controlling any bleeding; checking circulation, sensation, and movement above and below the injury site; dressing any wounds; considering the application of cold to the injury site; calming, comforting, and reassuring the patient; and splinting the injury as required.
- ❑ You should not move a patient with a musculoskeletal injury unless necessary. If bone ends are visible, you should not try to replace them. You should never attempt to straighten an angled or deformed extremity.
- ❑ Always immobilize the joint above and the joint below the site of injury. If the injured site is a joint, then immobilize the bone above and the bone below.
- ❑ It is important to assess the mechanism of injury with musculoskeletal injury. Patients with a concerning mechanism of injury should be suspected of having spinal injury.
- ❑ Signs and symptoms of possible spinal injury include concerning mechanism of injury, altered mental status, lack of responsiveness, loss of sensation or

Nuts and Bolts–continued

movement in any extremity, sensation of "pins and needles," pain or tenderness in neck or back, difficulty breathing, and loss of bladder or bowel control.

❏ If a patient has suspected spinal injury, apply manual stabilization of the head and neck, use a jaw thrust to open and maintain the airway, assist ventilations if necessary, and complete a detailed assessment as necessary.

❏ Head injuries can be either open or closed. Open injuries may involve profuse external bleeding. Closed injuries may involve internal bleeding.

❏ Signs and symptoms of possible head injury include pain, swelling, deformity, or open wounds to the head; altered mental status; loss of consciousness following trauma; an irregular breathing pattern; pupils that are unequal, slow, or nonreactive to light; loss of normal speech; weakness or paralysis of extremities; bleeding or fluid loss from the ears; exposed brain tissue; bruising around both eyes; and bruising behind one or both ears.

❏ If a patient has a suspected head injury, assume he or she also has a spinal injury, avoid probing open wounds or depressions in the skull, assist ventilations if necessary, provide supplemental oxygen if possible, control bleeding and dress wounds, and monitor mental status.

❏ Patients with suspected chest injury may have chest pain and significant difficulty breathing. Place patients in a position of comfort, assist ventilations if necessary, and provide supplemental oxygen if possible.

Key Terms

Appendicular skeleton The part of the skeleton consisting of the pelvis and the upper and lower extremities.

Axial skeleton The central skeleton consisting of the skull, spinal column, and thorax.

Cardiac muscle A type of involuntary muscle that is found only in the heart. Generates its own electrical impulse to contract and relax.

Closed injury An injury in which the skin remains intact.

Direct injury Injury as a result of force applied directly to the body or a body part.

Dislocation The separation of a bone from its normal position in a joint.

Fracture A broken bone.

Immobilize To prevent movement.

Indirect injury Injury as a result of a force applied to one part of the body, which transmits to and then injures another part.

Involuntary muscle Also called smooth muscle. Muscle that contracts or relaxes automatically.

Joint Where two or more bones come together. Allows movement of the body.

Ligaments Fibrous bands of tissue that connect bone to bone.

Open injury An injury in which the skin has been broken.

Skeletal muscle Also called voluntary muscle. Muscle connected to bone that requires an active thought process to contract or relax.

Smooth muscle Also called involuntary muscle. Muscle that contracts or relaxes automatically.

Splint A device used to immobilize injured bones or joints and prevent further damage.

Sprain An injury where ligaments are stretched or torn.

Strain A muscle pull around a joint.

Tendons Fibrous bands of tissue that connect muscle to bones.

Twisting injury Injury as a result of an extremity being twisted or pulled.

Voluntary muscle Also called skeletal muscle. Muscle connected to bone that requires an active thought process to contract.

First Responder NSC Objectives
COGNITIVE OBJECTIVES

- Describe the function of the musculoskeletal system.
- Differentiate between an open and a closed painful, swollen, deformed extremity.

- List the emergency medical care for a patient with a painful, swollen, deformed extremity.
- Relate mechanism of injury to potential injuries of the head and spine.
- State the signs and symptoms of a potential spine injury.
- Describe the method of determining if a responsive patient may have a spine injury.
- List the signs and symptoms of injury to the head.
- Describe the emergency medical care for injuries to the head.

AFFECTIVE OBJECTIVES

- Explain the rationale for the feelings of patients who need immobilization for a painful, swollen, deformed extremity.
- Demonstrate a caring attitude toward patients with musculoskeletal injuries who request emergency medical services (EMS).

- Place the interests of the patient with a musculoskeletal injury as the foremost consideration when making any and all patient care decisions.
- Communicate by showing empathy toward patients with musculoskeletal injuries and toward family members and friends of the patient.

PSYCHOMOTOR OBJECTIVES

- Demonstrate the emergency medical care of a patient with a painful, swollen, deformed extremity.
- Demonstrate opening the airway in a patient with suspected spinal cord injury.
- Demonstrate evaluating a responsive patient with a suspected spinal cord injury.
- Demonstrate stabilization of the cervical spine.

Check your understanding

Check your understanding

Please refer to p. 439 for the answers to these questions.

1. The disruption of a joint such that the bone ends are no longer in contact with each other is a:
   A. Dislocation
   B. Sprain
   C. Fracture
   D. Strain

2. The movable part of your jaw is called the:
   A. Maxilla
   B. Zygoma
   C. Orbit
   D. Mandible

3. Which of the following compose the shoulder?
   A. Radius, ulna, humerus
   B. Clavicle, radius, ulna
   C. Scapula, clavicle, humerus
   D. Humerus, scapula, tibia

4. Once an emergency first responder manually stabilizes the head and neck of a trauma patient, this manual stabilization must be maintained until _____.

5. If an unresponsive patient is suspected of having a cervical spine (neck) injury, the emergency first responder should prevent movement of the neck by opening the airway with a/an _____.

6. An injury to the spinal cord at the level of the cervical spine may paralyze the diaphragm, impairing the patient's ability to _____.

7. List five indications of a possible spinal injury.
   A. _____
   B. _____
   C. _____
   D. _____
   E. _____

8. Your assault patient has what you believe is a basal skull fracture, judging from the bloody fluid draining from his ears. The most appropriate management would include:
   A. Stopping the flow of the drainage by packing the ears with gauze
   B. Placing the patient in the Trendelenburg position, or with legs elevated
   C. Applying a C-collar, delivering oxygen
   D. Placing the patient in the recovery position

9. Matching: There are two terms from the list below that describe each section of the spine. Place the letters of the two terms that describe the section of the spine in the blanks next to the part of the spine. Some letters may be used more than once.

   (A) Tailbone, (B) 12 Vertebrae, (C) Neck, (D) 4 Vertebrae, (E) 7 Vertebrae, (F) Back, (G) Lower back, (H) 5 Vertebrae

   _____ _____ Cervical spine

   _____ _____ Thoracic spine

   _____ _____ Lumbar spine

   _____ _____ Sacrum

   _____ _____ Coccyx

10. The lower part of the sternum, which could cause damage to the liver if compressed during cardiopulmonary resuscitation (CPR), is called the: _____.
    A. Manubrium
    B. Sternal notch
    C. Body
    D. Xiphoid process

11. The two bones of the forearm are the: _____.
    A. Humerus and ulna
    B. Radius and ulna
    C. Tibia and fibula
    D. Radius and fibula

12. The large, strong bone of the thigh is called the: _____.
    A. Femur
    B. Fibula
    C. Patella
    D. Humerus

13. Which of the following bones, when fractured, can lead to massive internal bleeding, shock, and even death?
    A. Clavicle and scapula
    B. Tibia and fibula
    C. Femur and pelvis
    D. Humerus and ulna

14. The fibrous tissue that connects bone to bone is:
    A. Muscle
    B. Ligament
    C. Tendon
    D. Cartilage

15. Over which of the following muscle types can we exert conscious control?
    A. Involuntary
    B. Voluntary
    C. Smooth
    D. Cardiac

16. List four signs or symptoms of possible musculoskeletal injury.
    A. _____
    B. _____
    C. _____
    D. _____

17. The grinding, grating sound that may be noted when there is movement of a broken bone is called: _____.
    A. Osteoporosis
    B. Deformity
    C. Paralysis
    D. Crepitus

18. When should the emergency first responder attempt to straighten out an injured extremity that is abnormally angled or bent?
    A. Never
    B. Always
    C. When there is no pulse in the extremity
    D. When the extremity is numb

19. The best way for an emergency first responder to stabilize a musculoskeletal injury of an extremity until additional EMS resources arrive is to: _____.
    A. Apply a commercially made splint
    B. Apply an improvised splint, such as a rolled-up magazine
    C. Manually stabilize with the hands
    D. Apply an elastic wrap to the extremity

20. Which of the following is NOT an appropriate emergency first responder treatment of a conscious patient with a suspected rib injury?
    A. Position patient on the affected side
    B. Use of a combitube
    C. Begin chest compressions
    D. Allow the patient to stabilize or "self-splint" the injury

21. A traction splint is a special kind of splint that is only used for certain injuries of the: _____.
    A. Lower leg
    B. Upper arm
    C. Thigh
    D. Knee

22. Your patient is a forklift operator whose pelvis and legs were trapped under the forklift when it tipped over. Although additional help has not yet arrived, which of the following potential injuries is most life threatening to this patient?
    A. Injury of the lumbar spine
    B. Fracture of the tibia and fibula
    C. Considerable bruising of the thigh muscle
    D. Fracture of the pelvis

Check *your understanding*–continued

23. You are treating a crash victim who has an apparent open fracture of the L tibia. Which is the most appropriate course of action?
    A. Put the bone ends back into the wound
    B. Cover with a sterile dressing and control bleeding
    C. Wait for advanced life support (ALS) to apply a traction splint
    D. Help the patient walk to the ambulance

24. You respond to a motorcycle crash where a patient has sustained multiple injuries, including a fractured L forearm, road rash, multiple lacerations, and some facial swelling, particularly in the midface region, from trauma. Which of the injuries are you most concerned about?
    A. Lacerations
    B. Road rash
    C. Fractured L forearm
    D. Facial injuries

Chapter 13

Childbirth

LESSON GOAL

Thousands of babies are born each day and most of these babies arrive safely and in good health regardless of how we "help." As an emergency first responder, you may find yourself with the unique opportunity to assist with the birth of a child. If you know and have practiced the steps to assist with a normal delivery, you will be more confident and prepared should the need arise for you to help with a birth, whether it is normal or involves complications.

OBJECTIVES

1. Identify the following structures: birth canal, placenta, umbilical cord, and amniotic sac.
2. Define the following terms: crowning, bloody show, labor, and abortion.
3. State the indications of an imminent delivery.
4. State the steps in the predelivery preparation of the mother.
5. Establish the relationship between body substance isolation (BSI) and childbirth.
6. State the steps to assist in a delivery.
7. Describe care of the baby as the head appears.
8. Discuss the steps in delivery of the placenta.
9. List the steps in the emergency medical care of the mother postdelivery.
10. Discuss the steps in caring for a newborn.
11. Demonstrate the steps to assist in the normal cephalic delivery.
12. Demonstrate necessary care procedures of the fetus as the head appears.
13. Demonstrate the postdelivery care of the mother.
14. Demonstrate the care of the newborn.

In the Real World

While you are at a community picnic, your neighbor runs to you and breathlessly announces that his wife is in labor. Based on his wife's history of fast labor and delivery (this is her third child), the husband says they do not have enough time to travel to the hospital before the baby is born. He knows that you have taken an emergency first responder course, so he asks you for help. You run to your car to get your first-response kit and then join your neighbor, who is now sitting on the ground next to his wife. His wife is panting hard and says she feels an urge to go to the bathroom.

The process of birth is a normal and natural occurrence, and the labor process usually allows plenty of time for parents to get to the hospital or birth facility. Occasionally, however, a baby's arrival is unscheduled or early, or complications of pregnancy occur. At these times, as an emergency first responder you must know how to help. This chapter introduces you to the anatomy and physiology of pregnancy, the stages of labor and delivery, and care of the newborn. It also introduces some complications of pregnancy and delivery.

Anatomy and Physiology of Pregnancy

Pregnancy can be physically and psychologically stressful. The mother's body is undergoing many changes during all stages of the pregnancy and after delivery. This is often a happy time for a family but it can also be a time of unpredictability, stress, and difficulty depending on many factors. Understanding the anatomy and physiology of pregnancy and childbirth will help you assist in emergency medical care related to childbirth.

The female reproductive anatomy includes the ovaries, fallopian tubes, uterus, vagina, and the perineum (Fig. 13-1). The **ovaries** are a pair of almond-shaped organs located in the right and left lower quadrants of the abdomen. The ovaries function to release eggs and hormones. Once a month an egg is released from an ovary and travels through the **fallopian tube** to the uterus. A fallopian tube extends from each ovary and acts as a path for the egg to reach the uterus. The **uterus** is a pear-shaped muscular organ that houses the unborn infant. The neck of the uterus, the lower portion where it enters the vagina, is called the **cervix.** The cervix contains a mucous plug that acts as a barrier between the uterus and the vaginal opening during pregnancy. Once labor begins, the mucous plug will separate and be discharged from the vagina. This is sometimes termed **bloody show.** The **vagina,** or **birth canal,** is a sheath that encloses the lower portion of the uterus and extends down to the vaginal opening. The **perineum** is the area between the vaginal opening and the anus.

A fertilized egg implants in the uterus. For the first 8 weeks of pregnancy this fertilized egg is typically called an **embryo.** After 8 weeks and until birth the embryo is called a **fetus.** Pregnancy usually averages a span of 40 weeks that are divided into three 3-month intervals called trimesters.

The fetus grows and develops in the uterus and is linked to the mother via the **placenta.** Oxygen and nutrients from the mother's blood pass through the placenta and enters the circulatory system of the fetus through the **umbilical cord.** The fetus passes waste material back through the umbilical cord and placenta to the mother's circulatory system to be eliminated (Fig. 13-2).

During pregnancy the fetus is surrounded by a fluid-filled sac known as the **amniotic sac,** which helps to protect the developing fetus. Typically, the amniotic sac will rupture before the delivery of the fetus. This rupturing is called rupture of the membranes. Some mothers may refer to this as, "My water has broken."

Labor

The process that occurs when a woman is preparing to give birth is called **labor.** Labor can last from a few hours to many hours, or in some cases a day or more. The length of labor depends on several factors: the age of the mother, whether it is a first or subsequent pregnancy, the general health of the mother, and overall health of the fetus.

There are three stages of labor and in most cases an emergency first responder may give care from near the beginning of stage two or even later in stage two or stage three.

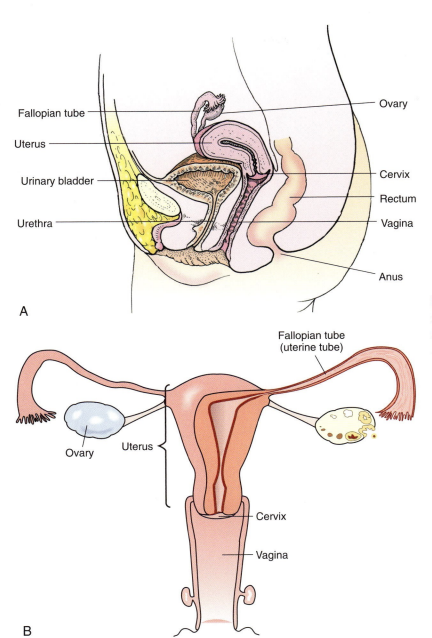

Fig. 13-1 Organs of the female reproductive system. (From McSwain N, Paturas J: *The basic EMT: comprehensive prehospital patient care,* 2003 ed 2, St Louis, 2003, Mosby.)

CAUTION!

False labor (or Braxton Hicks contractions) is a term used for irregular contractions that may be felt at any time during pregnancy but especially during the last month. These contractions are a result of the uterus changing shape and size in preparation for delivery of the fetus. It may be difficult to determine whether a mother is in false or true labor but in either case, as an emergency first responder, you should call 9-1-1 and arrange for Emergency Medical Services (EMS) to transport the mother to the hospital.

First Stage

The first stage of labor begins with the first **contraction** and ends when the cervix is fully dilated. A contraction is the hardening and tightening of the uterus or a muscular movement of the uterus. True contractions occur at regular intervals, which shorten as the fetus moves through the birth canal. Contractions are normally accompanied by pain; this pain and the intensity of the contraction increase as the time to birth is more imminent. Generally, contractions begin at approximately 30 minutes apart and become closer and closer until they are less than 3 minutes apart. Contractions are usually timed from the onset of the contraction until relaxation occurs.

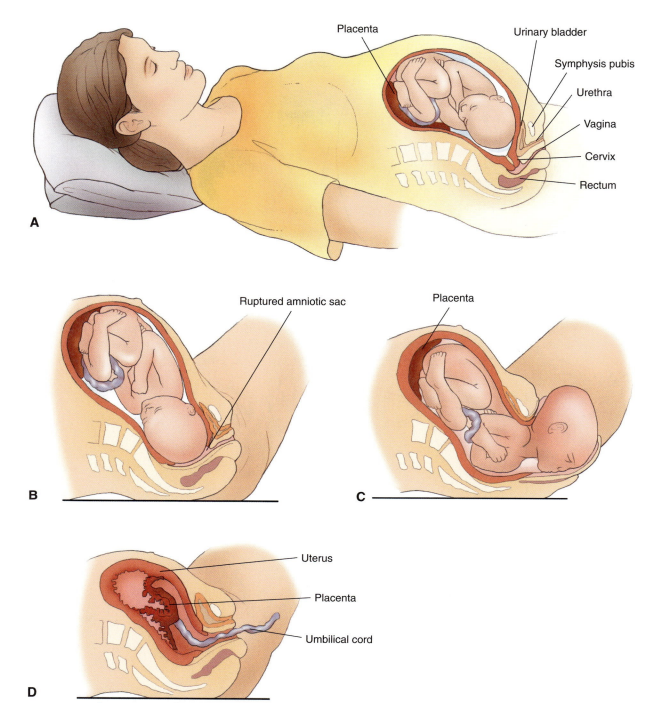

Fig. 13-2 A, The relationship of the fetus to the mother. **B,** The first stage of labor begins with the onset of contractions and ends with dilation of the cervix. **C,** The second stage of labor begins with the fully dilated cervix and ends with delivery of the infant. **D,** The third stage of labor begins with the delivery of the infant and ends with the delivery of the placenta. (From McSwain N, Paturas J: *The basic EMT: comprehensive prehospital patient care,* ed 2, St Louis, 2003, Mosby.)

This is called **contraction time. Interval time** is the time between contractions.

During the first stage of labor, vaginal discharge normally includes thin, bloody mucus and thin, bloody fluid.

Second Stage

The second stage of labor begins with the full dilation (opening) of the cervix and ends with the delivery of the baby. During this stage, the infant's head enters the vagina (birth canal). This increases the pain felt by the mother and also gives her the urge to bear down or feel as if she needs to move her bowels.

The part of the infant that appears first at the vaginal opening is called the **presenting part.** During a normal delivery the baby's head is the presenting part.

Third Stage

The third stage of labor starts after the baby is delivered and ends after the placenta (or afterbirth) is expelled from the mother's body.

Delivery

If you are called to assist a mother in the delivery of her baby, you and she first have to decide if you will need to deliver the baby at the scene or if there is time for the mother to reach the hospital. As birth nears, contractions will begin to last longer (up to 90 seconds) and become more intense. There will also be a shorter interval time between contractions. However, contractions are not always regular and evenly spaced, and the presence of contractions is not by itself a good indicator of whether the delivery is imminent. Several other indicators can also help you determine if delivery is imminent and may occur at the scene. You will need to ask specific questions about the mother's pregnancy and labor process during your SAMPLE history and perform a physical examination if necessary. Box 13-1 lists examples of specific questions for you to ask to determine if a delivery is imminent.

CAUTION !

When the baby's head passes through the **birth canal**, the mother's urge to push during contractions will be very strong. Do not let the mother go into the bathroom; the pressure she is feeling is the baby's presenting part, usually the head, in the birth canal. That pressure makes her feel like she needs to have a bowel movement.

If the patient is having contractions that are 3 minutes are less apart, states she needs to push or feels like she has to have a bowel movement, or has bloody show, or if the amniotic sac has ruptured, you should consider performing a visual inspection of the mother's perineum. A visual inspection is done by first having the patient lie on her back. You should then elevate her hips with some padding.

> **BOX 13-1   Questions to Help Determine If Delivery Is Imminent**
>
> - *Are you bleeding or having other kinds of vaginal discharge (bloody show)?* This may indicate the onset of labor or indicate a problem with the pregnancy if the bleeding or discharge is not normal.
> - *Do you feel like you need to have a bowel movement?* This indicates the infant has moved down into the birth canal.
> - *Do you feel increasing pressure in your vaginal area?* This indicates the infant has moved down into the birth canal.
> - *What is your due date?* It is important to note how far along in the pregnancy the mother is, not only to determine if the baby is ready to be born, but also to anticipate care of the newborn.
> - *Is there any chance of a multiple birth?* It is important to note in advance whether more than one baby is expected so that additional resources can be requested.
> - *Is this your first pregnancy?* Typically, labor for a first pregnancy lasts approximately 16 hours. This time is typically shortened with subsequent deliveries.
> - *How long have you been having contractions?* Contractions will increase in duration and intensity over time and as birth gets closer.
> - *How far apart are your contractions?* As birth is more imminent, the interval time will be shorter.
> - *Has your water broken (has the amniotic sac ruptured)?* If the membranes have ruptured, this means that birth may be imminent.

Her knees should be bent and the feet flat on the floor, and the knees should be spread apart for a visual inspection. Protecting the patient's modesty and privacy is essential. If after removing her undergarments you see that **bulging** of the vaginal opening or **crowning** is present, you will need to prepare for immediate delivery.

If possible, have another emergency first responder present when you perform a visual inspection to deter-

Fig. 13-3 Types of breech presentations. (From McSwain N, Paturas J: *The basic EMT: comprehensive prehospital patient care,* ed 2, St Louis, 2003, Mosby.)

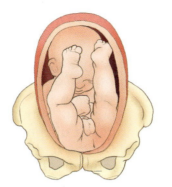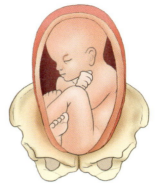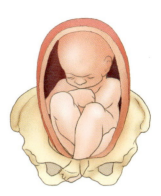

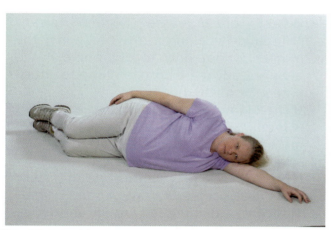

Fig. 13-4 Position a pregnant patient in the left lateral recumbent position.

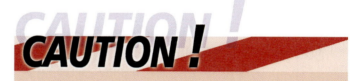

CAUTION!

Never hold or force the mother's legs together to try to prevent or delay delivery. This can be harmful or even cause death to the infant or mother.

mine if delivery is imminent. You should touch the vaginal area only during delivery and only when your partner is present. If you see bulging of the perineum or the baby's head at the vaginal opening, delivery is imminent. The term for the bulging perineum or seeing the head at the vagina is crowning. It is important to check for crowning during a contraction or you may be fooled into thinking that you have more time before the delivery.

If the baby's head is not the presenting part (i.e., the first part to emerge at the cervix), it is called a **breech birth** or a limb presentation and will be a complicated delivery (Fig. 13-3). In either situation, be sure EMS has been called if you have not already done so, and update the dispatcher or responding emergency medical technicians (EMTs) on the situation. You should encourage the mother not to push, and do what you can to calm and reassure her.

Remember that even if you are called upon to assist with a delivery, the mother will be doing most of the

work. Your role is in part to be a calming influence for the family during this unscheduled event. Pregnancy and delivery of a baby often involve the emotional reactions of fear, excitement, and anxiety, and you will need to provide emotional support and coaching throughout the process of delivery.

If the birth is not imminent, you should provide emotional support for the mother and bystanders, call for help, and continue to monitor the mother while you wait for EMS. You should position the mother on her left side while waiting or preparing for transport because this position relieves the pressure from the uterus and fetus on the mother's circulatory system (Fig. 13-4).

Supplies for Delivery

For your protection and the protection of the mother and newborn, it is essential to use proper body substance isolation (BSI). For childbirth it is recommended that each provider use gloves, a gown, a mask, and eye protection. You should also have a commercially prepared obstetrical kit or assemble the items you will need for this task. These items should include the following (Fig. 13-5):

- Gloves, gown, mask, and eye protection
- Clean, absorbent materials including sheets and towels

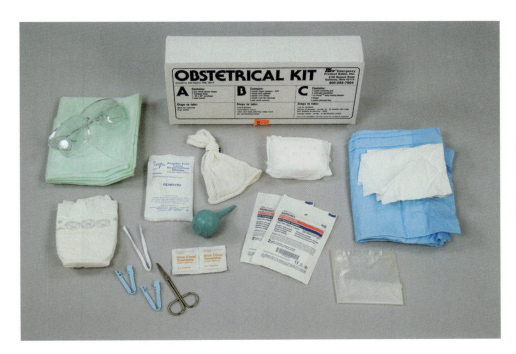

Fig. 13-5 Contents of an obstetrical kit. (McSwain N, Paturas J: *The basic EMT: comprehensive prehospital patient care,* 2003 edition, St Louis, 2003, Mosby.)

- Blankets
- Bulb syringe
- Sanitary napkins or bulky trauma dressings
- Scissors
- Gauze pads
- Rolled gauze, umbilical clamps
- Red plastic "medical waste" bags for soiled linen and disposable supplies
- Container for the placenta

Delivery Procedure

To prepare for delivery you will need to put on a gown, gloves, eye protection, and a mask and prepare your supplies and equipment to assist the mother with the delivery. You should try to provide reasonable privacy for the mother by asking unneeded bystanders to leave or have them turn their backs and look away from the mother to provide a privacy shield. You should have the mother remove her undergarments and lie on her back with her knees drawn up and spread apart. Provide help positioning her if needed. The mother's hips should be elevated by placing a small pillow or folded blankets under her buttocks, and clean, absorbent materials should be placed under her hips. A sheet should be placed across each leg and across the mother's abdomen (Skill 13-1).

As the baby moves down from the uterus into the birth canal, the mother's urge to push will be very strong. This is a natural process. Help her by reminding her not to arch her back. Her pushes will be more effective if she tucks her chin to her chest, grabs behind her knees, and curls her body forward. You can encourage the mother to hold her breath for 6 to 10 seconds as she bears down. Pushing for longer than 6 to 10 seconds can cause strain, rupture of blood vessels, exhaustion, and tearing of the perineum. The following steps outline the procedure for delivery once crowning has occurred.

CAUTION!

In some cases the umbilical cord may be around the baby's neck and can delay completion of the birth. It may even be wrapped tightly enough to prevent the baby from breathing. If you cannot loosen the cord, you will need to clamp and tie it and then cut the cord. To do this, clamp or tie the cord in two places a few inches apart and cut between the ties.

CAUTION!

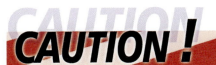

Remember that newborn babies are wet and very slippery! Support the baby around the neck and shoulders with one hand and use the other to firmly grasp the ankles and feet.

Skill 13-1

Normal Delivery

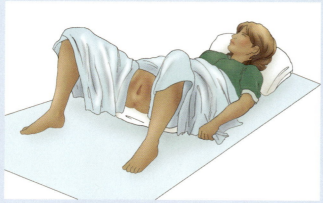

1. To prepare for delivery, position the mother on her back with her knees drawn up and spread apart. Elevate the hips with a pillow or folded blanket. Place clean, absorbent material under the hips and place a sheet across each leg and the mother's abdomen. (From McSwain N, Paturas J: *The basic EMT: comprehensive prehospital patient care,* ed 2, St Louis, 2003, Mosby.)

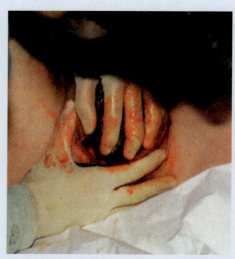

2. As the infant's head appears, place the palm of your hand on top of the baby's head and exert very gentle pressure to prevent an **explosive delivery,** in which the baby's head "explodes" through the birth canal quickly and causes extensive tearing at the vaginal opening.

3. If the amniotic sac is not yet broken, use your fingers to tear it and push it away from the infant's head and mouth. The baby's head is usually delivered face down.

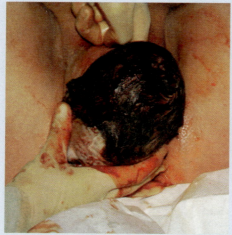

4. Support the baby's head and check around the baby's neck for the presence of the umbilical cord. If the cord is around the neck, instruct the mother not to push while you slide the cord down over the baby's shoulder or slip it up over the baby's head.

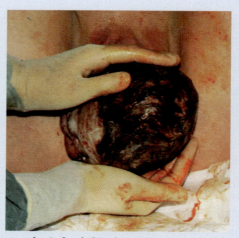

5. Support the infant's head as it rotates.

Skill 13-1

Normal Delivery—cont'd

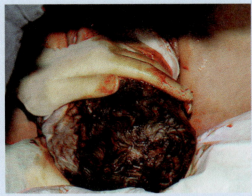

6. Guide the infant's head downward to deliver the anterior shoulder.

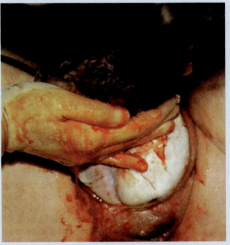

7. Guide the infant's head upward to release the posterior shoulder. (From McSwain N, Paturas J: *The basic EMT: comprehensive prehospital patient care,* ed 2, St Louis, 2003, Mosby.)

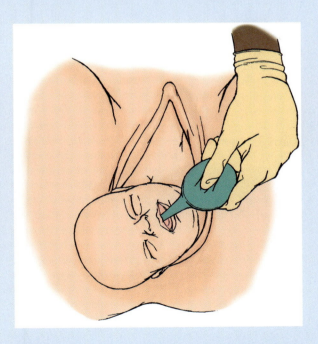

8. Suction the baby's mouth first and then the baby's nostrils two or three times with the bulb syringe. Hold the bulb syringe in your hand with your thumb on the large bulbous section so that it squeezes toward the narrow opening. Point the bulb syringe away from the patient, squeeze the air out, and hold it. Place the narrow end in the baby's mouth first; then release your thumb pressure. Point the bulb syringe away from the patient and squeeze it several times to eject the contents. The baby's mouth should be suctioned several times. This process is repeated with the narrow end of the bulb syringe placed in each nostril. Each nostril should be suctioned once or twice until reasonably clear. (Shade: Mosby's *EMT-intermediate textbook,* ed 2, St Louis, 2002, Mosby.)

Skill 13-1

Normal Delivery—cont'd

9. If you do not have a bulb syringe, the mouth and then the nose should be wiped with a gauze pad.

10. Support and assist in the delivery of the infant's shoulders. The rest of the baby will be born very quickly.

11. Once the infant is delivered, it is important to keep the infant at or around the level of the vagina until the umbilical cord has been cut.

12. When the umbilical cord stops pulsating you can tie it with gauze between the mother and the newborn. This is not a required procedure, and the umbilical cord may be left intact. The responding EMTs will have the proper equipment to clamp and cut the cord.

13. Wipe blood or mucus from the baby's mouth and nose with sterile gauze and suction the baby's mouth and nose again.

14. Dry and wrap the baby.

15. Stimulate the baby to breathe by rubbing its back or flicking the soles of its feet.

16. Position the baby on its side, with head slightly lower than the trunk, or place the baby on the mother's abdomen.

17. Record the time of delivery.

18. If there is a chance of multiple births, prepare for the second delivery.

19. Observe for delivery of the placenta. This could take up to 30 minutes.

20. When the placenta is delivered, wrap the placenta and approximately three fourths of the attached umbilical cord in a towel and place them in a plastic bag for transport to the hospital. If earlier you did NOT clamp and cut the umbilical cord, it should be tied and cut at this point if at all possible. If it is not possible, the baby should be kept at a level lower than the placenta to prevent backward flow of blood from the infant to the placenta.

21. Place a bulky pad over the vaginal opening, lower the mother's legs, and encourage her to hold her legs together. You should never place anything directly into the vagina.

In the Real World—continued

You check to ensure that the scene is safe for everyone. Your general impression of this woman lying on the ground is that she is awake and alert with an open airway and is breathing hard. You realize that she is in a late stage of labor and you ask someone to call 9-1-1.

You begin your care by asking questions to determine if you should help prepare her for transport or prepare to help deliver the baby in the park. Her answers lead you to believe that delivery is imminent. You get bystanders to provide privacy for her and tell her you need to look to see if the baby is coming. Your visual examination confirms that you will need to prepare for delivery here.

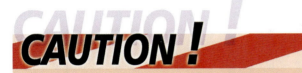

Never pull on the umbilical cord to hasten the delivery of the placenta. Over aggressiveness can cause life-threatening situations such as a torn placenta or uterine inversion.

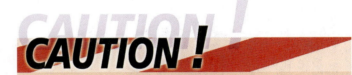

If the placenta has not been delivered by the time EMS has arrived, the EMTs will prepare the mother for transport.

Postdelivery Vaginal Bleeding

Vaginal and perineal bleeding is normal during and after the birth process. A mother's perineum tissue can tear during crowning and delivery of the head, causing moderate but not excessive bleeding. It is normal for the mother to lose between 300 and 500 milliliters (mL) of blood (from inside the uterus) after delivery. Do not be alarmed by this normal bleeding, but watch the mother closely for signs that bleeding is excessive (Box 13-2).

A new mother may be alarmed by the amount of bleeding. You should help calm her by reassuring her that the bleeding is normal. To help control excessive postdelivery bleeding and minimize the risk of shock, you can do the following:

- *Control bleeding by massaging the lower abdomen over the uterus.* You can ask the mother to massage her abdomen and you can assist her if she is unable. Uterine massage is done by placing the palm of your hand on the lower abdomen above the pubic bone and *gently* massaging or kneading the area (Fig. 13-6). The mother may experience slight cramping and a gush of blood as the massaging contracts the uterus. If the bleeding continues, you should check the massage technique because you may need to reposition your hands or change the intensity of the massage to stop the bleeding.

BOX 13-2   Signs of Excessive Postdelivery Bleeding

- Anxiety
- Changing level of consciousness or lethargy
- Rapid pulse
- Rapid respirations
- Bleeding that does not slow down or stop

- *Treat for shock.* If the bleeding continues, you should treat the mother for shock. You should provide the mother with oxygen if it is available and if you are trained in its administration. You should also try to maintain the mother's normal body temperature by covering her with a blanket.
- *Encourage breast-feeding.* If the mother plans to breast-feed her baby, you can encourage and help her to do so at this time because breast-feeding stimulates contraction of the uterus and may help control the rate of bleeding.

Postdelivery Care of the Mother

After the mother has delivered the baby, she will be excited but tired. Pregnancy, labor, and delivery of a baby evoke very strong emotions. It is important to provide psychological support for the mother and any family members and friends present throughout the birth and after delivery. After the mother has delivered, you should do the following:

- Continue to monitor the mother's breathing and pulse.
- Make the mother comfortable and monitor her for bleeding by replacing blood-soaked sheets, blankets, and pads with clean, dry ones.
- Maintain contact with the mother while awaiting her transport to the hospital.

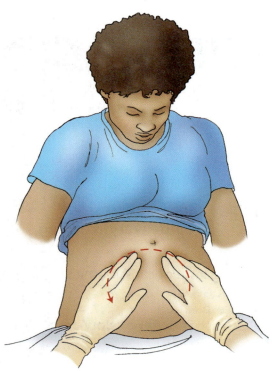

Fig. 13-6 To control postdelivery bleeding, you may need to massage the uterus. (From McSwain N, Paturas J: *The basic EMT: comprehensive prehospital patient care*, ed 2, St Louis, 2003, Mosby.)

Initial Care of the Newborn

Your initial assessment of the newborn baby is similar to that of any other patient. As discussed previously, during delivery you should clear the baby's airway and, once delivered, stimulate the baby to breathe (Fig. 13-7). Babies are bluish in appearance when first born and they begin to "pinken up" as their breathing becomes more regular. This is normal, and you should reassure the mother about anxieties she may have about her baby's appearance.

The most important steps in caring for a newborn are providing correct positioning, keeping the baby warm and dry by wrapping the baby in a blanket, placing the baby on the mother's abdomen, and continuing to stimulate breathing if needed. Following are the steps in the initial care of the newborn:

1. *Dry the baby*. It is important to dry the infant completely and keep the infant warm by wrapping the infant in a dry, warm blanket. Cover the infant's head to reduce heat loss.
2. *Clear the airway*. As soon as the newborn is delivered, clear the airway. Once delivered, the infant should be positioned on his or her side with the head slightly lower than the body. This position allows for drainage. As you did when the infant's head first appeared, you must wipe the mouth and then the nose with a gauze pad and, if available, use a bulb syringe to suction the mouth and then the nose (Fig. 13-8).
3. *Check for breathing*. Usually the act of drying the baby and clearing the airway will stimulate a newborn to breathe within the first 30 seconds of life. If the infant does not begin to breathe, you must provide stimulation to breathe. You can first try rubbing the infant's back in a vigorous yet gentle manner. If this does not stimulate breathing, you can flick the soles of the infant's feet. Once the infant begins breathing, you should check that

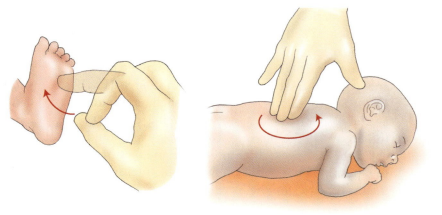

Fig. 13-7 After the baby is born you should stimulate breathing if necessary by rubbing the infant's back or flicking the soles of the feet. (From McSwain N, Paturas J: *The basic EMT: comprehensive prehospital patient care*, ed 2, St Louis, 2003, Mosby.)

he or she is breathing more than 40 breaths per minute and is awake and alert. Crying is normal for newborns. If the newborn does not begin to breathe or continues to have breathing difficulty, you should ensure an open airway and provide ventilation with the mouth-to-mask or bag-mask technique at a rate of 40 to 60 breaths per minute for approximately 30 seconds.

4. *Check circulation.* Check the newborn's circulation status by monitoring the pulse of the umbilical cord or the pulse at the brachial artery. The pulse rate should be more than 100 beats per minute. The baby should be "pinking up" in color. If there is no pulse, begin cardiopulmonary resuscitation (CPR). Chest compressions should be performed at a rate of 120 per minute, and 3 compressions should be given for every 1 ventilation. If there is a pulse, the action taken depends on the heart rate (Table 13-1).

The newborn should be assessed continually for the first few minutes after delivery. The APGAR scoring system is most commonly used. APGAR stands for **A**ppearance, **P**ulse, **G**rimace, **A**ctivity, and **R**espirations (Table 13-2).

Complications

Most unscheduled deliveries are routine and occur without problems or complications. Occasionally, however, things go badly during pregnancy, labor, or delivery. Problems can happen fast and be very distressing. Some of the problems that may occur include the following:

- Miscarriage or spontaneous abortion
- Multiple births
- Prolapsed cord
- A presenting part other than the baby's head

If a problem occurs, use the standard priorities for treatment. Conduct a scene size-up, call for additional help, perform an initial assessment, obtain the mother's history, perform a physical examination, and continue ongoing assessments. When those tasks are complete, you can begin to treat the specific situation as described in the following sections.

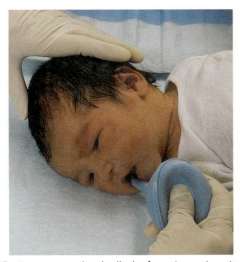

Fig. 13-8 Compress the bulb before inserting it into the mouth or nose. This removes air from the syringe so that it can remove the secretions. Do not compress the bulb while it is in the infant's mouth or nose or secretions will be expelled back into the mouth or nose. (From Murray SS, McKinney ES: *Foundations of maternal-newborn nursing,* ed 4, St Louis, 2006, Mosby.)

TABLE 13-1 The Newborn's Circulation Status and Appropriate Interventions

HEART RATE (BPM)	RESPIRATORY RATE	ACTION
>100	Breathing spontaneously	Continue to stimulate infant by rubbing back
>100	Inadequate breathing	Provide rescue breathing at a rate of 40-60 bpm and reassess after 30 seconds
60-80	Inadequate/absent after 30 seconds of rescue breathing	Continue rescue breathing
60-80	Inadequate/absent after 30 seconds of rescue breathing	Begin/continue CPR
<60	Inadequate/absent after 30 seconds of rescue breathing	Begin/continue CPR

bpm, Beats per minute.

TABLE 13-2   APGAR Scale

CATEGORY	0	1	2
Heart rate (bpm)	Absent	<100	>100
Respiratory effort	Absent	Slow	Good, strong cry
Muscle tone	Limp	Some flexion	Active motion
Reflex irritability	None	Grimace	Cry, sneeze, cough
Color	Blue, pale	Body pink, extremities blue	Completely pink

Miscarriage

For unknown reasons the mother's body sometimes rejects the developing fetus and expels the products of pregnancy. This is called a **miscarriage** or **spontaneous abortion** and it usually occurs before the twentieth week of pregnancy. Loss of the developing fetus can be emotionally and psychologically traumatizing for the mother and her partner. If you are called to the scene where a miscarriage has occurred, you should be prepared to offer comfort and psychological support in addition to physical care. The signs and symptoms of miscarriage or spontaneous abortion include bleeding, abdominal cramps or pain, and passing of pregnancy and fetal tissue. Following is the treatment for miscarriage or spontaneous abortion:

- Support the mother's airway, breathing, and circulation. Watch for bleeding and provide treatment for shock.

CAUTION!

If miscarriage or spontaneous abortion happens very late in the pregnancy, it can have a devastating psychological impact on the parents. Unless there are obvious signs of death, perform CPR, even if you strongly suspect that it will not resuscitate the baby. Your attempts may be your most compassionate offering (see Chapter 9).

- Save any passed blood or tissue for transport to the hospital.
- Provide oxygen if it is available and you are trained to use it.
- Arrange for transport.
- Provide psychological support.

Multiple Births

The steps for delivery of multiple babies are the same as those for a single birth. Most mothers expecting multiple-birth babies know this before the actual delivery and may tell you this when you arrive on the scene. Multiple-birth babies generally are more at risk for problems, and you should watch each infant closely for breathing difficulties and rapid cooling.

Things to remember with multiple births include the following:

- The mother is often not at full term when she goes into labor.
- Labor may not last as long.
- The babies often are smaller than a full-term baby, each baby typically less than or equal to 5½ pounds.

CAUTION!

When you assist in the unscheduled delivery of multiple-birth babies, you cannot know whether there is only one placenta for both babies (e.g., identical twins of the same sex), or a separate placenta for each baby (e.g., fraternal twins of either the opposite or the same sex). In these instances it is critical for the emergency first responder to clamp or tie *each* umbilical cord in two locations.

Prolapsed Cord

A prolapsed cord occurs when the umbilical cord is the presenting part in a delivery. The cord becomes pinched between the baby's head and the mother's birth canal, blocking the delivery of oxygen to the baby **(Fig. 13-9)**. You must quickly identify this situation to prevent harm to the baby. You should not attempt to push the cord

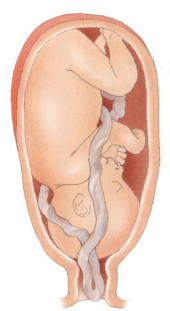

Fig. 13-9 Prolapsed cord. (From McSwain N, Paturas J: *The basic EMT: comprehensive prehospital patient care*, ed 2, St Louis, 2003, Mosby.)

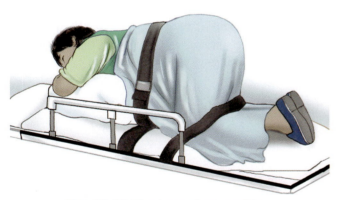

Fig. 13-10 The knee-chest position.

back into the birth canal but you should position the mother in a knee-chest position (Fig. 13-10). This position reduces the pressure on the umbilical cord. You should place wet dressings over the exposed umbilical cord, provide psychological support to the mother, and provide the mother with oxygen if it is available and you are trained to use it. Immediate transport is necessary.

Breech Birth

If the head is not the presenting part, it is called a breech birth. If the buttocks start to emerge first, labor and delivery may proceed normally; however, because the head is the largest part of the baby, it may take a little longer for the head to be born. In a breech birth situation, you should be prepared to support the infant during the delivery. If the head does not appear shortly after the rest

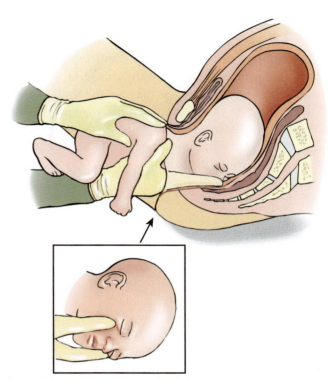

Fig. 13-11 During a breech birth you may need to create and maintain an airway for the infant.

of the body, you will need to create an airway for the baby. At the mother's next contraction support and raise the baby's body slightly upward to create a better angle for complete delivery of the baby's head. To create an airway while the baby's head is still in the birth canal, take the following steps (Fig. 13-11):

1. Support the baby's body on your forearm.
2. Do not pull on the baby to deliver the head.
3. Using the same hand that is supporting the baby's body, slide two gloved fingers into the mother's vagina and place them on each side of the baby's mouth. Rest your fingertips on each side of the baby's nose and bend your fingers slightly to create an air space for the baby as it tries to breathe. If oxygen is available and you are trained to use it, enrich the delivery area with blow-by oxygen. You may also help the mother by giving her oxygen.

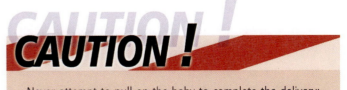

CAUTION!

Never attempt to pull on the baby to complete the delivery; doing so could harm both the baby and the mother.

If the presenting part is an extremity, this delivery will probably not occur out of the hospital. The mother will feel the urge to push, and all signs and symptoms will indicate an imminent delivery. In this case you must remain calm, and comfort and reassure the mother. Position the mother in a knee-chest position, place the mother on oxygen if it is available and you are trained to use it, and provide psychological support while waiting for her to be transported to the hospital.

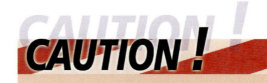

CAUTION !

In all situations with complications, remember that you have at least two patients: a mother and one or more babies. Abnormal deliveries can quickly escalate to emergencies; treat them accordingly. Be sure EMS has been called and continue to update the dispatcher or responding EMTs on changes.

Team Work

As part of the health care team, you may encounter additional complications of pregnancy. As an emergency first responder, it will be beneficial for you to understand some of these terms and potential complications to help you work with the mother and other advanced health care providers on the scene.

TOXEMIA

Toxemia is the term used to describe hypertension (high blood pressure) that occurs during pregnancy. These patients are usually confined to bed rest in an attempt to get the blood pressure under control. If the condition persists, the patient is at risk to develop eclampsia or seizures. This condition can be fatal for both the mother and the unborn child. These patients should be treated as any seizure patient.

ECTOPIC PREGNANCY

Occasionally pregnancies can occur outside of the uterus. Most commonly this occurs in the fallopian tube. When the fertilized egg implants in the fallopian tube, it will attempt to grow and develop in the tube; it will cause pain as it expands against the fallopian tube, and eventually the fallopian tube will rupture.

If you encounter a female patient of child-bearing age who complains of sharp abdominal pain, you should always suspect an ectopic pregnancy. Ruptured ectopic pregnancies can bleed profusely and result in death. Sudden onset of pain in pregnant patients should always be taken seriously and be evaluated by a physician.

PLACENTA PREVIA

In these patients the placenta is positioned over the opening at the base of the uterus, blocking the birth canal. This positioning prevents the infant from moving into the birth canal and therefore prevents a normal birth. If delivery progresses, the placenta may rupture, causing bleeding that can be fatal to both the mother and the child. The condition is characterized by painless, bright red bleeding without uterine contraction. Bleeding during the third trimester of pregnancy is an indication that placenta previa may be present, and the patient should be evaluated.

ABRUPTIO PLACENTA

In these patients the placenta abruptly detaches either completely or partially from the uterine wall before the birth of the infant. This detachment can be a result of trauma or can occur spontaneously. The amount of external bleeding may be minimal with these patients because much of the bleeding is concealed as internal bleeding. With this condition, pain is evident and is generally referred to as a "tearing pain." The condition may be fatal to the infant and the mother if bleeding persists.

PREMATURE BIRTHS

During the final weeks of pregnancy, the fetus undergoes important development of the respiratory system. A premature infant (an infant weighing less than $5\frac{1}{2}$ pounds at birth or born before the thirty-seventh week of pregnancy) may have complications attributable to the undeveloped respiratory system. These infants may need immediate artificial ventilation because they may be unable to breathe normally. Premature infants will also be more prone to hypothermia, so it is critical to keep these infants warm and dry.

In the Real World—Conclusion

With the help of another emergency first responder, using your combined first-response kits you take proper BSI precautions and assemble the needed equipment and supplies. You assist your neighbor in the normal delivery of a healthy baby girl before the EMTs arrive.

When the EMTs arrive, you assist them in transferring the mother and newborn baby to the stretcher. You provide your hand-off report, wish your neighbors well, and get ready to go home. Driving home you remember your emergency first responder training class. Helping a woman with an unscheduled delivery seemed a remote possibility back then, but now you are grateful that you learned about the process of childbirth. You are happy and confident that you assisted appropriately in your neighbor's delivery.

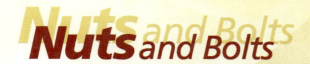

Nuts and **Bolts**

Critical Points

Remember that, in most instances, childbirth is a natural, normal process with few complications. Most deliveries occur in a hospital, at a birthing center, or at home under the care of a midwife or other attending medical personnel. If you are called to assist in a delivery, reassure the mother, prepare for delivery, assist the newborn in birth, and monitor the baby and mother for an open airway, effective breathing, and circulation after delivery. Remember that complications can occur, and when they do the situation can become very serious very quickly. Be prepared to act quickly and always remember to call for additional help immediately.

Learning Checklist

❑ The female reproductive system includes the ovaries, fallopian tubes, uterus, vagina, and the perineum.

❑ An egg is released from an ovary once a month and travels down the fallopian tube to the uterus. A fertilized egg will normally implant in the uterus to grow and develop.

❑ The fetus is linked to the mother via the placenta. Oxygen and nutrients pass from the mother to the fetus via the placenta. Waste materials are passed back to the mother from the fetus via the placenta.

❑ Labor is divided into three stages. The first stage begins with the onset of contractions and ends when the cervix is fully dilated. The second stage begins with the full dilation of the cervix and ends with the delivery of the baby. The third stage begins after the baby is delivered and ends after the placenta is delivered.

❑ It is important to ask the mother specific questions, such as the following: Are you bleeding or having any other kind of vaginal discharge? Do you feel like you need to have a bowel movement? Do you feel increasing pressure in your vaginal area? What is your due date? Is there any chance of a multiple birth? Is this your first pregnancy? How long and how far apart are your contractions? Has your water broken?

❑ Delivery is imminent if the mother is having regular contractions lasting up to 90 seconds each with a short interval time, if the mother feels the urge to go to the bathroom or push, and if there is bulging or crowning evident on visual inspection.

❑ A breech birth is when the presenting part is not the baby's head.

❑ Body substance isolation (BSI) to have during childbirth includes gloves, gown, eye protection, and a mask.

❑ Supplies to have on hand during childbirth include personal protection equipment; clean, absorbent materials (sheets, towels); blankets; a bulb syringe; sanitary napkins or bulky trauma dressings; scissors; gauze pads; rolled gauze; umbilical clamps; medical waste bags; and a container for the placenta.

❑ To prepare for delivery, provide privacy for the mother. Have the mother remove her undergarments and lie on her back with her knees drawn up and spread apart. The mothers' hips should be elevated with a small pillow or folded blanket under her buttocks and clean, absorbent material placed under the hips. A sheet should be placed across each leg and across the mother's abdomen.

❑ When the infant's head appears during delivery, gently exert pressure to prevent an explosive delivery. If the amniotic sac has not yet broken, you should break it. Support the baby's head and check around the neck for the umbilical cord, moving it from around the neck if necessary and possible. Suction the infant's mouth and then nose to clear the airway. Support and assist the delivery of the shoulders and the rest of the infant's body.

❑ Once the infant is born, dry and wrap the baby, clear the airway again, and, if necessary, stimulate the baby to breathe. Check breathing rate and circulation and resuscitate if necessary.

❑ When the placenta is delivered, wrap it in a towel and place it in a container for transport with the mother to the hospital. After the delivery, place a bulky pad over the vaginal opening, lower the mother's legs, and encourage her to hold her legs together.

❑ To help control excessive postdelivery bleeding, you should massage the uterus, treat for shock, and encourage breast-feeding.

❑ Postdelivery care of the mother includes monitoring the mother's vital signs; monitoring for blood loss

by replacing blood-soaked materials with clean, dry ones; and providing emotional support and comfort.
❏ Complications of pregnancy, labor, and delivery include miscarriage, multiple births, prolapsed cord, and breech birth.

Key Terms

Amniotic sac The "bag of waters" that surrounds and protects the developing fetus inside the uterus.

Birth canal During delivery this is the lower part of the uterus, the cervix, and the vagina.

Bloody show Blood and mucus discharged through the vagina; often the first sign of labor.

Breech birth A presenting part at the cervix other than the baby's head.

Bulging The "pushing out" of the perineum caused by the baby's head in the birth canal; this is a sign that delivery will occur very soon.

Cervix The muscular ring-like structure that forms the lowest part of the uterus; it shortens and dilates during labor.

Contraction The rhythmic tensing and relaxing of the uterine muscle that is critical for the expulsion of the fetus and the placenta from the womb.

Contraction time The time of a single contraction from the onset of the contraction until relaxation occurs.

Crowning The appearance of the first part of the infant during delivery.

Embryo The term for a fertilized egg for the first 8 weeks of pregnancy.

Explosive delivery An uncontrolled quick delivery of the baby's head.

Fallopian tube A tube that extends from each ovary to the uterus; provides a pathway for the egg to reach the uterus.

Fetus The term for the infant after 8 weeks of pregnancy and until the infant is born.

Interval time The time between contractions.

Labor The process of delivery from the first contraction through the delivery of the placenta.

Miscarriage Also called "spontaneous abortion," a miscarriage is the delivery of the products of conception before the fetus can survive on its own.

Ovaries A pair of almond-shaped organs located in the right and left lower quadrants of the abdomen of a female that function to release eggs and hormones.

Perineum The area between the mother's vaginal and rectal openings.

Placenta Structure in the uterus where nourishment and waste products are exchanged between the mother and the developing fetus; it is also called the "afterbirth".

Presenting part The part of the infant that appears first at the vaginal opening.

Spontaneous abortion Also called "miscarriage," a spontaneous abortion is the delivery of the products of conception before the fetus can survive on its own.

Umbilical cord An extension of the placenta; the actual structure that connects the fetus to the mother.

Uterus Also called the womb, a muscular structure where the fetus grows and develops.

Vagina Also called the birth canal, a sheath that encloses the lower portion of the uterus and extends down to the vaginal opening.

First Responder NSC Objectives
COGNITIVE OBJECTIVES

❏ Identify the following structures: birth canal, placenta, umbilical cord, amniotic sac.
❏ Define the following terms: crowning, bloody show, labor, abortion.
❏ State the indications of an imminent delivery.
❏ State the steps in the predelivery preparation of the mother.
❏ Establish the relationship between body substance isolation (BSI) and childbirth.
❏ State the steps to assist in delivery.
❏ Describe care of the baby as the head appears.
❏ Discuss the steps in delivery of the placenta.
❏ List the steps in the emergency medical care of the mother postdelivery.
❏ Discuss the steps in caring for a newborn.

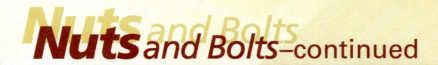

Nuts and Bolts–continued

AFFECTIVE OBJECTIVES

❏ Explain the rationale for attending to the feelings of a patient in need of emergency medical care during childbirth.

❏ Demonstrate a caring attitude toward patients who request Emergency Medical Services (EMS) during childbirth.

❏ Place the interests of the patient during childbirth as the foremost consideration when making any and all patient care decisions.

❏ Communicate by showing empathy toward patients during childbirth, and also toward family members and friends of the patient.

PSYCHOMOTOR OBJECTIVES

❏ Demonstrate the steps to assist in the normal delivery.

❏ Demonstrate necessary care procedures of the fetus as the head appears.

❏ Attend to the steps in the delivery of the placenta.

❏ Demonstrate the postdelivery care of the mother.

❏ Demonstrate care of the newborn.

Check your understanding
Check your understanding

Please refer to p. 439 for the answers to these questions.

1. A life-threatening condition in which a fertilized egg, implanted outside of the uterus, ruptures, resulting in severe abdominal pain and massive bleeding is:
   A. Prolapsed cord
   B. Placenta previa
   C. Ectopic pregnancy
   D. Miscarriage

2. The opening into the birth canal that dilates to allow for passage of the fetus is called the:
   A. Uterus
   B. Cervix
   C. Fundus
   D. Amniotic sac

3. List four indicators that should alert the emergency first responder to prepare to assist with the delivery of a baby at the scene.
   1. _____
   2. _____
   3. _____
   4. _____

4. When the baby's head can be seen in the opening of the vagina, either with contractions or constantly, this is called _____.

5. Appropriate BSI (body substance isolation) for assisting with childbirth includes _____.

6. The first part of the baby to emerge from the vagina in a normal birth is/are the _____.

7. A breech birth is when the baby's _____ or _____ emerges from the vagina first.

8. Describe the appropriate positioning for the mother in preparation for delivery.
   _____
   _____

9. As the baby's head begins to emerge from the vagina, the emergency first responder must control the emergence of the head by _____.

10. After the baby's head is delivered, the emergency first responder should clear the baby's airway by _____.

11. Before the umbilical cord is clamped or tied, the baby should remain at the level of _____.

12. The umbilical cord may be clamped or cut after it stops _____.

13. The newborn should be dried and wrapped in a blanket or towel because _____. When properly wrapped in a blanket, the only part of the baby that should be exposed is the _____.

14. Signs that the mother is having excessive bleeding following delivery include:
   _____
   _____
   _____

15. What are three ways in which the emergency first responder can treat excessive bleeding after delivery?
   1. _____
   2. _____
   3. _____

16. The loss of a pregnancy before 20 weeks of pregnancy is called a miscarriage or a/an _____.

17. List three special considerations in assisting with delivery for multiple births.
   1. _____
   2. _____
   3. _____

18. You are on scene of an imminent delivery when you see the umbilical cord protruding out of the vagina ahead of the baby. Your best course of action is to:
   A. Place mother in the knee-chest position
   B. Place mother in Trendelenburg's position
   C. Place mother in the prone position
   D. Place mother in the supine position

Check your understanding–continued

19. If a baby is born with the amniotic sac still intact, it will prevent the baby from breathing. The emergency first responder must _____ to remove it from the baby's face.

20. If the umbilical cord is wrapped around the baby's neck too tightly to slip over his or her head as he or she is born, the emergency first responder must:

    _____

    _____

    _____

21. If a newborn baby is not breathing or is only making weak efforts to breathe or cry, what is the first thing the emergency first responder should do?
    A. Stimulate the baby by rubbing his or her back.
    B. Start rescue breathing.
    C. Start CPR.
    D. Place the baby at the mother's breast to nurse.

22. CPR is indicated for a newborn when the pulse rate is less than:
    A. 10 per minute
    B. 60 per minute
    C. 50 per minute
    D. 100 per minute

23. In which of the following locations should the pulse of a newborn be checked?
    A. Inside of the upper arm
    B. The groin
    C. The wrist
    D. The neck

24. Which of the following descriptions of newborn appearance is cause for alarm?
    A. Body, face, and extremities are all pink
    B. Body and face are pink; extremities are slightly blue
    C. Body, face, and extremities are all blue
    D. Both B and C are cause for alarm

25. Match the terms with the correct definitions.
    A. Amniotic sac
    B. Birth canal
    C. Fetus
    D. Perineum
    E. Placenta
    F. Umbilical cord
    G. Uterus
    _____ A muscular structure in which the fetus grows and develops
    _____ Nourishment and waste products are exchanged here
    _____ The baby while still in the mother's womb
    _____ The actual structure connecting the fetus to the mother
    _____ Fluid-filled structure surrounding the developing fetus
    _____ Area between the mother's vaginal and rectal openings
    _____ The lower part of the uterus, cervix, and the vagina

Chapter 14

Infants and Children

LESSON GOAL

Infant and child patients challenge all levels of emergency care providers. A lack of experience in treating infants and children, the fear of failure, and concerns about legal issues can all cause anxiety when caring for an ill or injured infant or child. This chapter will familiarize you with the special issues and considerations important in the emergency care of infants and children.

OBJECTIVES

1. Differentiate between the anatomy and physiology of the infant, child, and adult patient.
2. Describe how assessment of the infant or child may be different from that of an adult.
3. Describe various causes of respiratory emergencies in infants and children.
4. Summarize emergency medical care strategies for respiratory distress and respiratory failure/arrest in infants and children.
5. List common causes of seizures in the infant and child patient.
6. Describe management of seizures in the infant and child patient.
7. Discuss emergency medical care of the infant and child trauma patient.
8. Summarize the signs and symptoms of possible child abuse and neglect.
9. Describe the medical-legal responsibilities in suspected child abuse.
10. Demonstrate assessment of the infant and child patient.

In the Real World

You are called to a scene where two children have collided on their bicycles. Heath is a 7-year-old boy with a significant laceration to his upper lip and multiple abrasions on his face and hands. The second patient, Kala, is a 5-year-old girl with abrasions on her hands and complains that her "tummy hurts." You note that both children are scared. You are the emergency first responder on the scene. You must assess the patients' conditions, treat their injuries, and prepare them for safe transport to the next level of care. You also know that you will need information about the scene, the patients, their parents. . . . You get started.

Sick and injured children are a unique patient population that requires special considerations in assessment and management. As an emergency first responder, it is important that you understand the anatomical, physiological, and developmental differences between infants, children, and adults. Through practice and continuing education, you should maintain a high level of comfort about working with pediatric patients. The **Emergency Medical Services for Children (EMSC)** is a nationally recognized organization that coordinates the development and implementation of educational programs and resources dealing with the care of children. The EMSC defines pediatric patients as those from birth to 21 years of age. Different jurisdictions may have different age limits to legally classify a patient as pediatric or a minor. This chapter focuses on the differences between infant, child, and adult patients and discusses special considerations in their emergency care.

Anatomical and Physiological Differences

Although children have the same basic anatomy as adults, they are far from simply being "small adults." In general, the following are true:

- *The variation in the sizes of infants and children can make assessment difficult.* It is important to realize that although guidelines are established by different age-groups, a 6-year-old patient may be the same size as another 9-year-old patient.
- Because of the lack of completely formed skeletal structures, muscles, ligaments, and tendons, *children are soft and can be easily damaged.* As an emergency first responder, you should not use excessive force or strength when treating a child.

- *A child's body surface area is greater per unit of weight than that of an adult.* This means that there is more surface area for heat to be lost in a child. A child may also not yet have fully developed thermoregulatory systems. Therefore children are more susceptible to heat and cold complications. This fact is an additional consideration and source of stress for pediatric patients who are already ill or injured.
- *Children are typically born strong and healthy and can compensate for many of the negative effects of illness and injury.* For example, children can increase their heart and respiratory rates in response to an increased need for oxygen, nutrients, or the removal of waste products. However, it is important to note that while this compensation is occurring, there may be few indications that a child is in trouble. This compensating ability can last only a short time before a child's body tires. Once this happens the child will *rapidly* begin to deteriorate.

Table 14-1 describes some of the relevant anatomical and physiological differences between pediatric and adult patients.

Family-Centered Care

One of the most dramatic changes in the prehospital environment is a focus on involving family members in the care of their children. This is called **family-centered care.** You may choose to use this approach in your care of infants and children. Imagine yourself as a pediatric patient or the parent of a pediatric patient. Think about what you would want to happen during this moment of crisis. Most patients prefer to have someone they know and trust with them during care, and this is especially true with children. Younger children may have violent reactions to being separated from their parents or caregivers.

TABLE 14-1 **Anatomical and Physiological Differences Between Children and Adults**

BODY AREA	DIFFERENCE
Head	• From the time of birth and for at least the first year of life, a child's brain is still developing. • Relative to the body, a child's head is proportionally larger and heavier. This makes head injuries one of the most common injuries in children. • An infant's skull has "soft spots." These spots (fontanels) provide a place where blood or other fluid can accumulate. A bulging soft spot may indicate bleeding or a buildup of fluid in the brain. A depressed soft spot may indicate dehydration or the loss of fluid from an infant. • The large occipital area of the skull causes infants and young children to assume a "chin-to-chest" position when placed on a flat surface. This may complicate airway control if it is not taken into consideration.
Airway	• The tongue is relatively large in comparison to the mouth. This can lead to airway blockage. • Positioning the airway in pediatric patients can be difficult because of the anatomical differences in the head. It is important to keep the head in a neutral position and not to hyperextend the neck. • The oral, nasal, and distal airway passages are smaller and quickly swell, causing an even smaller airway. • Infants and children tend to have more secretions, which can potentially block the smaller airway. • The short and narrow trachea makes foreign object obstructions a common problem in children.
Neck	• The muscles of the neck in a young child are weak and allow considerable movement. This can mean that it will allow more movement than an adult's neck, but it will also be more difficult to stabilize. • In the case of trauma, a child's short neck may make it impossible to properly fit a cervical collar. Other methods of cervical neck stabilization must be used.
Chest	• Children have a higher metabolic rate than adults, which requires more oxygen and nutrients. • Infants breathe through the nose almost exclusively. Therefore if the nose is plugged because of secretions or infection, the infant will be unable to breathe effectively. The infant may only be able to breathe through its mouth by crying. • Because the muscles of the chest are not well developed, infants and young children use their abdominal muscles as the primary breathing muscle. An inability to move the abdominal muscles, such as when the abdomen is constrained by gastric distention, straps, or restraints, will have a major negative impact on the child. • The heart, lungs, and great vessels are contained in a smaller area than in adults. This makes children more susceptible to major chest trauma. • The heart rate of a newborn is 140-160 beats per minute, compared to 60-80 beats per minute in an adult. When a child's body demands greater cardiac output, the heart rate will increase. In adults, the amount of blood pumped per beat (stroke volume) increases first and then the heart rate increases. A child's heart cannot increase the amount of blood pumped with each beat.

Continued

TABLE 14-1 Anatomical and Physiological Differences Between Children and Adults—cont'd

BODY AREA	DIFFERENCE
	• The bones of the chest have a higher percentage of cartilage at birth. As the child reaches puberty, the percentage of bone increases. Until then, the ribs are more flexible than an adult's and less likely to be fractured. This means that the internal organs of the chest may be significantly injured and there may be no external signs of injury.
Abdomen	• Because the abdominal wall is less developed, the child's internal organs in the abdomen are more susceptible to injury. This is especially true for the liver, spleen, and kidneys. • Children are often called "belly breathers" because they use their abdominal muscles to breathe. To assess breathing, it is easier to watch the abdomen than the chest.
Extremities	• The bones of newborns and younger children are softer, making them more flexible and more susceptible to fractures (the opposite situation of the chest bones).

Older children may become less cooperative. A common example is an asthmatic child in respiratory distress. If you remove the child from parents or caregivers, his or her anxiety often increases, and this typically causes even greater respiratory distress. On the other hand, sometimes a parent can create an environment in which you are less able to effectively treat the child. If a parent becomes emotional or agitated and interferes with your care of the child, you must remember that your priority is the patient.

Another challenging aspect of family-centered care is allowing the parents or caregivers to stay with their child during a resuscitation attempt. This may be important for the parents even though some providers may worry that the presence of family members increases the potential for legal actions if the outcome is not positive. Others believe the care the providers give may be compromised because of the family's presence. However, research in this area has demonstrated that neither of these concerns is generally true. Families who are allowed to view a pediatric resuscitation attempt are less likely to file legal action because they often leave the experience feeling the health care providers did everything possible to help their child. They leave the resuscitation with a greater understanding and appreciation of what was done for their child.

The third major aspect of family-centered care involves the care of children with special health care needs. More children with special needs are being cared for at home, many with complicated medical conditions.

This means that the parents or caregivers may have much more knowledge about their child's medical condition than you or other providers. As a professional, you should accept the knowledge and skill of others as you care for your patient.

As with other patients, when you work with children and their families your body language, verbal tone, and general appearance play a significant role in the overall outcome. As an emergency first responder, you should maintain a professional appearance, tone, mannerisms, and actions at all times.

Assessment

Assessment of pediatric patients requires special skills and knowledge. This section focuses on the different needs of infants, children, and adolescents during assessment.

Your assessment should begin when you first receive information about the pediatric patient. Starting to formulate a course of action before you reach the scene saves time that may be critical for the patient's ultimate outcome. You may learn whether a parent or adult family member is with the child. If one is not present, you will need to consider issues of consent for treatment. Use your judgment to involve parents in your assessment and management of the infant or child patient. Typically, if the parents are agitated the patient will be agitated, and if you can calm the patient you may calm the parents, and

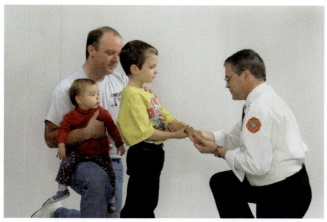

Fig. 14-1 When communicating with pediatric patients, get down to their level. Communicate with the patient directly if possible but involve the entire family.

vice versa. You should become familiar with the normal developmental characteristics to accurately assess infants and children. Table 14-2 describes the normal developmental aspects of pediatric patients and provides some tips on how to successfully intervene with them during your assessment. You should relate to children both physically and verbally at their level. You should never tower over them or talk down to them (Fig. 14-1). You should learn and use the patient's name and communicate directly with him or her, not just the caregiver, if it is age appropriate.

Primary Assessment

General Impression/Responsiveness

Begin your initial assessment by forming a general impression as you approach. A beneficial tool called the 20-foot rule states that a child who appears to be in a life-threatening crisis from 20 feet away probably is. A pediatric patient who is flaccid; is not interacting with the surroundings; has a fixed, glassy stare; and is silent or inconsolable is most likely critically ill or injured.

Responsiveness of the child should be immediately assessed using the AVPU tool (**A**lert, responds to **V**oice, responds to **P**ain, **U**nresponsive). The process for the primary assessment is the same for a pediatric patient as for an adult patient (see Chapter 8). The purpose is to assess and treat any life-threatening conditions.

Airway and Breathing

Essential airway management skills are described in Chapter 7. In this chapter, the emphasis is on differences related to infants and children. One of the differences between adults and children is that in general children have a higher metabolic rate and therefore a greater

demand for oxygen than adults. Children are also more sensitive to a lack of oxygen. Controlling the airway and providing adequate oxygenation and ventilation can mean the difference between life and death. Because of the anatomical differences in a child's airway, you will need to be gentle when performing the essentials of airway control. Proper airway positioning using the head-tilt/chin-lift or jaw-thrust method is a simple effective technique and may be all that is required to allow a pediatric patient to breathe. Remember to be gentle because you are much stronger than the patient. Infants' and children's necks lack full muscle development, and excessive force can cause hyperextension of the neck, leading to other problems including airway obstruction.

In a school-age or younger child, padding should be placed under the child to raise the body to an anatomical position. Because the **occipital skull** area is larger in young children, the natural position the child's body will assume when supine is "chin to chest." Padding from the shoulder to the lower torso usually eliminates this problem (Fig. 14-2). If you suspect a cervical spine injury, you should use padding that will not compromise any spinal immobilization efforts once the Emergency Medical Services (EMS) or ambulance personnel have arrived.

Chapter 7 describes the use of various airway adjuncts, including suctioning devices and oropharyngeal airways (OPAs). There are slight differences in technique for pediatric patients because a child's airways are smaller and more easily injured than those of an adult. For example, an OPA is inserted using the tongue blade method. In this method, the tongue is moved forward by depressing it with a tongue blade and the OPA is inserted in its anatomical position (Fig. 14-3). The type and technique for suction depend on the patient's condition and age. For example, an infant may require suction of the nose with a bulb suction (see Chapter 13), whereas an older child may require the use of a rigid suction catheter in the oropharynx (see Chapter 7).

When the airway is open and clear, you must check the quality of breathing. When hypoxia occurs in a child, the child's body compensates by increasing the respiratory rate and by using additional muscles to breathe. This increased effort can rapidly lead to fatigue, respiratory failure, respiratory arrest, and ultimately cardiac arrest. Signs of respiratory distress include the following:

- Increased respiratory rate
- Shallow breathing with minimal chest movement
- Head bobbing with each breath
- Gasping or grunting
- Stridor or snoring
- Retractions

TABLE 14-2 Developmental Stages of Children

AGE*	DEVELOPMENTAL ASPECTS OF A PEDIATRIC PATIENT	KEYS TO SUCCESSFUL INTERACTION
Newborn (0-3 mo)	• Normally alert, looking around • Focuses well on faces • Flexed extremities	• Likes to be held and kept warm • May be soothed by having something to suck • Avoid loud noises, bright lights
Infant (3-12 mo)	• Normally alert, looking around • Eyes follow examiner • Slightly flexed extremities • Can straighten arms and legs • Can sit unaided by 6-8 mo	• Likes to be held • May have separation anxiety • Recognizes parents' voices • Parents should be nearby • Examine from toes to head • Distract with a toy or penlight
Toddler (1-3 yr)	• Normally alert, active • Can walk by 18 mo, often earlier • Does not like to sit still • May grab at penlight or push hand away	• May have separation anxiety • Make a game of assessment • Distract with a toy or penlight • Examine from toes to head • Allow parents to participate in exam • Respect modesty, keep child covered when possible
Preschool (3-6 yr)	• Normally alert, active • Can sit still on request • Can cooperate with examination • Understands speech • Will make up explanations for anything not understood • May be uncomfortable around strangers	• Explain actions using simple language • May need to examine toe to head • Tell the child what will happen next • Tell the child just before procedure if something will hurt • Distract the child with a story • Respect modesty
School age (6-12 yr)	• Will cooperate if trust is established • Wants to participate and retain some control	• Respect modesty • Explain treatments and processes at a level child can understand • Be truthful; tell child when something will hurt and the true degree of the pain • Let child make treatment choices when possible • Allow child to participate in exam
Adolescent (12-21 yr)	• Has clear concepts of future • Can make decisions about care • Often expresses independence	• Explain the process as to an adult • Treat adolescents with respect • Respect modesty • Let adolescent make treatment choices when possible • Allow adolescent to participate in exam • Emancipated minors have right to accept or deny treatment

*Note that children who are frightened or in pain may act younger than their age.

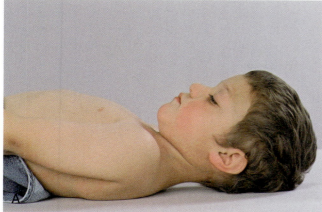

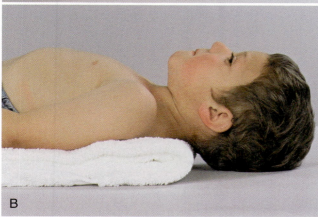

Fig. 14-2 A, Because the occipital skull area is larger in young children, the natural position the child's body will assume when supine is "chin to chest." **B,** Padding beneath the shoulders and torso will eliminate this problem. (From NAEMT: *PHTLS: Basic and advanced prehospital trauma life support*, ed 5, St Louis, 2003, Mosby.)

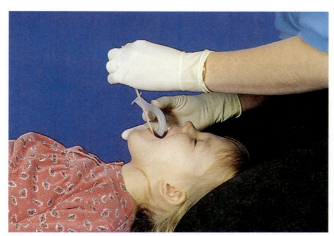

Fig. 14-3 The tongue-blade method is used in pediatric patients to insert an oropharyngeal airway. (From Shade B: *Mosby's EMT-intermediate textbook*, ed 2, St Louis, 2002, Mosby.)

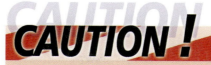

CAUTION !

As appropriate, let the parent or caregiver stay with the child throughout the assessment process. Remember that keeping the child and caregiver calm will help improve the patient's outcome.

If the child is having difficulty breathing, and if you are trained to do so, you can provide him or her with supplemental oxygen (Box 14-1). If the patient is not breathing, rescue breaths should be given at a rate of 12 to 20 breaths/minute (1 breath every 3 to 5 seconds), for children up to puberty or approximately the age of 12 (see Chapter 7).

Circulation

In the initial assessment you should check the pediatric patient's pulse and skin signs and check for signs of external bleeding. In a responsive infant a brachial pulse should be assessed initially. If there is no palpable brachial pulse, the femoral pulse should then be assessed. If the infant is nonresponsive and has no palpable brachial pulse, chest compressions should be initiated (see Chapter 9). In a responsive child, either the brachial or the radial pulse should be checked depending on the size of the patient (Fig. 14-4). In an unresponsive child, the carotid or femoral pulse should be assessed. If there is no pulse or if the pulse is less than 60 beats per minute accompanied with other signs of poor circulation, CPR should be started immediately (see Chapter 9).

The skin should also be assessed for color, temperature, and condition. Capillary refill time may also be assessed in younger children. Signs of reduced circulation include pale or cyanotic skin, increased capillary refill time (>2 seconds), and cool and clammy skin.

It is important to realize that a pediatric patient has less total blood volume than an adult. Therefore any major external bleeding should be quickly controlled.

Disability

An infant or child's responsiveness can be rapidly assessed using AVPU; however, the more detailed Glasgow Coma Scale (GCS) score should be calculated if possible. The GCS assessment is similar to that described for adults in

BOX 14-1   Blow-By Oxygen

Supplemental oxygen can be given via an oxygen mask or a bag-mask device at a flow rate of 10 to 15 liters per minute (LPM). You should not force oxygen on a child who resists. Placing a mask on a child's face may increase a child's anxiety level. Anxiety can then affect breathing rate and ultimately the oxygenation of the child. Instead, you can ask a parent or caregiver to hold the oxygen mask near the area of the child's face. This will still increase the oxygen in the air that the child is breathing but will be less intimidating for the child. This is called passive oxygenation or blow-by oxygenation (see figure). A common technique used by some prehospital care providers is to place oxygen tubing through a hole in the bottom of a paper cup. The child is then allowed to hold the cup and make-believe that they are drinking from it. There are also commercially available devices shaped like toys that can be connected to oxygen. Either technique distracts the child and accomplishes the goal of providing additional oxygen to the patient.

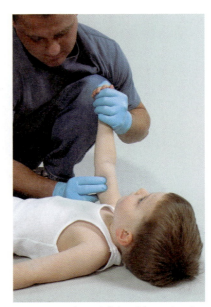

Fig. 14-4 In a responsive child, either the brachial or the radial pulse should be checked depending on the size of the child.

Chapter 8, but the verbal response section is modified for children under the age of 4 years (Table 14-3).

Priority

Most pediatric patients will not have a life-threatening illness or injury. Your assessment should focus on the most significant complaints and their likely causes. This process may be complicated by nonmedical issues such as the following common pediatric characteristics:

- Scared of strangers because of pain or the situation
- Crying, possibly inconsolably
- Moving excessively, "trying to escape"
- Inability to communicate or to communicate appropriately
- Failure to cooperate (e.g., will not follow requests)

If no immediate life-threatening conditions are present, or if they are quickly corrected, you should take a history and perform a physical examination on the patient.

The common signs and symptoms that a pediatric patient is in crisis include the following:

- Unresponsiveness
- Not breathing
- Breathing that is noisy: wheezing, stridor, croup, grunting

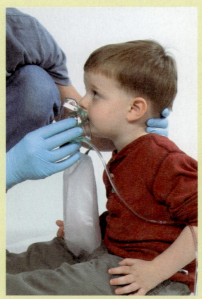

Blow-by oxygen administration.

TABLE 14-3 Glasgow Coma Scale (GCS) Score for Pediatric Patients

	POINTS
Eye Opening	
Spontaneous eye opening	4
Eye opening on command	3
Eye opening to painful stimulus	2
No eye opening	1
Best Verbal Response	
Appropriate words or social smile	5
Crying but consolable	4
Persistently irritable	3
Restless, agitated	2
Makes no response	1
Best Motor Response	
Follows command	6
Localizes painful stimuli	5
Withdrawal to pain	4
Responds with flexion to painful stimuli	3
Responds with extension to painful stimuli	2
Gives no motor response	1
Highest possible score	**15**
Critical patient	**≤13**

- Using accessory muscles to breathe: rib muscles, neck muscles, and stomach muscles; seeing retraction of intercostals, subclavicular, and substernal areas
- Flaring of the nostrils
- Bluish color or pale
- No pulse
- Excessive bleeding
- Pulses are too fast or too slow
- Altered mental status: "acting differently than normal," sleepy, unable to be comforted
- Change in muscle strength
- Uneven chest movement or expansion
- Failure to recognize parents
- Body temperature too high or too low

If any of these signs are present, this is a true emergency. Any life-threatening conditions should be treated as they are discovered and additional help should be requested without delay.

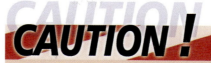

Even if a pediatric patient does not initially present as critical, it is important to closely monitor his or her condition. A pediatric patient's condition can quickly deteriorate and become critical.

Physical Assessment

With the more detailed physical examination (secondary assessment), it is sometimes better to begin with the child's feet rather than the head. This approach may allow the child to get used to you while providing you with critical information. Because young children (generally under the age of 2) use their abdominal muscles to breathe, you may see their respiratory effort better from near their feet. If a child has a palpable pulse in the feet, his or her circulatory status is probably adequate. The child may now be more accepting as you move to evaluate the face, head, and upper body.

First examine an area that is distant from where the child tells you it hurts. For example, in the opening scenario Kala says her "tummy hurts." Do not palpate this area first, but evaluate the rest of her and then the area around her abdomen. Avoid causing any more pain before you develop a rapport with the patient.

It is important throughout the physical examination to help maintain the child's temperature. Newborns and infants lose heat rapidly, especially from the head. They also may not be able to generate body heat to maintain their temperature. You should also support an older child's or adolescent's temperature. Providing a blanket or cover will offer more privacy to the patient.

Part of your physical examination may include taking vital signs. It is important to realize that normal vital signs for infants and children vary with age. As an emergency first responder, you should not try to memorize the average normal vital signs for children but carry a pocket guide or other tool that has this information. Table 14-4 outlines the normal ranges for the vital signs of different age-groups.

History

The detailed history may be taken at the scene or during transport if the patient is accompanied by a parent or

TABLE 14-4   Normal Respirations, Pulse, Blood Pressure

	AGE	RESPIRATORY RATE (breaths/min)	PULSE RATE (beats/min)	BLOOD PRESSURE* (mm Hg)
Newborn	Birth-6 wk	30-50	120-160	(74-100)/(50-68)
Infant	7 wk-1 yr	20-30	80-140	(84-106)/(56-70)
Toddler	1-2 yr	20-30	90-130	(98-106)/(50-70)
Preschool	2-6 yr	20-30	80-120	(98-112)/(64-70)
School age	6-13 yr	18-30	(60-80)-100	(104-124)/(64-80)
Adolescent	13-16 yr	(12-20)-30	60-100	(118-132)/(70-82)
Adult	>16 yr	12-20	60-100	(100-150)/(60-90)

*The normal systolic pressure in children ages 1 to 10 years can be calculated as 90 mm Hg + (child's age in years × 2) mm Hg. The lower systolic pressure in children ages 1 to 10 years can be calculated as 70 mm Hg + (child's age in years × 2) mm Hg.

caregiver. Communicating with the patient can be very challenging. Infants and children may be unable or unwilling to communicate with you. As an emergency first responder, you may have to rely on parents, caregivers, other family members, and bystanders for a history.

Reassessment

After gathering the history and performing a physical examination, give appropriate care. Continue treatments and make reassessments or ongoing assessments. Reassessment is a continuous process that includes repeating the initial assessment and the physical examination, and assessing the effectiveness of treatment. If the patient is stable and shows no signs of deteriorating, perform an ongoing assessment at least every 5 to 15 minutes. If the patient's condition is critical, repeat this process continuously.

Common Pediatric Conditions

Airway Obstructions

Foreign body airway obstructions (FBAOs) are more common in pediatric patients, especially in toddlers, for the following reasons:

- Children have smaller airway passages, which can be easily obstructed by swelling or food.
- The narrowest aspect of a child's airway is below the vocal cords.
- Children often eat while running, walking, or other active movement.
- Toddlers often place objects in their mouths to inspect.

In the Real World—continued

As you approach, the scene appears safe and without hazards. Heith, the 7-year-old boy, appears to be alert and coherent and has minor facial injuries. As you begin your assessment you quickly discover that he does not remember the collision or what has happened since. In addition, he is not able to tell you his address or birth date.

While you assess Heith, your partner begins assessment of Kala. She is alert and oriented and tells you that she hit her "tummy" on the handlebars when she collided with her brother. As you begin your assessment you discover that she has an abrasion on her abdomen and it is tender to palpation. Her pulse is 120 and her respiratory rate is 25 breaths per minute.

• Peanuts, hot dogs, and grapes (common causes of airway obstruction) are commonly given to children.

Partial Airway Obstructions

Once toddlers become mobile, they seem to remain in motion throughout their waking hours. Eating while moving increases the risk of airway obstruction. If the airway obstruction is incomplete or partial, the child is often found sitting upright, acting alert, and appearing scared or anxious. These children often have "noisy" respirations. Because some air is being exchanged, you may hear stridor (high-pitched inspiratory sounds), crowing, or noisy breathing. Look for chest wall retractions. Retractions occur when the patient attempts to take a breath. Because of the force needed to adequately inflate the lungs, the space between the ribs will be "sucked" inward. These are called intercostal retractions. As the patient has to increase the effort to breathe or becomes physically tired, you will also see an increased use of the neck muscles. Infants or children with partial airway obstruction may appear pink and have good peripheral perfusion because they are still capable of exchanging some air.

To treat an alert child with a partial airway obstruction, first determine if the obstruction can be removed by having the child cough. If the child can cough, ask him or her to keep coughing. If the child cannot cough, if coughing does not clear the obstruction, or if removing the obstruction does not clear the airway, you will need to take additional measures. In this situation you should allow the child to sit in a position of comfort. Do not force him or her to lie down. If oxygen is available and you are trained to use it, provide supplemental oxygen. If an infant, child, or adolescent with an obstruction becomes unconscious, immediately begin using the methods to clear a complete obstruction (see Chapter 7). This situation is a true life-threatening emergency.

Complete Airway Obstructions

For infants (younger than 1 year of age) you can confirm complete airway obstruction by observing inadequate respirations or an inability to cry. If a complete airway obstruction is present, follow the appropriate steps to clear the obstruction. The steps for clearing a complete airway obstruction are illustrated and listed in Chapter 7.

For children 1 year of age to adolescence, confirm a complete airway obstruction by observing for inadequate respirations or an inability to cry. You can ask older children if they can speak. If an airway obstruction is present and the child is conscious, follow the procedures illustrated and listed in Chapter 7 for complete airway obstruction.

For older children with a larger body size, the procedure for adults should be followed (see Chapter 7).

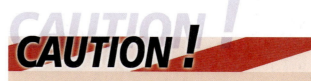

Be sure EMS has been called. Any child who has had difficulty breathing or has stopped breathing because of a foreign body obstruction must be evaluated by a physician to prevent potentially devastating consequences.

Respiratory Emergencies
Respiratory Distress

Respiratory distress is shortness of breath or a feeling of shortness of breath with labored breathing. You should assume a patient is in respiratory distress any time a child's respiratory rate is too fast or too slow or if the child appears to be working hard to breathe. Examples of possible respiratory distress include an infant with a respiratory rate of 70 breaths/min with retractions; a 4-year-old with a respiratory rate of 40 breaths/min and "noisy" respirations; and a 15-year-old with a respiratory rate of 30 breaths/min with wheezing. Although each of these has a different respiratory rate and associated problem, each must be treated and monitored closely. Table 14-5 lists respiratory rates that indicate respiratory distress at different ages.

Common signs of respiratory distress include nasal flaring during inhalation, intercostal retractions (between the ribs), supraclavicular retractions (around the collarbones), subcostal retractions (around the diaphragm), cyanosis, stridor, wheezing, grunting, and changes in

TABLE 14-5	Respiratory Rates Indicating Respiratory Distress
Infant	<20 or >60*
Toddler	<18 or >40
School-age child	<15 or >30
Adolescent	<12 or >25

*Breaths/min.

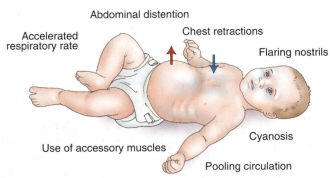

Abdominal distention

Accelerated respiratory rate

Chest retractions

Flaring nostrils

Use of accessory muscles

Cyanosis

Pooling circulation

Fig. 14-5 Common signs of respiratory distress in an infant or child. (From McSwain N, Paturas J: *The basic EMT: comprehensive prehospital patient care,* ed 2, St Louis, 2003, Mosby.)

mental status (Fig. 14-5). Each of the signs occurs as the infant or child attempts to make the airway bigger or to get more oxygen into the lungs. Each of these signs or a combination of them may occur in any child in respiratory distress. The more signs of distress observed, the greater the potential for respiratory failure or arrest.

A patient in respiratory distress should be helped into a comfortable position, often a sitting or tripod position, and provided with supplemental oxygen if it is available and you are trained to use it. Treat other life-threatening problems and ensure that additional medical help is on the way. Perform ongoing assessments, and calm and reassure the patient while waiting for EMS or ambulance personnel to arrive.

Respiratory Failure and Arrest

Respiratory failure is the inability to maintain adequate oxygen and carbon dioxide exchange. The patient may still be breathing, but the tissues are not being oxygenated adequately. **Respiratory arrest** means breathing has completely stopped. A patient in respiratory failure will progress into respiratory arrest unless life-saving treatment is started immediately. Respiratory failure and arrest often follow respiratory distress. Focus on the initial assessment and do not progress to a physical examination or history if the infant or child is in respiratory failure or arrest.

A rate of less than 20 breaths/min in an infant and less than 10 breaths/min in a child may indicate respiratory failure if other signs and symptoms are present. Remember the 20-foot rule in these situations. Children in respiratory failure may appear to be sleepy or even have a "death look" about them, may appear limp and unresponsive, and may be pale or cyanotic. Their eyes may be slightly open or closed and they may not respond immediately to your presence. If this is your general impression, the child is in critical condition and you should

begin treatment immediately. In your initial assessment you may find a slowed respiratory rate and heart rate. Immediate treatment and transport are imperative with respiratory failure and respiratory arrest. If oxygen is available and you are trained to use it, give high-flow, high-concentration oxygen with a bag-mask device. Rescue ventilations are usually needed because the patient has used almost all of his or her energy. If the child "fights" you during assisted ventilation, stop and switch to passive oxygenation using the pediatric bag-mask or a nonrebreather mask held several inches away from the child's face. If you do not have a bag-mask device, nonrebreather mask, or oxygen, use a barrier mask or device and provide ventilations. A child in respiratory arrest must be ventilated to provide a chance for recovery. Recall from Chapter 8 that cardiac arrest usually occurs in pediatric patients as a result of respiratory arrest. Although any respiratory emergency will be treated in the same way, the following are some specific conditions that may cause respiratory distress and consequently respiratory failure or arrest.

Asthma

A common cause of respiratory distress and failure in infants and children is **asthma.** Asthma affects more than 5 million children in the United States alone and is the most common chronic childhood illness (Centers for Disease Control and Prevention, Factbook, 2001). Asthma is an obstructive respiratory condition characterized by recurring attacks of difficulty breathing, coughing, and wheezing caused by constriction of the air passages in the lungs. Asthma attacks occur when the airway reacts to an allergen, similar to an allergic reaction. Ask asthma patients or their parents for information about their treatment and any medication they may be taking. Since asthma can be a manageable condition, a call for medical help signifies a serious situation.

Croup

Croup is a viral infection that usually affects infants and children 3 months to 3 years of age. A patient with croup generally has had symptoms of a cold or upper respiratory tract infection that has progressed into upper airway obstruction and respiratory distress. A child with croup has a characteristic "seal-like" bark or cough that is worse at night. Croup seems to be more common in the fall and early winter months (Fig. 14-6, *A*).

Epiglottitis

Epiglottitis is a bacterial infection of the upper airway that usually affects underimmunized children as well as adults. Epiglottitis is rare but is a life-threatening emergency. It is characterized by drooling, a sore throat,

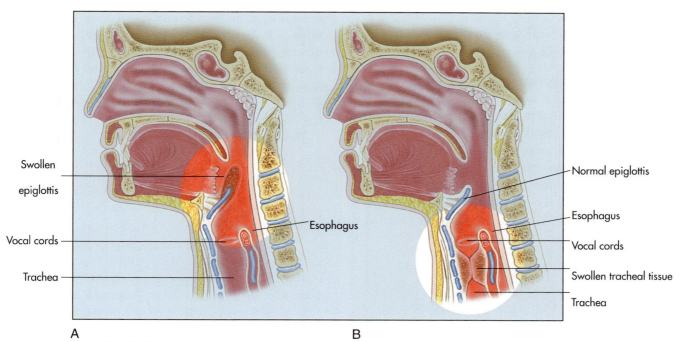

Swollen epiglottis

Vocal cords

Trachea

Esophagus

Normal epiglottis

Esophagus

Vocal cords

Swollen tracheal tissue

Trachea

A   B

Fig 14-6 A, Croup—note the normal esophagus size. **B,** Acute epiglottitis. (From Seidel H, Ball J, Dains J et al: *Mosby's guide to physical examination,* ed 6, St Louis, 2006, Mosby.)

difficulty swallowing or speaking, and a high fever. It is important to not examine the mouth or throat of a patient with epiglottitis because this may cause the airway to swell completely shut. The child should be transported as quickly as possible to the nearest hospital (**Fig. 14-6, B**).

Circulatory Failure (Shock)

Circulatory failure is the failure of the cardiovascular system to supply the body's cells with enough oxygenated blood to meet metabolic demands. Another name for circulatory failure is shock. The most common cause of shock in children is hypovolemia from either loss of blood or dehydration (loss of fluids). Although this complication is not unique to children, there are specials concerns for this population.

As with respiratory failure, use the 20-foot rule. Children in shock may appear to be sleepy or even have a "death look" about them, may appear limp and unresponsive, and may be pale or cyanotic. Their eyes may be slightly open or closed and they may not respond immediately to your presence. If this is your general impression, the child is in critical condition and must be treated immediately. In the initial assessment you may find the child has a heart rate that is either rapid or slowed, a respiratory rate that is altered or irregular, and a mismatch in quality of central and distal pulses. If the child's heart rate or respiratory rate is above normal, this may indicate an early stage of shock. When the heart begins

to slow, the child is starting to deteriorate. To treat a pediatric patient in shock you should ensure an open, clear airway and provide oxygenation and assisted ventilations. Perform chest compressions as needed, as outlined in Chapter 9. You should keep the patient warm and monitor the patient's vital signs frequently. When ambulance personnel arrive, you should help prepare the patient for transport and provide a detailed report on the patient.

Seizures

Seizures, including seizures caused by fever, should be considered potentially life threatening. Seizures are sudden, involuntary contractions of muscles as a result of an electrical discharge in the brain. This may cause the patient's mental status and level of consciousness to change. Many people are familiar with grand mal seizures or convulsions, but there are many other types of seizures. An estimated 5% of children will have at least one seizure by the age of 6 years. In children, seizures are often caused by trauma, a lack of oxygen (hypoxia), low blood sugar (hypoglycemia), fever (febrile state), and certain diseases.

Febrile seizures, caused by a *rapidly* rising body temperature, are probably the most common form of seizure in children. Febrile seizures usually last less than 15 minutes and are not associated with long-term brain injury or a disease process. The best course of action is to follow the steps listed in **Box 14-2** for seizure

---

BOX 14-2   Care of the Patient Having a Seizure

- Use the jaw-thrust method to open the airway.
- Never stick anything into the patient's mouth to pry the jaw open.
- If the patient's mouth is open, suction any fluids or foreign bodies; then provide supplemental oxygen if it is available and you are trained in its use. If the patient's jaw is clamped shut, provide supplemental oxygen in the area of the mouth and nose. Even if it appears that the child is not breathing, some respiratory action may be occurring. Increase the oxygen available to reduce the patient's risk of hypoxia.
- Protect patients from injuring themselves. Place the patient on the floor, remove any sharp objects, and place soft padding under the head to reduce blows against a solid floor. Loosen or remove tight clothing, especially around the neck.
- Protect the child's privacy and ask strangers to move back.

BOX 14-3   Questions to Ask When Treating a Seizure Patient

- "Has the child ever had a seizure before?" If the answer is yes:
  - H"Does she (or he) have a seizure disorder?"
  - "What medications is she (or he) taking?"
  - "Is this seizure different from others she (or he) has had?"
- "Has the child been injured recently?"
- "Has she (or he) recently had any head trauma?"
- "Is there any chance she (or he) has taken any other medication?"
- "Is there any chance she (or he) has used drugs or alcohol?"
- "Is the child diabetic?"

---

management. In an attempt to cool the obviously hot patient, you may consider (in certain situations) re-moving layers of clothing down to the diaper or underclothes.

Seizures that last more than 10 minutes, or repetitive seizures in which the child does not completely "wake up" between the seizures, are called **status epilepticus,** or status seizures. Status seizures are a true emergency. Regardless of the type of seizure, the treatment is the same (see Box 14-2).

Attempt to get a complete history from the parent or caregiver (Box 14-3). Document all answers and relay this information to EMS personnel when they arrive.

After the seizure, conduct an initial assessment, gather the history, and perform a physical examination and ongoing assessments. Most patients will be sleepy or confused after a seizure. This period, known as the postictal phase, may last from minutes to hours. In addition to the medical care you provide, you should comfort and reassure the child. You should protect the patient from bright or flashing lights because patients are often extremely sensitive to light after a seizure. After the seizure, the child should be placed in the recovery position or in whatever position he or she seems most comfortable, and suctioning equipment should be kept nearby. Any child who has had a seizure needs to be evaluated by a physician, and you should ensure that a transporting agency is on the way.

Altered Mental Status

Altered mental status in a child is any state of awareness that differs from what is usual for the child. The best way to interpret whether a child's behavior is usual is to accept what the parent or caregiver says about how the child is acting.

The main causes of altered mental status in children include the following:

- Trauma, such as head injury and blood loss
- Hypoxia resulting from an obstructed airway or chemical exposure
- Ingestion or absorption of a known or unknown chemical or medication (poisoning/overdose)
- Drug or alcohol use
- Hypoglycemia (diabetes)
- Seizure
- Severe infection
- Heat exhaustion
- Dehydration

As an emergency first responder, your role will be to support the patient who has an altered mental status. Open the patient's airway and provide supplemental oxygen if available and you are trained in its use. If the patient is unresponsive and breathing and you suspect no trauma, you should position the patient in the recovery position to protect the airway until additional help arrives. If trauma is suspected, you should use a jaw thrust to maintain an open airway and keep the patient supine while maintaining manual stabilization of the head and neck.

Sudden Infant Death Syndrome (SIDS)

Sudden infant death syndrome (SIDS) is the sudden and unexpected death of an apparently normal, healthy infant, typically during the first year of life. The death usually occurs during sleep and with no physical or autopsy evidence of disease. SIDS is a devastating situation for both the family and the emergency first responder.

SIDS typically results in a call to a home where a child is found "not breathing." As an emergency first responder, you should first ensure the scene is safe. Sometimes a parent's extreme emotions can be misdirected into physical violence against the responders. As with any other patient, you should perform an initial assessment. You should ask the parents about recent history such as whether the infant has had a "cold" or the "flu" recently. The parents or caregivers may have checked on the infant very recently without noticing anything unusual. Comfort, calm, and reassure the parents while waiting for the arrival of additional EMS personnel. You should attempt to resuscitate the patient unless the infant is obviously stiff. In a SIDS situation, the parents are usually in great emotional distress and you should be careful not to make any comments that might suggest they are in any way to blame.

An infant still in the crib may have bruised areas on the parts of the body in contact with the bed. This is called postmortem lividity, which is caused by venous blood pooling because of gravity after death. Postmortem lividity is normal and not a sign of abuse. Blood-tinged fluids may be present about the mouth and nose. If the infant has been dead more than 30 minutes, the body may be cold to the touch and have rigor mortis or stiffness of the muscles. But if the child was found soon after the heart stopped, follow full resuscitation procedures and perform CPR as described in Chapter 9. The infant's only chance for survival is prompt resuscitation.

You should know that despite prompt and effective resuscitation, an infant found not breathing and without a heartbeat will likely not survive. According to the National Center for Health Statistics, approximately 4500 infants die every year from SIDS in the United States.

SIDS cases sometimes involve a choice between two distinctly different courses of action. Some professionals suggest that rescuers should begin full resuscitation regardless of the patient's status and the parents' or caregivers' wishes. According to this school of thought, the parents or caregivers will be better able to mourn the death of their child and heal if they believe that everything that could be done was done.

The other school of thought is that if the parents or caregivers acknowledge that the infant has died before the rescuer's arrival, the parents or caregivers themselves are now the patients, not the deceased infant. If you start resuscitative measures in this case, you might give the parents or caregivers false hope, causing them to be devastated a second time. According to this school of thought, rescuers should respond to the parents' needs, including contacting clergy or other emotional support personnel.

No book can tell you which path to follow in any situation. As an emergency first responder, you should look at each individual situation and to your medical director, your local or state SIDS foundation, and local social services for more insight and information. You should find resources and think about this situation before you respond to your first "baby not breathing" call (Box 14-4).

An infant's death has a traumatic impact on everyone involved. In these types of situations it is critical to know and use your local critical incident stress management (CISM) resources (see Chapter 2). CISM teams often exist within the fire department or local hospital.

Trauma

Trauma is a leading cause of death in all pediatric age-groups. Each age-group is susceptible to certain types of trauma, but vehicular trauma is a leading cause of death at all ages. Your responsibility with pediatric patients, as with adult patients, is to treat life-threatening injuries first, care for non–life-threatening injuries, and ensure that your actions cause no further harm.

Specific types of trauma have typical patterns of injury. Unrestrained children in vehicle collisions often have head and neck injuries, while restrained children have abdominal and lower spine injuries. Infants in improperly restrained safety seats often have head and neck injuries. School-age children struck by vehicles typically sustain head, thorax, and extremity injuries.

Infants and toddlers are very susceptible to head injuries. A toddler who falls down a set of stairs most likely has a head injury. The toddler's head is proportionally larger than the rest of the body, making the child top heavy. If a child has fallen or was ejected, treat for a head injury until you can prove otherwise.

Neck injuries from falls are common in adolescents. Diving injuries have a mechanism of injury consistent with neck trauma and head injuries. Adolescents are also

BOX 14-4   Risk Factors for SIDS

Several factors have been identified that increase an infant's risk for SIDS.

1. **Tummy (prone) or side sleeping**
   Infants who are put to sleep on their tummy or side are more likely to die from SIDS than infants who sleep on their backs.

2. **Soft sleep surfaces**
   Sleeping on a waterbed, couch, sofa, or pillows, or sleeping with stuffed toys has been associated with an increased risk for SIDS.

3. **Loose bedding**
   Sleeping with pillows or loose bedding such as comforters, quilts, and blankets increases an infant's risk for SIDS.

4. **Overheating**
   Infants who overheat because they are overdressed, are covered by too many blankets, or are in a room that is too hot are at a higher risk of SIDS.

5. **Smoking**
   Infants born to mothers who smoke during pregnancy are at increased risk of SIDS. Also, infants exposed to smoke at home or at daycare are more likely to die from SIDS.

6. **Bed sharing**
   The safest place for an infant to sleep is in his or her own crib or other separate safe sleep surface next to the parent or caregiver's bed.

7. **Preterm and low-birth-weight infants**
   Infants born premature or with low birth weight are more likely to die from SIDS.

(Data from Centers for Disease Control and Prevention, Department of Health and Human Services, updated 3/15/08; accessed 7/24/08 at www.cdc.gov/SIDS/riskfactors.htm.)

commonly injured in organized sports. Head and neck injuries are common in football; extremity injuries are common in soccer and basketball. The mechanism of injury can help you determine any potential injuries.

In adults, some blunt trauma forces may be absorbed by the rigid structure of the rib cage and the density of chest soft tissues (muscles and fat). Younger children and infants have soft, pliable ribs and little soft tissue and are more susceptible to internal organ damage caused by blunt trauma. Trauma forces can move through the chest wall and impact the heart, lungs, and great vessels. This can cause life-threatening bruising or tearing of those organs. You should always look for signs of shock when you assess these patients.

Like the chest, the abdominal wall in younger children is poorly developed and easily transmits forces to internal organs. Blunt trauma can cause solid organs (liver, spleen, and kidney) to fracture and hollow organs (stomach, intestine, and bladder) to rupture.

According to the American Academy of Pediatrics (AAP) fires and burns are the fourth most common cause of unintentional injury-related deaths. Every year about 4000 children under age 15 die from burns. Burns can be more serious for children than for adults. Even a superficial burn like sunburn can be life-threatening for a toddler if it covers a large surface area. The loss of body fluid and the effects of dehydration can be serious. Burns to the face, hands, genitalia, and feet are considered critical because of their life-threatening or life-altering potential. Burns covering large surface areas and partial- or full-thickness burns are very serious for children. See Chapter 11 for more information on the treatment of burns.

Child Abuse and Neglect

Child abuse is defined as the situation in which a caregiver (parent, guardian, teacher, or other) intentionally causes a child physical or emotional injury. Child neglect is defined as the situation in which a child's physical, mental, or emotional condition is impaired or endangered because the parents or guardians fail to provide for the child's basic needs including food, clothing, shelter, education, and medical care.

About 650,000 cases of child abuse are confirmed each year and many more cases are unreported. As an emergency first responder, you will likely encounter child abuse. There are four types of child abuse: physical abuse, physical neglect (including medical neglect), emotional abuse, and sexual abuse. Sometimes the abuse or neglect is obvious; other times it is not. Whenever you feel uncertain about a child's situation, you should consider the possibility of abuse or neglect. Emergency first responders have a unique opportunity to assess the child's environmental conditions and the family's interactions for signs of abuse or neglect. You should maintain a high index of suspicion and should report any suspicions to the appropriate authorities as designated by your local protocols. Do not confront the caregivers with your suspicions. Table 14-6 outlines the signs of potential child abuse or neglect.

TABLE 14-6 Signs of Potential Child Abuse or Neglect

Environment	• Unsanitary conditions • Unsafe conditions • Lack of heat in cold weather or cooling in warm weather • Child wearing inappropriate clothing for weather • Parent ignores child or appears incapable of caring for child (e.g., intoxicated)
General impression of child (20-foot rule)*	• Thin to point of starvation • Stares blankly, does not interact with parent or emergency first responder • Appears fearful of parents
Initial assessment	• Child has signs of critical illness or injuries that have not been treated
History	• Inadequate or conflicting explanation for injury • No explanation for injury • Explanation for injury does not match physical findings • Explanation for injury exceeds child's capabilities • Accusation of abuse made by the child or an adult • Unexplained delay in seeking treatment for injury • History of previous injuries without reasonable explanation • Parents unconcerned about a major injury • Parents overly concerned or defensive about a minor injury • Parents' unpredictable schedules, frequent parental absences, or inappropriate supervision • Lack of routine well-child care • Vulnerable child: premature baby, child with developmental delay, child with special health care needs, or child of an estranged parent
Physical examination	• Multiple bruises of different colors • Old scars • Deformed extremities suggesting poorly healed fractures • Swollen or deformed ears (cauliflower ear) • Broken teeth • Bruising or trauma to face, including slap marks • Head trauma • Burns or bruises in unusual locations such as inner thigh, buttocks, or genitals • Scald burns, especially on hands, feet, or buttocks • Pattern burns that appear to be caused by a manufactured object • Multiple burns on hands, fingers, or genitals • Rope burns around neck, wrists, or ankles • Whip marks • Pinch marks or human bite marks

*The 20-foot rule states that a child who appears to be in a life-threatening situation from 20 feet away, probably is.

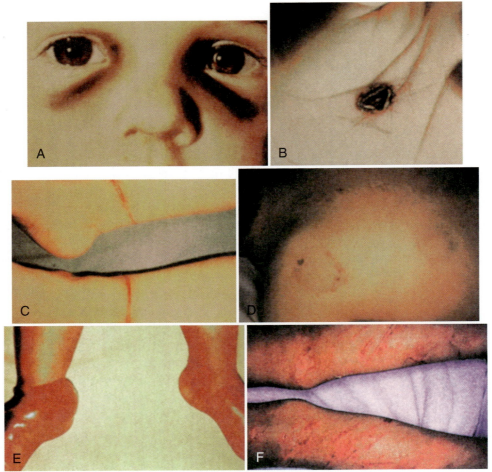

Fig. 14-7 Indicators of possible abuse. **A,** "Raccoon eyes" or bruising around the eyes. **B,** Cigarette burn to the palm. **C,** Abrasions from restraint injury. **D,** Human bites. **E,** "Dunking" burns to the feet. **F,** Welts and abrasions to legs as a result of abuse with an electrical cord. (From NAEMT: *PHTLS: basic and advanced prehospital trauma life support,* ed 5, St Louis, 2003, Mosby.)

If your initial assessment finds the child is medically stable, you should gather the history, perform a physical examination as appropriate, and conduct ongoing assessments. During the examination you should observe the child's skin for any signs of abuse or neglect such as burns, scalding, whip marks, bruises at different stages of healing, cigarette burns, bite marks, or severe diaper rash (Fig. 14-7).

Shaken baby syndrome is a specific type of abuse in infants and children under the age of 2 years. It occurs when violent shaking of an infant leads to severe head injuries, damage to nerve tissue deep within the brain, tearing of the veins between the brain and the skull lining, and rupture of retinal blood vessels. There may be no external evidence of trauma, and altered mental status may be the only sign of the injury.

As an emergency first responder, you may be legally required to report suspected abuse to a local authority. Understand your local laws pertaining to child abuse. As an emergency first responder, you should always report your suspicions in your hand-off report to another care provider.

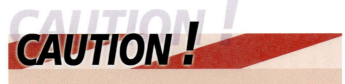

CAUTION!

Children, especially young children, seldom experience genital injuries. Consider genital injuries suspicious if they are unexplained or are inconsistent with the explanation from parents or guardians.

Team Work

One of the most important things that emergency first responders can do to affect the care of infants and children in their community is to become involved in injury prevention programs. Educating families to create a safer environment for children will decrease the number of childhood deaths attributable to illness and injury. Emergency first responders can provide education on some of the following subjects:

- Helmet safety
- Proper car seat and restraint use for children
- Smoke detectors and carbon monoxide detectors
- Childproof containers for hazardous household materials
- Storing firearms in locked containers
- Water safety (e.g., pools, beaches, and bathtubs)
- Escape routes in case of a fire
- Cardiopulmonary resuscitation (CPR)

The emergency first responder is in a unique position to see different patients in different environments. It is up to all emergency first responders to come together as a team to implement educational strategies and lobby for law changes to make the world a safer place for children.

In the Real World—Conclusion

Despite Heath's seemingly normal appearance, your assessment reveals that he has an altered mental status and signs of injury to his head. You reassess the scene and discover that Heath was not wearing a bike helmet. You know he needs to be evaluated at the Emergency Department and you call for immediate transport. Unlike her brother, Kala was wearing a helmet. Although she appears normal, the mechanism of her injury suggests she has a potentially serious abdominal injury. She too must be transported to the Emergency Department for further evaluation.

While you wait for additional EMS responders, you continue ongoing assessments and comfort, calm, and reassure the patients. You ask questions of the parents about the children's histories, allergies, and preexisting conditions. You and your partner prepare a hand-off report for the EMS providers.

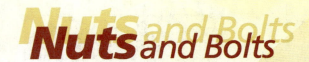

Critical Points

An understanding of the developmental stages and the anatomical and physiological differences in a child compared to an adult is vital to assess and treat pediatric patients. A child can compensate for illness and injury and can go from a seemingly normal state to a critical state very rapidly. The emergency first responder needs to recognize the importance of family-centered care with pediatric patients. It could make a difference in the patient's outcome. Recognize the signs of abuse and report your suspicions to the appropriate authorities.

Learning Checklist

❏ Emergency Medical Services for Children (EMSC) is a nationally recognized organization that coordinates the development and implementation of educational programs and resources dealing with the care of children.

❏ The variation in the sizes of infants and children can make assessment difficult. You should base your management more on the size of the patient than on the patient's age.

❏ A child's body surface area is greater per unit of weight than an adult's. This means there is more surface area for heat to be lost.

❏ Children can compensate well for illness and injury but this can only last for a short time. A child can rapidly deteriorate.

❏ A child's tongue is relatively large compared to the mouth, which can lead to airway blockage.

❏ Compared to an adult, a child has a shorter, narrower trachea and air passages; therefore foreign body airway obstruction (FBAO) can be a common problem.

❏ The 20-foot rule states that a child who appears to be in a life-threatening crisis from 20 feet away probably is.

❏ A pediatric patient who is flaccid; is not interacting with the surroundings; has a fixed, glassy stare; and is silent or inconsolable is most likely critically ill or injured.

❏ Signs of respiratory distress in children include increased respiratory rate, shallow breathing with minimal chest movement, head bobbing with each breath, gasping or grunting, stridor or snoring, and retractions.

❏ A brachial pulse should be assessed in an infant. The brachial or radial pulse should be assessed in a responsive child. The carotid or femoral pulse should be assessed in the unresponsive child.

❏ The following are common signs and symptoms that a pediatric patient is in crisis: unresponsiveness, no breathing, evidence of respiratory distress, no pulse, excessive bleeding, pulses that are too fast or too slow, altered mental status, and body temperature that is too high or too low.

❏ Using a toe-to-head approach to physical examination may be appropriate with children. This allows the child to get used to the provider.

❏ Examine away from the area that hurts first and then focus on the area that is injured.

❏ Common pediatric conditions include airway obstruction, respiratory emergencies, shock, seizures, and altered mental status.

❏ In children, seizures are often caused by trauma, hypoxia, hypoglycemia, fever, and certain diseases.

❏ Emergency care of a seizure includes opening the airway, suctioning the airway if needed, providing oxygen if available, protecting the patient from injury, and protecting the child's privacy.

❏ Causes of altered mental status include trauma, hypoxia, poisoning or overdose, drug or alcohol use, hypoglycemia, seizure, infection, heat exhaustion, and dehydration.

❏ Emergency care of altered mental status is mainly supportive. Keep the airway open and provide oxygen if available.

❏ Sudden infant death syndrome (SIDS) is the sudden and unexpected death of an apparently normal, healthy infant.

❏ Trauma is a leading cause of death in all pediatric age-groups. An emergency first responder's responsibility is to assess and treat life-threatening injuries.

❏ Child abuse is any situation in which a caregiver intentionally causes a child physical or emotional injury.

❏ Child neglect is any situation in which a child's physical, mental, or emotional condition is impaired or endangered because of failure to provide for the child's basic needs.

❏ Emergency first responders should maintain a high index of suspicion for situations of child abuse and neglect during their assessment of children and report any suspicions to the appropriate authorities.

Key Terms

Asthma An obstructive respiratory condition characterized by constriction of the airways.

Croup A viral infection that can lead to upper airway obstruction and respiratory distress.

Emergency Medical Services for Children (EMSC) A nationally recognized organization that coordinates the development and implementation of educational programs and resources dealing with the care of children.

Epiglottitis A bacterial infection of the upper airway.

Family-centered care Involving family members in the care of their children.

Febrile seizure A seizure caused by a rapidly rising body temperature.

Occipital skull The back part of the head.

Respiratory arrest The cessation of breathing.

Respiratory distress Shortness of breath with labored breathing.

Respiratory failure The inability to maintain adequate oxygen and carbon dioxide exchange.

Shaken baby syndrome A specific form of child abuse that occurs when violent shaking of an infant leads to severe head injuries, damage to the brain, and tearing of blood vessels in the head.

Status epilepticus A seizure that lasts more than 15 minutes, or repetitive seizures in which the person does not completely regain consciousness between seizures.

Sudden infant death syndrome (SIDS) The sudden and unexpected death of an apparently normal, healthy infant; typically occurs during the first year of life.

First Responder NSC Objectives
COGNITIVE OBJECTIVES

- Describe differences in the anatomy and physiology of the infant, child, and adult patient.
- Describe assessment of the infant or child.
- Indicate various causes of respiratory emergencies in infants and children.
- Summarize emergency medical care strategies for respiratory distress and respiratory failure/arrest in infants and children.
- List common causes of seizures in infants and children.
- Describe management of seizures in infants and children.
- Discuss emergency medical care of the infant and child trauma patient.
- Summarize the signs and symptoms of possible child abuse and neglect.
- Describe the medical/legal responsibilities in suspected child abuse.
- Recognize the need for emergency first responder debriefing following a difficult infant or child transport.

AFFECTIVE OBJECTIVES

- Attend to the feelings of the family when dealing with an ill or injured infant or child.
- Understand the provider's own emotional response to caring for infants or children.
- Demonstrate a caring attitude toward infants and children with illness or injury who require EMS.
- Place the interests of the infant or child with an illness or injury as the foremost consideration when making any and all patient care decisions.
- Communicate by showing empathy toward infants and children with an illness or injury, and toward family members and friends of the patient.

PSYCHOMOTOR OBJECTIVES

- Demonstrate assessment of the infant and child.

Check your understanding

Check your understanding

Please refer to p. 439 for the answers to these questions.

1. To gain the trust of a pediatric patient and minimize his or her fear, how should the emergency first responder position himself or herself in relation to the child during the assessment?

   _____

   _____

2. To minimize patient anxiety when assessing a pediatric patient who does not have an immediately life-threatening problem, the emergency first responder should start the assessment at the patient's _____, instead of at the patient's _____, as he or she would do when assessing an adult patient.

3. List five common signs of respiratory distress in a child.
   1. _____
   2. _____
   3. _____
   4. _____
   5. _____

4. List four causes of altered mental status in a child.
   1. _____
   2. _____
   3. _____
   4. _____

5. List five injuries that are suspicious for child abuse.
   1. _____
   2. _____
   3. _____
   4. _____
   5. _____

6. Often, the only indication of illness or injury is a decrease or change in the infant's _____.

7. Which of the following injuries is the usual result of shaken baby syndrome?
   A. Lung injuries
   B. Spleen injuries
   C. Brain injuries
   D. Broken bones

8. Which of the following is a leading cause of death in children?
   A. Trauma
   B. SIDS
   C. Infectious disease
   D. Birth defects

9. A child who is restrained only by a lap belt in a motor vehicle crash (MVC) is most likely to have which of the following injuries?
   A. Leg injuries
   B. Abdominal injuries
   C. Chest injuries
   D. Head injuries

10. In caring for an ill or injured child, which of the following actions is the highest priority?
   A. Allowing the child to bring along a favorite toy to the hospital
   B. Keeping the parents calm
   C. Keeping the heart rate at 100 to 120 beats per minute
   D. Managing airway and ventilation

11. Which of the following statements regarding differences in the physiology of children, as compared with adults, is correct?
   A. Children are unlikely to become dehydrated when ill.
   B. Children are not as prone to airway obstruction.
   C. Children lose body heat more quickly.
   D. The onset of decompensated shock is more gradual.

12. Which of the following actions is most appropriate for attaining proper airway management positioning in a child?
    A. Placement of a folded towel under the shoulders
    B. Hyperflexion of the neck (bringing the chin toward the chest)
    C. Hyperextension of the neck (tipping the chin up so that it points toward the ceiling)
    D. Placement of a pillow under the head

13. Which of the following statements concerning vital signs in children is correct?
    A. Blood pressure is higher than in adults.
    B. Breathing is slower than in adults.
    C. Pulse (heart rate) is faster than in adults.
    D. Body temperature is higher than in adults.

14. Which of the following should be done by the emergency first responder for an infant with a complete airway obstruction?
    A. Chest thrusts and finger sweeps
    B. Abdominal thrusts and finger sweeps
    C. Back blows and abdominal thrusts
    D. Back blows and chest thrusts

15. When should the emergency first responder perform a finger sweep on an infant with an obstructed airway?
    A. Only if the object can be seen in the mouth
    B. Only if the infant is still breathing
    C. After every attempt to ventilate
    D. Only if the infant's heart stops

16. Which of the following actions is appropriate for a child who has a complete airway obstruction?
    A. Blind finger sweeps
    B. Abdominal thrusts
    C. Chest thrusts
    D. Back blows

17. Which of the following is the most common cause of seizures in children?
    A. Poisoning
    B. Lack of oxygen
    C. Fever
    D. Low blood sugar

18. Sudden infant death syndrome (SIDS) occurs in which of the following age-groups?
    A. 6 to 18 months
    B. 0 to 2 years
    C. 0 to 1 year
    D. 1 to 2 years

19. When assessing a child it is important to remember that at a certain age children will make up "magical" explanations for things they do not understand. This commonly occurs in which of the following age-groups?
    A. Toddler (1 to 3 years)
    B. Preschooler (3 to 6 years)
    C. School-age child (6 to 12 years)
    D. Adolescent (12 to 21 years)

20. During the assessment of a 2-year-old child, which of the following behaviors would be of greatest concern medically?
    A. Trying to escape from the emergency first responder
    B. Showing fear of the emergency first responder
    C. Refusal to cooperate with the assessment
    D. Inattentive to environmental stimuli (people, noises, and other)

21. You are on scene with a near-drowning of a 4-year-old girl. She has been pulled from the pool and is breathing at 10/minute. What is your best course of action?
    A. Check a blood pressure.
    B. Apply oxygen via nasal cannula.
    C. Get a medical history.
    D. Assist ventilations with bag-mask device.

Chapter 15

Operations

LESSON GOAL

Being proficient in nonmedical operational skills is as critical as being competent in patient care skills. As an emergency first responder, you have learned the fundamentals of patient care. This chapter describes the operational skills required for all phases of an emergency first responder response. You must be prepared to fulfill your role in each phase and each type of emergency response.

OBJECTIVES

1. Differentiate the phases of a prehospital call.
2. Discuss the medical and nonmedical equipment needed to respond to a call.
3. Identify the major components of an Incident Command System.
4. Discuss your role in extrication.
5. List various methods of gaining access to the patient.
6. Distinguish between simple and complex access.
7. Describe what you should do if there is reason to believe that there is a hazard at the scene.
8. State the role you should perform until appropriately trained personnel arrive at the scene of a hazardous materials situation.
9. Describe the criteria for a multiple-casualty situation.
10. Discuss your role in the multiple-casualty situation.
11. Summarize the components of basic triage.
12. Given a scenario of a multiple-casualty incident, perform triage.
13. Identify signs of an event of terrorism and take appropriate action to ensure personal and crew safety.

In the Real World

You have just finished the second-shift roll call. You and the other state troopers in your squadron are standing behind your police cruisers with the trunks open. You must check your medical supplies and the automated external defibrillator (AED) as carefully as you check your weapon, your Kevlar vest, and your vehicle. You check the batteries and operation of the AED. You ensure you have adequate medical supplies for any emergency care you may have to render in the emergency first responder role. Soon your daily checks of your vehicle, medical supplies, personal protection equipment (PPE), and AED are complete.

Satisfied that you and your equipment are ready, you call dispatch to inform them that you will soon be at your assigned patrol area. Within minutes you are dispatched to a single-vehicle rollover on the interstate. You are told that the number of occupants is unknown at this time and that Emergency Medical Services (EMS) has been dispatched with an ETA of 8 minutes. You are less than 5 minutes from the scene. You will be arriving as an emergency first responder and you are confident and ready to assume that role.

As an emergency first responder, you are part of a team of specialists—specialists in rescue, law enforcement, fire suppression, hazardous materials, and confined space and prehospital medical specialists like other emergency first responders, emergency medical technicians (EMTs), and paramedics. To participate effectively as a team member, you will need to be familiar with prehospital operations. In this chapter you will learn how the call for aid is answered and coordinated.

Phases of a Prehospital Response

A typical prehospital response has the following nine stages:

1. Preparation for a call
2. Dispatch
3. En route to the scene
4. Arrival at the scene
5. Transferring the patient to the ambulance
6. En route to the receiving facility
7. Arrival at the receiving facility
8. En route to the station
9. The post-run phase

Emergency first responders usually are not involved in stages 6 through 8, which apply to other transporting personnel, so those stages are not discussed in this chapter. However, if you are involved in transport, you must clearly understand your local protocols and receive additional education in these stages as well.

Preparation for a Call

The preparation phase is the period before a call for aid. Preparation for response to a call includes the following:

- Inspecting supplies and equipment in emergency first responder kits or gear bags and in emergency vehicles (Box 15-1)
- Checking that mechanical equipment, such as the AED, is operating properly
- Making sure your vehicle is fueled, fluid levels are correct, and it is operating properly

As important as having your supplies and vehicle ready is your own preparation. You have a responsibility to yourself, your family, and most importantly to your patient, to be mentally and physically fit. Exercise and a balanced diet, as described in Chapter 2, are essential to physical and mental fitness. To be prepared, you must also practice the skills and review the knowledge you learned in your emergency first responder program.

Your vehicle, whether it is an EMS response vehicle, a squad car, or your own private vehicle, must be equipped to respond to any emergency call. You should always keep it stocked with both medical and nonmedical supplies and the medical equipment you are trained and authorized to use. Your Emergency Medical Services (EMS) system, following state and local regulations, determines the equipment you should have in the vehicle. Most EMS systems and other emergency first responder agencies equip emergency vehicles (e.g., ambulance, fire apparatus, and police squad car) with basic medical supplies.

BOX 15-1   Emergency Vehicle Equipment

- Basic supplies
- Airways and masks (barrier devices)
- Artificial ventilation devices
- Suction equipment
- AED
- Basic wound care supplies

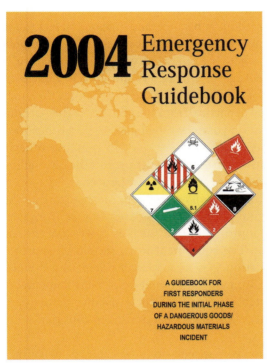

Fig. 15-1 The U.S. DOT *Emergency Response Guidebook.*

You should also have other personal protection equipment (PPE) such as gloves, gowns, masks, and protective eyewear. Your PPE may also include gear based on your work environment to assume your role in the rescue or extrication of a patient. Many state and local governments require emergency first responders to use certain PPE and safety equipment. Other supplies and equipment that are helpful include street maps, preplanned routes, patient care reports, the U.S. DOT *Emergency Response Guidebook,* a protocol book **(Fig. 15-1),** and flashing lights or flares.

As part of being prepared, you should know your role in the local EMS system. You may be the third pair of hands in the responding vehicle if you are an emergency first responder working with EMS or the fire service. You may have some other job, you may be a volunteer in your community, or you may simply happen to be first on the scene of an emergency. Whatever your role, you must be prepared to respond to an emergency at any time. You should be familiar with your local process for requesting additional resources and assistance.

Continuing education is essential at all levels of EMS. You may, for example, attend additional classes, conferences, or symposiums offered by hospitals, EMS services, and EMT associations. You can also increase your patient care knowledge by talking about patient care experiences with fellow emergency first responders and advanced care providers. All members of the response team must be aware of and adaptable to procedures in the rapidly changing field of prehospital emergency care.

Dispatch

Dispatch is a critical phase of emergency response. Most jurisdictions have a central access number, usually 9-1-1. In areas where this access number is not available (mostly rural areas), another well-publicized number is usually available to the public to reach the public safety system. The dispatch or communication center is staffed 24 hours a day with personnel who may be able to provide emergency medical instructions to the caller before EMS or emergency first responders arrive. This system may allow family members, friends, or bystanders to begin basic emergency care while help is en route. Many systems allow dispatchers to use computer-assisted dispatch (CAD) programs or Cardex systems to select the dispatch unit(s) based on patient information.

As an emergency first responder, you should receive detailed information from the dispatcher when you receive a call. You need to know the location of the patient and the mechanism of injury or nature of the illness. The dispatcher should also provide the caller's name, location, and call-back number. In systems with enhanced 9-1-1, the address and phone numbers are automatically displayed on the dispatcher's computer screen. Additional information such as the following may be provided at the time of dispatch or while en route: the number of patients, the severity of injuries, whether the patient is breathing or responsive, and other special problems or complications at the scene. Reviewing dispatch information and considering whether more resources, such as law enforcement or firefighters, may be needed should be a part of your initial scene size-up.

En Route to the Scene

You must arrive at the scene safely to effectively assist patient care. You should know and follow all state and local regulations and laws regarding the use of emergency warning devices. Following simple actions such as not running to the vehicle or to the scene will minimize your risk of injury. You should always notify the dispatch center once you are en route.

Safe driving is an important part of emergency response. Whether you are in your personal vehicle or an emergency vehicle, it is important to promote safe driving and not create an even greater emergency by getting into a collision. When driving, you should do the following:

- Wear a seat belt. Seat belts must be worn by everyone in the response vehicle.
- Pay attention to weather and road conditions.
- Keep your speed within your ability to control the vehicle. (Could you stop suddenly if it was necessary?)
- Reduce speed for curves.
- Monitor all traffic around you and note the following:
- Is crossing traffic stopping?
- Is the traffic behind you too close if you have to stop suddenly?
- Are you too close to the traffic in front of you if they were to stop suddenly?

If you are driving an emergency vehicle, it is important for you to know your local and state guidelines for emergency vehicles. At the very least, the law will call for you to exercise "due regard" for the safety of others in the operation of your vehicle. In effect, you are requesting traffic to yield to you and let you pass. Some motorists may not hear or see you coming and may dart in front of you at any moment. Plan to adjust your speed to your ability to stop when a vehicle cuts in front of you. With 1 out of 10 emergency vehicles likely to be involved in a collision, it is important to note that the majority of these collisions occur at intersections. Always wait for traffic to stop for you before proceeding through intersections.

The preceding list is just a few driving tips. Many departments conduct safe driving courses that include a practical session on a course. Specific training on driving emergency vehicles is available and can improve your driving skills specific to emergency vehicles.

In addition to driving safely, you should be sure you understand the nature and location of the call while en route. If you are not the driver, obtain additional information from the dispatcher to help prepare for your scene size-up. Write down as much information as you can from dispatch, assign specific duties, and consider special equipment needs. If possible, select and prepare the initial equipment you will take to the scene even if you only do it mentally. Planning ahead will save time at the scene. Take into consideration the time of day and usual traffic patterns when planning your route. Emer-

gency driving is tough enough without the distractions and frustrations of heavy traffic. Another driving safety problem can arise if you do not know where you are going. If you are not sure of your route, take a look at the map book or GPS before leaving the garage.

Arrival at the Scene

When you arrive on the scene, be sure to notify dispatch. As you approach the scene and before you step out of your vehicle, size up the scene and check that it is safe. Park your vehicle safely and appropriately at the scene. Safety considerations include parking uphill or upwind from any hazardous substance, and at least 100 feet (30 meters) from any wreckage or unknown spillage. Local policy will dictate whether to park the vehicle in front of or beyond the wreckage or spillage. Position your vehicle to allow room for safe loading of the patient into the ambulance and easy departure from the scene. Use the parking brake and turn on your warning lights to alert other vehicles of your presence. After dark, avoid blinding other drivers approaching the scene by turning off the headlights unless they are needed to illuminate the scene.

Remember, *safety first!* This means sizing up the scene *before* entering it and protecting yourself from harm. Put on the appropriate PPE, such as gloves, goggles, or turn-out gear. The equipment worn should be appropriate to the situation. If you suspect a potential for violence or danger, wait for additional help from law enforcement, firefighters, and/or EMS for assistance before approaching. The following is a list of risks to consider:

- Do you need body substance isolation (BSI) precautions?
- Is there a hazardous spill or vapor?
- Are there downed power lines?
- Is there fire?
- Is it safe to approach the patient?
- Is it necessary to move the patient(s) to remove them from some hazard?

Next, note the mechanism of injury or the nature of the illness. Determine the number of patients and whether it is a **multiple-casualty incident (MCI).** An MCI is a situation that overwhelms available resources. Additional resources and triage may be necessary if there are more patients than you or others present can handle. The principles of triage are discussed later in this chapter. After the scene size-up, you begin patient care with your initial assessment.

The emergency first responder is responsible for caring for the patient until the transporting agency arrives.

In the Real World—continued

While driving on the highway, you review in your mind the types of injuries expected from a vehicle rollover. You notify the dispatch center that you are en route and expect to be on scene in approximately 3 minutes. You pull up at a safe distance from the rollover and leave your emergency lights on as a warning to traffic. You quickly survey the scene: Is the vehicle on fire? Is gasoline leaking? Is there a downed power line?

You step from your vehicle, grab your emergency first responder kit from the trunk, and walk carefully down the slightly sloping shoulder of the roadway. There appears to be no fire, spilled gasoline, or downed power lines. As you approach the vehicle you repeat your scene size-up. You look to see if anyone has been ejected from the vehicle, count the number of patients, and determine if air medical transport is required. You see one passenger in the driver's seat and no one else in the vehicle. The vehicle is upright on all four wheels and the rear left door has sprung open.

Transferring the Patient to the Ambulance

Once the transporting agency arrives, the emergency first responder may be called upon to assist in activities varying from administering life-saving care to immobilization of the patient and physical transport to the transporting vehicle.

To help the transporting crew prepare the patient for transport, you should ensure that all dressings, bandages, and splints are secure. You should also cover patients to protect them from the elements and use the principles from Chapter 6 to assist the transporting crew in lifting and transferring the patient to the transporting vehicle. Be sure the patient is secured to the appropriate lifting and moving device. EMS personnel should be given a thorough account of the events from your arrival until their arrival.

The Post-Run Phase

After the run you should prepare for the next call by checking your vehicle's fuel levels, restocking supplies and equipment, and cleaning and disinfecting the equipment and the inside of the response vehicle. Once you have completed these tasks, you are ready for the next call and should notify dispatch of your availability. Complete and file all paperwork from the call as required by your service or agency.

Incident Command System

Disaster responses, multiple-casualty incidents, or any situation that calls for numerous resources to respond requires an organized system to manage the incident.

The standard for disaster management is the **Incident Command System (ICS).** The ICS defines a chain of command, lines of communication, and organization of efforts that allows numerous resources to be used in a coordinated response (**Fig. 15-2**).

Once a large-scale emergency is identified, the responder in charge of the scene should establish command, size up the scene, request additional resources, and begin triage. The structure of the ICS at an emergency will depend on the nature of the event. For instance, sectors responsible for fire suppression, triage, rehabilitation, and staging may be set up and all report to incident command (**Fig. 15-3**).

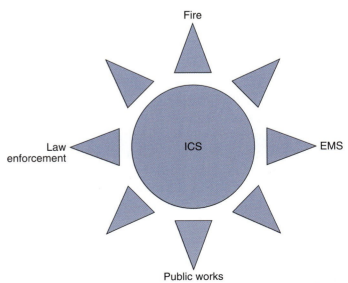

Fig. 15-2 Different sectors involved in an Incident Command System.

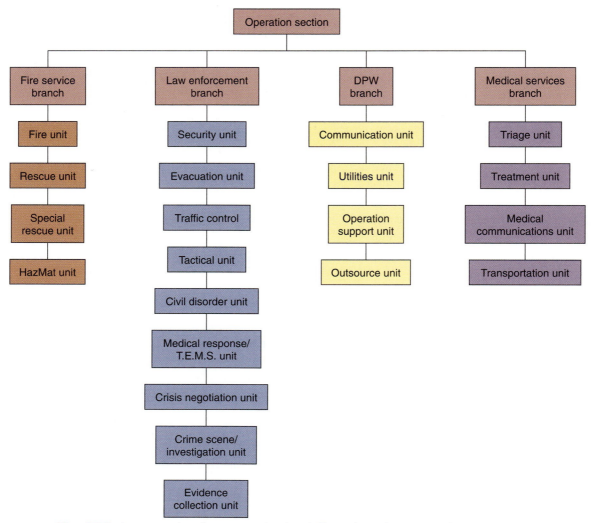

Fig. 15-3 An example of an organizational flow chart for an Incident Command System.

Within each of the sectors, commanders will direct the activities of personnel to specific tasks. For instance, the triage sector may request vehicles for transport from command; command will call upon staging to send vehicles forward to take on patients.

Some events do not require a variety of resources, but rather a number of responses from a single sector. For instance, a food poisoning outbreak will not necessarily require police and fire support but a large number of ambulances are a critical need. Incident command will make the requests to agencies to respond, assign them to a staging area, and coordinate transferring them to the triage area to pick up their patients.

Emergency first responders will most likely find themselves assigned to tasks within one of the sectors. Emergency first responders should know where they fit into their area's disaster response planning. In order to under-

stand and participate in an ICS structure, specific training is necessary.

An emergency first responder trained in incident command, when first on the scene, should establish incident command. When passing command to another with equal or higher rank and/or training, it will be important to report on the nature of the problem, the potential hazards, the number of patients, the time elapsed since the emergency began, and what has already been done. This includes the resources on hand and still needed.

Multijurisdictional or large-scale natural disasters or terrorist attacks call for an expansion of the ICS. The Unified Command System gathers command personnel from all of the agencies that will have to work together to provide a sustained response to a large event (Fig. 15-4). Emergency managers will bring together fire, police, public health, public works, utility companies,

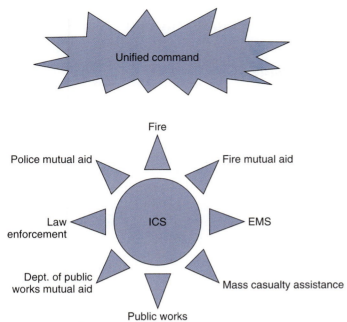

Fig. 15-4 Unified command system.

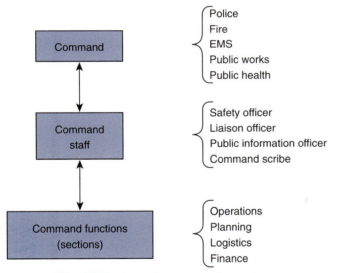

Fig. 15-5 Unified command structure.

and a variety of other resources into a combined command structure to coordinate the response to a catastrophe. Emergency operation centers can be in fixed locations or can be mobile (in which communications capabilities allow information to flow to and from operational divisions to command personnel) (Fig. 15-5). Planning and training exercises ensure that these diverse groups are able to work together to meet the needs of the situation.

National Incident Management System (NIMS)

In March of 2004, the **National Incident Management System**, or NIMS, was instituted by the Department of Homeland Security. NIMS serves as a national framework for response to mass casualty incidents, such as natural disasters or terrorist events. NIMS includes all levels of responders and all levels of government—federal, state, and local. All agencies are to be credentialed NIMS compliant per a governmental directive. As an emergency first responder, you will need to complete certain NIMS training courses set forth by the Department of Homeland Security to meet compliance regulations.

As you can imagine, at a response involving hundreds of patients and numerous agencies, it is imperative that all levels of response work together as an effective team. NIMS provides common terminology, resource classification, and a unified command structure. NIMS can be thought of as the ultimate example of interoperability. The major components of NIMS are listed and discussed in the next section.

Command/Management

- **Incident Command System (ICS)**—The ICS defines the operating characteristics, components, and structure of incident management organizations. ICS is discussed in detail below.
- **Multi-agency Coordination (MAC) System**—The MAC system defines the organizational structure of supporting entities when dealing with large or wide-scale emergencies. One common component found here is the Emergency Operations Center, or EOC. The EOC is a vital part of ICS in that representatives from responding or involved agencies, both public and private, are present to make informed decisions about such things as resource allocation.
- **Public Information Systems**—The public information systems described in NIMS are designed to effectively manage public information at an incident, regardless of the size and complexity of the situation or the number of entities involved in the response. The importance of the release of sometimes sensitive or time-critical information in the event of a major response or natural disaster cannot be overemphasized. The public is dependent upon such information for evacuation, notification, and protection. In order for everyone to receive the same accurate and timely information, NIMS has created a division to focus solely on information,

not having to worry about response, operations, or resources, for example.

Preparedness

Preparedness includes all actions required to establish the level of capability necessary to execute incident management operations. Simply put, organizations must plan, train and educate, remediate, and develop mutual-aid agreements in order to be ready to implement NIMS principles when responding to a large event. Staging annual or semi-annual MCI drills is a good way to practice and prepare for setting up a NIMS response, as roles within the system often change.

Resource Management

NIMS requires "resource typing." It makes sense to categorize resources in plain language and into groups of measurable standards of performance and capability. For example, if you need a generator, you need to know where you can get the size you need and that the generator will be able to perform the required task. The same principle holds true for personnel. If you need someone to operate heavy equipment, you need to know that the operator indeed is credentialed to perform such tasks. This credentialing takes place before the incident, as it is part of the planning and typing of resources. Resource management also provides a means for inventorying, mobilizing, dispatching, and returning resources after the incident. Resource management is all about preplanning and knowing what resources are available and how to procure them.

Communications and Information Management

NIMS provides for standardization of all communication, information, and information-sharing among all levels of incident management. A unified message is the goal of this component of NIMS. It makes resource allocation and other decisions easier when everyone is looking at the same picture of the incident, which is made possible by Communications and Information Management.

Supporting Technologies

To effectively communicate with other responding agencies, or in the event of a massive power or phone outage, the technology infrastructure must be robust. This may mean an upgrade in radios, cellular technology, portable computing, or mobile command centers equipped with state-of-the-art communications technology and power.

Ongoing Management and Maintenance

The NIMS Integration Center (NIC) was created to provide direction and oversight to the NIMS process. The NIC is responsible for maintaining preparedness standards, defining training requirements, and reviewing and approving emergency response equipment lists that meet national standards.

It is important to recognize that NIMS implementation is a dynamic system, and the philosophy and implementation requirements will continue to change as our prevention, preparedness, response, and recovery capabilities improve and our homeland security landscape changes. New personnel will continue to need NIMS training, and NIMS processes will have to be exercised in future years.

Air Medical Considerations

You may be required to decide whether to request air medical transport in consultation with medical control. Standing orders, guidelines, and protocols determine how helicopter transport is used in your region. You should be familiar with the policies in your area to request a helicopter when appropriate. Arriving EMS personnel may also decide to call for helicopter transport (Fig. 15-6).

In general, you should consider air medical transportation in the following situations:

- The patient's condition warrants it and significant time can be saved.
- The patient must be transported to a special care facility (e.g., trauma center, burn center, neonatal center).
- A remote or hazardous site limits ambulance access.

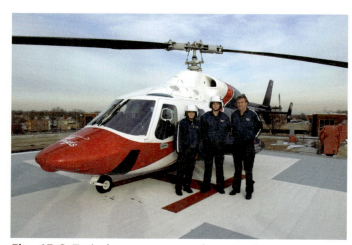

Fig. 15-6 Typical nurse, paramedic, pilot flight crew configuration.

Remember that helicopter transport may not be available at all times. For example, helicopters cannot fly in certain weather conditions and they may be unavailable because of maintenance requirements.

As an emergency first responder, you may be asked to help prepare the patient for air medical transport. This may include such actions as securing the patient to the cot, protecting the patient from the elements, or helping to carry the patient to the helicopter.

Landing Zone

Preparation of the helicopter landing zone requires following established protocols and additional personnel and equipment. If trained staff is present, one person should be identified as the communication person. This person should have a good sense of direction, be familiar with the area around the landing zone, and not be directly involved with patient care. If in radio or cell phone contact with the air medical dispatch center, the communication person should provide essential information to the air medical dispatch center. This information includes the following:

- The unit or individual making the call, with any call sign
- The radio frequency
- The number of patients
- A request for more aircraft, if appropriate
- The location of the incident
- A description of prominent landmarks in the area

The landing zone should be established by trained personnel. Specific requirements vary from place to place and the following instructions are only general guidelines. If you will be involved in helicopter transport, be sure you understand the appropriate specifications and protocol in your area. Considerations for a landing zone include the following:

- Establish the landing zone a safe distance from the scene. Generally the landing zone should be at least 500 feet away from the scene to compensate for the helicopter rotor wash and noise.
- The minimum acceptable dimensions of a landing zone are 60 feet by 60 feet (18 meters [m] by 18 m) during daylight and 100 feet by 100 feet (30 m by 30 m) during the night hours (Fig. 15-7).
- The landing zone should be free of debris, obstructions, overhead wires, trees, or fences.
- Ideally an area should be chosen where the ground does not slope.
- Each corner should be marked with an independent light source such as flares, light sticks, adequately secured cones, emergency vehicle(s), or private vehicles.
- Vehicle headlights should point to the center of the landing zone.
- At night, turn headlights off when the helicopter makes its final descent into the landing zone to prevent blinding or distracting the pilot.

A communication person should be in contact with the helicopter service to describe the area as the helicopter is trying to land. Descriptive landmark information such as directions relative to water (lakes, rivers, pools) or major roadway intersections should be provided. Details about the surface of the landing zone should be given to the pilot in advance of the final approach. Boundary information is also important, including trees, buildings, wires, fences, and towers. The proximity of power lines is critical information. If possible, you should illuminate potential hazards at night.

Safety

Safety is extremely important around a helicopter. All personnel must understand their role in and responsibility for ensuring safe operations. You should always keep

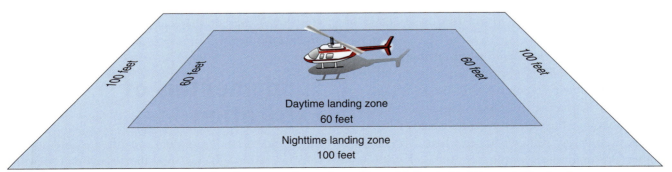

Fig. 15-7 Minimum landing zone dimensions. (From McSwain N, Paturas J: *The basic EMT: comprehensive prehospital patient care,* ed 2, St Louis, 2003, Mosby.)

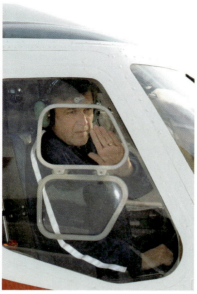

Fig. 15-8 Do NOT approach the aircraft until the pilot indicates that it is safe to do so.

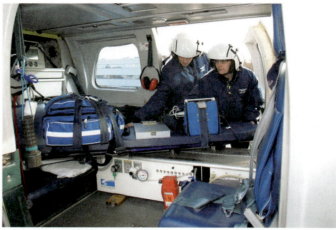

Fig. 15-10 Flight crew removing a stretcher from a helicopter.

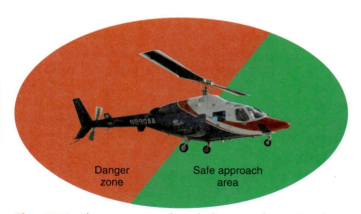

Danger zone

Safe approach area

Fig. 15-9 Always approach a helicopter from the front where the pilot can see you. Never approach from the rear.

a safe distance from the helicopter's blades, keeping vehicles 30 feet (9 m) from the landing zone and crowds at least 100 feet (30 m) away. Do not run or smoke in or around the landing zone.

As a general rule, *you should never approach the helicopter unless directed by the pilot and always approach from the front so that the pilot can see you* (Fig. 15-8). The tail section of a helicopter is especially dangerous for ground personnel because the tail rotor blade is usually lower to the ground and very difficult to see when it is rotating. Whether the engine is running or not, *all* personnel should avoid the tail section (Fig. 15-9). You should never attempt to take shortcuts under the body, the rear

section, or the tail boom. *Do not* attempt to operate any of the aircraft doors.

It is important to stay low when approaching the helicopter because wind gusts can unexpectedly change the height of the blades. Do not carry equipment above your head, and be aware that hats or loose equipment can be blown by the wind from the rotor blades. If the helicopter parks on a slope, approach from the downhill side since the main rotor blade is lower to the ground on the uphill side. It is important to remember that the flight crew is in charge of activity around the helicopter and you must follow their directions on your approach to and departure from the aircraft (Fig. 15-10). Do not touch or step on any part of the helicopter unless directed by the flight crew. Because of winds or obstacles, the pilot may choose a different departure route and the helicopter may turn while still close to the ground. It is therefore critical that *all* personnel and equipment be clear of the landing zone.

Take advantage of continuing education courses offered by local flight crews. Additional information on EMS helicopters is available from the Association of Air Medical Services, the National EMS Pilots Association, your local EMS air medical provider, and other similar organizations.

Fundamentals of Extrication

Emergency first responders are often called to motor vehicle crashes (MVCs) or other situations in which a patient is trapped (Fig. 15-11). Personal safety is very important in these situations. An emergency first

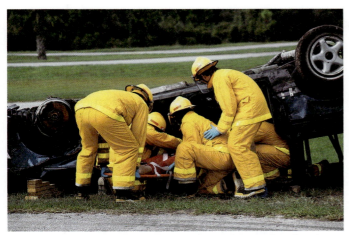

Fig. 15-11 A motor vehicle crash is an example of a situation requiring extrication. (From McSwain N, Paturas J: *The basic EMT: comprehensive prehospital patient care,* ed 2, St Louis, 2003, Mosby.)

BOX 15-2 Personal Protection Equipment

- Protective eyewear should have an elastic strap and vents to prevent fogging. The shield on a helmet is not considered protective eyewear.
- Impact-resistant protective helmet with ear protection and chin strap.
- Lightweight, puncture-resistant turnout coat.
- Leather gloves.
- Boots with steel insoles and steel toes.
- Lightweight, puncture-resistant turnout pants.

responder who becomes injured cannot help the patient and will then require additional EMS or rescue resources. Many emergency first responders have special training in rescue techniques. Rescue may be handled by the fire service, a special rescue squad, or law enforcement personnel; therefore it is important to know the system in your area and seek additional training as necessary. You should understand your role and those of all personnel at crash scenes, structural collapses, industrial incidents, and other settings of entrapment. You may perform rescues or provide assistance, depending on the guidelines of your system.

Everyone's actions are directed by an ICS. The designated incident commander coordinates the efforts of medical, rescue, and transport personnel and assigns tasks as necessary. Teamwork and accountability are essential in these operations. Successful extrication depends on the knowledge, skills, and equipment of rescue personnel. As an emergency first responder, you must cooperate with rescuers and ensure that rescue activities do not compromise patient care.

Extrication is the process of safely and appropriately removing a patient entrapped in a motor vehicle or other situation. Sometimes the extrication process must begin with the removal of structures or obstructions from around the patient. This part of the process, called disentanglement, requires special equipment, tools, and training.

Critical emergency care may need to be provided before and during the extrication process. Work with the rescue crew to remove the patient in a way that minimizes the risk of further injury to either the patient or the rescuers. In all cases of entrapment, critical patient care starts first unless a delay in extrication would endanger the life of the patient or rescue crew. Extrication begins immediately if the patient or rescue crew is endangered. While the rescue crew works, you should prepare the equipment necessary to give care such as airway management and bleeding control. Rescuers must cooperate with emergency first responders providing medical care to ensure the patient is removed in a way that minimizes the risk of further injury.

Safety and equipment are critical elements in the extrication process. Your own safety is your first priority. Personal safety applies to *all* workers involved in rescue activities or medical care. The Occupational Safety and Health Administration (OSHA) and the National Fire Protection Association (NFPA) have issued guidelines for personal safety equipment that are followed by many services. Many state agencies mandate the use of specific PPE. Box 15-2 suggests PPE for emergency first responders working around vehicle collisions.

Once you ensure that medical and rescue personnel are safe, you should consider the safety of the patient and the bystanders. Always explain the extrication process to the patient, including loud or sudden noises that will occur. Cover patients with blankets or tarps to protect them from glass, sharp metal, and other hazards and keep the patient warm and dry. Ensure that bystanders stay clear of the scene because they present an additional risk of injury. Potential hazards at the scene of an extrication may include the following:

- *Hazardous materials.* Hazardous materials are often present at motor vehicle collisions (MVCs) or other rescue situations. These may prevent you from gaining access to a patient.

- *Fire.* Fire at a crash scene is another potential hazard. If you can do so safely, turn off the ignition of the vehicle. Prohibit cigarette smoking at the scene and use a fire extinguisher to prevent the spread of a small fire. Do not attempt to extinguish a vehicle fire unless you have had special training in vehicle firefighting.
- *Downed power lines.* Downed power lines present a risk of electrical shock. Only utility or rescue workers who are trained to handle live power lines should approach downed power lines to secure them. A patient inside a vehicle in contact with or under a downed power line should be advised to remain there. If you cannot approach the vehicle because of downed lines, use a bullhorn or a public address system to speak to the patient. If the scene is unsafe, make it safe or do not enter. If you are unable to make the scene safe, call the appropriate agency.
- *Unstable vehicles.* Unstable vehicles pose an additional safety concern. An unstable vehicle can shift, roll, or fall and possibly injure you, the patient, or other personnel. Ensure that the vehicle is stabilized before you care for the patient.

The safety of a rescue scene must be carefully managed. If there are enough personnel, the incident commander should appoint a safety officer. Someone not directly involved in patient care or the rescue operation should assume this responsibility. This individual should be an objective observer and must continually watch for safety concerns and additional hazards, including the development of fire(s), movement of vehicle(s), or unsafe acts by anyone at the scene. The safety officer can also rotate in fresh rescuers during prolonged extrication when other rescuers become tired or dehydrated.

Accessing the patient during extrication can be simple or complex. Emergency first responders can perform simple access by opening a door, rolling down a window, or unlocking a door. Complex access requires additional training, skills, equipment, and personnel.

If you are interested in or required to become a specialized rescue technician, investigate rescue programs available locally, statewide, or regionally. Such programs may include vehicle rescue, water rescue, confined building/structure rescue, high-angle rescue, and trench rescue.

Once you have accessed the patient, he or she must be removed or extricated. Be sure there are enough personnel to maintain spinal stabilization. Work with additional EMS personnel to ensure that the spine is immobilized by using a short spine board or other immobilization device. A patient should never be moved without spinal stabilization unless there is immediate danger to the patient or rescuers.

Before removing the patient, perform the initial assessment and critical interventions. Remember to pick up the patient, not the immobilization device, unless the device is designed to be lifted. Choose a clear path and use enough personnel to safely remove the patient from the scene. Protect the patient from hazards, ensure an open airway, and maintain spinal stabilization.

Hazardous Materials

Any substance or material that poses a risk to health, safety, or property is considered a **hazardous material.** In your emergency first responder career you will likely respond to a hazardous material incident. Training specific to hazardous materials is necessary to ensure the safety of responders. There are several levels of training available that are specific to the job requirements of the responder. These training levels include the following:

- *Hazardous Materials Awareness.* This training level prepares the emergency first responder to identify a hazardous materials event and take precautions to isolate bystanders and rescuers from exposure while notifying the Office of Hazardous Materials Safety (HAZMAT) specialists to respond.
- *Hazardous Materials Operations.* This level of training prepares initial responders to set up perimeters and safety zones while limiting the spread of the event.
- *Hazardous Materials Technician.* This level of training prepares responders to stop the release of hazardous materials and get control of the exposure.
- *Hazardous Materials Specialist.* This is an advanced level of training that allows the responder to provide command and support skills to a hazardous materials event.

At a minimum, a Hazardous Materials Awareness level education program is recommended for emergency first responders.

Safety is a major concern in scenes involving hazardous materials. Although people often think of hazardous materials in the context of vehicle collisions, many chemicals, pesticides, and other compounds found in the home and industrial sites can also cause a hazardous materials situation. A spill or leak of chemicals, gas, or vapor is a potential hazardous materials incident. If the public, the emergency first responder, or the environment is exposed, this is a hazardous materials situation.

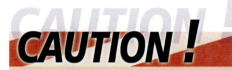

CAUTION !

Remember the scene size-up rule: if the scene is not safe, make it safe or do not enter. A highly trained HAZMAT team has the expertise to make the scene safe. Do not enter the scene unless you are trained to handle hazardous materials and to use the necessary equipment.

Safe management of hazardous materials incidents requires knowledge of the material involved and the appropriate response. If possible, seek additional information from the dispatcher while en route to help you reduce the risk to rescuers and prepare your response. The United States Department of Transportation (U.S. DOT) publishes a reference titled the *Emergency Response Guidebook (ERG)*, which lists hazardous materials and the appropriate emergency procedure (see Fig. 15-1). The *ERG* should be in every emergency first responder, EMS, fire service, or response vehicle.

If you determine that the scene may involve hazardous materials based on dispatch information or your observation of the scene, follow these important safety guidelines as you approach the scene:

- Ensure the scene is secure.
- Stage (wait) upwind and upgrade a safe distance from the scene.
- Use binoculars if necessary to observe the scene.
- Deny entry.
- Wait for HAZMAT team arrival.
- Approach the patient only when the scene is safe.

If the scene involves a hazardous materials incident, you should try to identify the extent of the problem. For instance, determine the number of potential patients and the size and shape of the container of hazardous materials. This information helps the hazardous materials team quickly identify the materials. The U.S. DOT has devised a **placard** system to identify hazardous materials that are being transported (Fig. 15-12). The placard has a four-digit number that identifies the class of material or the material itself. The *Emergency Response Guidebook* is then

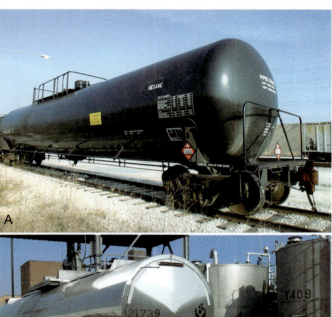

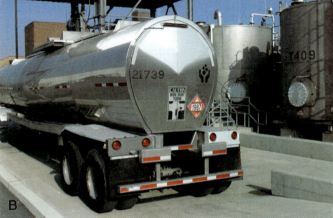

Fig. 15-12 A, U.S. DOT placard on a railcar. **B,** U.S. DOT placards visible on the back of a transportation truck.

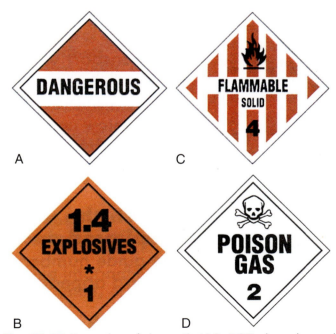

Fig. 15-13 Examples of domestic U.S. DOT placards used on transportation vehicles. (From McSwain N, Paturas J: *The basic EMT: comprehensive prehospital patient care,* ed 2, St Louis, 2003, Mosby.)

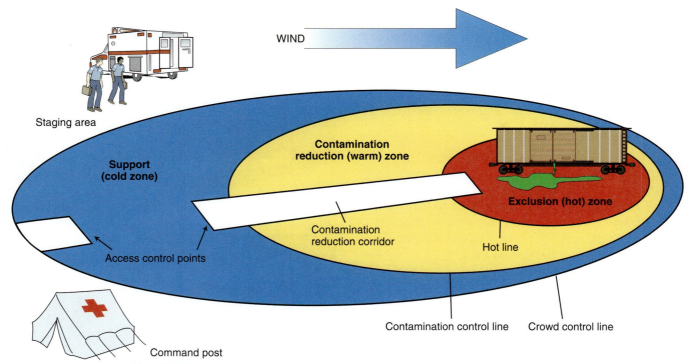

WIND

Staging area

Support
(cold zone)

Contamination
reduction (warm) zone

Exclusion (hot) zone

Contamination
reduction corridor

Hot line

Access control points

Contamination control line   Crowd control line

Command post

Fig. 15-14 The "zones" established during a hazardous materials incident.

used to look up the placard numbers. Once the material is identified, the *ERG* also identifies the hazards presented by the material and gives guidance on suppression, evacuation zones, and medical concerns (Fig. 15-13). With this information, HAZMAT teams will set up control zones (Fig. 15-14). The hot zone will be where the exposed material is located, and only trained personnel in full protective gear appropriate to the exposure can enter. The warm zone is a buffer between the hazardous material and the surrounding community. Specially trained personnel in protective clothing will work to prevent spread of the material and perform life-saving care. The cold zone is free of contaminants and is the location where support personnel and equipment are gathered to receive decontaminated patients, prepare personnel for entry into the scene, and remove clothing from responders leaving the hot and warm zones.

Stationary hazardous materials, such as chemicals in a grocery store, are identified by an NFPA placard (Fig. 15-15). The NFPA placard identifies the material as a health hazard, reactivity hazard, flammability hazard, or any other specific hazard. The hazards are color coded and rated numerically from 0 through 4, where 0 is no hazard and 4 is the highest hazard level. Fig. 15-16 identifies an NFPA placard and its components.

Other resources available to you are the shipping papers, located inside the vehicle. These can provide

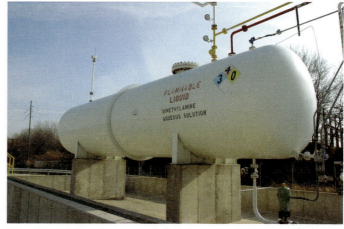

Fig. 15-15 Fixed storage of a flammable liquid identified with an NFPA placard.

important information, but you should retrieve them only if it is safe to do so. Your *ERG* is a resource for possible interventions. The local hazardous materials response team is also a resource. Another resource is the Chemical Transportation Emergency Center (CHEMTREC), a service of the Chemical Manufacturers Association. This public service agency can provide immediate online advice to emergency and rescue personnel at the scene of hazardous materials incidents. CHEMTREC is available 24 hours a day, 7 days a week, through an emergency phone number (1-800-424-9300). Involve CHEM-TREC as early as possible. Provide as much information as possible about the incident. Include the name of the material, its identification number, and a description of the incident. CHEMTEL is another emergency response center that is available in North America 24 hours a day. CHEMTEL can be reached at 1-800-255-3924 or 1-813-979-0626.

OSHA, the NFPA, and local or state agencies publish guidelines for public safety and other health care personnel in hazardous materials incidents.

Multiple-Casualty Incidents

A multiple-casualty incident (MCI) is a situation that overwhelms available resources. If there are more patients than you and other responding units can safely and efficiently handle, the Incident Command System should be activated.

Natural Disasters

A **natural disaster** is a calamity or catastrophe caused by a natural occurrence such as a thunderstorm, tornado,

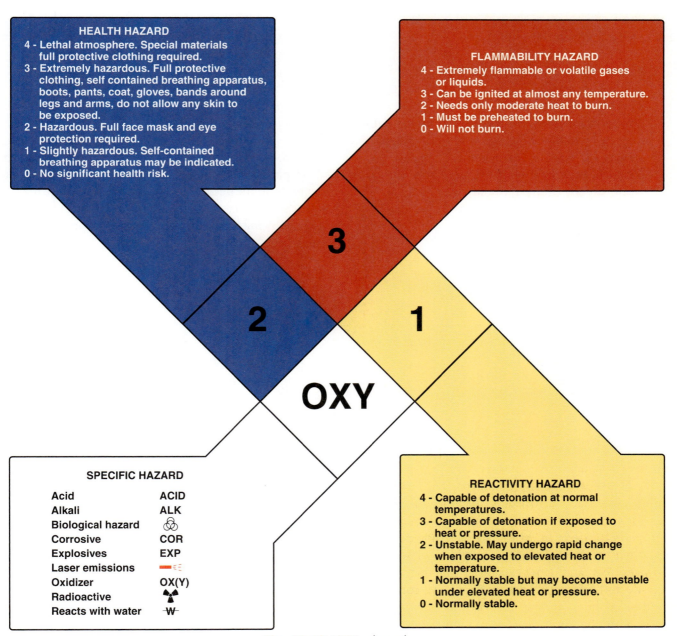

HEALTH HAZARD
4 - Lethal atmosphere. Special materials full protective clothing required.
3 - Extremely hazardous. Full protective clothing, self contained breathing apparatus, boots, pants, coat, gloves, bands around legs and arms, do not allow any skin to be exposed.
2 - Hazardous. Full face mask and eye protection required.
1 - Slightly hazardous. Self-contained breathing apparatus may be indicated.
0 - No significant health risk.

FLAMMABILITY HAZARD
4 - Extremely flammable or volatile gases or liquids.
3 - Can be ignited at almost any temperature.
2 - Needs only moderate heat to burn.
1 - Must be preheated to burn.
0 - Will not burn.

SPECIFIC HAZARD
Acid	ACID
Alkali	ALK
Biological hazard	⚛
Corrosive	COR
Explosives	EXP
Laser emissions	▬◄
Oxidizer	OX(Y)
Radioactive	☢
Reacts with water	‒W‒

REACTIVITY HAZARD
4 - Capable of detonation at normal temperatures.
3 - Capable of detonation if exposed to heat or pressure.
2 - Unstable. May undergo rapid change when exposed to elevated heat or temperature.
1 - Normally stable but may become unstable under elevated heat or pressure.
0 - Normally stable.

Fig. 15-16 NFPA placard.

or earthquake that results in a disruption of the normal functioning of the response system, facility, or infrastructure. On the serious end of the spectrum, there could be large-scale destruction and loss of life. Related to natural disasters could be unforeseen occurrences such as water line breaks, boiler explosions, gas line leaks, power failure, and fires, for example, which may have the same effects as a natural disaster. Events such as tornadoes, hurricanes, floods, and earthquakes are common examples of natural disasters. Remember that during a natural disaster, local resources will be involved in the event, not just responding as usual. Your agency should have a contingency plan for those situations where they are unable to adequately respond because of a disaster situation. This is just one of the problems that NIMS addresses with mutual-aid agreements. Natural disasters are likely to result in the following conditions:

1. **Inconvenience occurrences:** Included are power failures, water line breaks, air conditioning failure, hazardous materials, etc.
2. **Property destruction:** Included is minor damage such as window breakage and roof damage, to damage as extensive as structural damage.
3. **Physical injury or death:** Conceivably, this could occur on any of the above levels.

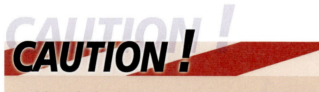

CAUTION!

While involved in disaster operations, remember to think of safety first. Do not get caught up in the moment and take an unnecessary risk. As has been mentioned before, do not become part of the problem!

Terrorism

There are many definitions of **terrorism.** For the purposes of this text we will use the U.S. Department of Defense definition that states terrorism is "the unlawful use of—or threatened use of—force or violence against individuals or property to coerce or intimidate governments or societies, often to achieve political, religious, or ideological objectives." We can further categorize that definition into domestic and international terrorism if we consider the definition of international terrorism as "terrorism conducted with the support of a foreign government or organization and/or directed against foreign nationals,

institutions or governments," while domestic terrorism is "groups or individuals operating entirely inside the US, attempting to influence the US government or population to effect political or social change by engaging in criminal activity" (FBI). When responding to a large-scale event, the possibility that it was an act of terrorism should cross your mind. Remember, your safety is your biggest concern when responding to any scene, terrorist acts included. You must be aware and alert that someone or a group of terrorists may still be on scene, waiting for the emergency first responder to arrive. The intent may be to injure or kill those responding to the incident, furthering the severity and magnitude of the original event. Even if all of those responsible for the attack are gone, your safety is not guaranteed. There have been incidents where a secondary explosive device, or as it is sometimes referred to, a "sucker-punch," was set to detonate when the responders arrive and begin their work.

High-Risk Locations

Your first clue that you may be responding to an act of terrorism may be the location of the incident. Recent history has shown us that those responsible for terrorist acts choose targets to incite fear in an attempt to further their political or religious agendas. The target chosen depends on the desired objective. Is the objective to debilitate the financial system, or crash the computer network? The following lists are some examples of potential terrorist targets:

- Infrastructure—power plants, data networks and computers, and transportation such as bridges, tunnels, and ports
- Civilian—schools, shopping centers, churches, sporting events, and festivals
- Symbolic—National monuments or historically significant buildings

Regardless of the location, you must remain vigilant in your pursuit of personal and crew safety. Survey the scene for anything seemingly out of place or odd. When that little voice tells you that something is not right, learn to listen and take appropriate action.

Weapons of Mass Destruction (WMD)

WMD include any weapons or devices that are intended, or have the capability, to cause death or serious bodily injury to a significant number of people through the release of toxic or poisonous chemicals or their precursors, a disease organism, or radiation or radioactivity as defined by the U.S. Department of Defense.

Types of Agents Used in Terrorist Attacks

As an emergency first responder, you will be trained to recognize and take precautions against many common hazards, such as pesticides, anhydrous ammonia, fire, and explosions. Terrorists use many of the same substances with which you are familiar. We can remember the commonly used weapons in terrorist attacks with the help of the mnemonic B-NICCE.

- Biological
- Nuclear
- Incendiary
- Chemical
- Cyber/Technological
- Etiological

Biological Agents

A naturally occurring substance that produces disease is a biological agent. Although potent and effective, biological agents are not so easily dispersed upon a large population. We have seen throughout the course of history examples such as the plague, hemorrhagic fever, anthrax, smallpox, and ricin (Fig. 15-17). Ricin is a toxin that can be made from the waste left over from processing castor beans. It is one of the most toxic and easily produced plant toxins. If injected, as little as 500 micrograms of ricin could be enough to kill an adult; some animal research indicates that similar amounts could be lethal, if inhaled. A 500-microgram dose of ricin would be about the size of the head of a pin (OSHA). While responsible for many deaths, these diseases were not immediately fatal. If the agent was released on day 1, people may not become ill and seek medical attention until day 3. This time from exposure to symptoms is known as the incubation period, and varies with each agent. This presents a challenge to the emergency first responder and the health care system as a whole. How do you begin to put the pieces of a biological attack together? The ability to communicate and share information is absolutely crucial in containing a biological incident. Have you responded to a number of calls with similar complaints and similar time frames? If so, notify the hospital or health department of your concerns.

Nuclear/Radiological Agents

There is the possibility that a terrorist could use a "dirty bomb" to spread radioactive material over an area. Exposure to ionizing radiation occurs daily in hospitals and clinics all over the world. What, then, is the difference? Why do you not become ill after getting an x-ray? Remem-

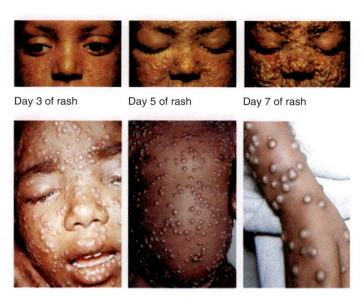

Day 3 of rash   Day 5 of rash   Day 7 of rash

On any part of the body, all lesions are in the same stage of development.

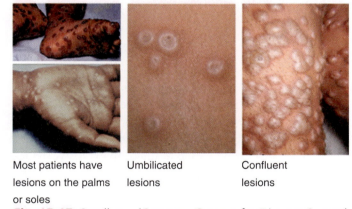

Most patients have lesions on the palms or soles   Umbilicated lesions   Confluent lesions

Fig. 15-17 Smallpox. (Courtesy Centers for Disease Control and Prevention, Atlanta, Ga.)

ber, the lead apron they make you wear protects you from the radiation. Also, you are only exposed for a very short time. Those who work in radiology wear dosimeters, or devices that measure the level of radiation exposure. There are safe levels of exposure, and then there are levels of exposure found at a radiological incident. At an incident where there has been a release of radioactive material, your exposure lasts as long as you participate, and you do not usually respond in lead gear. You cannot see, smell, or otherwise sense radiation in the environment without the use of a dosimeter or similar equipment. In an attempt to minimize your exposure to radiation, remember the following three items; time, distance, and shielding. Of these, distance offers the most protection because of the inverse square law. This means that if you double your distance from the source, your exposure is decreased by a factor of 4. It is also very important to always wear appropriate BSI as it will afford you some initial exposure protection.

There are different symptoms for different levels of exposure, from nausea, vomiting, and diarrhea at low doses; to burns, genetic mutation, and hair loss at moderate levels; to severe burns, cancer, and death at high doses.

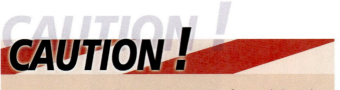

CAUTION !

Your agency should have a response plan for a radiological event, especially if you live near a nuclear power generating station. Take the opportunity to participate in radiological drills to become familiar with procedures, safety equipment, and local decontamination procedures.

Incendiary Devices

Explosives are a common weapon used by terrorists to incite fear and inflict horrific damage, in terms of both property and loss of life. Look at the size of the craters left at bombing sites, such as Oklahoma City. Many different substances can be used to make an explosive device and they can be hidden in any conceivable place. When you are on scene at a suspected act of terrorism, scan the scene for things that may look out of place or just do not seem right. As mentioned, terrorists may hide "secondary" devices in cars, backpacks, or even on other human beings in the case of suicide attacks. While the concussion of the explosion does the major structural damage, these devices are often filled with marbles, nails, and other projectiles meant to injure or kill as many people as possible. These devices may also start fires, making the response inherently more dangerous. Be aware that there may be structural instability involved in these types of responses. Make sure the scene is safe before beginning any rescue efforts.

Chemical Agents

As you have been made aware by the news media, a wide variety of chemicals have been intentionally released in terrorist incidents. While these chemicals are dangerous and destructive, Emergency Medical Services personnel are trained in HAZMAT operations and understand how to protect themselves and the public on such occasions. Chemical agents are generally classified by their mechanism of action, or the effects on the body and systems.

These divisions can be easily remembered by the mnemonic (IMNBC; or I am in BC):

INSECTICIDES

These are commonly used chemicals that are inhaled or absorbed through the skin. Because of the fact that they are commonly used in agriculture, they remain readily available for terrorist use. The most popular type of chemical found in this group is *organophosphates*. Exposure to organophosphates causes a cascade of symptoms known as DUMBELS:

- **D**iaphoresis and diarrhea
- **U**rination
- **M**iosis (pinpoint pupils)
- **B**radycardia, bronchorrhea (excessive secretions/mucus), bronchospasm
- **E**mesis (vomiting)
- **L**acrimation (secretion of excess tears)
- **S**alivation

As you can see, these symptoms involve the release and leaking of body fluids. You can appreciate the concern for ABC management with the bradycardia and airway secretions. Most people who are exposed will have symptoms 12 to 24 hours postexposure. Management of this patient is aimed at reversing the fluid leakage and bradycardia. However, remember that you should not begin care for this patient until the patient has been decontaminated appropriately by trained personnel. This is another example of how preparedness training and drilling make responding to such incidents easier and safer. Position your vehicle and personnel uphill and upwind from the release to minimize exposure.

METABOLIC

These agents hinder the body's ability to use oxygen at the cellular level. The most common agent in this group is something most firefighters have probably been exposed to in a fire—cyanide. Cyanide gas is produced from the burning of plastics and textiles; it is also used in photography and gold/silver mining. The following is a list of symptoms associated with exposure to cyanide:

- Difficulty breathing
- Tachycardia
- Flushed or red skin
- Seizures/coma
- Cardiac arrest

Emergency treatment of someone exposed to cyanide consists of oxygen administration, ABC support, and the administration of a cyanide antidote kit, containing amyl nitrate, sodium nitrite, and sodium thiosulfate. The amyl nitrate is to be inhaled, while the two sodium substances are injected.

NERVE

Those terrorists who want to inflict maximum damage with minimum dosage will usually choose a nerve agent. It takes a very small amount of some agents to cause cardiac arrest. In 1995 there was an incident in the subway system of Tokyo with the release of sarin gas. There were only 12 deaths, but more than 1000 people were temporarily affected and sought medical care. Management of a casualty with nerve agent intoxication consists of decontamination, ventilation, administration of the antidotes, and supportive therapy. The condition of the patient dictates the need for each of these and the order in which they are done. Although extremely lethal, antidotes exist for those exposed to nerve agents. The most common kits are the DuoDote, which is the new version of the MARK 1, and the NAAK (nerve agent antidote kit) (Fig. 15-18).

BLISTER

Like their name implies, these agents cause burnlike blisters to the area of exposure. If these agents are inhaled, they may cause severe respiratory compromise. Other symptoms of exposure to blister agents may include eye and skin irritation along with coughing. As a responder, if you are involved in an incident where you begin to experience these symptoms, leave the area immediately and notify the HAZMAT team. Unless you are properly trained and have access to self-contained breathing apparatuses (SCBAs) and proper attire, do not enter or re-enter an area of chemical exposure. Everyone exposed in the incident will need to be decontaminated. Examples of blister agents include lewisite and sulfur mustard.

CHOKING (PULMONARY)

You can find these agents in the industrial and even home settings. Chlorine gas can be found commonly in manufacturing facilities as well as pools and hot tubs. Phosgene gas is a byproduct of burning Freon, which is found in air conditioners. You are familiar with the smell of bleach, which could indicate a chlorine-rich environment, as well as the smell of freshly-cut grass, indicative of phosgene. Exposure to agents in this category causes significant respiratory distress and pulmonary edema. After inhaling the vapors, the lung tissue breaks down and leaks fluid into the lungs, causing pulmonary edema and death if not corrected. Other symptoms of a pulmonary agent exposure include airway irritation, coughing, choking, or gasping.

Etiological Agents

Etiological agents are those microorganisms and microbial toxins that cause disease in humans and include bacteria, bacterial toxins, viruses, fungi, and parasites. These disease-causing microorganisms may also be referred to as infectious agents. Arthropods and other organisms that transmit pathogens to animals (including humans) are called vectors (CDC). There are strict regulations on the importation of exotic animals, bats, snails, and other organisms in an attempt to keep unwanted and potentially destructive diseases away from the domestic population. Although you may not respond to an etiological agent incident, it bears notice that this is a potential delivery method of disease, and you would be wise to constantly communicate with those in your area about symptom trends.

Emergency First Responder's Response to an Act of Terrorism

Regardless of the agent used, the following are some of the clues to an attack of this type:

- Number of casualties—at a large-scale event this would be easy to spot; however, at a more widespread event, such as the release of a respiratory agent, you may not see large numbers of casualties in one place, as the agent has carried and drifted away from the release location. In this case, interoperability and effective communications are extremely important to alert and attempt to minimize the severity of the incident.
- Debris field—assess the breadth and magnitude of any damage or destruction.
- Unusual signs/symptoms
- Dead or dying animals
- High-risk location of the incident—government buildings, power plants, large public gatherings
- Responder casualties
- Severe structural damage
- Infrastructure system failures
- Unusual odors (cut grass, chlorine, almonds), colors of smoke, and vapor clouds
- Take note of the date of the attack. Is this a historically significant date? Is it an anniversary of a previous event, such as the Oklahoma City bombing or the terror attacks of September 11, 2001?

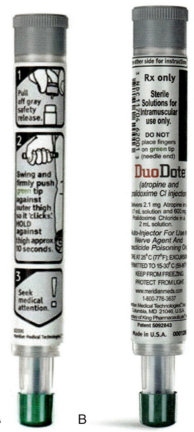

A   B

Fig. 15-18 DuoDote (front and back). (Courtesy Meridian Medical Technologies, Inc., Columbia, Md.)

Auto-injector procedure:

Important: Do not remove Gray Safety Release until ready to use.

CAUTION: Never touch the Green Tip (Needle End)!

1. Tear open the plastic pouch at any of the notches. Remove the DuoDote™ Auto-Injector from the pouch.
2. Place the DuoDote Auto-Injector in your dominant hand. (If you are right-handed, your right hand is dominant.) Firmly grasp the center of the DuoDote Auto-Injector with the Green Tip (Needle End) pointing down.
3. With your other hand, pull off the Gray Safety Release. The DuoDote Auto-Injector is now ready to be administered.
4. The injection site is the mid-outer thigh area. The DuoDote™ Auto-Injector can inject through clothing. **However, make sure pockets at the injection site are empty.**
5. Swing and firmly push the Green Tip straight down (a 90° angle) against the mid-outer thigh. Continue to firmly push until you feel the DuoDote Auto-Injector trigger.

IMPORTANT: After the auto-injector triggers, hold the DuoDote Auto-Injector in place against the injection site for approximately 10 seconds.

After Injecting

6. Remove the DuoDote™ Auto-Injector from the thigh and look at the Green Tip. If the needle is visible, the drug has been administered. If the needle is not visible, check to be sure the Gray Safety Release has been removed and repeat the previous steps beginning with Step 4, but push harder in Step 5.
7. After the drug has been administered, push the needle against a hard surface to bend the needle back against the DuoDote Auto-Injector.
8. Put the used DuoDote Auto-Injector back into the plastic pouch, if available. Leave used DuoDote Auto-Injector(s) with the patient to allow other medical personnel to see the number of DuoDote Auto-Injectors administered.
9. Immediately move yourself and the patient away from the contaminated area and seek definitive medical care for the patient.

Functions of the Emergency First Responder at a Multiple Casualty Incident (MCI)

Regardless of the scale of the event, the role of the First Responder is to first address your safety and the safety of your crew. By becoming familiar with NIMS, you can see that you may be asked to perform a number of functions at a large event. You may be directly involved in patient care, you may become involved in triage, or you may be involved in staging and transport, or any other area found at an MCI. No two responses are the same, nor are the roles you might play from call to call. Once the event has been accurately identified, quick and decisive actions by emergency responders can mitigate and isolate existing hazards. It is easy to become overwhelmed very rapidly once patient care begins. Request assistance and delegate duties among responding members before beginning patient care activities whenever possible.

The following is a list of actions to be considered upon initial arrival at the scene of an emergency:

- Ensure the safety of response personnel (do not become part of the problem).
- Take personal protective measures.
- Ensure life/property safety.
- Identify the nature of the incident.
- All First Responders should be aware of the threat of a possible secondary device when responding to a suspected terrorist event. If at all possible, hasty perimeter sweeps should be conducted to ensure the safety of all First Responders.
- Protect/isolate the scene.
- Initiate the Incident Command System.
- Establish a command post.
- Identify the incident commander.
- Secure safe response routes for additional responding resources.
- Identify staging areas.
- Notify adjacent communities regarding potential hazard.
- Evaluate need for additional response resources.
- Position response vehicles uphill and upwind from hazard area.
- Look for physical indicators and other outward signs of biological, nuclear, chemical, and explosive events.
- Treat affected area as a crime scene.

- Deny entry for other than life safety measures.
- Identify and separate witnesses.

Emergency Medical Services (EMS)

General functions for all EMS are the following:

- Identify hazards if they are present.
- Use appropriate self-protection measures.
- Provide prehospital medical triage.
- Treat affected patients using existing EMS protocols.
- Provide support to fire and rescue agencies.
- Initiate or participate in the Incident Command System.
- Never transport contaminated patients. All potentially contaminated victims should be decontaminated before being transported.
- Notify local hospitals of potential large number of incoming patients.
- Treat as a multiple casualty incident.

Triage

The first priority in an MCI, after safety, is patient triage. **Triage** is the process of categorizing patients into treatment and transportation priorities. Triage is a dynamic process and patients' categories may change between the initial assessment and subsequent assessments.

Several commercial triage tagging systems are used in different systems to designate the triage category of each patient. In most systems there are four priority levels: immediate, delayed (secondary), minor (delayed), and deceased (dead). Box 15-3 describes these priority levels.

BOX 15-3 Triage Priorities

Highest Priority (Immediate)
- Airway and breathing difficulties
- Uncontrolled or severe bleeding
- Decreased mental status

Second Priority (Delayed)
- Burns without airway problems
- Major or multiple-extremity injuries
- Back injuries

Lowest Priority (Minor)
- Minor extremity injuries
- Minor soft tissue injuries

Deceased
- Death

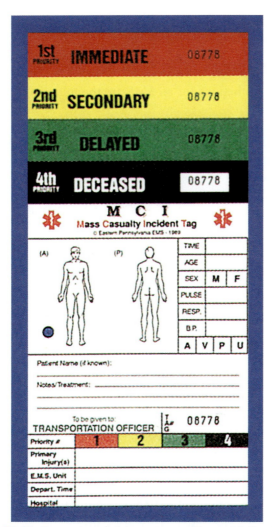

Fig. 15-19 Example of triage tags. (From McSwain N, Paturas J: *The basic EMT: comprehensive prehospital patient care,* ed 2, St Louis, 2003, Mosby.)

Color-coded and numbered tags are most commonly used (Fig. 15-19). You should be familiar with the tags used in your local system.

START (Simple Triage and Rapid Treatment) is one example of a commercially available triage system. The START system incorporates a 60-second assessment of respirations, perfusion, and mental status. Fig. 15-20 outlines the process used by START to categorize patients as immediate, delayed, minor, or deceased.

The triage officer should be the emergency first responder or EMS provider who is on scene and the most knowledgeable in the areas of patient assessment and intervention. Responders with higher levels of training relieve the triage officer as they become available at the scene. During scene size-up, additional assistance is requested if needed. The triage officer confirms the nature of the incident and establishes a command post. The officer then performs a quick initial assessment of all patients. Care is *not* provided during triage *except* to correct immediate life-threatening conditions such as airway blockage or major bleeding. As triage progresses, tags are applied to patients to indicate their triage treatment categories. Next, available personnel are assigned to the highest-priority patients. Tagged patients are moved to the appropriate treatment area for further evaluation and interventions. Patients are then moved to a waiting area for transport to a receiving facility. As with treatment priorities, transportation decisions are based on patient triage. Other considerations include the receiving hospital's capability and transportation resources.

After all patients have been triaged, the triage officer notifies the incident commander. The triage officer remains at the scene to assign and coordinate personnel, supplies, and vehicles.

As an emergency first responder in the role of triage officer, you will have to make difficult decisions. You must be able to quickly prioritize patients during triage to provide effective care. Your skill can maximize the number of patients receiving appropriate quality care during an MCI. It is important to receive triage training and to continually practice your triage skills using your local triage system to prepare you for a real MCI situation.

In any MCI situation, as an emergency first responder, you should immediately report to the incident commander or command post when you arrive at an established MCI scene. Identify yourself and your level of training and follow the directions of the incident commander.

Your role as an emergency first responder at an MCI or terrorist event may take on many forms, but the expectations are the same, no matter what your role in each incident. You are expected to act quickly, decisively, and professionally. Given the many possible roles you may play in an incident, it makes sense that you seek out any education and training opportunities available for dealing with MCIs. The more you practice and drill, the more comfortable you will feel when you respond to a real MCI. As an emergency first responder, you may truly be the first one on scene! Do not let the magnitude or severity of the incident stop you from taking care of the basics: personal and crew safety, hazard identification and notification, setting up incident command, and triage.

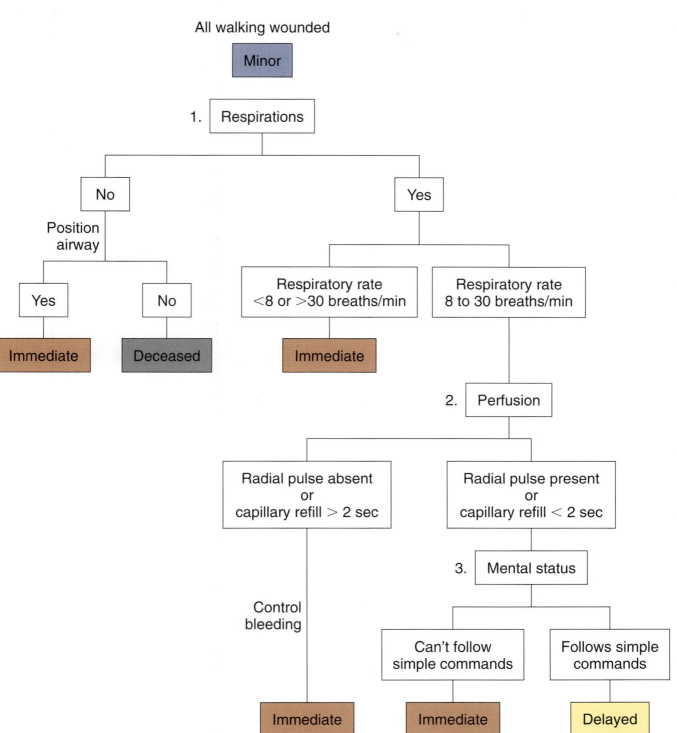

Fig. 15-20 START system. (Adapted from the Simple Triage and Rapid Treatment [S.T.A.R.T.] algorithm developed by Hoag Hospital and Newport Beach Fire Department, Newport Beach, Calif.)

Team Work

PREPARING FOR INTERFACE WITH TRANSPORT AGENCIES

Although emergency first responders may not work for transporting agencies, many of your patients will require transport to a hospital. It will be important for you as an emergency first responder to facilitate the arrival of incoming transport agencies and to promote a smooth transition of care from the scene to the transporting team.

It is important to give the responding transport team information that will prepare them to care for your patient. Relay your exact location and the best access to where you are in a facility. You should also give information about the mechanism of injury or particular illness of your patient along with your general impression of the patient's condition.

If there are special considerations at the scene, such as hazards or entry points to the facility, have someone meet the transport agency at the street to guide them to your location. Those that are assigned to meet the responding unit should also ensure that they have clear access to the site and ample space to park the vehicle and exit the site. It will be important that someone give the team some sense of how far they will have to travel on foot and how difficult it will be to get to you because they may be bringing equipment to your location.

Once the team reaches you and your patient, give them a detailed hand-off report. This report should include a history of your patient's emergency, the results of your history and physical examination, any treatment you may have done, and how your patient's condition may have changed since you have been on scene.

In the Real World—Conclusion

As the EMS unit pulls away you finish your patient care report and inventory your medical supplies. You review the entire rescue scenario and realize you performed all the tasks you were taught in your emergency first responder class. You participated in all the phases of a response except transferring the patient to the hospital. After notifying dispatch that you are back in service, you head back to headquarters to restock your supplies.

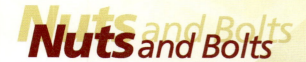
Nuts and Bolts

Critical Points

Emergency first responders are usually involved in all phases of EMS response except transporting the patient to the receiving facility. Your safety, the patient's safety, and the safety of bystanders must be your main priorities in each phase of any emergency. Always wear appropriate PPE, and use body substance isolation (BSI) techniques.

Emergency care is a team effort from beginning to end. The team includes emergency first responders, dispatch, EMTs and paramedics, fire service, law enforcement, air medical services, specialty rescue teams, trauma centers, and hospitals. Each component has its own role and responsibility. All fit together in the system called Emergency Medical Services (EMS).

Education and training must be an ongoing process. Each specialty and higher level in EMS requires more training and education. The EMS system continues to grow with medical and scientific advances occurring frequently. To ensure the optimal quality of care, every provider must stay up to date.

Learning Checklist

❏ A typical EMS response has eight stages: preparation for a call, dispatch, en route to the scene, arrival at the scene, transferring the patient to the ambulance, en route to the receiving facility, en route to the station, and the post-run phase.

❏ Emergency first responders are generally involved in only in six stages: preparation for a call, dispatch, en route to the scene, arrival at the scene, transferring the patient to the ambulance, and the post-run phase.

❏ The preparation phase includes inspecting and checking supplies, equipment, and vehicle operation.

❏ The dispatch phase is when information is received about the call from a dispatcher.

❏ Safe driving is an important aspect of the en route to the scene phase.

❏ Arrival at the scene includes parking your vehicle safely and appropriately and assessing the safety of the scene. This phase also includes patient care.

❏ You may be expected to help prepare the patient for transport in the transferring of the patient to ambulance phase.

❏ The post-run phase involves checking the vehicle, supplies, and equipment again to prepare for the next call.

❏ The standard for disaster management is the Incident Command System (ICS).

❏ The ICS is a chain of command and organization of efforts that allows numerous resources to be used in a coordinated response. It involves the coordination of agencies such as police, fire, EMS, and public works.

❏ Air medical transportation may be considered when the patient's condition warrants such transport and significant time can be saved, the patient must be transferred to a special care facility, or a remote or hazardous site limits ambulance access.

❏ Establish a landing zone approximately 500 feet away from the scene.

❏ A landing zone should be a minimum of 60 feet by 60 feet during daylight and 100 feet by 100 feet at night.

❏ Keep a safe distance from the helicopter's blades and keep vehicles 30 feet and crowds at least 100 feet away from the landing zone. Do not run or smoke in the landing zone area.

❏ Never approach an aircraft unless directed to do so by the pilot.

❏ Extrication is the process of safely and appropriately removing a patient entrapped in a motor vehicle or other situation.

❏ Simple access to a patient is performed by opening a door, rolling down a window, or unlocking a door. Complex access involves additional training, skills, equipment, and personnel.

❏ Potential hazards at an extrication scene may include hazardous materials, fire, downed power lines, and unstable vehicles.

❏ Any substance or material that poses a risk to health, safety, or property is considered a hazardous material.

❏ Emergency first responders should be specially trained to the Hazardous Materials Awareness level.

❏ The U.S. DOT requires transportation vehicles carrying hazardous materials have placards and labels with four-digit numbers that correspond to specific material information in the *Emergency Response Guidebook*.

Nuts and Bolts–continued

❏ Stationary hazardous materials are identified by an NFPA placard that identifies the health, reactivity, and flammability hazards as well as any other specific hazards.

❏ Resources to use in a hazardous materials situation include U.S. DOT placards, the *Emergency Response Guidebook*, the local hazardous materials team, CHEMTREC, and CHEMTEL.

❏ A multiple-casualty incident (MCI) is a situation that overwhelms available resources. In such situations the ICS should be activated.

❏ The National Incident Management System (NIMS) was developed to improve the response to a large-scale incident, and courses like NMS 100 and 700 will be necessary to get everyone on the same page.

❏ The First Responder's role at an act of terrorism is to first ensure personal safety, survey the scene for secondary hazards, and then provide appropriate patient care or perform other tasks as assigned by incident command.

❏ Triage is the process of categorizing patients into treatment and transportation priorities. Usually patients are classified into one of four levels: immediate, delayed, minor, or deceased.

❏ As an emergency first responder, if you arrive at an established MCI scene, you should report to the incident commander or command post, identify yourself and your level of training, and follow their direction.

Key Terms

Biological agent A naturally occurring substance that produces disease.

Extrication The process of removing a patient from entanglement in a motor vehicle or other situation in a safe and appropriate way.

Hazardous material Any material or substance that can cause an unreasonable risk to a person's safety or health or to property.

Incident Command System (ICS) A protocol or system for coordinating procedures to assist in the command, control, direction, and coordination of emergency response resources.

Multiple-casualty incident (MCI) A situation that overwhelms available resources.

Natural disaster A calamity or catastrophe brought about by a natural occurrence such as a thunderstorm, tornado, or earthquake that results in a disruption of the normal functioning of the response system, facility, or infrastructure.

NIMS National Incident Command System.

Placard An informational sign with various symbols and numerals to help identify the hazardous material or class of material.

Terrorism Unlawful use of, or threatened use of, force or violence against individuals or property to coerce or intimidate governments or societies, often to achieve political, religious, or ideological objectives.

Triage The process of sorting or categorizing patients into treatment and transport priorities in a multiple casualty situation.

Weapon of mass destruction (WMD) Any weapon or device that is intended, or has the capability, to cause death or serious bodily injury to a significant number of people.

First Responder NSC Objectives
COGNITIVE OBJECTIVES

- Discuss the medical and nonmedical equipment needed to respond to a call.
- List the phases of an out-of-hospital call.
- Discuss the role of the emergency first responder in extrication.
- List various methods of gaining access to the patient.
- Distinguish between simple and complex access.
- Describe what the emergency first responder should do if there is reason to believe that there is a hazard at the scene.
- State the role the emergency first responder should perform until appropriately trained personnel arrive at the scene of a hazardous materials situation.
- Describe the criteria for a multiple-casualty incident (MCI).

- Discuss the role of the emergency first responder in an MCI.
- Describe some identifying characteristics that may be indicative of an act of terrorism.
- Discuss the role of the emergency first responder at an act of terrorism.
- Summarize the components of basic triage.

AFFECTIVE OBJECTIVES

- Explain the rationale for having the unit prepared to respond.

PSYCHOMOTOR OBJECTIVES

- Given the scenario of an MCI, perform triage.

Check your understanding

Please refer to p. 439 for the answers to these questions.

1. The first phase of an EMS response is _____.

2. List at least four actions the emergency first responder should take in order to be prepared to respond to calls.
   1. _____
   2. _____
   3. _____
   4. _____

3. List four actions to reduce the risk of injury when driving to a call.
   1. _____
   2. _____
   3. _____
   4. _____

4. List at least three considerations in deciding where and how to park at the scene.
   1. _____
   2. _____
   3. _____

5. What are the critical tasks an emergency first responder must carry out after a call in order to be prepared for the next response?

   _____
   _____
   _____

6. The organized system of management implemented at the scene of large-scale incidents or disasters is called the _____.

7. List at least four considerations for preparing a landing zone for a medical transport helicopter.
   1. _____
   2. _____
   3. _____
   4. _____

8. The emergency first responder should not approach the helicopter unless directed to by the _____.

9. The process used to free a patient from entrapment in a vehicle is called _____.

10. Any substance that poses a risk to health, safety, or the environment is considered to be a/an _____.

11. The U.S. Department of Transportation publishes a reference guide to hazardous materials that should be carried in every emergency first responder's vehicle. This reference is called _____.

12. The diamond-shaped emblem on a container or vehicle carrying a hazardous material is called a/an _____.

13. Which of the following is the most dangerous direction from which to approach a helicopter?
    A. The front
    B. The rear
    C. The right side
    D. The left side

14. Which of the following is the term for a situation in which the number of patients overwhelms the available resources?
    A. Triage
    B. Incident Command System
    C. Confined space rescue
    D. Multiple-casualty incident

15. You are the first to arrive at a farmer's co-op where there has been a leak of anhydrous ammonia from a tank. You can see as you approach that there are several people in distress in the parking lot. Which of the following is the best course of action?
    A. Wait for arrival of a hazardous materials team so they can bring the patients to you.
    B. Stay in your vehicle with the windows up and quickly drive over to pick up the people in the parking lot to get them to safety.
    C. Use standard precautions, including a HEPA mask, for protection as you approach the patients.
    D. Take a position downwind from the location of the incident.

16. A patient who is complaining of an ankle injury at the scene of a multiple-casualty incident would be classified as which of the following?
    A. Immediate
    B. Delayed
    C. Minor
    D. Deceased

17. You have been assigned as the triage officer for 15 victims on an overturned bus. After making sure the scene is safe, which of the following would you perform during your initial triage?
    A. Administer oxygen.
    B. Open the airway.
    C. Splint injuries.
    D. Perform a detailed exam.

Chapter 16

Environmental Emergencies

LESSON GOAL

As an emergency medical responder (First Responder), you may find yourself confronted with patients who are suffering illness or injury caused by their environment. In this chapter, we will describe different environments and the harm they can cause along with descriptions of the care you can provide to improve your patients' chances at a positive outcome. We will look at heat and cold injuries, poisons bites, and stings as well as allergic reactions and anaphylaxis.

OBJECTIVES

1. Describe heat loss.
2. List the signs and symptoms of cold exposure.
3. Describe assistance that can be given to victims of cold exposure.
4. List the signs and symptoms of exposure to heat.
5. Describe assistance that can be given to victims of heat exposure.
6. List the signs and symptoms of drowning and near-drowning.
7. Describe the assistance that may be given to victims of drowning or near-drowning.
8. Describe the types of bites and stings that may cause illness in patients.
9. Describe the assistance that can be given to victims of bites and stings.

In the Real World

You are called to assist a "man down" in an alley on a cold November evening. The ground is covered with 1 to 2 inches of snow. You arrive to find an unresponsive man who is lying among some flattened boxes in the alley. He is very cold to the touch and it is difficult to feel a pulse, but he is breathing very slowly. What is happening to this man and what can you do for him as you await the ambulance?

Environmental emergencies are situations in which the external environment surrounding a person makes the person ill. Exposure usually results in illness or injury but can cause death in extreme cases. Two common examples of environmental emergencies are those caused by exposure to heat or cold. Individuals exposed to extremes of heat or cold can have mild to severe effects, and even relatively short periods of lighter exposure can cause harm to patients who are otherwise compromised by illness or injury.

Thermoregulation

Thermoregulation refers to the way the body creates and releases heat.

Knowledge of this process will help you understand how people respond to extreme changes in temperature. First, the body creates heat through cellular metabolism. As fuel and oxygen enter the cells of the body, CO_2 (carbon dioxide) waste and heat are generated. Generally, the heat generated is sufficient to keep the body's temperature in optimal operating ranges. If the heat generated is more or less than the body requires, it is either released from or absorbed into the body.

Heat Transfer

Heat transfer is the way that needed heat is moved into the body or how excess heat is released from the body. This transfer is accomplished through one or more of the following mechanisms (**Fig 16-1**):

- Conduction
- Convection
- Evaporation
- Respiration
- Radiation

Conduction

Conduction is the direct transfer of heat from a warmer object to a cooler object. This means conduction causes you to lose body heat when you sit or lie on a surface cooler than your body temperature. An example would be a patient lying on the ground during cold weather. Because the ground temperature is lower than the patient's body temperature, heat from the patient will be transferred to the ground and your patient's body temperature will drop. In contrast, if your patient is lying on a surface with a temperature greater than the patient's body temperature, the heat from the surface will transfer to the patient's body. In certain cases if the temperature differences are extremes, burns can occur. Certain materials conduct heat better than others. Metal conducts heat faster than most other materials and can cause the local injury of burn or frostbite to patients.

Convection

Convection is heat loss through the heating of cooler water or air as it passes over a warmer surface such as the skin. As the heated air or water moves away from the body, cooler air or water moves in to take its place and the body continues to lose additional heat to the new air or water. The body will lose heat 25 times faster in water than in air. Convection heat loss of the body to cooler air is the basis for wind chill. A windbreaker or a wet suit helps to decrease or prevent convection heat loss. Wrapping your patient in an outer layer of plastic may help to prevent heat loss caused by convection. In cool weather, this kind of outer wrapping may also help to prevent heat loss caused by evaporation.

Evaporation

Evaporation is the loss of heat that occurs when water or the moisture from perspiration on the skin is converted to water vapor. Evaporation can be the cause of large amounts of body heat loss.

Radiation

Radiation is the term for the direct transfer of energy without an external medium such as wind or water. Any object warmer than the external environment gives off

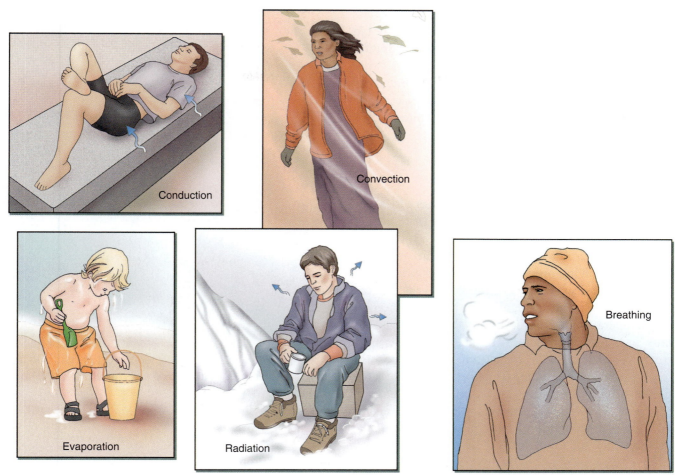

Fig. 16-1 Five mechanisms of heat loss in a patient. (From McSwain N, Paturas J: *The basic EMT: comprehensive prehospital patient care,* ed 2, St Louis, 2003, Mosby.)

heat in the form of infrared radiation. Keeping skin covered helps to prevent loss of body heat from radiation. The head and neck are major sources of infrared radiation heat loss in cold weather.

Respirations

Respirations can also be a source of heat loss if the external air is cooler than the body's temperature. Cooler outside air is inhaled and then warmed to the body's internal temperature. Once the warmed air is exhaled it takes the increased heat with it, causing a decrease or drop in the body's temperature. Also, during respirations body water is lost and can contribute to dehydration.

Cold-Related Emergencies

Exposure to a cold environment can result in a localized cold emergency (**frostbite**) or a generalized cold emergency (**hypothermia**). When exposed to cold it is important to keep yourself and your patient dry, avoid direct contact with items colder than yourself, and dress in layers that will trap dry air, which will assist in maintaining body heat. These layers should be made of a material that will wick (pull) moisture away from the body and retain the ability to insulate if it gets wet. Materials such as wool, polypropylene, pile, and fleece (not sweatshirt fleece) are good examples of material that can provide wicking and insulation. You should wear an outer layer that will keep air from blowing through your clothing and removing body heat. You should also wear a hat to prevent heat loss from your head. At the same time, however, you should not allow yourself to overheat during a rescue. If you sweat, for example, the moisture will be retained in your clothing and you will have to expend energy to keep this water as warm as your body. If you dress in layers, then as you warm up hiking into a rescue, you can remove layers to prevent overheating and sweating. Once on scene, you can spend the first minute layering up with extra clothing (this can be done while surveying the scene for safety and mechanism of injury) so that as you get involved in patient care and cool off, you will remain warm. Proper nutrition gives you a better chance at conserving heat and you should remember to drink plenty of water because dehydration can prevent the body from producing heat. Stay away from caffeine and alcohol, sources of fluid that dehydrate. Stay away from nicotine products, which will constrict blood vessels and therefore increase the risk of frostbite.

Local Cold Emergencies
Frostbite

The freezing or near-freezing of a body part is a localized cold emergency, or **frostbite.** Unprotected, inadequately protected, or wet skin is the most likely area for a localized cold exposure. Frostbite can be classified as either superficial (involving only the top layers of the skin) or deep (involving deeper layers of the skin). Frostbite can occur with or without generalized cooling of the core body temperature (hypothermia). Frostbite typically occurs in exposed extremities because these areas are further from the central circulation. Fingers, toes, the face, ears, and the nose are frequent frostbite sites. You can often see a line of demarcation (a clear line of color separation) separating the frostbitten area from undamaged tissue. Other signs and symptoms of localized cold injuries include the following (Fig. 16-2):

SUPERFICIAL FROSTBITE

- Blanching (whitening) of the skin
- Loss of sensation in the injured area
- Skin that is soft to the touch
- If the area is rewarmed, complaints of a tingling sensation

DEEP FROSTBITE

- White, waxy skin
- Skin that is firm or feels frozen to the touch
- Swelling
- Blisters
- If thawed or partially thawed, the skin may appear flushed with areas of purple and blanching or may be mottled and bluish

Management of Local Cold Emergencies

Emergency management of a localized cold injury should focus on getting the patient out of the cold environment to prevent further injury and progression from a localized cold injury to a generalized cold emergency (hypothermia). Follow the usual sequence for assessment. Wet or restrictive clothing should be removed from the patient because its presence may continue to decrease body temperature through evaporation. The frostbitten part should

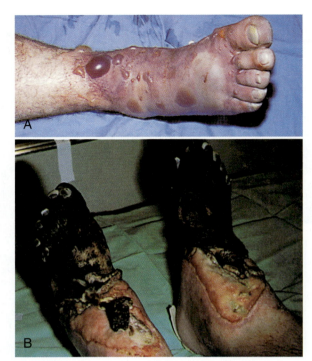

Fig. 16-2 A, Swelling and blister formation with frostbite injury. **B,** Feet of patient 6 weeks after frostbite injury. (From McSwain N, Paturas J: *The basic EMT: comprehensive prehospital patient care,* ed 2, St Louis, 2003, Mosby.)

be warmed quickly, but through passive means such as placing the cold body part next to a warm body part (e.g., putting the patient's hands in their armpits). You should not try to actively warm the body part by rubbing the injured part or applying direct heat because this may cause further injury to the patient. Remember to comfort, calm, and reassure the patient until the ambulance arrives. Special considerations for the assessment and treatment of patients with localized cold injuries are detailed in Box 16-1.

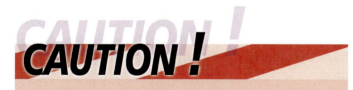

CAUTION !

Elderly patients are more susceptible to heat and cold emergencies for several reasons. They may be taking medication that alters their circulation and their nervous system may have deteriorated, inhibiting their ability to feel heat and cold and their ability to regulate body temperature. They may also have circulatory disease that will predispose them to complications.

BOX 16-1 Care for a Patient with a Localized Cold Injury (Frostbite)

- Complete a scene size-up.
  - Establish a safe environment for rescuers, patient(s), and bystanders.
  - Remove patient from cold environment.
  - Request additional resources as needed.
- Perform an initial (primary) assessment.
  - Identify and treat any life-threatening conditions.
- Obtain vital signs and SAMPLE history.
- Treat the patient's signs and symptoms as indicated.
  - Remove wet clothing—wet clothing promotes heat loss.
  - Maintain body heat.
  - Active rewarming techniques are not recommended.
    - Do not massage cold/frozen extremities—this can cause tissue destruction.

- Do not apply direct heat.
  - Protect the injured extremity.
- Frostbitten extremities have decreased sensation (prone to further injury).
- Consider splinting the extremity.
- Remove jewelry.
- Separate fingers and toes if possible with dressings.
- Perform a detailed physical examination (secondary assessment) as indicated.
- Maintain patient comfort.
- Calm and reassure patient as needed.
- Perform reassessments as indicated.
- Report any changes in the patient's condition.

Generalized Cold Emergencies

Hypothermia

A generalized cold emergency occurs when a patient's core (internal) body temperature drops from a normal 98.6° to below 95° Fahrenheit (F). This condition is called **hypothermia** (low temperature). A number of factors can make a patient susceptible to having a low body temperature, including the following:

- Prolonged exposure to a cold or wet environment
- Being very old or very young
- Underlying medical conditions
- Alcohol use or abuse
- Certain medications or drugs

Hypothermia can occur even in normal external temperature environments. An example would be a situation where the outside temperature is 70°F and individuals are swimming in water that is below 70°F. Because of convection the body can rapidly lose a great amount of heat to the low-temperature water, causing hypothermia. Hypothermia can be present with or without localized cold injury (frostbite). Patients may become hypothermic for an obvious reason, such as being stranded in the snow, but they may also develop hypothermia for more subtle reasons. For example, an elderly patient whose internal thermostat is not maintaining a normal body temperature can become hypothermic at normal room temperatures. The following are predisposing factors for hypothermia:

- The patient's age (the very old and the very young are at higher risk)
- A preexisting illness or medical condition
- Use of certain medications or the abuse of some drugs

These factors can inhibit the body's ability to conserve heat.

Primary hypothermia refers to the body's core temperature dropping below 95°F (35° Centigrade [C]) because of an environmental exposure. **Secondary hypothermia** occurs when illness, alcohol, or aging influences the body's ability to retain heat. This is sometimes referred to as urban hypothermia. More commonly this affects patients at age extremes. Underlying medical conditions such as hypothyroidism can also make patients susceptible to secondary hypothermia.

Hypothermia is also classified by severity levels. Mild hypothermia occurs with body temperatures of 95° to 89.6°F (35° to 32.2°C), moderate hypothermia with body temperatures from 89.6° to 78.8°F (32.2° to 28°C), and severe hypothermia with body temperatures below 78.8°F (28°C).

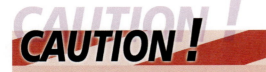

CAUTION!

Hypothermia does not only happen in the winter or outside. Consider an elderly patient that falls and breaks her hip and spends the night on a tile bathroom floor that is 68° F. This patient will become hypothermic as well.

CAUTION!

Remember that the first priority in environmental emergencies is to get the patient out of the problematic environment.

Signs and Symptoms

Signs and symptoms of generalized hypothermia include the following (Fig. 16-3):

- *Cool or cold skin temperature.* You should place the back of your hand between the clothing and the patient's abdomen to check for cool or cold abdominal skin temperature.
- *Shivering.* Shivering is the body's attempt to generate heat and raise the body temperature.
- *Decreasing mental status or motor function.* As the degree of hypothermia worsens (the body temperature continues to lower), it can cause poor motor coordination, memory disturbances or confusion, reduced or loss of touch sensation, mood changes, reduced communication, or speech difficulty.
- *Poor judgment.* With the decrease in mental status, the patient may show poor judgment by removing his or her clothing while still in the cold environment.
- *Dizziness.*
- *Stiff or rigid posture.* In addition, the patient may complain of joint or muscle stiffness.

Management of Generalized Cold Emergencies

The emergency management of a hypothermic patient includes a scene size-up and initial assessment. As the patient's body temperature lowers, the respiratory rate and pulse rate will slow and eventually stop. Pulses may be especially difficult to assess because all of the patient's blood will be flowing to vital internal organs such as the brain and the heart and not to the skin or surface level organs. It is therefore important that breathing and circulation be assessed for 30 to 45 seconds before starting rescue breathing or cardiopulmonary resuscitation (CPR). As with the emergency management of frostbite, the hypothermic patient needs to be warmed gently through passive means such as blankets. You should avoid rough handling of a hypothermic patient because exertion and movement may cause the sensitive heart to change to a lethal rhythm or even cardiac arrest. You should never give the patient anything by mouth. Consuming coffee, tea, alcohol, or nicotine can further impair the patient's circulation and worsen the patient's condition. Special considerations for the assessment and treatment of hypothermic patients are listed in Box 16-2 (see Fig. 16-4).

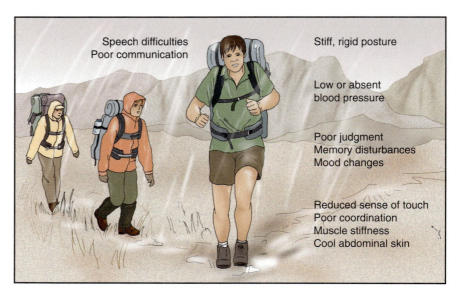

Fig. 16-3 Signs and symptoms of a generalized cold emergency. (From McSwain N, Paturas J: *The basic EMT: comprehensive prehospital patient care,* ed 2, St Louis, 2003, Mosby.)

BOX 16-2 Care of the Patient with Hypothermia

- Complete a scene size-up.
  - Establish a safe environment for rescuers, patient(s), and bystanders.
  - Remove patient from cold environment.
  - Request additional resources as needed.
- Perform an initial (primary) assessment.
  - Identify and treat any life-threatening conditions.
  - For nonresponsive patients, check breathing and carotid pulse for 30 to 45 seconds. If there is no breathing, start rescue breathing. If there is no pulse, start CPR.
  - The AED may not be effective with a hypothermic patient until the core body temperature has been elevated; however, defibrillation should be attempted regardless.
- Obtain vital signs and SAMPLE history.
- Treat the patient's signs and symptoms as indicated.
  - Remove wet clothing; wet clothing promotes heat loss.
- Maintain body heat (e.g., with blankets).
- Avoid active rewarming techniques.
  - Do not massage cold/frozen extremities—this can cause tissue destruction.
  - Active rewarming techniques can cause the circulatory system to rapidly move cold blood into the vital organs, worsening the patient's hypothermic state.
- Avoid rough handling of the patient.
  - Rough handling or sudden movement of the patient may cause the heart's electrical system to produce a lethal rhythm or cardiac arrest.
- Do not allow hypothermic patients to exert energy.
- Perform a detailed examination (secondary assessment) as indicated.
- Maintain patient comfort.
- Calm and reassure patient as needed.
- Perform reassessments as indicated.
- Report any changes in the patient's condition.

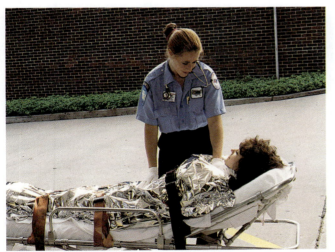

Fig. 16-4 Hypothermia wrap. (From NAEMT: *PHTLS: Basic and advanced prehospital trauma life support*, ed 6, St Louis, 2007, Mosby.)

Heat-Related Emergencies

The patient's external environment and level of physical activity are the primary factors that lead to heat-related emergencies. Normally the body tries to maintain a tem-perature of 98.6° F. If the body temperature starts to rise, the body uses thermoregulation methods to get rid of the excess heat. For example, when the air temperature is cooler than a person's body temperature, the body can lose heat through the skin to the environment. The body can also cool itself through sweating. The sweat evaporates (along with the heat) into the relatively dryer air. A very active person can lose more than 1 L of sweat in 1 hour.

In addition to exposure to heat, other factors may predispose a patient to heat-related emergencies, including the following:

- The patient's age (the very old and the very young are at higher risk)
- A preexisting illness or medical condition
- Use of certain medications or the abuse of some drugs

These factors may inhibit the body's ability to dissipate heat.

Excessive exposure to heat can lead to one of three types of heat-related emergencies: **heat cramps, heat exhaustion,** and **heat stroke** (Table 16-1).

TABLE 16-1   Signs and Symptoms of Heat-Related Illness

	GENERAL WEAKNESS	MUSCLE CRAMPS	RESPIRATORY RATES	PULSE RATES	SKIN CONDITION	SWEAT	LOSS OF RESPONSIVENESS
Heat cramps	Yes	Yes	Vary	Vary	Normal	Heavy	Seldom
Heat exhaustion	Yes	No	Rapid, shallow	Weak	Cold, clammy	Heavy	Sometimes
Heat stroke	Yes	No	Deep, then shallow	Full, rapid	Dry, hot	Little or none	Often

Heat Cramps

Heat cramps are muscle cramps that are usually limited to the patient's legs and abdominal area. The muscle cramps are a result of fluid and salts being lost from the body through sweating. Besides muscle cramps, the patient may also complain of exhaustion, dizziness, or periods of faintness.

Heat Exhaustion

Heat exhaustion is the term used when the circulatory system fails to adequately maintain its normal function because of the excessive loss of fluids and salts from the body. The signs and symptoms of heat exhaustion include the following:

- Rapid, shallow breathing
- Excessive sweating
- Total body weakness
- Dizziness

Heat Stroke

Heat stroke is a *true life-threatening emergency*. It is the result of the body's inability to cool itself. This causes the body's core temperature to rise (hyperthermia). The body temperature can increase so much that brain damage can occur. The signs and symptoms of heat stroke include the following:

- Deep breathing followed by periods of shallow breathing
- Rapid, strong pulses followed by rapid, weak pulses
- Dry, hot skin
- Dilated pupils
- Loss of consciousness
- Muscle twitching or seizures

As patients progress from heat exhaustion to heat stroke, the most important sign or symptom is the changing level of consciousness. The patient may still have moist skin.

As an emergency first responder, you are not expected to definitively distinguish between the specific types of heat-related emergencies. Instead you should look for and control factors that can lead to a worsening heat-related emergency. For example, heat exhaustion may become heat stroke if not recognized early (Fig. 16-5).

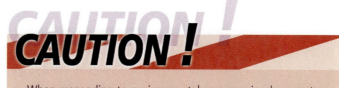

CAUTION!

When responding to environmental emergencies, be sure to protect yourself from the environment. For example, wear proper clothing and consume appropriate nutrition when working in the cold and always be properly hydrated while working in the heat.

Management of Heat Emergencies

The steps for emergency care for a patient with exposure to heat are detailed in Box 16-3 and Fig. 16-6.

Poisonings

A **poison** is any substance that can be potentially harmful to the body. Poisons can enter the body through one of four routes: ingestion, inhalation, absorption, or injection (Fig. 16-7).

- *Ingestion.* Poisoning by ingestion occurs when a toxic substance is taken by mouth and enters the

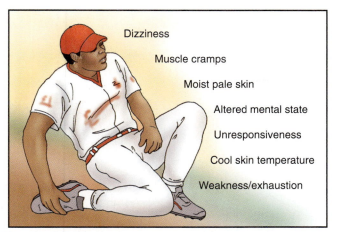

Fig. 16-5 Signs and symptoms of a heat-related emergency. (From McSwain N, Paturas J: *The basic EMT: comprehensive prehospital patient care,* ed 2, St Louis, 2003, Mosby.)

Labels in figure:
Dizziness
Muscle cramps
Moist pale skin
Altered mental state
Unresponsiveness
Cool skin temperature
Weakness/exhaustion

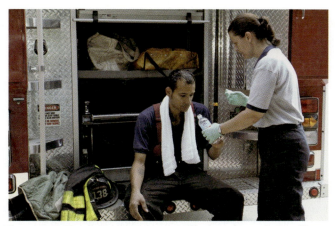

Fig. 16-6 Cooling a patient suffering from heat illness. (From Chapleau W, Pons P: *Emergency medical technician, making the difference,* St Louis, 2007, Mosby.)

BOX 16-3 Care of the Patient with a Heat-Related Emergency

- Complete a scene size-up.
  - Establish a safe environment for rescuers, patient(s), and bystanders.
  - Remove the patient from heat into a cool or shaded environment.
  - Request additional resources as needed.
- Perform an initial (primary) assessment.
  - Identify and treat any life-threatening conditions.
- Obtain vital signs and SAMPLE history.
- Treat the patient's signs and symptoms as indicated.
- Consider the recovery position for spontaneously breathing patients who are not suspected of having spinal injury.
- Perform a detailed physical examination (secondary assessment) as indicated.
- Maintain patient comfort.
- Calm and reassure patient as needed.
- Perform reassessments as indicated.
- Report any changes in the patient's condition.

---

digestive system. Types of poison that can be ingested include drugs, plants, alcohol, and household products. Food poisoning also occurs by ingestion. A patient who has ingested poison may have discoloration, burning, or swelling in the mouth and throat, which can compromise the airway. Other signs and symptoms include nausea and vomiting, diarrhea, and abdominal pain.

- *Inhalation.* Poisons can also be inhaled by patients. The poisonous substance is brought into the body through the lungs during breathing. One example of an inhaled poison is carbon monoxide, a colorless, odorless gas that is present in smoke. When carbon monoxide enters the blood through the lungs, it displaces oxygen and leads to a respiratory emergency. Cyanide is another poisonous gas that

can be inhaled. Cyanide prevents the use of oxygen by the cells. Other examples of inhaled poisons include drugs or fumes from household cleaners. The signs and symptoms of an inhaled poison include headache, nausea, coughing, difficulty breathing, altered mental status, and loss of consciousness.

- *Absorption.* Poisons that can be absorbed through the skin include insecticides or toxins from poisonous plants such as poison ivy. The signs and symptoms of an absorbed poison can be local to the affected area of skin or the poison may have a more generalized effect on the body. The signs and symptoms of an absorbed poison include itching, rashes, burning, redness of the skin, shock, nausea, and vomiting.

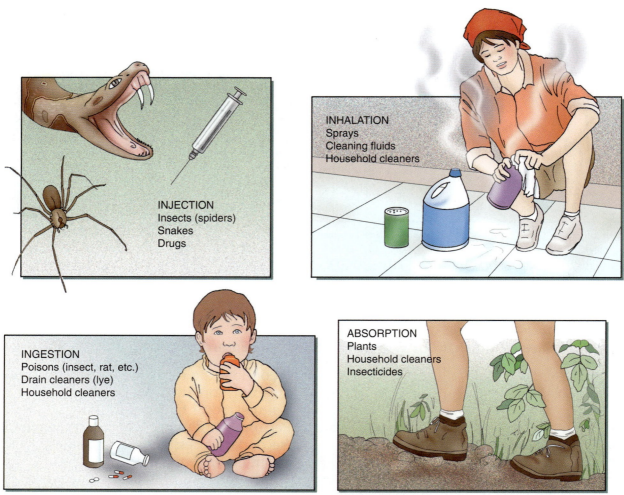

Fig. 16-7 How poisons enter the body. (From McSwain N, Paturas J: *The basic EMT: comprehensive prehospital patient care,* ed 2, St Louis, 2003, Mosby.)

- *Injection.* Poison can be injected directly through the skin, causing a local reaction, or it can enter the circulatory system. Examples of this type of poisoning include intravenous (IV) drug use and bites or stings from animals such as insects or snakes (**see Fig. 16-7**). The signs and symptoms of an injected poison include an obvious puncture site where the substance bypassed the skin, redness and itching, tenderness, swelling, and pain at the injection site.

Management of Poisoning

No matter what the cause of the poisoning, as an emergency first responder, you should always call 9-1-1 and the Poison Control Center. If you are part of the 9-1-1 response and transport is available, the Poison Control Center can be contacted while the patient is en route to the hospital by EMS or the receiving hospital's staff. Your assessment of the patient should include a thorough SAMPLE history to determine what has occurred, what type of poison the patient may have contacted, when the

poison may have been taken, and how much may have been taken.

Emergency management of poisons will depend on the type of poison ingested. As an emergency first responder, you should do a scene size-up, ensuring that the patient is moved to a safe area if needed. An initial assessment should be done and any life-threatening conditions treated. The patient should be watched carefully for signs and symptoms of shock and treated accordingly. You should always try to identify the poisonous substance without delaying transport, and you should save any material that the patient vomits. All material should be transported with the patient to the hospital whenever possible without compromising the safety of the individuals providing transportation.

Allergic Reactions

An **allergic reaction** is the response the body makes to a foreign substance such as insect venom, food, medication, animal dander, or pollen. Reactions can be as simple as a local skin reaction or as complex as respiratory difficulty and shock. A typical allergic reaction involves hives and reddened, itchy skin. The reaction may also cause the airways to swell and constrict, resulting in an asthma-like response. When the airway is involved the patient will present with wheezing and difficulty breathing.

Anaphylaxis

The most severe allergic reaction is termed *anaphylaxis.* **Anaphylaxis** occurs when the patient's body is overwhelmed by the allergic substance and the reaction intensifies into shock. This is triggered by swelling and constriction of the airways and dilation of the blood vessels, which causes inadequate circulation. Patients who have allergies, particularly if they have had significant reactions in the past, may carry medication to attempt to control the reaction. Anaphylaxis is a life-threatening emergency that requires medical attention as soon as possible. As an emergency first responder you should provide supportive care by maintaining the airway and breathing assistance as necessary while waiting for EMS to arrive.

Water-Related Emergencies
Decompression Sickness (Dysbarism)

Altitude-related illnesses arise with decreases in atmospheric pressure. However, increases in pressure also can cause problems. This most often occurs when a person goes scuba diving. Scuba diving involves breathing oxygen and other gases from a container while underwater. As a diver descends deeper in the water, the weight of the water compresses any gases the diver inhales. As a result, gases that normally do not cross from the lungs into the blood readily go into solution. When the diver ascends to the surface, the gas expands. Gas that was in solution in the blood and tissues expands to form bubbles. Bubbles in the joints exert a painful pressure, which forces the individual to bend the joints. This is called **decompression sickness,** commonly referred to as **the bends.** Decompression sickness can develop days after a dive and may not show up until a patient has returned from vacation. Bubbles can also form in the blood and can block blood vessels to the heart or brain, causing a heart attack or stroke. If the diver is holding his or her breath, a pneumothorax may result from the expanding air in the lungs.

Management of Decompression Sickness

Administration of high-flow oxygen with a nonrebreather mask is very important for patients with decompression

sickness. Try to gather the history of the dive, such as the number of dives, the length and depth of each dive, when the signs and symptoms first started, and whether the patient has flown in an airplane since the dive. Make sure the hospital staff knows that this may be a scuba diving illness. Definitive care of this type of emergency often involves treating the patient in a hyperbaric chamber. Local protocols may dictate direct transport of these patients to a hospital with such a chamber.

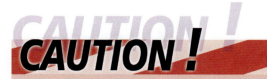

CAUTION !

In water-related emergencies, if the patient is in the water, only trained rescuers should approach the patient. The rule of "reach, throw, row, and only then go" should always be used, which means unless you are trained to do water rescue, you should only attempt to assist from shore.

Drowning

A far more common water-related emergency is drowning. **Drowning** is defined as suffocation that occurs from submersion in a liquid. The term *near-drowning* is commonly used, but it is no longer the recommended term; *submersion incident* is preferred. It is estimated that 80,000 submersion incidents occur each year in the United States, with about 9000 deaths. Worldwide more than a half a million drowning deaths are reported annually. This number is thought to be significantly lower than the actual drowning deaths due to underreporting of drownings.

It is particularly important to ensure rescuer safety in water incidents. EMS personnel as well as bystanders may also become victims if they are not well trained in water rescue and protected by personal flotation devices (PFDs) when appropriate. If rescue is to be attempted, every effort must be made by the rescuer to stay out of the water or away from a struggling, awake victim. More tragic than an unnecessary drowning is the double drowning of a victim and a potential rescuer. The following rule is important: *Reach, throw, row, and only then go.* This means that rescue should first be attempted by extending your reach to a victim using a pole, a branch, or an article of clothing. Most drownings occur while the patient is within reach of safety. If the victim cannot be reached safely, throw an item that will float and can support the individual. The item should be soft, if possible, and should have a rope attached for retrieval. If the individual is too far from the shore for these measures, a boat-based rescue is preferable to a swimming rescue. All these rescue techniques require practice to be done safely. They should be drilled frequently if water rescue or water hazards are part of the responders' responsibilities (Fig. 16-8).

Drowning does not occur only around large bodies of water. Washing machines, bathtubs, and even 5-gallon buckets are particularly dangerous to one of the age-

groups at highest risk for drowning: children under 5 years of age. Indeed, only a few ounces could cause the airway to close and cause suffocation. Teenagers and people who have been drinking alcohol are also well represented among victims of submersion incidents. Several preventative measures can be taken that may lower the incidence of drowning, which is the third most common cause of unintentional death in the United States. These

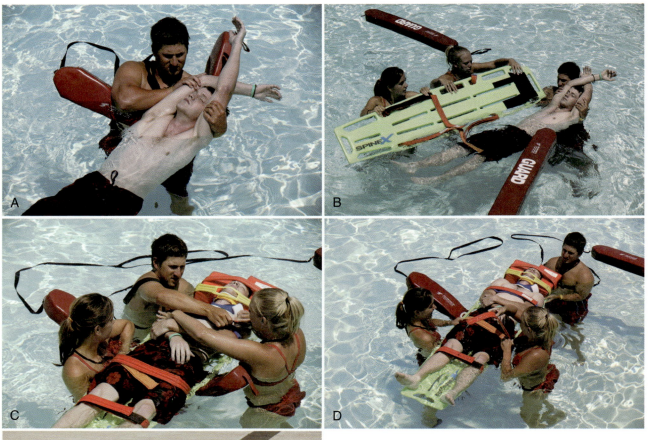

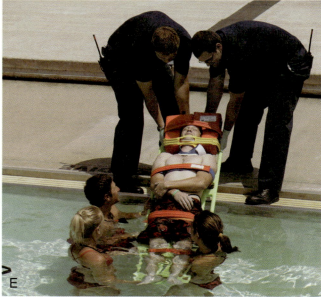

Fig. 16-8 Water rescue requires special training. **A,** Lifeguards find an unresponsive person floating face down in a community pool. One lifeguard reaches the victim, secures the man's head and neck between his arms, and rolls the patient's face out of the water. **B,** Two other lifeguards bring a backboard, a cervical collar (C-collar), and head blocks to the first lifeguard and the patient. **C,** The backboard is floated under the patient, and the patient is secured to it. **D,** After the patient has been secured to the backboard, the lifeguards float the patient to the side of the pool, where emergency personnel are waiting. **E,** Emergency personnel help remove the patient from the pool. (From Chapleau W, Pons P: *Emergency medical technician, making the difference,* St Louis, 2007, Mosby.)

measures include erecting fences around swimming pools, having rescue equipment readily accessible, and using water motion alarms.

Survival after submersion is primarily related to the duration of the submersion. The longer the patient is without oxygen, the smaller the chance of survival. Therefore the sooner artificial ventilation can be started, the better. This may mean starting ventilations while the patient is still in the water. It is recommended that chest compressions be started only after the patient is on a firm surface. Another factor that affects survival is the purity of the water. The more polluted the liquid, the worse the potential outcome. A much discussed factor is the temperature of the water. Water temperature may be a protective factor for young patients if the water temperature is below 70° F (21° C).

Another concern in submersion incidents is the risk of trauma. If a diving board is present or if the patient may have dived or fallen into the water from a height, spinal precautions should be taken when turning the patient over in the water and when removing the patient from the water on a backboard. This technique requires practice in both shallow and deep water before it is attempted on actual patients. Submersion patients or patients found in the water also may have other traumatic injuries, such as fractures or soft tissue injuries resulting from boat versus boat or boat versus swimmer collisions.

Lightning and Electrocution

Lightning kills about 200 people per year. Many more people are struck every year and not killed. Only 20% to 30% of those struck are killed. In addition, about 800 people per year are electrocuted by human-made sources of electricity. Lightning is a hazard to responders on search and rescues and there are many stray sources of electricity in the aftermath of a disaster that can pose a danger. The most dangerous time for a lightning strike is actually before the storm hits. Lightning can travel horizontally in front of a storm as far as 6 miles. During lightning storms, stay away from high geographic points or high trees (including ridges or antennas). Stay out of water and caves when possible. Patients struck by lightning are not burnt to a crisp when struck; lightning actually travels mostly over (not through) the body. This flow of lightning may blow the clothing right off the patient. However, there is often internal damage to patients of high-voltage electrocution (such as lightning strikes), even without external burns. If the patient is not in cardiac or respiratory arrest immediately, internal injuries may exist that may not be evident for hours. Light-

ning strike patients may pass in and out of cardiac or respiratory arrest repeatedly, and must be watched closely. You should use extreme caution when assessing and treating a victim of a lightning strike or electrocution. Lightning strike patients are not electrified and can be touched safely. However, you should always make sure that victims of human-made electricity are disconnected from the source before you attempt to render care. This may include disconnecting or turning off the power source. Avoid contact with electrical devices during rescue. Do not handle or stand near metal objects.

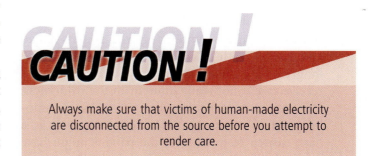

CAUTION !

Always make sure that victims of human-made electricity are disconnected from the source before you attempt to render care.

Emergencies in the Wilderness

Emergencies in the wilderness can be challenging. Rescuers must protect themselves and be prepared for injuries and illness common to the particular environment. There are standards of care for these types of emergencies.

Special Protocols

The Wilderness Medical Society and the National Association of Emergency Medical Services Physicians have each published position papers detailing the care of patients in extended care situations for the following areas:

- *Discontinuation of CPR.* The *Emergency Cardiovascular Care Guidelines* for starting and stopping CPR assume a traditional progression of bystander CPR within 4 to 6 minutes and defibrillation and advanced life support within 8 minutes. Even with this "best of all worlds" progression, only 30% to 60% survival has been shown. After 20 minutes of CPR alone, almost no survival has ever been demonstrated. Therefore the protocols mentioned previously suggest that after 30 minutes of CPR without effect, efforts should be discontinued. The exceptions include hypothermic patients and lightning strike patients. In these circumstances, prolonged CPR may be effective. CPR should not be started in the first place in cases of hypothermia without any sign of life nor in the cold patient with an incompressible chest. CPR should not be started if the patient has been submersed for more than 60 minutes, regardless of the temperature of the water. CPR should not be started in wilderness trauma patients. CPR should not be started if performing it could cause any danger to the rescuer. CPR during evacuation by litter or sled or even in most helicopter situations is difficult if not ineffective.

- *Spinal immobilization.* It is difficult to improvise a spinal immobilization device that actually works. In a disaster, maybe a door removed from its hinges and padded with a blanket would work. But how long can a patient lie on this hard surface and receive care if not really injured? In the wilderness, it is even more difficult to improvise spinal immobilization. Therefore, if a small group such as a hasty search team believes the patient might have a spinal injury, they must send for a litter team. However, if the patient is conscious and alert with full pain-free range of motion in the spine, with no pain or deformity to palpation, and with normal spine length and normal sensation and motor function, then it is unlikely that the patient has a spinal injury.

- *Wound care.* After stopping bleeding with direct pressure, the next concerns with soft tissue wounds are function of the affected part, infection, and cosmetic result. Because of pain, swelling, and stiffness, soft tissue wounds can incapacitate a patient, preventing him or her from helping with evacuation. High-risk wounds such as human or animal bites, open fractures, wounds with exposed tendons or ligaments, large or ragged wounds, contaminated wounds, wounds with dead tissues, or wounds entering into a body cavity must be treated with particular care. In the extended care situation, these wounds should be cleaned by pressure irrigation with sterile water. A sterile water–like solution can be created for emergency use by boiling regular water and letting it cool before use. An alternative is to add 1% povidone-iodine to the water if the patient is not allergic to iodine or shellfish. The same solution can be used directly in high-risk wounds. Large wounds can be packed and covered with sterile bandages. Swelling should be kept to a minimum with cold application and elevation above the level of the heart. Impaled objects should be cut as close as possible to the skin. If an impaled object

is made of metal, then in a cold environment it will act as a heat sink, conducting heat out of the patient rapidly, and must be removed to prevent hypothermia and frostbite.

Altitude

As you travel up from sea level, the weight of the blanket of air gets thinner and thinner as the barometric pressure decreases. The percentage of oxygen in the air remains the same (21%), but as the overall weight of air decreases, the partial pressure of oxygen also decreases. At 10,000 feet, the air pressure is two thirds of that at sea level. At 18,000 feet, just above the highest permanent human habitation, the air pressure is half of that at sea level. This means the pressures pushing oxygen out of the lung and into the blood are only two thirds and one half, respectively, of those at sea level. This causes a number of problems, particularly if you travel quickly to altitude without time to adjust (e.g., if you arrive on a mountain top in a rescue helicopter).

Acute mountain sickness (AMS) can occur in these situations. Signs of AMS include headache, apathy, insomnia, lightheadedness, loss of appetite, and nausea. In severe cases, vomiting and shortness of breath on exertion are present. AMS can occur at altitudes as low as 6500 feet if you travel to that altitude too fast. Ascending slowly and keeping hydrated may prevent AMS on rescues; however, following these precautions is not always possible.

High-altitude pulmonary edema (HAPE) and high-altitude cerebral edema (HACE) may result if AMS is not treated or if the patient ascends even higher, usually above 10,000 to 12,000 feet. HAPE and HACE are life-threatening and require immediate treatment. HAPE is characterized by cough, increasing distress, chest pain, and fluid in the lungs. The fluid can be heard by using a stethoscope or by placing your ear against the patient's chest. HACE is characterized by altered mental status and lack of coordination. The treatment for all altitude illness is to take the patient to a lower altitude. Oxygen administration may buy some time, but treatment is to take the patient to lower altitude.

Blisters

Blisters may seem like a minor annoyance, but they can stop a Search and Rescue (SAR) team or interrupt a wildland fire response. Prevention with well-fitting, double-layer socks and properly fitted, broken-in boots is preferable to treatment. It is also better to treat hot spots caused by chaffing than to let them develop into blisters. Put some tape or moleskin over the hotspot. Once a blister develops but is not yet broken, it should be protected intact. The intact blister is not an open wound; therefore it is less likely to become infected. Protect it from popping by putting several layers of tape over a lower layer with a hole cut in it to fit around the blister. Some recommend putting a lubricant such as petroleum jelly in the "doughnut" of the lower layer of tape. If the blister opens or must be drained because of location, treat it like any other open wound. Wash the area thoroughly and keep it clean with frequent dressing changes. To drain, use a sterilized needle under the edge.

Poison Ivy

Poison ivy causes an allergic reaction spread by an oil in the stems, leaves, and roots of the plant. About 25% of the American population is immune to the oils from poison ivy, and the rest of the population is susceptible. Poison ivy is the leading reason for workers' compensation cases in the forest service. In smoke, it can be life-threatening if inhaled. The oil's binding to the skin can be prevented through the use of several blocking agents that are commercially available. If it is known that someone is exposed, it may be possible to prevent the rash by washing the area thoroughly with cool water and strong soap within 20 minutes of exposure. Once the rash is visible, it is bound to the skin and (despite the popular myth to the contrary) is not communicable to other people or other parts of the body. The itching can be reduced by use of topical hydrocortisone.

Bites and Stings

Patients that are bitten or stung can become ill because of an allergic response or because the animal secretes or inject toxins into the wound. Bites and stings are also prone to infection.

Insects

Bees, wasps, and spiders can all cause reactions whether or not they inject toxins. Bee sting allergies are common and allergic patients should carry antidote kits that can keep the reaction from becoming fatal. In fact, bee and wasp stings cause the majority of serious reactions. All spiders have venom, although only the black widow and brown recluse are considered toxic to the point of being poisonous (Fig. 16-9).

Mammals

Dog and cat bites are common and the injury can be severe with damage to soft tissues and muscles. Infection is always a concern, and rabies should always be considered particularly if the vaccination status of the animal cannot be determined.

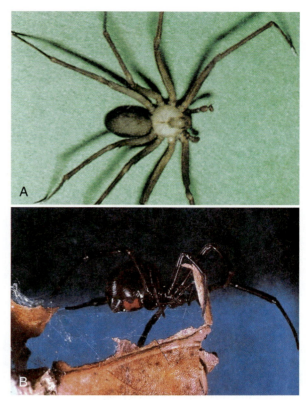

Fig. 16-9 A, Brown recluse spider. **B,** Black widow spider. (From Sanders MJ: *Mosby's paramedic textbook,* revised ed 3, St Louis, 2007, Mosby.)

Snakes

Snake bites are actually uncommon and envenomation rarely occurs. For instance, there were fewer than 10 deaths attributable to snake bites in all of 2003. In the United States, the most common bites capable of envenomation come from rattlesnakes and copperheads, but exotic snake bites occur as people bring snakes into the country as pets or they stow away on shipments of fruits and vegetables. Coral snakes often hitch rides and they are poisonous (Fig. 16-10).

Marine Animals

Jellyfish sting is the most common poisoning by marine animals. The most common reaction to a jellyfish sting is a local skin reaction with red, raised lesions (Fig. 16-11).

Management of Bites and Stings

Treatment of bites in general is supportive; that is, you should cleanse the wound and apply cold compresses for comfort. There are some things specific to the responsible animal that you may be able to do, such as scraping the stingers of bees from the skin and immobilizing snake-bitten extremities. Beyond that, particularly if the patient

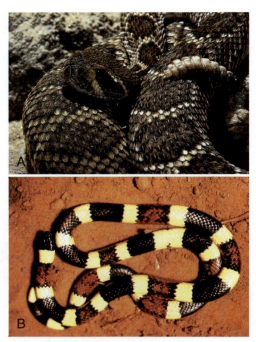

Fig. 16-10 A, Pit viper. **B,** Coral snake. (**A** from Sanders MJ: *Mosby's paramedic textbook,* revised ed 3, St Louis, 2007, Mosby; **B** from Chapleau W, Pons P: *Emergency medical technician, making the difference,* ed 1, St Louis, 2007, Mosby.)

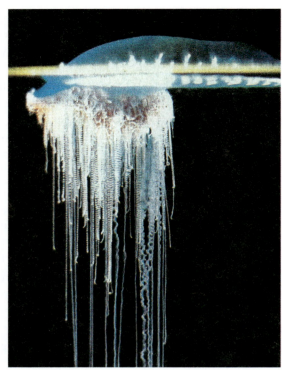

Fig. 16-11 Man-of-war jellyfish. (From Sanders MJ: *Mosby's paramedic textbook,* revised ed 3, St Louis, 2007, Mosby.)

delayed seeking treatment, you should monitor the patient's level of consciousness and be prepared to maintain airway and ventilations with oxygen.

Summary

Environmental emergencies require that the emergency medical responder understands and anticipates the environment as well as its consequences on the patient. This knowledge will help prevent the emergency first responder from suffering the same consequences as the patient. Helping patients to conserve or dissipate heat will aid patients and give them the best chance for recovery. By recognizing allergic or toxic reactions, the emergency first responder can help prepare other health care professionals to administer the correct medication that will help the patient recover.

In the Real World—Conclusion

After moving your patient out of the cold and into a nearby grocery store, his wet clothes were removed and he was covered with dry towels. It was difficult to feel a radial pulse but a carotid pulse of 60 was obtained, and the patient is now breathing at a rate of 12 times per minute. The ambulance is en route and while the patient is not responsive as yet, as he warms his pulse and breathing have improved and he is beginning to move around. The ambulance arrives and as they leave for the hospital, you can hear the patient making an attempt to speak.

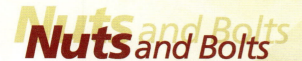

Nuts and Bolts

Critical Points

As emergency medical responders, you should recognize the signs and symptoms of heat and cold exposure and understand the predisposing factors that can increase the potential for hypothermia or hyperthermia.

Emergency medical responders must recognize the risks in environmental emergencies and remember that special training and equipment are required to work in certain environments.

Learning Checklist

❏ Environmental extremes are a danger to the patient and the rescuer.
❏ Hypothermia can occur indoors and in relatively warm environments.
❏ The elderly and the very young are particularly vulnerable to environmental exposure injuries of all kinds.
❏ Smaller parts of the body with more outside surfaces relative to the interior mass (such as fingers, ears, or the tip of the nose) are the most common sites of cold injury.
❏ Frostbite is the most common form of local cold injury.
❏ Heat injury ranges from heat cramps to severe and life-threatening heat stroke.
❏ The most important distinction between heat exhaustion and heat stroke is the deteriorating level of consciousness.
❏ Whether climbing to higher altitudes or descending into the depths, the rate of ascent or descent can create problems for the patient.
❏ Thousands of drownings occur in the United States every year.
❏ Water emergencies call for understanding the limits of the rescuer's ability. "Reach, throw, and go" means first attempt to assist from shore and only enter the water if trained to do so.

Key Terms

Anaphylaxis A severe, life-threatening allergic reaction.

Conduction The transfer of heat energy from a warmer object to a cooler one as a result of direct contact.

Convection The transfer of heat through a gas or liquid by the circulation of heated particles.

Decompression sickness A painful and sometimes fatal condition caused by the formation of nitrogen bubbles in the tissues of divers, caisson workers, and aviators who move too rapidly from a higher to a lower atmospheric pressure.

Drowning Asphyxiation caused by submersion in a liquid.

Evaporation Change in a substance from a liquid to a gas.

Frostbite The traumatic effect of extreme cold on skin and subcutaneous tissues exemplified by pallor of exposed skin surfaces, particularly of the fingers, nose, ears, and toes.

Heat cramps Painful spasms of muscles in the arms, legs, or abdomen that occur after several hours of sustained activity in hot environments.

Heat exhaustion A heat-related illness that occurs when the circulatory system fails to adequately maintain its normal function because of excessive loss of fluids and salts.

Heat stroke The most severe form of heat exposure illness; prolonged exposure to high temperatures causes failure of body's temperature-regulating capacity.

Heat transfer The mechanism by which needed heat is moved into the body or how excess heat is released from the body.

Hypothermia A dangerous condition in which the body temperature falls below 95°F (35°C) and the body's normal functions are impaired.

Poison Any substance that can be potentially harmful to the body.

Radiation Heat that moves across a space from one object to another. Also describes pain that moves from one site to another part of the body.

Thermoregulation The control of heat production and heat loss.

Nuts and *Bolts*–continued

First Responder NSC Objectives

COGNITIVE OBJECTIVES

- Describe the various ways the body loses heat.
- List the signs and symptoms of exposure to cold.
- Explain the steps of providing emergency care to a patient exposed to cold.
- List the signs and symptoms of exposure to heat.
- Explain the steps of emergency care to a patient exposed to heat.
- Recognize the signs and symptoms of patients involved in water-related emergencies.

- Explain the complications of near-drowning.
- Discuss the medical care of bites and stings.
- Recognize the signs and symptoms of allergic reactions.
- Recognize the signs and symptoms of anaphylaxis.

PSYCHOMOTOR OBJECTIVES

- Demonstrate the assessment and emergency care of patients exposed to cold.
- Demonstrate the assessment and care of patients exposed to heat.
- Demonstrate the assessment and care of near-drowning patients.

Check your understanding

Check your understanding

Please refer to p. 439 for the answers to these questions.

1. On a hot summer day, sitting in front of a fan provides cooling by which of the following methods?
   A. Conduction
   B. Convection
   C. Radiation
   D. Respiration

2. You are treating a patient from a motorcycle collision who is lying on the hot blacktop. You should be concerned with heat transfer by which of the following mechanisms?
   A. Conduction
   B. Convection
   C. Radiation
   D. Evaporation

3. Which of the following should be your main concern while on scene at any temperature-related emergency?
   A. Obtaining vital signs
   B. Performing a detailed exam
   C. Moving the patient out of the current environment
   D. Giving the patient cool or warm water to drink

4. You are called to the local high school football field where a player has become ill during the mid-day summer practice. Coaches tell you the player became dizzy, developed rapid breathing, and was noted to have extreme weakness. This player is most likely suffering from:
   A. Heat cramps
   B. Heat exhaustion
   C. Sun stroke
   D. Heat stroke

5. Which of the following findings would indicate your patient has progressed from heat exhaustion to heat stroke?
   A. Sweating
   B. A decrease in mental status
   C. Normal vital signs
   D. Ambient temperature

6. When attempting to rescue and provide care for a near-drowning victim, which of the following needs to be your first priority?
   A. ABC's
   C. CPR
   C. Safety
   D. Immobilization

7. You are treating an anxious 42-year-old male with numerous bee stings when he tells you he had a "very bad" reaction last time he was stung, during which he almost died. Your care of this patient should focus on which of the following?
   A. Vital signs
   B. Removing the stingers
   C. Cooling and relieving the itching
   D. Airway and breathing status

8. You are treating a 23-year-old female hiker with complaints of redness and itching to both lower legs. Your exam reveals a significant case of poison ivy. Which of the following identifies the route of exposure?
   A. Injection
   B. Ingestion
   C. Inhalation
   D. Absorption

9. A small child has ingested a large amount of a cleaning solution. Which of the following is most appropriate?
   A. Put a sample of the liquid in a cup and bring it with you to the Emergency Department.
   B. Leave the liquid on scene as it poses a risk to responders.
   C. Take the liquid's original container with you to the Emergency Department.
   D. Induce vomiting.

10. You respond to a golf course for a report of someone struck by lightning. Your greatest concern should be for which of the following?
    A. Burn care
    B. Trauma from the fall
    C. Vital signs
    D. Cardiac arrhythmias/cardiac arrest

Check your understanding–continued

11. You are caring for a victim of a construction mishap in which your patient was electrocuted. After shutting down the power, your next step would be to:
    A. Measure vital signs
    B. Apply AED
    C. Provide wound care
    D. Perform ABC assessment

Chapter 17

Special Populations

LESSON GOAL

As an emergency first responder, you will encounter patients who require special considerations for assessment and treatment. Patients with physical disabilities, patients who are dying or chronically ill, and elderly patients all require these special considerations. This chapter describes how to identify, assess, and treat patients in these special populations.

OBJECTIVES

1. Define the term *disabled*.
2. State the major challenges in assessing and treating patients who are physically impaired.
3. Identify major concerns of critically ill or dying patients.
4. Describe special considerations for the assessment and treatment of geriatric patients.
5. Identify signs of elderly abuse.
6. List potential resources that provide services to special populations.

In the Real World

You are called to the scene of an elderly patient who dialed 9-1-1 and asked for help but could provide no other information. Dispatch sends you to a single-family dwelling 5 minutes away. A neighbor is at the door, apparently responding to the wailing heard from inside the house. You knock and call out but hear no response other than sobbing. The neighbor informs you that Mr. Harfield lives alone, is kind-spirited but frail, and has an occasional daytime nurse looking after him. You enter the door and find him sobbing by the side of his bed, clutching his left leg.

As an emergency first responder, you will encounter patients who require special considerations for assessment and treatment. Patients with disabilities, critically or chronically ill patients, and elderly patients are just some examples. This chapter describes special considerations to identify, assess, and treat patients in these special populations.

Patients with Disabilities

Persons with physical impairments that limit one or more major life activity are considered **disabled.** As an emergency first responder, you should understand that patients with disabilities may require special techniques for assessment and treatment. For example, patients with visual or hearing disabilities will require special methods of communication and patient assessment. It is important to note that *disability* as described in the assessment chapter refers to mental status and not to a disabling condition. You should assess and treat persons with disabilities as you would any other patient while keeping in mind certain special considerations. Physical disabilities may include the following:

- Deafness or hearing impairment
- Blindness or visual impairment
- Impaired mobility such as paralysis or other muscular disorders

Hearing-Impaired Patients

Patients who are deaf or hearing impaired may be especially frightened during an emergency. They may be unable to understand what is occurring without someone to assist them with communication.

If a patient does not answer your questions or follow basic directions, he or she may have a hearing impairment. It is important to establish that the patient has a

CAUTION!

Individuals with physical impairments may have service animals that are specially trained to assist them with daily activities. If you, as an emergency first responder, encounter a patient with a service animal, allow the patient to utilize the animal where appropriate. Recognize that a special bond often exists between a person and his or her animal. Whenever possible, the patient and the animal should remain together. Occasionally a service animal may exhibit signs and symptoms of aggression when you try to assess or treat the patient. Recognize that this is a protective mechanism. If the patient cannot help to control the situation, you may need to enlist the help of other family members, bystanders, or specially trained individuals (e.g., animal control).

hearing impairment and to assess the communication problem. With any patient you should determine the patient's ability to understand, speak, and communicate. For example, you can find out from family members or caregivers if the patient can lip-read, read written words, or use sign language. If you know some basic **American Sign Language (ASL)** signs, you could ask, "Where do you hurt?" or "Where are you sick?" or "How can I help?" Even without knowing these ASL signs, you may still be able to communicate through gestures, expressions, or writing.

When you speak to a person with a hearing impairment, you should face the patient so that he or she can see you. Speak slowly and clearly; identify yourself and let the patient know you are there to help. When you first encounter the patient, you may have to get his or her attention by doing such things as waving your hands, blinking overhead lights, or turning your flashlight on and off. You should not shout or exaggerate your lip movements but simply slow your rate of delivery and separate your words. Try to establish eye contact and watch the patient's facial expressions.

If verbal communication is not effective, you can supplement your efforts with other methods. Write out important words, use signs and gestures, and keep checking that the patient understands you. With any patient who has a hearing impairment, you should allow more time for each communication. You may also want to keep paper and a writing instrument ready and if it is necessary and possible, let the patient write down the answers to your questions.

Visually Impaired Patients

Patients who are blind or visually impaired are also likely to be frightened in an emergency. The patient's impairment may be a total vision loss from birth, the vision loss may have resulted from disease or trauma later in life, or the patient may have a partial loss of vision or cloudy vision, such as caused by cataracts. Patients with visual impairments often adapt effectively to their regular environment, but in an emergency, different sounds, smells, and other external stimuli may confuse or disorient them. The patient's visual condition may alter his or her ability to manage an emergency.

You should establish physical contact with a patient who is blind or visually impaired. Place your hand on the patient's shoulder and maintain physical contact during emergency medical care to reassure him or her. Explain what is going on and what care you will give. Speak slowly and listen carefully to understand your patient's needs. Effective, reassuring verbal communication is essential for the effective assessment and treatment of patients with a visual impairment.

To prevent frightening a visually impaired patient, you should refrain from touching or grabbing him or her without first stating your intention. If the patient is required to move, offer your assistance. The patient may wish to place a hand on your shoulder or elbow and allow you to guide him or her.

Patients with Mobility Disabilities

Patients with problems that limit their ability to move may present assessment and treatment challenges. It is important to note that although a patient may have a physical impairment, you should not associate this with a mental impairment. Unless it is established otherwise, you should assume that a patient with a physical disability can understand you. You may encounter, for example, a patient who has a wasting illness (**atrophy**). A patient

may have reduced muscle size and strength resulting from **muscular dystrophy** or a degenerative illness, from paralysis related to nervous system defects, or from trauma. Damage to the spinal cord may result in paralysis of one or more limbs. You may need to use special procedures to effectively and appropriately assess and treat patients with mobility disabilities. For example, a patient with spinal cord damage causing paralysis of all four extremities, or **quadriplegia,** has no sensation in any extremity. Therefore, these patients are susceptible to burns or other traumatic injuries because they will not feel them occurring. When you assess a patient with severe atrophy of leg muscles, you may need to establish what is normal for that patient, which may be very different from that of a patient without a disability. When you move a person who uses a wheelchair, you may encounter tension in affected muscle groups or braces that help the patient walk or stand.

A patient's splints and other supportive devices can be helpful when managing musculoskeletal injuries, but if they interfere with emergency care, particularly airway management or bleeding control, they must be removed. If the patient is in a wheelchair, you may need to remove the patient from the chair to render care (Fig. 17-1).

Some patients may have **ostomy** appliances or collection devices. An ostomy is a surgical opening made from the urinary bladder, small intestine, or large intestine as a temporary or permanent pathway for urine or feces to reach a collection bag outside the body. If the patient's family members or caregivers are present, ask them for assistance in rendering care. They usually know how to use and remove the device (Fig. 17-2).

Cerebral Palsy

Cerebral palsy (CP) is a motor function disorder caused by a brain defect or lesion present at, or shortly after, birth. A person with CP has difficulty controlling muscular movement, and the person's extremities may be held in characteristic positions. It is important with these patients to be gentle during the physical examination and not force movement if an extremity will not easily move to a desired position (Fig. 17-3). For example, it may not be possible to position an arm to take a blood pressure. If neither arm can be used, you should document why a blood pressure could not be obtained and continue with your assessment.

Patients with CP may also be at increased risk for airway obstruction because they may have more difficulty swallowing food or secretions. These patients may also be on different types of medication to help relieve their symptoms.

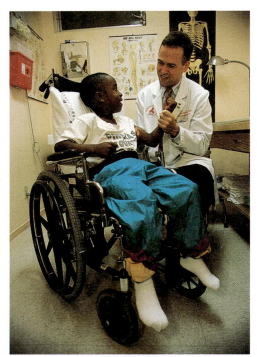

Fig. 17-1 If a patient is in a wheelchair, you may need to remove the patient from the chair to render care. (From McSwain N, Paturas J: *The basic EMT: comprehensive prehospital patient care,* ed 3, St. Louis, 2003, Mosby.)

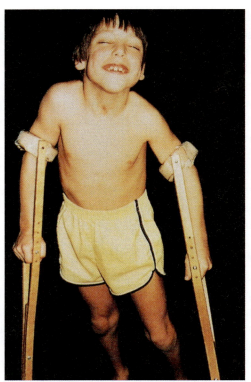

Fig. 17-3 Cerebral palsy is a motor function disability that consists of difficulty controlling voluntary muscles as a result of damage to a portion of the brain. (From McSwain N, Paturas J: *The basic EMT: comprehensive prehospital patient care,* ed 3, St. Louis, 2003, Mosby.)

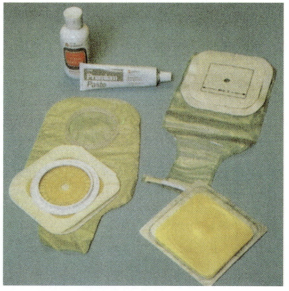

Fig. 17-2 Ostomy pouches. (From McSwain N, Paturas J: *The basic EMT: comprehensive prehospital patient care,* ed 3, St. Louis, 2003, Mosby.)

Critically Ill and Injured Patients

Critically ill and injured patients make up a special population that requires additional care. As with all patients, you should introduce yourself and let the patient know your level of training and that you are there to help. Let patients know that you are attending to their immediate needs and that these are your primary concerns. Continually explain what is occurring because this may decrease the patient's confusion, anxiety, and feelings of helplessness. You, other medical providers, and family and friends should not make any grim comments about the patient's condition. Such remarks may depress the patient, reduce hope, and possibly compromise recovery.

Lights, sirens, smells, and unknown personnel can confuse a patient. Help the patient stay oriented to the situation. Give simple explanations such as "Mr. Smith, you've been hurt, the police are here, and I'm now splinting your arm. My name is John. I am an emergency first responder. I'm here to help you, and I'll stay with you until the ambulance arrives." Use your judgment to be honest with patients without unnecessarily shocking or confusing them. If a patient refuses emergency medical care or asks that you leave him or her alone, explain the seriousness of the condition and your ability to help. Do not try to persuade the patient by communicating undue alarm, and do not say, "Everything will be okay" when it's obvious that the situation is serious. If a patient refuses emergency care, document this in your report and if possible have the patient sign a refusal-of-care form (see Chapter 3).

Patients may ask you if they are going to die. You may feel at a loss for words if you know that the prognosis is poor. But it is not your responsibility, nor perhaps even your right, to tell a patient that death is imminent. Instead, make honest but helpful statements such as "I don't know if you are going to die, but let's fight this together" or "I'm not going to give up on you, so don't give up on yourself." Offer hope and show your conviction to do everything possible to save the patient's life.

Often patients will ask you to contact family members or someone else. The patient may or may not be able to assist with phone numbers or other information. Assure the patient that you or someone else will attempt to locate the person.

Chronically Ill Patients

Any condition that is present over a long period of time is called **chronic.** This is different from an **acute** illness, which has a sudden onset of symptoms. There are many different types of chronic conditions including asthma, diabetes, or seizures, which are covered elsewhere in this text. Other examples include cancer or heart disease. It is important to determine in your focused history whether a patient has a chronic illness and to make note of any medications, side effects, and the usual routine or condition of the patient compared to the signs and symptoms of the chief complaint.

Hospice Patients

Hospice patients are a special category of patients that you may encounter as an emergency first responder. Hospice is family-centered care designed to assist patients who have a terminal illness to be comfortable and to maintain quality of life through the last phases of life.

Hospice care includes home visits, professional medical help available on call, and teaching and emotional support of the family regarding the physical care of the patient. Some hospice programs provide care in a center, and others provide care in the patient's home. The number of hospice patients being cared for either at home or at a hospice center is increasing annually. As an emergency first responder, your chance of responding to a call for a hospice patient is also increasing.

Once you identify that you are caring for a hospice patient, you should check to see if the patient's hospice representative has been notified. You should then try to determine if the reason you were called is related to the patient's terminal health condition. If the complaint is not directly related to the patient's underlying medical condition, it should be managed as you would with any other patient.

Acquiring a detailed history for a hospice patient is of great importance. The patient's current medical condition and medications may cause a significant change in the traditional treatment modality. The best source for a hospice patient's current medical status is the hospice representative. If the hospice representative is not readily available, you should seek the help of a family member and the patient. Because hospice is family- and patient-oriented care, both the patient and the immediate family members are usually quite knowledgeable of the current medical condition, treatment, and medications.

It is not unusual for hospice patients to have a physician's order that will limit or remove resuscitation efforts. Physician orders that withhold resuscitation efforts are generally referred to as do not attempt resuscitation (DNAR) orders. DNAR orders do not mean withholding "comfort care," which could include providing oxygen, suctioning the airway, controlling external bleeding, or other such care. In certain circumstances you may encounter physician orders that may limit resuscitation efforts to certain forms of care such as CPR and drugs without intubation. Again, the patient, hospice representative, or family member will be your best source of information. It is extremely important that you are respectful of the patient's choices and honor the patient's wishes whenever possible. Additional emotional support may also be needed for the patient's family members. **Box 17-1** summarizes some special considerations that should be used for all patients with disabilities.

Geriatric Patients

People over 65 years of age are considered the elderly. This age group represents the fastest-growing population

In the Real World—continued

You introduce yourself and ask Mr. Harfield if his leg is hurting him. He continues sobbing and does not respond. You place a hand on his shoulder, introduce yourself again, and point to his leg. You ask slowly, while facing him, if his leg is hurt. He screams, "It's broken again!" You ask him to show you where it hurts and to tell you when he hurt it before. He points to his hip and shows you a recent scar across his left outer hip and thigh. You help him into a position of comfort, do an initial assessment, perform a physical examination and ongoing assessments, and calm and reassure him while you wait for the ambulance. During your examination you notice a deep bruise on each forearm and one on his ankle.

BOX 17-1   Special Considerations for Patients with Disabilities

- *Use "person first" language.* For example, a patient should be described as "a person with a physical disability" rather than a "disabled person."
- *Focus on a patient's abilities—not disability.* Ask about the patient's usual activities and avoid using words such as "normal" and "abnormal."
- *Develop creative means of communication.* Do not assume that a patient cannot understand what you are saying. If, through your usual assessment, you realize that the patient requires a different communication method, you should alter your method and ensure that the patient understands what you are saying.
- *Use the caregiver as a resource.* The caregiver or family members of patients with special needs are experts in the care of the patient. Use them as a resource for information, to assist in care, or to communicate with the patient.
- *Treat the patient with respect.* Just like any other patient, a person with a disability deserves your respect during your assessment and treatment.

Geriatric patients experience changes in physical structure, body composition, and organ function that you must consider when giving emergency medical care.

Changes That Occur with Aging

Aging is a natural process in which the body gradually declines over a number of years. Persons of older age are generally more fragile, have decreased energy and increased susceptibility to illness and injury, and show physical signs that may limit functional ability, such as arthritis. Following is a systematic look at the anatomical and physiological changes that occur with aging.

- *Respiratory system.* As a person ages, the chest wall stiffens and there is a decrease in the ability of the thoracic cavity to expand and contract. An older person may also have impaired cough and gag reflexes and be at a higher risk for airway obstruction and aspiration. As a person ages, his or her spinal curvature may also change, which may further compress the lungs and affect the respiratory system and breathing.
- *Cardiovascular system.* As a person ages, there is a decrease in arterial elasticity, which can lead to circulatory problems. Atherosclerosis, narrowing of the blood vessels from fatty deposits, is a condition that can develop over time and may result in high blood pressure (hypertension) or other cardiac problems. These types of changes all lead to a decreased ability for the elderly patient to compensate for such things as blood loss. The elderly patient is at more risk for shock.
- *Nervous system.* The patient's mental status may also be a major factor as you attempt to find out the patient's emergency problem. As a person ages, the brain mass decreases as does the speed at which nerve impulses are conducted. As changes occur in the brain, memory can be affected or behavioral changes may be noticed.

in the nation. The elderly currently constitute 12% of the population of the United States, or approximately 34 million persons. It is projected that by 2030, the elderly will constitute 18% of the U.S. population.

- *Sensory system.* As a person ages, he or she is more likely to experience vision and hearing difficulties. The elderly may also not perceive pain in the same ways as younger patients. They may experience a decreased sense of balance, diminished pain perception, an inability to differentiate between hot and cold, or a decreased tolerance of hot or cold conditions.
- *Musculoskeletal system.* The loss of bone as a person ages can result in osteoporosis. Osteoporosis is excessive loss of bone density and deterioration of bone tissue. Osteoporosis occurs more frequently in women of postmenopausal age and results in a higher risk for fractures. Osteoarthritis is another condition that can be found in the elderly. It is characterized by stiff, deformed, swollen joints that can limit movement and change posture. Gait is also affected as a person ages because of the inability to flex joints as well or because of curvature of the spine that may occur.
- *Digestive system.* As a person ages, it is common to see an increase in digestive system changes. Some common changes include difficulty in chewing or swallowing, difficulty with digestion, and constipation.
- *Urinary system.* Aging will also cause the kidneys to atrophy, the bladder to become less elastic, and weakening of the bladder muscles. This change can cause the sensation to urinate to become delayed, resulting in urinary incontinence. As a consequence, some patients may limit their fluid intake and become dehydrated.
- *Skin.* As a person ages, the skin thins and loses elasticity. These changes lead to an increased risk of infection. Although there is an increased risk of infection, there is usually a decrease in the signs and symptoms of the infection. Elderly patients often cannot thermoregulate as well as younger patients and can be at increased risk of heat- or cold-related injuries.

Fig. 17-4 illustrates other changes caused by aging.

Risk of Illness and Injury

It is important to note that some elderly individuals have minimal medical problems, whereas others may have had prolonged illnesses. Those who have been ill may deteriorate more rapidly in an emergency medical situation. The elderly may be more susceptible to disease and injury because of the changes that occur with aging. An acute illness or trauma may occur on top of a chronic disease. Illness and trauma are also more likely to affect multiple organ systems in geriatric patients. The following are health risk factors for elderly patients:

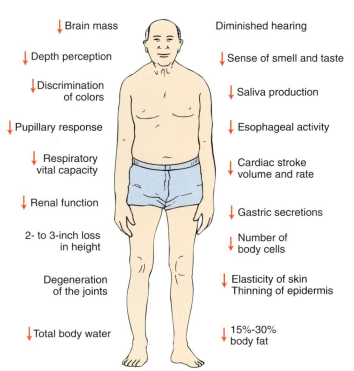

Fig. 17-4 Changes caused by aging. (From NAEMT: *PHTLS: Basic and advanced prehospital trauma life support,* ed 5, St. Louis, 2003, Mosby.)

- Being over 75 years of age
- Living alone
- Experiencing the recent death of a significant other
- Having recently been hospitalized
- Being unable to hold urine or feces (incontinence)
- Being immobile
- Having an unsound mind (dementia)

Mechanisms of Injury

The leading cause of death in the elderly is cardiovascular disease, such as heart disease and stroke. Trauma deaths commonly occur with the following:

- *Falls.* Falls are the leading cause of death as a result of trauma in those over 75 years of age. Most falls occur because of the changes in posture and gait and visual acuity that occur with aging. However, the most important variables contributing to falls can be prevented. These include such things as slippery floors, throw rugs, stairs, poor-fitting shoes, and poor lighting.
- *Vehicular trauma.* Motor vehicle collisions (MVCs) are a leading cause of trauma death in the geriatric population. This is a result of a physiological inability to compensate for trauma, changes in memory and

reaction time, and impairment in vision and hearing. Elderly patients are also frequently involved in pedestrian fatalities. They may require more time to cross streets, and visual and hearing impairment may prevent them from moving out of the path of a vehicle.

Mental Health Considerations

Approximately 10% of those in the elderly population require professional mental health services. There are elderly patients who have developed senile dementia or other disorders like Alzheimer's disease. However, when you are assessing an elderly patient, you should always assume that an altered mental status is a result of something like hypoxia, shock, or brain injury unless proven otherwise.

Assessment

When you are caring for geriatric patients, you should tailor your assessment and treatment to their needs and anticipate complications in care. Assessment may take longer and be more challenging because of sensory deficits (e.g., hearing or vision impairments), senility, and physiological changes. You should consider the possibility of other medical conditions when performing your assessment. Other factors to consider include the following:

- Failure of the heart to provide adequate circulation
- Auditory and visual loss
- Reduced red blood cells (anemia)
- Respiratory insufficiency

Communication

Be respectful when addressing elderly patients. Address all patients by their last name unless they invite you to use their first name. For example, "Mrs. Doe, my name is Jack. How would you like to be called?" Try to relieve their anxiety by stating, "I am John, a trained emergency first responder, and I am here to help you." Sit close to the patient and ask, "May I shake your hand?" Communicate your compassion and express your friendliness. Reassure your patient honestly and appropriately. Talk more slowly and allow more time for the patient's answers. Remember to consider that the patient may have a hearing deficit. Talk to the "better" ear, and face the patient. Box 17-2 summarizes a list of common complaints with elderly patients.

When assessing a geriatric patient, ask specific questions. Some elderly patients tend to respond "yes" to all

---

BOX 17-2 **Common Complaints in Elderly Patients**

- Alcoholism
- Constipation or diarrhea
- Dementia
- Depression
- Dizziness, fainting
- Difficulty eating
- Difficulty breathing
- Falls
- Fatigue and weakness
- Headache
- Incontinence or inability to void
- Musculoskeletal stiffness
- Poor nutrition, loss of appetite
- Sleep disorders
- Visual disorders

---

questions. You should avoid open-ended questions, and give details to choose from when describing his or her problem. For example, "Describe the pain in your hip" is an open-ended request and may not effectively provide information. Questions such as the following are more likely to yield useful information: "Is the pain in your hip sharp, stabbing, or dull?" "On a scale of one to 10, 10 being the most intense, what number is your pain?" If the patient has a history of difficulty breathing, ask precise questions such as "Do you have to stop and rest when walking to the kitchen?" Ask a friend, caregiver, or spouse to help provide relevant information if the patient allows. Some elderly patients may be reluctant to give information unless a relative or support person assists them.

Respect the patient's privacy when gathering information. Geriatric patients often have sensory deficits. Their hearing, vision, balance, and senses of smell, taste, and touch may be compromised. Maintain eye contact, speak slowly and loudly enough, and listen closely to gather patient information. Family or friends may have important insights into the patient's condition or care.

Neurological disorders ranging from mild confusion to profound dementia may affect a geriatric patient's ability to communicate and comprehend your questions. The patient may be restless or combative. Be sure all patients understand your questions and your intent, and remind them you are there to help.

Primary Assessment

Your primary assessment with elderly patients should be the same as what you would do with any other patient. Assess the patient's responsiveness, airway, breathing, circulation, and mental status (disability) and give care as needed.

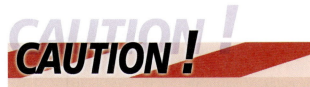

Elderly patients may not want anyone else present while you do your assessment and provide care, for several reasons, one of which may be abuse. A geriatric patient may fear punishment if the abuser is present and the patient shows or tells the emergency first responder about suspicious bruises.

During your assessment of elderly patients, you may need to consider certain specific factors such as the presence of dentures, preexisting diseases that affect the airway or respiration, degenerative arthritis, and neurological deficits.

Dentures may affect airway management. Usually you should leave dentures in place, because creating a seal with a mask around the patient's mouth is more difficult without dentures in place. If partial dentures (plates) become dislodged during an emergency and occlude or partially block the airway, remove them.

Preexisting disease of upper or lower airway structures may affect airway management. Elderly patients who have had laryngectomies (partial or full removal of voice box structures), chest surgery, or a lateral curvature of the spine may have respiratory difficulty.

The chest walls and cartilage are often stiffer in elderly patients, and they also may have reduced chest wall muscle power. This reduces the lung volume and increases the need for respiratory support in many geriatric patients.

Protection of the cervical spine, particularly in trauma patients with multiple system injuries, is a standard of care. Apply the same standard to elderly patients in trauma situations and in the treatment of acute medical problems when you must maintain an open airway. Even when there is no traumatic injury, degenerative arthritis may cause changes in spine shape and deformities. Maneuvering the neck may cause spinal cord injury to the cervical spine.

Bleeding in elderly trauma patients is managed the same ways as with other patients, but you should be aware of a greater risk of shock in geriatric patients.

Many geriatric patients have a decreased level of consciousness. Ask about the patient's use of medications for sleeping disorders, depression, or cardiovascular diseases such as high blood pressure.

It is sometimes difficult to assess neurological deficits in elderly patients because of preexisting conditions. You may have difficulty determining whether an elderly patient's neurological deficit is the result of a previous stroke or the current trauma or illness. An elderly patient's medications may interfere with central nervous system functions in times of trauma or acute medical illness. Perform a rapid neurological evaluation using the AVPU scale (see Chapter 8) and the Glasgow Coma Scale (GCS) score. Any decrease in the level of consciousness should be assumed to be from a decreased flow of oxygen to the brain or inadequate circulation.

Secondary Assessment

After completing your primary assessment, you should continue with your SAMPLE history (see Chapter 8) and physical examination. Some general considerations in assessment are as follows:

- Allow more time than usual for gathering information and taking a history.
- Be patient when accommodating for hearing or visual deficits.
- Express empathy and compassion.
- Do not underestimate the patient's intelligence merely because communication is difficult or absent.
- If close friends or relatives are present, ask them to help provide or validate information.
- Obtain a list of medicines and drugs the patient is using, and give it to the responding emergency medical services (EMS) unit. Many elderly persons participate in the "VIAL OF LIFE" or a similar program, in which a listing of drugs is kept in a vial in the refrigerator.
- Make sure the patient can hear you. Stand directly in front of the patient so that the patient can see you speaking.
- Repeat questions if you are not sure if an elderly patient can hear you.
- Conduct your physical examination as you would for other patients, but be mindful of potential physical disabilities or medical conditions.

Abuse of the Elderly

Reports and complaints of abuse and neglect of the elderly are increasing in the United States, although the exact extent remains unknown because abuse of the elderly has been largely hidden from society's view. Abuse and neglect are defined in varying ways that affect how incidents are reported. Patients may be afraid to report the problem to law enforcement agencies or social welfare personnel. If the abuser is the patient's child, the elderly parent may feel ashamed or guilty. Elderly women are often hesitant to report incidents of sexual assault to law enforcement agencies. The victim may also be traumatized and may be afraid of reprisal by the abuser. Some jurisdictions do not have a formal reporting mechanism, and some areas have no statutory requirements for reporting elder abuse.

The physical and emotional signs of abuse, rape, spouse beating, or nutritional deprivation are often overlooked or misidentified. Sensory deficits, senility, drug-induced depression, and other forms of altered mental status may make it nearly impossible for an elderly patient to report maltreatment.

Abuse includes actions that take advantage of an elderly person's property or that disrespect the patient's physical or emotional needs. The abuser may be the victim's relative, roommate, housekeeper, caretaker, or anyone else on whom the elderly person relies. Characteristics that make the elderly particularly susceptible to abuse include the following:

- Being over 65 years of age
- Being a female over 75 years of age
- Being frail, with multiple chronic medical conditions
- Having dementia
- Having impaired sleep cycle, sleepwalking, or loud shouting during the nighttime
- Being incontinent of feces, urine, or both
- Being dependent on others for activities of daily living

The elderly also experience abuse in nursing homes and convalescent and continuing care centers. Some care providers in these environments may consider the elderly to be obstinate, undesirable, or problem patients. Common situations and characteristics of elderly abusers include the following:

- Household conflict
- Marked fatigue
- Underemployment or unemployment
- Financial difficulties
- Substance abuse
- Previous history of being abused

Categories of Abuse

Forms of abuse include physical, psychological, and financial abuse. Physical abuse may include assault, withholding food, and lack of basic hygiene, shelter, and necessities (Fig. 17-5). Psychological abuse may include neglect, verbal abuse, being treated like an infant, and deprivation of sensory stimuli. Financial abuse may include having money embezzled, valuables stolen, or information about their income withheld.

When you treat elderly patients, you should maintain a high index of suspicion for the possibility of abuse. Look for obvious signs, such as bruises and wounds, and for more subtle signs, such as undue fear or malnutrition. Remember that abused patients may be afraid to tell you about the abuse for fear of retribution. In addition to the

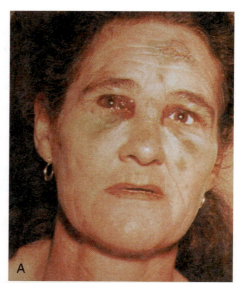

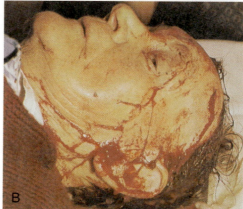

Fig. 17-5 Signs of physical abuse in the elderly. **A,** Bruising caused by a punch. **B,** Wound of the scalp. (From NAEMT: *PHTLS: basic and advanced prehospital trauma life support,* ed 5, St. Louis, 2003, Mosby.)

medical care you give, your thorough assessment may also identify trauma resulting from abuse. Reporting the abuse can lead to the patient benefiting from the protective services of human, social, and public safety agencies. See Chapter 3 for further discussion on special reporting requirements.

Resources and Agencies for Assistance

When appropriate, you should contact a service agency for a patient with a disability. This agency may assist directly with the care you provide or give you information about the specific disability related to treatment. As an emergency first responder, you should become familiar with the special service resources and agencies in your community or state.

Additional resources you can use to gather more information on disabilities include social services, medical specialists, child-life services, and physical and occupational therapists. It is also important to realize that the caregivers and family are important resources for obtaining information.

Team Work

Patients with chronic illness may also present with different types of medical equipment and supportive devices. As an emergency first responder, you are not expected to know how to operate and manage these different devices, but you should be able to recognize and work around technological aids as part of the health care team.

Tracheostomy

A tracheostomy is an opening in the trachea that provides a person with an airway to breathe through. A tracheostomy tube is an airway device similar to an endotracheal tube (but much shorter) that is placed into the stoma in the neck (Fig. 17-6). Patients with a tracheostomy tube may be more susceptible to airway obstruction as a result of secretions blocking the tube. It is important to note with these patients that ventilation will not occur as with other patients. They will require ventilation with a bag-mask device through the tracheostomy tube or through a mask placed over the stoma (see Chapter 7).

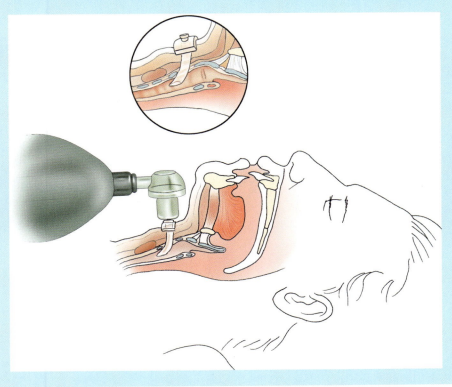

Fig. 17-6 A tracheostomy is an opening in the trachea through which a tube may be inserted. (From McSwain N, Paturas J: *The basic EMT: comprehensive prehospital patient care,* ed 3, St. Louis, 2003, Mosby.)

Team Work—cont'd

Apnea Monitor

Premature infants often have respiratory disorders and may require the use of an apnea monitor at home. An apnea monitor is hooked up to pads placed on the infant; it alarms if the infant stops breathing for a specified period of time (Fig. 17-7).

Gastrostomy Tube

A gastrostomy tube or button is put in place for patients who cannot eat and digest food in the usual manner over an extended period of time. You may see this device in patients with a chronic illness, a nervous disorder, or disorders of the gastrointestinal system. As an emergency first responder, you should be aware of this device and work around it. You should also notify other health care providers about its location (Fig. 17-8).

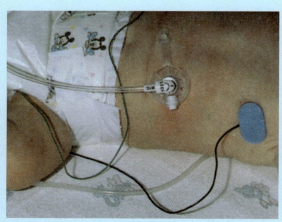

Fig. 17-8 A gastrostomy is the surgical creation of an artificial opening in the stomach to provide a means of feeding a patient. In this patient, a feeding tube is connected to a gastrostomy button. (From McSwain N, Paturas J: *The basic EMT: comprehensive prehospital patient care*, ed 3, St. Louis, 2003, Mosby.)

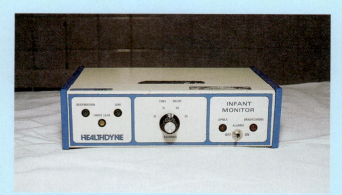

Fig. 17-7 An apnea monitor. (From McSwain N, Paturas J: *The basic EMT: comprehensive prehospital patient care*, ed 3, St. Louis, 2003, Mosby.)

In the Real World—Conclusion

You ask Mr. Harfield about who helps to care for him. He looks around carefully and whispers that an aide, Ronnie, comes in twice a day but isn't here now. You ask Mr. Harfield about the bruises on his arms and ankle, and he tells you that Ronnie sometimes ties him to his bed. He had to get up this morning to go to the bathroom and fell when he was twisting out of the cloth strips used to tie him. He asks you not to tell Ronnie that he told you this. When the ambulance arrives, you provide your hand-off report and pass on this information. Before the end of your shift, you check with your medical supervisor to be sure you have provided all the necessary notifications.

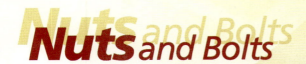
Nuts and **Bolts**

Critical Points

Patients who are physically challenged, critically or chronically ill, or elderly may require special skills for effective assessment and treatment. The basic skills are the same as for other patients, but you have additional considerations for these special populations. Understanding the needs of patients who are physically challenged will help you provide better care. When you care for a patient who is critically ill, your understanding of common emotional reactions will help you communicate honestly and empathetically. Remember that family members of a critically ill patient may also require your support. Elderly patients may have more complicated reactions to trauma or illness because of their age or previous illnesses. Consider their special issues and needs when assessing and treating them. Attend seminars and classes to learn more about special care populations so that you can provide the best care possible for every patient.

Learning Checklist

❑ Persons with physical impairments that limit one or more major life activity are considered disabled.
❑ Physical disabilities may include impaired mobility, visual impairment, and hearing impairment.
❑ If a patient is hearing impaired, you should face him or her so he or she can see you. Speak slowly and clearly, and find out if you can communicate through sign language, writing, or lip-reading.
❑ You should establish physical contact with a visually impaired person and explain what is going on around him or her. You should verbalize your movements before you do them.
❑ A patient's splints or other supportive devices can be helpful when managing musculoskeletal injuries, but if they interfere with emergency care, particularly

airway management or bleeding control, they must be removed.
❑ Critically ill and injured patients should be communicated with, and you should explain what is occurring around them because this may decrease the patient's confusion, anxiety, and feelings of helplessness.
❑ It is important to find out during your assessment if a patient has any chronic illnesses and to make note of any medications, side effects, and the usual routine of the patient compared to the signs and symptoms of the chief complaint.
❑ The elderly, those aged 65 and older, constitute 12% of the population of the United States.
❑ Health risk factors for elderly patients include being over 75 years of age, living alone, experiencing the recent death of a significant other, having recently been hospitalized, being incontinent, being immobile, and having an unsound mind.
❑ The leading cause of death in the elderly is cardiovascular disease. The leading causes of death resulting from trauma are falls and vehicular trauma.
❑ The body undergoes natural changes when it ages. It is important to be aware of these changes and how they can affect assessment of a trauma patient.
❑ Special considerations during assessment of a geriatric patient include the presence of dentures, preexisting diseases that affect airway or respiration, degenerative arthritis, and neurological deficits.
❑ Allow more time for taking a history with a geriatric patient. Ask specific questions rather than open-ended questions. Express empathy and compassion, and be patient when accommodating needs based on physical deficits.
❑ Maintain a high index of suspicion for elder abuse. Abuse can be physical, psychological, or financial.

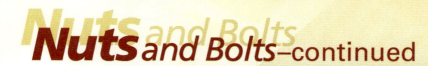

Nuts and Bolts–continued

Key Terms

Acute An illness or condition that has a sudden onset of symptoms.

American Sign Language (ASL) A method of communication for the hearing impaired or deaf. Involves speaking through hand gestures.

Atrophy The wasting away or loss in size of part of the body as a result of disease or lack of use.

Chronic Any condition or disease that is present over a long period of time.

Disabled Persons with physical impairments that limit one or more major life activity.

Muscular dystrophy A group of diseases characterized by weakness and wasting away of skeletal muscles. The cause is unknown.

Ostomy A surgical opening made into the urinary bladder, small intestine, or large intestine as a temporary or permanent pathway for urine or feces to reach a collection bag outside the body.

Quadriplegia Paralysis of all four extremities.

Check your understanding

Please refer to p. 439 for the answers to these questions.

1. An individual who has a physical limitation that interferes with one or more major life activities is considered to be _____.

2. When a spinal cord injury causes loss of function of both arms and both legs, the patient is said to be a:
   A. Paraplegic
   B. Quadriplegic
   C. Hemiplegic
   D. Biplegic

3. The wasting away of muscle tissue that often accompanies chronic illness is:
   A. Hypertrophy
   B. Apathy
   C. Atrophy
   D. Consolidation

4. A surgical opening in the body created for the purpose of allowing the products of elimination to be collected in a bag on the outside of the body is called a/an:
   A. Tracheostomy
   B. Tracheotomy
   C. Colonostomy
   D. Appendectomy

5. List four factors that put the elderly at greater risk for health problems.
   A. _____
   B. _____
   C. _____
   D. _____

6. When providing rescue breathing for an elderly patient with dentures, under what circumstances should the emergency first responder remove the dentures?
   A. _____
   B. _____

7. List four general considerations in the assessment of elderly patients.
   A. _____
   B. _____
   C. _____
   D. _____

8. True or False: Elderly patients who have difficulty sleeping at night are at an increased risk for abuse by a caregiver or family member.

9. True or False: The elderly are more susceptible to illness and injury than are younger patients.

10. True or False: When a disabled patient has a service animal, the emergency first responder should confine the animal to another room when assessing the patient.

11. When communicating with a person who has impaired hearing, which of the following is recommended?
    A. Exaggerate your lip movements so the patient can read your lips.
    B. Shout near the patient's "good" ear.
    C. Write your questions down for the patient.
    D. Assume the patient is not competent to refuse treatment.

12. When assessing a patient with impaired vision, which of the following is recommended?
    A. Speak loudly.
    B. Use American Sign Language.
    C. Allow extra time for the patient to answer questions.
    D. Explain what you are going to do before touching the patient.

13. Which of the following is the fastest-growing population in the United States?
    A. Pediatric
    B. Geriatric
    C. Male
    D. Female

Check your understanding–continued

14. Which of the following is the most common cause of death in the elderly?
   A. Heart disease
   B. Cancer
   C. Motor vehicle crashes
   D. Broken bones

15. Which of the following would be the most effective way to ask about an elderly patient's pain?
   A. "Does your hip hurt?"
   B. "What does the pain feel like?"
   C. "On a scale of 1 to 5, with 5 being the worst, how would you rate your amount of pain?"
   D. "How much does your hip hurt?

16. Which of the following represents the most appropriate way to address an elderly patient?
   A. "Hello, grandmother."
   B. "Let me help you with that, sweetie."
   C. "Hello, Mrs. Cunningham."
   D. "What's the matter today, Velma?"

17. An elderly man has tripped over some tools in his garage on Christmas Day and been lying on the floor for 6 hours, unable to get up. Along with your assessment for traumatic injuries, you should be alert for signs of which of the following?
   A. Medication reaction
   B. Hypothermia
   C. Hyperglycemia
   D. Dependent adult abuse

18. An elderly female has been struck by a car while crossing the street. The vehicle was traveling approximately 30 mph. Which of the following is correct when dealing with trauma to the elderly?
   A. The elderly compensate well and therefore do very well with shock and injury.
   B. The medical history has nothing to do with the reaction to traumatic injury.
   C. The elderly trauma patient only requires oxygen via nasal cannula.
   D. The medication that they take may actually mask signs and symptoms of shock and injury.

19. You are treating an elderly male who has injuries that are inconsistent with the history you receive from the son with whom the patient lives. You have a feeling that this may be a case of dependent adult abuse. What should you do?
   A. Tell the son to be more careful and vigilant with the medical care, and transport to the hospital.
   B. Tell the transporting agency about your findings, and alert them to the possibility of an abuse case.
   C. Tell no one, as the information is confidential.
   D. Alert the transporting agency about your abuse suspicions, and promptly complete an abuse report.

ANSWERS TO
Check your understanding

Chapter 1 Introduction to EMS Systems

1. False
2. False
3. Emergency Medical Services system
4. Medical oversight
5. First Responder
6. Trauma center
7. Poison control center
8. Patient assessment
9. Personal health and well-being, Personal behavior, Self-composure, Professional appearance
10. Abandonment
11. Good Samaritan
12. D. Control of bleeding
13. A. EMT-Paramedic
14. C. Personal safety
15. A. Physician
16. B. Check to see that the vehicle is in *Park*. The safety of the responder always comes first. Kneeling in front of the vehicle to assess the patient could result in injury if the driver, after realizing he or she struck someone, gets out of the vehicle, forgetting to put it in *Park*.
17. C. Indirect Medical Control

Chapter 2 Well-Being of the Emergency First Responder

1. Mass casualty incidents, Pediatric (child) patients, Death, Amputation, Violence, Abuse, Death or injury of a public safety worker
2. Anxiety, Anger, Hostility, Depression, Guilt, Dependency, Denial
3. Decreasing caffeine intake, Moderation in alcohol drinking, Quitting smoking, Regular exercise, Decreasing intake of sugars and fats
4. Critical incident stress
5. Critical incident stress debriefing
6. Decontamination
7. Body substance isolation (Universal Precautions, Standard Precautions)
8. Personal protection equipment
9. Power lines, Fuel spills, Unstable vehicles, Broken glass, Sharp metal, Traffic, Hazardous materials, Violent patients
10. Hazardous materials
11. B. The patient is found outdoors in cold weather.

12. D. Denial
13. B. Spending more time than usual with friends
14. B. Frequent hand washing with soap and water
15. D. Tuberculosis (TB)
16. C. Begin your assessment and treatment of the patient, explaining to the family that you are not permitted to act on a DNR unless you are able to see the DNR to verify its existence and authenticity.
17. A. Reassure the patient that you will do everything you can to take good care of her; however, don't give promises that the patient knows are unreasonable (B). It is also important not to unduly alarm the patient (C) or to decrease the patient's confidence in your abilities (D).
18. D. Personal Safety

Chapter 3 Legal and Ethical Issues

1. False
2. Standard of care
3. Scope of practice
4. Competence
5. Implied
6. Advance directive
7. Durable power of attorney for health care
8. Assault
9. Negligence
10. Protocols; Standing orders
11. C. Patient is a pregnant 18-year-old who is not married
12. A. Confidentiality
13. B. EMS agencies generally have policies and procedures related to the release of patient information. Requests such as those should be handled by the person specifically assigned the responsibility for doing so.
14. A. Treat as you would any patient with oxygen and comfort care.
15. A. Scope of Practice

Chapter 4 Communications and Documentation

1. B. Encoding
2. Feedback
3. Use plain English, do not interrupt others, treat others with respect, use alternative methods of communications (writing, signing, interpreters)

4. "Sounds like you are . . .", "I can imagine that must be . . .", I understand that must make you feel . . ."
5. Interference
6. Clenched fists, Wringing of hands, Pointing, Loud speech, Pacing, Aggressive stance
7. C. Getting on their level, palms open
8. B. Closed-ended questions
9. Age, sex, chief complaint, current condition, HPI(history of present illness), any major medical history, vital signs, pertinent exam findings, care given and response to care given
10. B. Writing responses/questions
11. C. HIPAA
12. D. Objective observations
13. So all agencies can easily understand what is necessary. Many agencies that don't always work together need to be able to communicate as easily as possible.
14. B. FCC
15. B. Mobile radio

Chapter 5 The Human Body

1. C, E, D, H, A, G, B, F
2. LUQ, RUQ, LUQ, RUQ, RLQ

3.

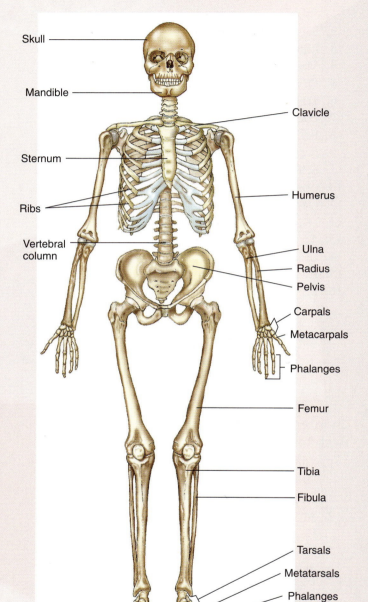

4. Epiglottis
5. Larynx
6. Diaphragm
7. Carotid arteries
8. Left
9. Coronary
10. Brachial
11. Femoral
12. Capillaries
13. Left ventricle
14. Right ventricle
15. Brain, Spinal cord
16. Peripheral
17. Sensory, Motor
18. Involuntary, Voluntary
19. Cardiac
20. Integumentary
21. C. Epidermis
22. D. Pancreas
23. B. Alveoli
24. D. On the posterior side, proximal to the elbow
25. D. Radius and ulna
26. B. Spleen

Chapter 6 Lifting and Moving Patients

1. Legs shoulder width apart, Knees bent, Lift with the leg muscles, Keep the back straight, Keep the weight close to the body
2. Immediate danger (or potential for immediate danger), such as fire or explosion; unable to assess a critically injured patient without moving a first patient; unable to perform life-saving care unless the patient is moved.
3. Worsening the injuries
4. Recovery; Left side
5. Long back board (long spine board)
6. Stair chair
7. C. Position of comfort for the patient
8. D. Disturbing the sleep of those who would be called to help
9. A. Allow her to remain in a position of comfort, but continue to monitor her condition. A calm explanation to the husband of the benefits of his wife being as comfortable as possible should gain his cooperation.

Chapter 7 Airway Management and Ventilation

1. A. Chest rise and fall
2. Esophagus
3. Epiglottis
4. Trachea
5. Alveoli
6. Inspiration (Inhalation)
7. Oxygen; Carbon dioxide
8. Tongue
9. D. Head tilt–chin lift maneuver
10. C. Begin abdominal thrusts
11. Oropharyngeal airway
12. B. Nasopharyngeal (NP)
13. C. Stridor
14. Dyspnea
15. A. Apneic
16. C. Bag-mask device
17. Partial/Incomplete
18. Abdominal thrusts
19. Place a folded towel under the patient's shoulders
20. Dual lumen airway device
21. Bag-valve-mask device
22. Nonrebreather
23. C. Check that the head is in the proper position to open the airway

Chapter 8 Patient Assessment

1. B. Scene size-up
2. U, U, S, U, S, U
3. B. Mechanism of injury
4. B. Life-threatening conditions
5. C. Symptom
6. A—The patient is ALERT
   V—The patient is not alert, but responds to a VERBAL or VOICE stimulus
   P—The patient is not alert and doesn't respond to voice, but responds to a PAINFUL stimulus
   U—The patient is UNRESPONSIVE to all stimuli
7. Choice A = V(erbal); Choice B = U(nresponsive); Choice C = P(ainful); Choice D = A(lert)
8. Decreased responsiveness; Cyanosis (bluish discoloration) of the skin or mucous membranes; Respirations are too fast or too slow; Respirations are noisy; Use of accessory muscles; Respirations are too shallow

9. I, I, A, I, I, A
10. D. Pulse
11. D. Supine with the legs elevated
12. D—Deformities
 O—Open wounds/injuries
 T—Tenderness
 S—Swelling
13. S—Signs and Symptoms of illness or injury
 A—Allergies to medications or other substances, such as bees or food items
 M—Medications that the patient takes, including both prescription and over the counter
 P—Past medical history (chronic illness, major surgeries)
 L—Last oral intake (the last time the patient had anything to eat or drink)
 E—Events leading up to the call for help (for example, if the patient fell, or suddenly became short of breath while climbing stairs)
14. 15; 5
15. 12-20
16. 60-100
17. Wrist; Neck
18. B. Bag valve mask device
19. B. Dry, pale mucous membranes
20. Triage
21. D. Apply direct pressure to the bleeding arm wound to control hemorrhage
22. C. Painful
23. B. Pulse, respirations, blood pressure

Chapter 9 Cardiopulmonary Resuscitation and AED

1. Atria; Ventricles
2. Capillaries
3. Arteries; Veins
4. C. Cardiac arrest
5. Brain
6. CPR (cardiopulmonary resuscitation)
7. Early recognition, early CPR, early defibrillation, and early advanced life support care
8. Defibrillation
9. B. Squeezing too quickly and forcefully
10. Decreases
11. 1
12. Pulse

13. Agonal
14. D. 52 y/o pulseless and apneic male
15. B. Carotid
16. A. On the inside of the upper arm (brachial pulse)
17. C. Make sure that someone is calling 9-1-1. (This is nearly simultaneous with beginning the initial patient assessment.)
18. D. Nipple line
19. C. Pulse, normal breathing, coughing, movement
20. D. Open his airway
21. D. Make sure all are clear of the patient

Chapter 10 Medical Emergencies

1. B. Sweating
2. C. Chest Pain
3. Mental status
4. Recovery
5. Facial droop, speech, palmar drift
6. Pulmonary edema (CHF)
7. B. Taking too much insulin
8. Identify yourself; State that you are there to help; Explain what you are doing; Use a calm, reassuring voice; Ask what happened; Don't be judgmental; Repeat/rephrase the patient's statements to show you are listening and to check understanding; Acknowledge the patient's feelings.
9. Weapons are involved, There are hostages, Physical violence has already occurred, There is a large gathering of people (e.g., a demonstration or rally), Certain sporting events, Involvement of drugs or alcohol
10. Not enter the scene (or leave the scene if he or she has already entered)
11. D. Inability to speak
12. A. Move objects away from the patient
13. C. Administer oxygen, obtain a history, call ALS
14. B. Airway management
15. B. Hypoglycemia
16. C. "Do you have any medical problems?"
17. B. Pain that radiates down the arm.
18. Onset, Provocation, Quality, Radiation, Severity, Time
19. D. Non-rebreather mask
20. A. Stroke
21. E, F, D, B, A, C

ANSWERS TO
Check your understanding—continued

Chapter 11 Bleeding, Soft Tissue Wounds, and Shock Management

1. Hemorrhage
2. Shock
3. C. Femur
4. Vein
5. (1)Direct pressure, (2) Pressure bandage, (3) Elevation, (4) Arterial pressure points
6. Apply more dressing material and bandage over the original bandage (should not remove the saturated dressing)
7. Rapid pulse; Rapid breathing; Pale, cool, sweaty skin; Altered mental status; Low blood pressure; Thirst; Obvious bleeding
8. Mental status
9. C. Cover with dry, sterile dressings
10. C. Managing the airway
11. E, D, F, G, C, A, B
12. B. The patient's heart may have stopped
13. D. Stabilizing the screwdriver in place
14. C. Giving her oxygen

Chapter 12 Musculoskeletal Injuries

1. A. Dislocation
2. D. Mandible
3. C. Scapula, clavicle, humerus
4. It is taken over by another EMS worker or until the patient is completely secured to a long back board.
5. Jaw-thrust maneuver
6. Breathe
7. Mechanism of injury; Unresponsive patient; Neck pain or tenderness; Deformity of cervical spine; Paralysis, weakness, or tingling of extremities
8. C. C-Collar application, oxygen delivery
9. Cervical spine—C, E
   Thoracic spine—B, F
   Lumbar spine—G, H
   Sacrum—G, H
   Coccyx—A, D
10. D. Xyphoid process
11. B. Radius and ulna
12. A. Femur
13. C. Femur and pelvis
14. B. Ligament
15. B. Voluntary

16. Pain; Swelling; Deformity; Open wound; Tenderness, bruising or discoloration; Inability to move the injured part; Crepitus (grating sound as bone ends move against each other); Exposed bone; Numbness or tingling; No pulse in the injured part
17. D. Crepitus
18. A. Never
19. C. Manually stabilize with the hands
20. D. Allowing the patient to stabilize or "self-splint" the injury
21. C. Thigh
22. D. Fracture of the pelvis
23. B. Cover with a sterile dressing and control bleeding
24. D. Facial trauma (airway involvement)

Chapter 13 Childbirth

1. C. Ectopic pregnancy
2. B. Cervix
3. Contractions are frequent and strong, The mother has an urge to push or a sensation as if she needs to have a bowel movement, The perineum (area of the female genitalia surrounding the vagina) is bulging, The baby's head is visible at the vaginal opening (crowning)
4. Crowning
5. Gown, Gloves, Eye protection, Face mask (optional)
6. Head
7. Feet or buttocks
8. The mother should be on her back with her head and shoulders supported by pillows or significant other; her knees should be bent and feet apart. There should be a folded towel or blanket under the buttocks.
9. Placing a gloved hand over the baby's head and applying gentle pressure to allow the head to emerge slowly
10. Using a bulb syringe to suction first the baby's mouth, then the nostrils
11. The mother's vagina
12. Pulsating
13. Newborns lose heat very easily; Face
14. Noticeable, significant bleeding (more than 1 cup, or 8 ounces, of blood); Anxious; Pale; Diaphoretic; Increased pulse; Thirst; Decreased blood pressure;

Increased respirations; Decreased level of Consciousness

15. Encouraging the mother to allow the baby to breast-feed, Placing a sanitary napkin over vaginal opening, Massaging the uterus while supporting it just above the pubic bone.
16. Spontaneous abortion
17. The babies are smaller, May be born earlier, Delivery may take place more rapidly, The babies are more prone to heat loss
18. A. Place mother in the knee-chest position
19. Tear it away
20. Clamp or tie the cord securely in two places and cut the cord between the two clamps or ties before the baby's body is delivered.
21. A. Stimulate the baby by rubbing his back
22. B. 60 per minute
23. A. Inside of the upper arm
24. C. Body, face, and extremities are all blue
25. G, E, C, F, A, D, B

Chapter 14 Infants and Children

1. The First Responder should position himself or herself at the child's eye level, for example, by kneeling next to a chair in which the child is sitting.
2. Feet; Head
3. Flaring of the nostrils, Cyanosis, Wheezing or stridor (abnormally noisy breathing), Retractions of the intercostal muscles (muscles between the ribs), Chest does not rise and fall normally with breathing, Decreased responsiveness, Abnormally increased or decreased rate of breathing.
4. Trauma (such as head injury or blood loss); Lack of oxygen caused by obstructed airway, respiratory distress, or poisons that affect breathing and oxygen delivery to the body; Poisoning; Overdose; Drugs; Alcohol; Seizure; Infection; Dehydration; Low blood sugar; Heat-related emergencies (such as being left in a vehicle on a hot day)
5. Multiple bruises of different colors (except on the shins); Presence of many old scars; Deformed extremities; Swollen or deformed ears; Broken teeth, bruising, or trauma to the face; Head trauma; Burns and bruises in unusual/unlikely places; Scald burns—especially those with a clear line of demarcation; Burns that appear to be caused by specific objects; Bite or pinch marks; Whip or belt marks; Rope burns or impressions around neck, wrists, or ankles

6. Level of consciousness (or mental status)
7. C. Brain injuries
8. A. Trauma
9. B. Abdominal injuries
10. D. Airway management and ventilation
11. C. Children lose body heat more quickly
12. A. Placing a folded towel under the shoulders
13. C. Pulse (heart rate) is faster than in adults
14. D. Back blows and chest thrusts
15. A. Only if the object can be seen in the mouth
16. B. Abdominal thrusts
17. C. Fever
18. C. 0 to 1 year
19. B. Preschooler (3 to 6 years)
20. D. Inattentive to environmental stimuli
21. D. Assist ventilations with a bag-mask device

Chapter 15 Operations

1. Preparation for the call
2. Make sure equipment and supplies are stocked in First Responder kits and emergency vehicles, Check that mechanical equipment is operating properly, Make sure the vehicle is well-maintained, Take good care of oneself through diet and exercise, Maintain the skills and knowledge learned in the First Responder training program
3. Be aware of weather and road conditions, Drive at speeds at which you can maintain control of the vehicle, Reduce speed for curves, Pay attention to traffic around you, Take an emergency vehicle operations course
4. Park upwind or uphill from any hazardous substance spills, Allow room for EMS personnel to load the patient into the ambulance and to depart the scene, Use the parking brake, Use warning lights, Turn off headlights if not needed for illumination of the scene
5. Check fuel level, Restock supplies, Clean and disinfect equipment, Complete paperwork, Notify the dispatch center of your availability
6. Incident Command System
7. Landing zone should be at least 60 feet × 60 feet (day) or 100 feet × 100 feet (night); Area should

be free of loose debris, obstructions, overhead wires, trees, or fences; The ground should not slope; Each corner of the zone must be marked; At night vehicle headlights should point to the center of the zone; Turn lights off as the helicopter makes its final descent.

8. Pilot
9. Extrication
10. Hazardous material
11. *The Emergency Response Guidebook*
12. Placard
13. B. The rear
14. D. Multiple-casualty incident
15. A. Wait for the hazardous materials team. Maintain your own safety.
16. C. Minor
17. B. Open the airway

Chapter 16 Environmental Emergencies

1. B. Convection
2. A. Conduction
3. C. Moving the patient out of the current environment
4. B. Heat exhaustion
5. B. A decrease in mental status
6. C. Safety
7. D. Airway and breathing status
8. D. Absorption
9. C. Take the liquid's original container with you to the Emergency Department
10. D. Cardiac arrhythmias/cardiac arrest
11. D. ABC assessment

Chapter 17 Special Populations

1. Disabled
2. Quadriplegia

3. Atrophy
4. Ostomy
5. Age greater than 75, Living alone, Recent loss of loved one, Recent hospitalization, Incontinence, Immobility, Altered mental status
6. If they become dislodged
7. Allow more time than usual to assess the patient and obtain a history, Be patient, Express empathy and compassion, Do not underestimate the patient's intelligence or level of awareness of what you are saying, Validate information with friends and family, Obtain a list of medications to be given to transporting EMS personnel, Look for "VIAL OF LIFE," Make sure the patient can see your face when you are speaking, Be patient when repeating questions
8. True
9. True
10. False
11. C. Write your questions down for the patient
12. D. Explain what you are going to do before you touch the patient
13. B. Geriatric
14. A. Heart disease
15. C. "On a scale of 1 to 5, with 5 being the worst, how would you rate your pain?"
16. C. "Hello, Mrs. Cunningham."
17. B. Hypothermia
18. D. The medication they take may actually mask the signs and symptoms of shock and injury.
19. D. Alert the transporting agency about your abuse suspicions and promptly complete an abuse report.

Glossary

Abandonment Leaving a patient before another health care provider has assumed responsibility for that patient or before you have delivered the required standard of care.

ABC The mnemonic used to help rescuers remember the sequence for the assessment and treatment of respiratory and cardiac emergencies. A is for airway, B is for breathing, and C is for circulation.

Abdomen The part of the body between the hips and the chest.

Abdominal guarding A characteristic fetal-like position that someone with acute abdominal pain may take to help alleviate the pain.

Abrasion Injury from a scraping force involving the outermost layer of skin.

Acute An illness or condition that has a sudden onset of symptoms.

Advanced care (also called *advanced life support, or ALS*) The use of sophisticated emergency equipment including airway management and medications to help stabilize a patient.

Agonal breaths Often called "dying breaths." These breaths are weak, ineffective, gasping attempts that cannot sustain life. Rescue breathing is needed.

Altered mental status A sudden or gradual decrease in a patient's level of responsiveness or understanding.

American Sign Language (ASL) A method of communication for the hearing impaired or deaf. Involves speaking through hand gestures.

Amniotic sac The "bag of waters" that surrounds and protects the developing fetus inside the uterus.

Amputation An extremity or other body part that is completely severed from the body.

Anaphylaxis A severe, life-threatening allergic reaction.

Anatomy The structure of the body.

Angina Chest pain caused by a lack of oxygen to the heart tissue.

Anterior Toward the front of the body.

Appendicular skeleton The part of the skeleton consisting of the pelvis and the upper and lower extremities.

Arterial bleeding Blood loss from the arteries.

Arteries Blood vessels that carry blood away from the heart.

Asthma A disease that causes reversible narrowing and spasm of the bronchi and excessive mucus production.

Atrophy The wasting away or loss in size of part of the body as a result of disease or lack of use.

Auscultation The process of listening with a stethoscope.

Automated external defibrillator (AED) A simple, lightweight, computerized device used to stop deadly heart rhythms.

AVPU The mnemonic for the scale used to determine a patient's level of response (A, Alert; V, Verbal; P, painful; U, unresponsive).

Avulsion A type of wound that occurs when a piece of skin or soft tissue is either partially torn loose or pulled completely off.

Axial skeleton The central skeleton consisting of the skull, spinal column, and thorax.

Bag-mask device A mechanical resuscitation device consisting of a self-inflating bag, one-way valve, reservoir, and a mask. Squeezing the bag results in positive pressure (a breath) being delivered to the patient.

Bandage An object that holds a dressing in place.

Barrier device A resuscitation device that places a layer of thin film with either a filter or a one-way valve between you and a patient.

Base station A radio located at a fixed location, such as a hospital, dispatch center, or emergency services station. This is usually the most powerful radio within the EMS communication system.

Basket stretcher A device that a patient can be placed into and then lifted over rough terrain or to different levels.

Behavior The way a person acts or performs, or a person's physical and mental activities.

Behavioral emergency A situation in which a patient exhibits behavior that is unacceptable or intolerable to the patient, family, or community.

Biological agent A naturally occurring substance that produces disease.

Birth canal During delivery, this is the lower part of the uterus, the cervix, and the vagina.

Blood pressure The pressure the blood exerts on the arteries as the blood flows through the vessels.

Bloody show Blood and mucus discharged through the vagina; often the first sign of labor.

Body mechanics The movement and positioning required to make a physical movement. Using proper body mechanics can prevent injury.

Body substance isolation (BSI) An infection control method that is based on the assumption that all body fluids are infectious.

Breech birth A presenting part at the cervix other than the baby's head.

Bulging The "pushing out" of the perineum caused by the baby's head in the birth canal; this is a sign that delivery will occur very soon.

Burn centers Provide specialized care for victims of thermal, chemical, electrical, and radiation burns.

Capacity A medical determination of a person's ability to make an informed decision.

Capillaries Microscopic blood vessels that connect arteries to veins.

Capillary bleeding Blood loss from the capillaries.

Capillary refill time The time it takes for color (blood) to return to the skin or nail bed after it has been squeezed to blanch the area; normal capillary refill time is less than 2 seconds.

Cardiac arrest When the heart stops beating and a pulse cannot be felt.

Cardiac muscle A type of involuntary muscle that is found only in the heart. Generates its own electrical impulse to contract and relax.

Cardiopulmonary resuscitation (CPR) The combination of artificial ventilation (rescue breathing) and chest compressions given to an unresponsive patient with no breathing or signs of circulation.

Centers for Disease Control and Prevention (CDC) A federal agency of the U.S. government that provides resources and equipment for the investigation, identification, prevention, and control of infectious disease.

Cerebral Vascular Accident (CVA) A disruption of blood flow to the brain caused by an occluded or ruptured artery. Also called a stroke.

Cervix The muscular ring-like structure that forms the lowest part of the uterus; it shortens and dilates during labor.

Chain of survival A term coined by the American Heart Association (AHA) to describe the sequence of events that increases survival rates from sudden cardiac death when performed rapidly. Early access, early CPR, early defibrillation, and early ACLC are links in the adult chain of survival. The links in the pediatric chain of survival are prevention, early BLS rescue, early EMS access, and early ACLS.

Chemical burns Burns produced by chemical substances.

Chief complaint The patient's initial or primary statement of the problem.

Chronic Any condition or disease that is present over a long period of time.

Chronic bronchitis An inflammation and irritation of the bronchi causing excessive production of mucus.

Chronic obstructive pulmonary disease (COPD) A collection of diseases that cause obstruction of the airways and make breathing difficult.

Circulation The movement of blood to allow for the exchange of nutrients and waste products through the body.

Cleaning Washing something thoroughly with soap and water.

Closed-ended questions Questions that can be answered with a yes or no answer. In other words, these are questions that require specific responses using the answer choices you provide.

Closed injury An injury in which the skin remains intact.

Communication Any act by which one person gives to or receives from another person information about that person's needs, desires, perceptions, knowledge, or affective states. Communication may be intentional or unintentional, may involve conventional or unconventional signals, may take linguistic or nonlinguistic forms, and may occur through spoken or other modes.

Compensation The body's response to try to stop shock from developing.

Conduction The transfer of heat energy from a warmer object to a cooler one as a result of direct contact.

Contraction The rhythmic tensing and relaxing of the uterine muscle that is critical for the expulsion of the fetus and the placenta from the womb.

Contraction time The time of a single contraction from the onset of the contraction until relaxation occurs.

Contusion A bruise. A type of closed wound.

Convection The transfer of heat through a gas or liquid by the circulation of heated particles.

Convulsions Severe, violent muscle contractions that can occur during a seizure.

Crackles Low-pitched bubbling sounds produced by fluid in the lower airways.

Crepitus A sound or a feeling of bone ends grating against one another or air trapped between tissue layers; feels like bubble wrap popping.

Cricoid pressure A technique that collapses the esophagus between the trachea and cervical spine; used to prevent air from entering the stomach and the patient from vomiting during ventilation.

Critical incident stress A stress reaction normally exhibited after experiencing a particularly difficult situation.

Critical incident stress debriefing (CISD) A function of the critical incident stress management system that uses specific techniques such as debriefings to help people express their feelings and recover from a stressful incident faster.

Critical incident stress management (CISM) A comprehensive system devised to help professionals recover from critical incidents.

Croup A viral infection that can lead to upper airway obstruction and respiratory distress.

Crowning The appearance of the first part of the infant during delivery.

Debriefing A review of a stressful event to allow discussion between the people involved. Usually held within 24 to 72 hours of the event.

Decoding The process by which the intended receiver interprets the meaning of a message sent by another.

Decompression sickness A painful and sometimes fatal condition caused by the formation of nitrogen bubbles in the tissues of divers, caisson workers, and aviators who move too rapidly from a higher to a lower atmospheric pressure.

Defibrillation The application of sufficient energy to the fibrillating heart muscle to stop all activity, with the hope that normal activity will return.

Defusing A shorter and less formal review of stressful events to allow discussion between the people involved. Usually held within a few hours of the event.

Diaphragm The dome-shaped muscle that is largely responsible for ventilation.

Diastolic blood pressure The pressure the blood exerts on the blood vessels when the heart is relaxed.

Direct injury Injury as a result of force applied directly to the body or a body part.

Direct medical control Real-time communication between prehospital care personnel and medical control. This can take place in person, on the phone, or over the radio. Also called online medical control.

Disabled Persons with physical impairments that limit one or more major life activity.

Disinfecting In addition to cleaning something, using alcohol or bleach to kill contaminants.

Dislocation The separation of a bone from its normal position in a joint.

Dispatch center A centralized location that obtains information about and assigns resources to an incident.

Distal Away from the trunk of the body.

Do not attempt resuscitation (DNAR) order A written order by a physician instructing health care providers not to provide medical care to a patient who is clinically dead.

DOTS A mnemonic (*Deformities, Open* wounds, *Tenderness, Swelling*) for observations to make in the physical examination.

Dressing A protective or supporting covering that is placed over an injured site.

Drowning Asphyxiation caused by submersion in a liquid.

Dual lumen airway An advanced airway device that has two separate ports for the delivery of oxygen; can be inserted into either the trachea or the esophagus.

Durable power of attorney A legal document that designates another individual to make health care decisions for the person who signed the document once that person becomes incapacitated.

Duty to act The legal obligation to provide medical care.

Dyspnea Difficulty in breathing.

Electrical burns Burns produced by electricity.

Emancipated minor A minor who has been determined by a court to be legally capable of making adult decisions including consenting to or refusing medical treatment.

Embryo The term for a fertilized egg for the first 8 weeks of pregnancy.

Emergency An unexpected situation that arises and threatens the life of one or more people.

Emergency medical services (EMS) system The network of services that handles prehospital medical and trauma emergencies. These systems are organized at a local, regional, state, or national level.

Emergency first responder One of the four training levels of EMS. The new terminology was created to better describe the position of First Responder as written by the 2005 National Scope of Practice.

Emergency Medical Services for Children (EMSC) A nationally recognized organization that coordinates the development and implementation of educational programs and resources dealing with the care of children.

Emergency medical technician (EMT) A medical provider who performs prehospital care. Typically refers to the EMT-Basic level but may be used to denote any level of prehospital care. Part of the organized EMS system.

Emergency move Any move that is initiated because there is an immediate danger to the patient and provider.

Empathy One's ability to recognize, perceive, and feel directly the emotion of another.

Encoding The process by which the sender of a message places the message into a format that the receiver can understand.

Emphysema A lung disease that causes destruction of the alveoli, making it difficult to exchange oxygen and carbon dioxide.

Endotracheal tube An advanced airway device that is inserted directly into the trachea.

Epiglottitis A bacterial infection of the upper airway.

Evaporation Change in a substance from a liquid to a gas.

Evisceration A laceration through the abdominal muscle wall that allows organs to protrude from the abdomen.

Explosive delivery An uncontrolled quick delivery of the baby's head.

Expressed consent Written or verbal consent from a patient that tells you he or she has consented to medical care.

Extrication The process of removing a patient from entanglement in a motor vehicle or other situation in a safe and appropriate way.

Fallopian tube A tube that extends from each ovary to the uterus; provides a pathway for the egg to reach the uterus.

Family-centered care Involving family members in the care of their children.

Febrile seizure A seizure caused by a rapidly rising body temperature.

Federal Communications Commission (FCC) An agency of the federal government that is responsible for governing all radio transmissions in the United States.

Feedback The component of communication that indicates whether the message received was actually the message that was intended.

Fetus The term for the infant after 8 weeks of pregnancy and until the infant is born.

First Responder The initial person at the scene of a medical or trauma emergency who has been trained in medical care. Part of the organized EMS system.

Focused history Information regarding the patient's medical problems, medications, and other information pertinent to the injury or illness.

Foreign body airway obstruction (FBAO) An obstruction of the airway caused, for example, by choking on food or other foreign material or by bleeding into the airway or vomiting.

Fracture A broken bone.

Frostbite The traumatic effect of extreme cold on skin and subcutaneous tissues exemplified by pallor of exposed skin surfaces, particularly of the fingers, nose, ears, and toes.

Full-thickness burn A burn involving all layers of the skin.

Gag reflex A response to stimulation of the posterior oropharynx causing gagging and vomiting in many people. Generally, unconscious patients do not have a gag reflex.

General impression A quick evaluation of the scene to determine what has happened and the seriousness of the scene.

Glucose Sugar used by the cells for energy.

Hand-off report Verbally delivering information to another medical provider who is taking over the care of a patient.

Hazardous material Any material or substance that can cause an unreasonable risk to a person's safety or health or to property.

Head-tilt/chin-lift A manual maneuver used to open someone's airway. The head is tilted back with one hand while the chin is lifted up with the other.

Heat cramps Painful spasms of muscles in the arms, legs, or abdomen that occur after several hours of sustained activity in hot environments.

Heat exhaustion A heat-related illness that occurs when the circulatory system fails to adequately maintain its normal function because of excessive loss of fluids and salts.

Heat stroke The most severe form of heat exposure illness; prolonged exposure to high temperatures causes failure of the body's temperature-regulating capacity.

Heat transfer The mechanism by which needed heat is moved into the body or how excess heat is released from the body.

Hemoglobin A molecule that carries oxygen in the blood.

Hemorrhage The loss of blood, or bleeding.

High-efficiency particulate air (HEPA) mask A special mask designed to decrease the spread of infection of airborne diseases such as tuberculosis.

Hyperglycemia High blood sugar.

Hypoglycemia Low blood sugar.

Hypoperfusion Also called shock. A condition caused by decreased circulation of the blood.

Hypothermia A dangerous condition in which the body temperature falls below 95°F (35°C) and the body's normal functions are impaired.

Hypoxia A condition in which there is lack of oxygen to the cells of the body.

Immobilize To prevent movement.

Implied consent A legal definition that assumes a person unable to give consent because of his or her injury would want medical care if he or she could give that consent. Also refers to consent based on "lack of protest" from the patient when medical care is given.

Incident Command System (ICS) A protocol or system for coordinating procedures to assist in the command, control, direction, and coordination of emergency response resources.

Incompetence The state of a patient who is unable to understand your questions or understand the implications of the decisions he or she may be making.

Indirect injury Injury as a result of a force applied to one part of the body, which transmits to and then injures another part.

Indirect medical control The use of standing orders or written protocols to provide care. This type of medical control does not involve actual communication with a medical director at the time of the incident. Also called offline medical control.

Inferior Toward the feet or bottom of the body.

Insulin Hormone produced by the pancreas that allows the cells to properly metabolize sugar.

Interference Any disruption or distraction in the communication process.

Internal bleeding Blood loss inside the body.

Interval time The time between contractions.

Involuntary muscle Also called smooth muscle. Muscle that contracts or relaxes automatically.

Jaw thrust A manual maneuver used to open the airway of a trauma patient. The patient's jaw is thrust forward without tilting the head back, which could potentially cause further injury to the spine.

Joint Where two or more bones come together. Allows movement of the body.

Labor The process of delivery from the first contraction through the delivery of the placenta.

Laceration A break in the skin of varying depth and damage.

Lateral Away from the midline of the body.

Ligaments Fibrous bands of tissue that connect bone to bone.

Living will A written document that describes an individual's wishes for lifesaving measures if certain medical conditions occur.

Log roll A technique for moving a patient by rolling him or her onto the side to insert a device underneath the patient or to move the patient from a prone position to a supine position.

Long backboard A device that is long enough for a person's entire body to be completely immobilized as a single unit.

Mechanism of injury An impact or other cause of a patient's injury.

Medial Toward the midline of the body.

Medical director A physician who develops guidelines and protocols for the prehospital treatment of patients. The medical director is responsible for the prehospital medical care delivered by the EMS service.

Medical insignia Any identification device worn by patients to identify certain preexisting medical conditions.

Medical patient A patient who appears to have an illness or complains of symptoms of an illness.

Midline An imaginary vertical line drawn through the middle of the body.

Minor A person not yet of a predefined age to make legal decisions.

Miscarriage Also called "spontaneous abortion," a miscarriage is the delivery of the products of conception before the fetus can survive on its own.

Mobile radio A radio that is mounted in a vehicle.

Multiple-casualty incident (MCI) A situation that overwhelms available resources.

Muscular dystrophy A group of diseases characterized by weakness and wasting away of skeletal muscles. The cause is unknown.

Myocardial infarction (MI) Also called heart attack. A condition in which part of the heart muscle dies because of inadequate supply of oxygen.

Nasal cannula An oxygen delivery device that consists of two prongs that go into a patient's nose; delivers a low concentration of oxygen.

Nasopharyngeal airway (NPA) A mechanical device inserted into the nostril and used to prevent the tongue from obstructing the airway.

Nature of illness A determination of the patient's illness from findings.

Negligence The act of failing to provide the expected standard of care to a patient, which leads to further injury to the patient.

NICS National Incident Command System.

Nonemergency move The type of move that is designed to provide the best care of the patient in a controlled, safe environment.

Nonrebreather mask An oxygen-delivery device used to deliver higher concentrations of oxygen; consists of a mask, one-way valve, and a reservoir bag.

Nonverbal communication A component of communication in which messages are relayed through movements, postures, gestures, and the eyes.

Normal anatomical position The position of a human body standing upright, facing forward, with arms at the side and the palms turned forward.

Occipital skull The back part of the head.

Occlusive dressing A dressing that is airtight and nonporous.

Occupational Health and Safety Administration (OSHA) A federal agency that has developed guidelines to protect health care workers.

Open injury An injury in which the skin has been broken.

Open-ended questions Questions that cannot be answered with yes or no answers. These questions allow patients to put their situations in their own words and provide the most information. These questions also allow an opportunity to identify nonverbal communication clues.

Oropharyngeal airway (OPA) A mechanical device inserted into the mouth and used to prevent the tongue from obstructing the airway.

Ostomy A surgical opening made into the urinary bladder, small intestine, or large intestine as a temporary or permanent pathway for urine or feces to reach a collection bag outside the body.

Ovaries A pair of almond-shaped organs located in the right and left lower quadrants of the abdomen of a female that function to release eggs and hormones.

Palpate To feel a part of the body to identify injury, pain, or tenderness.

Paramedic The most advanced level of prehospital emergency medical care. Part of the organized EMS system.

Partial-thickness burn A burn involving the outer and middle layers of the skin.

Patent Open (e.g., a patent airway is an open and functioning airway).

Pathogen A microorganism capable of causing disease.

Patient care report The standard form used to document patient care in emergency medical systems.

Pelvis The lower part of the trunk of the body.

Penetration/puncture wound A wound caused by a sharp, pointed object and with varying degrees of blood loss.

Perineum The area between the mother's vaginal and rectal openings.

Personal protection equipment (PPE) Equipment used to isolate a health care worker from a patient's body substances. Also refers to specialty equipment that emergency providers use during the course of a rescue or a fire.

Physical examination Assessing a patient to identify signs or symptoms of an illness or injury.

Physiology The function of the body.

Placard An informational sign with various symbols and numerals to help identify the hazardous material or class of material.

Placenta The structure in the uterus where nourishment and waste products are exchanged between the mother and the developing fetus. It is also called the "afterbirth."

Pocket mask A mask that can be used to deliver mouth-to-mask ventilation.

Poison Any substance that can be potentially harmful to the body.

Poison control center A service that provides data on all aspects of poisonings, keeps records of poisonings, and refers patients to treatment centers.

Portable radio A radio that an emergency first responder can carry wherever he or she goes. Although very convenient and necessary, these radios have a limited transmission distance.

Portable stretcher A piece of equipment that can easily carry patients down stairs or over rough terrain.

Posterior Toward the back of the body.

Power grip A way to hold your hands on something that you are lifting to have the most effective lifting technique.

Power lift A lifting technique used to lift heavy objects. The positioning emphasizes proper body mechanics.

Presenting part The part of the infant that appears first at the vaginal opening.

Pressure dressing A special dressing that places pressure over a wound site.

Primary assessment The first evaluation of the patient, to identify life-threatening problems.

Protocols Written instructions to carry out care for certain medical symptoms or conditions.

Proximal Toward the trunk of the body.

Proximate cause A legal term meaning one's actions or inactions were in fact the cause of a patient's injuries.

Quadriplegia Paralysis of all four extremities.

Radiation Heat that moves across a space from one object to another. Also describes pain that moves from one site to another part of the body.

Rapid extrication The rapid removal of a critical patient out of a vehicle; requires at least three providers.

Reassessment The reevaluation of the patient's initial assessment and problems.

Recovery position Position that places a patient on his or her side, keeping the airway open and allowing easy access to the airway. Unresponsive, breathing, nontrauma patients are placed in this position.

Refusal Declined medical treatment.

Rescue breathing Artificial ventilation provided to a patient who cannot breathe on his or her own.

Respiratory arrest The cessation of breathing.

Respiratory distress Shortness of breath with labored breathing.

Respiratory failure The inability to maintain adequate oxygen and carbon dioxide exchange.

Responsiveness The patient's neurological status, described by how and to what type of stimuli a patient reacts.

Rule of nines An assessment tool that allows a quick calculation of the extent of a burn.

SAMPLE A mnemonic used to collect a patient history (*Signs/symptoms, Allergies, Medications, Pertinent* past medical history, *Last* oral intake, *Events* leading to the injury or illness).

Scene safety Evaluating the scene of an incident or illness for potential hazards to the emergency first responder, patient, crew, or bystanders.

Scene size-up The process of looking at the scene to determine safety factors and the mechanism of injury or nature of illness.

Scoop stretcher A patient-lifting device that can be separated into two halves and placed under the patient and then reconnected.

Seizure A sudden attack that usually results from a nervous system malfunction resulting in varying levels of altered mental status.

Shaken baby syndrome A specific form of child abuse that occurs when violent shaking of an infant leads to severe head injuries, damage to the brain, and tearing of blood vessels in the head.

Shock Also called hypoperfusion. A condition caused by decreased circulation of the blood.

Short backboard Device that allows immobilization of the spine of a patient who is in a sitting position.

Sign A finding you can hear, see, feel, or measure during the physical examination.

Skeletal muscle Also called voluntary muscle. Muscle connected to bone that requires an active thought process to contract or relax.

Smooth muscle Also called involuntary muscle. Muscle that contracts or relaxes automatically.

Specialty centers Cater to specific needs with specialized equipment and trained personnel.

Sphygmomanometer A device used to evaluate blood pressure; also called a blood pressure cuff.

Splint A device used to immobilize injured bones or joints and prevent further damage.

Spontaneous abortion Also called "miscarriage," a spontaneous abortion is the delivery of the products of conception before the fetus can survive on its own.

Sprain An injury in which ligaments are stretched or torn.

Stair chair A device that facilitates moving a patient down stairs.

Standard of care The care you are expected to give based on your level of training and experience.

Standing order Patient care instructions, in writing, that authorize specific steps in patient assessment and treatment without contacting medical control.

Status epilepticus A seizure that lasts more than 15 minutes, or repetitive seizures in which the person does not completely regain consciousness between seizures.

Sterilizing The use of chemicals and superheated steam to kill all microorganisms.

Stethoscope An instrument used to hear sounds within the body such as breath sounds or the blood pressure.

Strain A muscle pull around a joint.

Stridor A high-pitched, whistling sound that occurs when a patient breathes in if there is an obstruction (foreign body or tissue swelling) in the upper airway (between the pharynx and the vocal cords).

Stroke A disruption of blood flow to the brain caused by an occluded or ruptured artery. Also called a cerebral vascular accident.

Sucking chest wound A penetrating/puncture chest wound that is deep enough to penetrate the lungs, allowing air to escape the body through the wound.

Sudden infant death syndrome (SIDS) The sudden and unexpected death of an apparently normal, healthy infant; typically occurs during the first year of life.

Superficial burn A burn that involves only the outer layer of skin.

Superior Toward the head or top of the body.

Symptom A problem or condition that a patient describes.

Systolic blood pressure The pressure the blood exerts on the blood vessels when the heart is contracted.

Tendons Fibrous bands of tissue that connect muscle to bones.

Terrorism Unlawful use of—or threatened use of—force or violence against individuals or property to coerce or intimidate governments or societies, often to achieve political, religious, or ideological objectives.

Thermoregulation The control of heat production and heat loss.

Thorax The chest.

Trauma center A specialized hospital equipped with personnel and resources to immediately care for a critically injured trauma patient.

Trauma chin lift Also called tongue-jaw lift. A manual maneuver used to open the airway and keep the tongue from obstructing the airway. Used to inspect the airway or to do finger sweeps of the airway.

Trauma patient A patient who has sustained an injury as a result of an external force.

Trauma system A system to help identify the appropriate hospital or specialized center for a trauma patient to be transported to.

Triage The process of sorting or categorizing patients into treatment and transport priorities in a multiple-casualty situation.

Twisting injury Injury as a result of an extremity being twisted or pulled.

Umbilical cord An extension of the placenta; the actual structure that connects the fetus to the mother.

Uterus Also called the womb, a muscular structure where the fetus grows and develops.

Vagina Also called the birth canal, a sheath that encloses the lower portion of the uterus and extends down to the vaginal opening.

Veins Blood vessels that carry blood toward the heart.

Venous bleeding Blood loss from the veins.

Ventilation The mechanical movement of air being inhaled and exhaled; also refers to the artificial breathing given to a patient through a mask or your mouth.

Ventilation The mechanical process of moving air in and out of the lungs.

Ventricular fibrillation A lethal heart rhythm. Produces chaotic electrical activity in the heart, resulting in no blood flow out from the heart (cardiac arrest). Treated with defibrillation.

Vest-type device A device that can be strapped to a patient to immobilize the spine. It fits like a vest around the patient.

Vital signs The patient's pulse rate, respiratory rate, skin signs, pupils, and blood pressure.

Voluntary muscle Also called skeletal muscle. Muscle connected to bone that requires an active thought process to contract.

Weapon of mass destruction (WMD) Any weapon or device that is intended, or has the capability, to cause death or serious bodily injury to a significant number of people.

Wheeled stretcher A device that allows a patient to recline while being transported. Generally used in ambulances.

Wheezing A high-pitched sound that occurs when air moves through narrowed airways; usually occurs on exhalation and generally indicates obstruction of the lower airways.

Xiphoid process The lowest part of the base of the sternum. It is to be avoided during chest compressions.